CURRENT MANAGEMENT

OF ARRHYTHMIAS

Medical Titles in the Current Therapy Series

CURRENT MANAGEMENT

OF ARRHYTHMIAS

Edited by

LEONARD N. HOROWITZ, M.D.

Clinical Professor of Medicine
University of Pennsylvania School of Medicine

Co-Director, Philadelphia Heart Institute
Presbyterian Medical Center
Philadelphia, Pennsylvania

B.C. Decker, Inc. • Philadelphia • Hamilton

Publisher

B.C. Decker Inc
1 James Street, South
Hamilton, Ontario L8P 4R5

B.C. Decker Inc
320 Walnut Street
Suite 400
Philadelphia, Pennsylvania 19106

Sales and Distribution

United States and Puerto Rico
Mosby–Year Book Inc.
11830 Westline Industrial Drive
Saint Louis, Missouri 63146

Canada
Mosby–Year Book Ltd.
5240 Finch Ave. E., Unit 1
Scarborough, Ontario M1S 5A2

Australia
**McGraw-Hill Book Company
Australia Pty. Ltd.**
4 Barcoo Street
Roseville East 2069
New South Wales, Australia

Brazil
Editora McGraw-Hill do Brasil, Ltda.
rua Tabapua 1.105, Itaim-Bibi
Sao Paulo, S.P. Brasil

Colombia
Interamericana/McGraw-Hill de Colombia, S.A.
Carrera 17, No. 33-71
(Apartado Postal, A.A., 6131)
Bogota, D.E., Colombia

Europe
McGraw-Hill Book Company GmbH
Lademannbogen 136
D-2000 Hamburg 63
West Germany

France
MEDSI/McGraw-Hill
6, avenue Daniel Lesueur
75007 Paris, France

Hong Kong and China
McGraw-Hill Book Company
Suite 618, Ocean Centre
5 Canton Road
Tsimshatsui, Kowloon
Hong Kong

India
**Tata McGraw-Hill Publishing
Company, Ltd.**
12/4 Asaf Ali Road, 3rd Floor
New Delhi 110002, India

Indonesia
Mr. Wong Fin Fah
P.O. Box 122/JAT
Jakarta, 1300 Indonesia

Italy
McGraw-Hill Libri Italia, s.r.l.
Piazza Emilia, 5
1-20129 Milano MI
Italy

Japan
Igaku-Shoin Ltd.
Tokyo International P.O. Box 5063
1-28-36 Hongo, Bunkyo-ku,
Tokyo 113, Japan

Korea
Mr. Don Gap-Choi
C.P.O. Box 10583
Seoul, Korea

Malaysia
Mr. Lim Tao Slong
No. 8 Jalan SS 7/6B
Kelana Jaya
47301 Petaling, Jaya
Selangor, Malaysia

Mexico
**Interamericana/McGraw-Hill
de Mexico,
S.A. de C.V.**
Cedro 512, Colonia Atlampa
(Apartado Postal 26370)
06450 Mexico, D.F., Mexico

New Zealand
McGraw-Hill Book Co. New Zealand Ltd.
5 Joval Place, Wiri
Manukau City, New Zealand

Portugal
Editora McGraw-Hill de Portugal, Ltda.
Rua Rosa Damasceno 11A–B
1900 Lisboa, Portugal

South Africa
Libriger Book Distributors
Warehouse Number 8
"Die Ou Looiery"
Tannery Road
Hamilton, Bloemfontein 9300

Singapore and Southeast Asia
McGraw-Hill Book Company
21 Neythal Road
Jurong, Singapore 2262

Spain
McGraw-Hill/Interamericana de Espana, S.A.
Manuel Ferrero, 13
28020 Madrid, Spain

Taiwan
Mr. George Lim
P.O. Box 87–601
Taipei, Taiwan

Thailand
Mr. Vitit Lim
632/5 Phaholyothin Road
Sapan Kwai
Bangkok 10400
Thailand

United Kingdom, Middle East and Africa
McGraw-Hill Book Company (U.K.) Ltd.
Shoppenhangers Road
Maidenhead, Berkshire
SL6 2QL England

Venezuela
Editorial Interamericana de Venezuela, C.A.
2da. calle Bello Monte
Local G-2
Caracas, Venezuela

NOTICE

The authors and publisher have made every effort to ensure that the patient care recommended herein, including choice of drugs and drug dosages, is in accord with the accepted standards and practice at the time of publication. However, since research and regulation constantly change clinical standards, the reader is urged to check the product information sheet included in the package of each drug, which includes recommended doses, warnings, and contraindications. This is particularly important with new or infrequently used drugs.

Current Management of Arrhythmias

ISBN 1-55664-154-0

Library of Congress catalog card number: 89-81841

10 9 8 7 6 5 4 3 2

CONTRIBUTORS

MASOOD AKHTAR, M.D.

Professor of Medicine and Associate Chief, Cardiovascular Disease Section, University of Wisconsin Medical School, Milwaukee Clinical Campus, Milwaukee, Wisconsin
Paroxysmal Atrioventricular Reentrant Tachycardia: Pharmacologic Therapy

HUANLIN AN, M.D.

Research Fellow in Electrophysiology, University of Medicine and Dentistry of New Jersey—New Jersey Medical School and Eastern Heart Institute, Newark, New Jersey
Preexcitation Syndromes: Nonpharmacologic Management

JEFFREY L. ANDERSON, M.D.

Professor of Medicine (Cardiology), University of Utah School of Medicine; Chief, Cardiology Division, LDS Hospital, Salt Lake City, Utah
Flecainide

JOHN D. ARNETT, M.D.

Fellow, Cardiac Electrophysiology, Louisiana State University Medical Center, Shreveport, Louisiana
Automatic Atrial Tachycardia and Nonparoxysmal Atrioventricular Junctional Tachycardia

LOU-ANNE M. BEAUREGARD, M.D.

Assistant Professor of Medicine, University of Medicine and Dentistry of New Jersey—Robert Wood Johnson Medical School; Director, Heart Station, Cooper Hospital/University Medical Center, Camden, New Jersey
Calcium Antagonists

SALLY G. BEER, M.D.

Fellow in Cardiology, Philadelphia Heart Institute; Clinical Associate of Medicine, University of Pennsylvania School of Medicine, Philadelphia, Pennsylvania
Endocrine Disease

BERNARD BELHASSEN, M.D.

Associate Professor of Cardiology, Sackler School of Medicine, Tel-Aviv University; Director, Cardiac Electrophysiology Laboratory, Ichlov Hospital, Tel-Aviv, Israel
Adenosine Triphosphate and Adenosine

DAVID G. BENDITT, M.D.

Associate Professor of Medicine, and Director, Clinical Arrhythmia Service, University of Minnesota School of Medicine, Minneapolis, Minnesota
Bretylium

ROBERT C. BERNSTEIN, M.D.

Assistant Professor of Medicine, Eastern Virginia Medical School; Staff Electrophysiologist, Sentara Norfolk General Hospital, Norfolk, Virginia
Sustained Ventricular Tachycardia

J. THOMAS BIGGER, JR., M.D.

Professor of Medicine and Pharmacology, Columbia University College of Physicians and Surgeons; Attending Physician, Presbyterian Hospital, New York, New York
Ventricular Arrhythmias: Classification and General Principles of Therapy

STEVE Z. BINENBAUM, M.D., PH.D.

University of Medicine and Dentistry of New Jersey—New Jersey Medical School, Newark; Staff Cardiologist, Veterans Affairs Medical Center, East Orange, New Jersey
Accelerated Idioventricular Rhythm

K. ATTA BOAHENE, M.D.

Assistant Professor, Baylor College of Medicine; Attending Physician, Methodist Hospital, Houston, Texas
Atrial Fibrillation in the Wolff-Parkinson-White Syndrome

MARTIN BORGGREFE, M.D.

Consultant Cardiologist, Medical Hospital of the University of Münster, Münster, Germany, F.R.
Catheter Ablation

GÜNTER BRIETHARDT, M.D.

Professor of Cardiology, Medical Hospital of the University of Münster, Münster, Germany, F.R.
Catheter Ablation

SUSAN C. BROZENA, M.D.

Assistant Professor of Medicine, Temple University School of Medicine; Co-Medical Director, Heart Failure and Transplantation Center, Temple University Hospital, Philadelphia, Pennsylvania
Cardiomyopathy and Congestive Heart Failure

MICHAEL E. CAIN, M.D.

Associate Professor of Medicine, and Director, Clinical Electrophysiology Laboratory, Washington University School of Medicine, St. Louis, Missouri
Preexcitation Syndromes: Diagnostic and Management Strategies

DAVID S. CANNOM, M.D.

Clinical Professor of Medicine, University of California, Los Angeles, School of Medicine; Medical Director of Cardiology, Hospital of The Good Samaritan, Los Angeles, California
Automatic Implantable Cardioverter Defibrillator

AGUSTIN CASTELLANOS, M.D.

Professor of Medicine, University of Miami School of Medicine; Director, Clinical Electrophysiology, University of Miami/Jackson Memorial Medical Center, Miami, Florida
Intraventricular Conduction Disturbance and Atrioventricular Block

DANIEL S. CONTRAFATTO, M.D.

Assistant Professor of Medicine, Temple University School of Medicine; Director, Clinical Cardiac Electrophysiology, Temple University Hospital, Philadelphia, Pennsylvania
Lidocaine

JAMES L. COX, M.D.

Evarts A. Graham Professor of Surgery, and Chief, Division of Cardiothoracic Surgery, Washington University School of Medicine; Cardiothoracic Surgeon-in-Charge, Barnes Hospital, St. Louis, Missouri
Antiarrhythmic Surgery: Ventricular Arrhythmias

JOHN P. DiMARCO, M.D., Ph.D.

Professor of Medicine, University of Virginia School of Medicine; Director, Clinical Electrophysiology Laboratory, University of Virginia Hospital, Charlottesville, Virginia
Quinidine

LIONEL FAITELSON, M.D.

Assistant Professor of Medicine, University of Arizona College of Medicine, Tucson, Arizona
Arrhythmogenic Right Ventricular Dysplasia

LAMEH FANANAPAZIR, M.D.

Senior Investigator, and Director, Clinical Electrophysiology Laboratory, National Institutes of Health, Bethesda, Maryland
Arrhythmias in Hypertrophic Cardiomyopathy

T. BRUCE FERGUSON Jr., M.D.

Assistant Professor of Surgery, Division of Cardiothoracic Surgery, Washington University School of Medicine; Attending Surgeon, Barnes Hospital, St. Louis, Missouri
Antiarrhythmic Surgery: Ventricular Arrhythmias

PEDRO FERNANDEZ, M.D.

Assistant Professor of Medicine, University of Miami School of Medicine; Director, Pacemaker and Arrhythmia Center, University of Miami/Jackson Memorial Medical Center, Miami, Florida
Intraventricular Conduction Disturbances and Atrioventricular Block

JOHN D. FISHER, M.D.

Professor of Medicine, Albert Einstein College of Medicine; Director, Arrhythmia Service, and Director, Cardiology Division, Montefiore Hospital, Bronx, New York
Antitachycardia Pacing

RICHARD N. FOGOROS, M.D.

Director, Cardiac Electrophysiology, Allegheny General Hospital, Pittsburgh, Pennsylvania
Phenytoin

JAMES R. FOSTER, M.D.

Professor of Medicine, and Director, Cardiac Arrhythmia Service, University of North Carolina at Chapel Hill School of Medicine, Chapel Hill, North Carolina
Exercise and Catecholamine-Induced Ventricular Arrhythmia

WILLIAM H. FRISHMAN, M.D.

Professor of Medicine, Albert Einstein College of Medicine; Director of Medicine, Hospital of the Albert Einstein College of Medicine, Bronx, New York
Beta-Adrenergic Blocking Agents

OSAMU FUJIMURA, M.D.

Staff Cardiologist, University of Kentucky Medical Center, Lexington, Kentucky
Atrial Fibrillation in the Wolff-Parkinson-White Syndrome

HASAN GARAN, M.D.

Associate Professor of Medicine, Harvard Medical School; Co-Director, Cardiac Arrhythmia Service, Massachusetts General Hospital, Boston, Massachusetts
Sotalol

ARTHUR GARSON JR., M.D.

Professor of Pediatrics and Medicine, Baylor College of Medicine; Chief of Pediatric Cardiology, Texas Children's Hospital, Houston, Texas
Supraventricular Tachycardia in Pediatric Patients

FREDRIC GEREWITZ, M.D.

Clinical Instructor, University of Pennsylvania; Interventional Cardiac Fellow, Philadelphia Heart Institute, Philadelphia, Pennsylvania
Cardiac Catheterization and Coronary Angioplasty

BERNARD J. GERSH, M.B., CH.B., D.PHIL.

Professor of Medicine, Mayo Medical School; Consultant, Division of Cardiovascular Diseases and Internal Medicine, Mayo Clinic and Mayo Foundation, Rochester, Minnesota
Hypersensitive Carotid Sinus Syndrome

PAUL C. GILLETTE, M.D.

Professor of Pediatrics and Surgery, Division of Pediatric Cardiology, Medical University of South Carolina; Director, Division of Pediatric Cardiology, Medical University of South Carolina Children's Hospital, Charleston, South Carolina
Cardiac Pacing in Children and Young Adults

MARY ANN GOLDSTEIN, M.D.

Staff Pediatrician, Emergency Services, Minneapolis Children's Medical Center, Minneapolis, Minnesota
Bretylium

J. ANTHONY GOMES, M.D.

Professor of Medicine, and Director, Section of Electrocardiography and Electrophysiology, Mount Sinai School of Medicine, New York, New York
Ventricular Premature Complexes and Unsustained Ventricular Tachycardia: Invasive Approach

CHARLES D. GOTTLIEB, M.D.

Assistant Professor of Medicine, University of Pennsylvania School of Medicine; Associate Director of Cardiac Electrophysiology, Philadelphia Heart Institute, Philadelphia, Pennsylvania
Torsades de Pointes and Multiform Ventricular Tachycardia

ALLAN M. GREENSPAN, M.D.

Associate Professor of Medicine, Temple University School of Medicine; Co-Director, Clinical Cardiac Electrophysiology Laboratory and Heart Station, Philadelphia, Pennsylvania
Procainamide

JERRY C. GRIFFIN, M.D.

Associate Professor of Medicine, University of California San Francisco, School of Medicine; Associate Chief, Electrocardiography and Clinical Cardiac Electrophysiology Section, Moffitt-Long Hospitals, San Francisco, California
Paroxysmal Atrioventricular Reentrant Supraventricular Tachycardia: Nonpharmacologic Therapy

GERARD M. GUIRAUDON, M.D.

Professor of Surgery, University of Western Ontario Faculty of Medicine; Surgeon, Division of Cardiovascular and Thoracic Surgery, University Hospital, London, Ontario, Canada
Antiarrhythmic Surgery: Supraventricular Arrhythmia in Patients with Preexcitation

CHARLES I. HAFFAJEE, M.D.

Associate Professor of Medicine, Tufts University School of Medicine; Director of Cardiac Electrophysiology and Pacing, St. Elizabeth's Hospital, Boston, Massachusetts
Amiodarone

ROBERT M. HAMILTON, M.D.

Duncan L. Gordon Fellow, The Hospital for Sick Children, Toronto, Ontario, Canada; Fellow in Pediatric Cardiology, Texas Children's Hospital, Houston, Texas
Supraventricular Tachycardia in Pediatric Patients

STEPHEN C. HAMMILL, M.D.

Associate Professor of Medicine, Mayo Medical School; Consultant, Division of Cardiovascular Diseases and Internal Medicine, Mayo Clinic and Mayo Foundation, Rochester, Minnesota
Hypersensitive Carotid Sinus Syndrome

WILHELM HAVERKAMP, M.D.

Resident, Medical Hospital of the University of Münster, Münster, Germany, F.R.
Catheter Ablation

WALTER R. HEPP, M.D.

Fellow, Clinical Cardiac Electrophysiology, Philadelphia Heart Institute, Philadelphia, Pennsylvania
Ambulatory Electrocardiographic Monitoring

GERHARD HINDRICKS, M.D.

Resident, Medical Hospital of the University of Münster, Münster, Germany, F.R.
Catheter Ablation

LEONARD N. HOROWITZ, M.D.

Clinical Professor of Medicine, University of Pennsylvania School of Medicine; Co-Director, Philadelphia Heart Institute, Philadelphia, Pennsylvania
Ambulatory Electrocardiographic Monitoring
Atrial Fibrillation
Acute Myocardial Infarction
Endocrine Disease
Cardiac Arrhythmias in Pulmonary Disease
Infective Endocarditis
Cardiac Surgery and Cardiac Trauma
Digitalis Intoxication

EDWARD C. HUYCKE, M.D.

Division Surgeon, Irwin Army Community Hospital, Fort Riley, Kansas
Paroxysmal Reentrant Supraventricular Tachycardia Without Preexcitation: Pharmacologic Therapy

ALBERTO INTERIAN JR., M.D.

Assistant Professor of Medicine, and Director, Electrophysiology Laboratory, University of Miami School of Medicine, Miami, Florida
Ventricular Flutter and Ventricular Fibrillation

AMI E. ISKANDRIAN, M.D.

Clinical Professor of Medicine, University of Pennsylvania School of Medicine; Director, Noninvasive Cardiac Imaging, and Co-Director, Philadelphia Heart Institute, Philadelphia, Pennsylvania
Sinus Tachycardia

ROBERT M. JERESATY, M.D.

Professor of Medicine, University of Connecticut School of Medicine, Farmington, Connecticut; Director, Section of Cardiology, St. Francis Hospital and Medical Center, Hartford, Connecticut
Ventricular Arrhythmias in Mitral Valve Prolapse

MARIELL JESSUP, M.D.

Associate Professor of Medicine, Temple University School of Medicine; Medical Director, Heart Failure and Transplantation Center, Temple University Hospital, Philadelphia, Pennsylvania
Cardiomyopathy and Congestive Heart Failure

JOHN A. KASTOR, M.D.

Theodore E. Woodward Professor of Medicine, and Chairman, Department of Medicine, University of Maryland School of Medicine; Physician-in-Chief, University of Maryland Hospital, Baltimore, Maryland
Supraventricular Tachyarrhythmias: Classification and General Principles of Therapy

RAJ R. KAUSHIK, M.D.

Clinical Fellow, University of Western Ontario Faculty of Medicine; Clinical Fellow, Division of Cardiovascular and Thoracic Surgery, University Hospital, London, Ontario, Canada
Antiarrhythmic Surgery: Supraventricular Arrhythmia in Patients with Preexcitation

HAROLD R. KAY, M.D.

Associate Clinical Professor of Surgery, University of Pennsylvania School of Medicine; Attending Physician, Department of Cardiothoracic Surgery, Presbyterian Medical Center, Philadelphia, Pennsylvania
Permanent Pacemakers: Techniques of Implantation

ROBERT S. KIEVAL, V.M.D.

Research Fellow, University of Pennsylvania School of Veterinary Medicine, Philadelphia, Pennsylvania
Mechanisms of Arrhythmias and Basis of Antiarrhythmic Drug Action

GEORGE J. KLEIN, M.D.

Professor of Medicine, University of Western Ontario Faculty of Medicine; Director, Arrhythmia Service, and Director, Electrophysiology Laboratory, University Hospital, London, Ontario, Canada
Atrial Fibrillation in the Wolff-Parkinson-White Syndrome
Antiarrhythmic Surgery: Supraventricular Arrhythmia in Patients with Preexcitation

HARRY A. KOPELMAN, M.D.

Medical Director, Cardiac Electrophysiology, St. Joseph's Hospital of Atlanta, Atlanta, Georgia
Proarrhythmia

PHILLIP A. KOREN, M.D.

Fellow in Cardiology, Philadelphia Heart Institute; Clinical Associate of Medicine, University of Pennsylvania School of Medicine, Philadelphia, Pennsylvania
Digitalis Intoxication

JOHN KRATZ, M.D.

Associate Professor, Division of Surgery, Medical University of South Carolina, Charleston, South Carolina
Cardiac Pacing in Children and Young Adults

STEVEN P. KUTALEK, M.D.

Assistant Professor of Medicine and Clinical Pharmacology, Hahnemann University School of Medicine; Director, Clinical Cardiac Electrophysiology, Hahnemann University Hospital, Philadelphia, Pennsylvania
Temporary Pacemakers

MARIE-NOELLE S. LANGAN, M.D.

Fellow in Cardiology, Philadelphia Heart Institute; Clinical Associate of Medicine, University of Pennsylvania School of Medicine, Philadelphia, Pennsylvania
Cardiac Surgery and Cardiac Trauma

JONATHAN J. LANGBERG, M.D.

Assistant Professor of Medicine, University of California, San Francisco, School of Medicine; Director of Cardiac Electrophysiology Research, Moffitt-Long Hospitals, San Francisco, California
Paroxysmal Atrioventricular Reentrant Supraventricular Tachycardia: Nonpharmacologic Therapy

BRUCE D. LINDSAY, M.D.

Assistant Professor of Medicine, and Associate
Director, Clinical Electrophysiology Laboratory,
Washington University School of Medicine, St.
Louis, Missouri
*Preexcitation Syndromes: Diagnostic and Management
Strategies*

FRANCIS E. MARCHLINSKI, M.D.

Associate Professor of Medicine, University of
Pennsylvania School of Medicine; Co-Director,
Electrophysiology Laboratory, and Director,
Arrhythmia Evaluation Center, Hospital of The
University of Pennsylvania, Philadelphia,
Pennsylvania
Sustained Ventricular Tachycardia

FRANK I. MARCUS, M.D.

Professor of Medicine, University of Arizona
College of Medicine; Director of Electrophysiology,
University of Arizona Health Sciences Center,
Tucson, Arizona
Arrhythmogenic Right Ventricular Dysplasia

BARRY J. MARON, M.D.

Senior Investigator, National Institutes of Health,
Bethesda, Maryland
Arrhythmias in Hypertrophic Cardiomyopathy

BRIAN A. McGOVERN, M.D.

Assistant Professor of Medicine, Harvard Medical
School; Co-Director, Cardiac Arrhythmia Service,
Massachusetts General Hospital, Boston,
Massachusetts
Sotalol

T. JOHN MERCURO, M.D.

Fellow in Cardiology, Philadelphia Heart Institute;
Clinical Associate of Medicine, University of
Pennsylvania School of Medicine
Infective Endocarditis

SIMON MILSTEIN, M.D.

Assistant Professor of Medicine, University of
Minnesota School of Medicine; Director, Clinical
Electrophysiologic Laboratory, University of
Minnesota Hospital, Minneapolis, Minnesota
Bretylium

E. NEIL MOORE, D.V.M., Ph.D.

Professor of Physiology in Medicine, University of
Pennsylvania School of Medicine and School of
Veterinary Medicine, Philadelphia, Pennsylvania
*Mechanisms of Arrhythmias and Basis of Antiarrhythmic
Drug*

JOEL MORGANROTH, M.D.

Clinical Professor of Medicine, University of
Pennsylvania School of Medicine; Director, Center
of Excellence for Cardiovascular Studies, The
Graduate Health System, Philadelphia, Pennsylvania
*Ventricular Premature Complexes and Unsustained
Ventricular Tachycardia: Noninvasive Approach*

ROBERT J. MYERBURG, M.D.

Professor of Medicine and Physiology, and Director,
Division of Cardiology, University of Miami School
of Medicine; Director, Division of Cardiology,
University of Miami Jackson Memorial Medical
Center, Miami, Florida
*Intraventricular Conduction Disturbances and
Atrioventricular Block*
Ventricular Flutter and Ventricular Fibrillation

GERALD V. NACCARELLI, M.D.

Associate Professor of Medicine, and Director,
Clinical Electrophysiology, University of Texas
Medical School at Houston, Houston, Texas
*Paroxysmal Reentrant Supraventricular Tachycardia
Without Preexcitation: Nonpharmacologic Therapy*

STEVEN J. NIERENBERG, M.D.

Assistant Clinical Professor of Medicine, University
of Pennsylvania School of Medicine; Associate
Director, Cardiac Electrophysiology Laboratory,
Philadelphia Heart Institute, Philadelphia,
Pennsylvania
Electrophysiologic Techniques

CHARLES NYDEGGER, M.D.

Assistant Professor of Medicine, Hahnemann
University School of Medicine; Clinical Cardiac
Electrophysiology, Hahnemann University Hospital,
Philadelphia, Pennsylvania
Temporary Pacemakers

PAUL OSLIZLOK, M.D.

Fellow and Clinical Instructor, Division of Pediatric
Cardiology, Medical University of South Carolina,
Charleston, South Carolina
Cardiac Pacing in Children and Young Adults

JAMIE D. PARANICAS, M.D.

Clinical Cardiology Fellow, Albert Einstein Medical
Center, Philadelphia, Pennsylvania
Procainamide

PHILIP J. PODRID, M.D.

Associate Professor of Medicine, Boston University
School of Medicine; Director of Arrhythmia
Service, University Hospital, Boston, Massachusetts
Exercise Testing
Propafenone

CRAIG M. PRATT, M.D.

Associate Professor of Medicine, and Director,
Clinical Cardiology Research, Baylor College of
Medicine; Director, Coronary Care Unit, Methodist
Hospital, Houston, Texas
Moricizine

MAURICE PYE, M.B.

Research Fellow, Department of Medical
Cardiology, Royal Infirmary, Glasgow, United
Kingdom
Disopyramide

ALAN P. RAE, B.Sc., M.D.

Consultant Cardiologist, Department of Medical
Cardiology, Royal Infirmary, Glasgow, United
Kingdom
Disopyramide

C. PRATAP REDDY, M.D.

Professor of Medicine, Louisiana State University
School of Medicine; Associate Director, Cardiology
Section, and Director, Clinical Cardiac
Electrophysiology Laboratory, Louisiana State
University Medical Center, Shreveport, Louisiana
*Automatic Atrial Tachycardia and Nonparoxysmal
Atrioventricular Junctional Tachycardia*

JAMES A. REIFFEL, M.D.

Professor of Clinical Medicine, Columbia University
College of Physicians and Surgeons; Attending
Physician, and Associate Director, Arrhythmia
Control Unit, Presbyterian Hospital, New York,
New York
*Sinus Node Dysfunction: Sinus Bradyarrhythmias and
the Brady-Tachy Syndrome*

WALTER REYES, M.D.

Research Associate, University of Minnesota
Hospital, Minneapolis, Minnesota
Bretylium

DAN M. RODEN, M.D.

Professor of Medicine and Pharmacology, and
Director, Arrhythmia Unit, Vanderbilt University
School of Medicine, Nashville, Tennessee
Tocainide

RODOLPHE RUFFY, M.D.

Associate Professor of Internal Medicine, University
of Utah School of Medicine; Director, Arrhythmia
Service, University of Utah Medical Center, Salt
Lake City, Utah
Patients at High Risk of Sudden Cardiac Death

JEREMY N. RUSKIN, M.D.

Associate Professor of Medicine, Harvard Medical
School; Director, Cardiac Arrhythmia Service,
Massachusetts General Hospital, Boston,
Massachusetts
Sotalol

SANJEEV SAKSENA, M.D.

Clinical Associate Professor of Medicine, and
Director, Arrhythmia and Pacemaker Service,
University of Medicine and Dentistry of New
Jersey—New Jersey Medical School, Newark, New
Jersey
*Preexcitation Syndromes: Nonpharmacologic
Management*

MAGDI SAMI, M.D.

Associate Professor, McGill University Faculty of
Medicine; Associate Physician,
Medicine/Cardiology, and Director, Pacemaker and
Arrhythmia Service, Royal Victoria Hospital,
Montreal, Quebec, Canada
Encainide

MELVIN M. SCHEINMAN, M.D.

Professor of Medicine, University of California, San
Francisco, School of Medicine; Chief,
Electrocardiography and Clinical Cardiac
Electrophysiology Section, Moffitt-Long Hospitals,
San Francisco, California
*Paroxysmal Atrioventricular Reentrant Supraventricular
Tachycardia: Nonpharmacologic Therapy*

DAVID LEE SCHER, M.D.

Fellow in Cardiology, Philadelphia Heart Institute;
Clinical Associate of Medicine, University of
Pennsylvania School of Medicine, Philadelphia,
Pennsylvania
Cardiac Arrhythmias in Pulmonary Disease

PETER J. SCHWARTZ, M.D.

Professor of Medicine, University of Milan, Italy;
Chief, Cardiac Arrhythmias Unit/Department of
Medicine 2, University of Milan, Italy.
Long Q-T Syndrome

WILLIAM SCOTT, M.D.

Assistant Professor of Medicine, University of
Arizona College of Medicine, Tucson, Arizona
Arrhythmogenic Right Ventricular Dysplasia

BERNARD L. SEGAL, M.D.

Clinical Professor of Medicine, University of
Pennsylvania School of Medicine; Director,
Philadelphia Heart Institute, Philadelphia,
Pennsylvania
*History and Physical Examination of Patients with
Arrhythmia*

ARJUN D. SHARMA, M.D.

Volunteer Faculty, University of California, Davis, School of Medicine; Director, Interventional Electrophysiology, Sutter Memorial Hospital; Co-Director, Electrophysiology, Mercy General Hospital, Sacramento, California
Atrial Fibrillation in the Wolff-Parkinson-White Syndrome
Antiarrhythmic Surgery: Supraventricular Arrhythmia in Patients with Preexcitation

MARIUS SHARON, M.D.

Fellow in Cardiology, Philadelphia Heart Institute; Clinical Associate of Medicine, University of Pennsylvania School of Medicine, Philadelphia, Pennsylvania.
Acute Myocardial Infarction

ROSS J. SIMPSON, JR., M.D.

Associate Professor of Medicine, University of North Carolina at Chapel Hill School of Medicine; Director, Coronary Care Unit, North Carolina Memorial Hospital, Chapel Hill, North Carolina
Exercise and Catecholamine-Induced Ventricular Arrhythmia

MICHAEL B. SIMSON, M.D.

Associate Professor of Medicine, University of Pennsylvania School of Medicine; Director, Cardiac Care Unit, Hospital of the University of Pennsylvania, Philadelphia, Pennsylvania
Signal-Averaged Electrocardiography

JOSEPH F. SPEAR, PH.D.

Professor of Physiology, University of Pennsylvania School of Veterinary Medicine, Philadelphia, Pennsylvania
Mechanism of Arrhythmias and Basis of Antiarrhythmic Drug Action

SCOTT R. SPIELMAN, M.D.

Associate Professor of Medicine, Temple University School of Medicine; Co-Director, Clinical Cardiac Electrophysiology Laboratory and Heart Station, Albert Einstein Medical Center, Philadelphia, Pennsylvania
Permanent Pacemakers: Indications for Placement and Device Selection

CLIFFORD S. STRAUSS, D.O.

Cardiology Fellow, Albert Einstein Medical Center, Philadelphia, Pennsylvania
Permanent Pacemakers: Indications for Placement and Device Selection

RUEY J. SUNG, M.D.

Professor of Medicine, University of California, San Francisco, School of Medicine; Director, Cardiac Electrophysiology, San Francisco General Hospital, San Francisco, California
Paroxysmal Reentrant Supraventricular Tachycardia Without Preexcitation: Pharmacologic Therapy

BORYS SURAWICZ, M.D.

Senior Research Associate, Krannert Institute of Cardiology, Indiana University School of Medicine, Indianapolis, Indiana
Electrolyte Solutions

WILLIAM J. UNTEREKER, M.D.

Director, Cardiac Catheterization Laboratory, Philadelphia Heart Institute, Philadelphia, Pennsylvania
Cardiac Catheterization and Coronary Angioplasty

RICHARD L. VERRIER, PH.D.

Professor of Pharmacology, Georgetown University School of Medicine, Washington, D.C.
Autonomic Influences and Cardiac Arrhythmias

VICTORIA L. VETTER, M.D.

Associate Professor of Pediatrics, University of Pennsylvania School of Medicine; Senior Cardiologist, and Director, Electrophysiology and Electrocardiology Laboratories, Children's Hospital of Philadelphia, Philadelphia, Pennsylvania
Ventricular Arrhythmias in Pediatric Patients With and Without Congenital Heart Disease

KENT J. VOLOSIN, M.D.

Assistant Professor of Medicine, University of Medicine and Dentistry of New Jersey—Robert Wood Johnson Medical School; Director, Electrophysiology Laboratory, Cooper Hospital/ University Medical Center, Camden, New Jersey
Calcium Antagonists

ALBERT L. WALDO, M.D.

Walter H. Pritchard Professor of Cardiology and Professor of Medicine, Case Western Reserve University School of Medicine; Chief, Section of Cardiac Electrophysiology, University Hospitals of Cleveland, Cleveland, Ohio
Atrial Flutter

JAMES B. WATERS, M.D.

Fellow in Cardiovascular Disease, St. Elizabeth's Hospital, Boston, Massachusetts
Amiodarone

HARVEY L. WAXMAN, M.D.

Professor of Medicine, University of Medicine and Dentistry of New Jersey—Robert Wood Johnson Medical School; Head, Division of Cardiology, Cooper Hospital/University Medical Center, Camden, New Jersey
Calcium Antagonists

CHARLES R. WEBB, M.D.

Assistant Clinical Professor of Medicine, University of Michigan Medical School, Ann Arbor; Director, Cardiac Electrophysiology, Henry Ford Hospital, Detroit, Michigan
Wide QRS Complex Tachycardia

JAN RICHARD WEBER, M.D.

Clinical Assistant Professor of Medicine, University of Pennsylvania School of Medicine; Director, Cardiac Ultrasound Laboratory, Philadelphia Heart Institute, Philadelphia, Pennsylvania
Pregnancy
Management of Arrhythmias in Athletes

ISAAC WIENER, M.D.

Associate Clinical Professor of Medicine, University of California, Los Angeles, School of Medicine, Los Angeles; Associate Director of Cardiology, Valley Presbyterian Hospital, Van Nuys, California
Anesthesia and Surgery

DANIEL V. WILKINSON, JR., M.D.

Director of Electrophysiology, Swedish Hospital Medical Center, Seattle, Washington
Supraventricular (Atrial and Junctional) Premature Complexes

JOHN S. WILSON, M.D.

Instructor, Boston University Medical School; Chief Resident, University Hospital, Boston, Massachusetts
Propafenone

STEPHEN L. WINTERS, M.D.

Assistant Professor of Medicine, Mount Sinai School of Medicine; Director, Arrhythmia Clinic, Mount Sinai Medical Center, New York, New York
Ventricular Premature Complexes and Unsustained Ventricular Tachycardia: Invasive Approach

ALAN WOELFEL, M.D.

Assistant Professor of Medicine, and Director, Clinical Cardiac Electrophysiology Laboratory, University of North Carolina at Chapel Hill, Chapel Hill, North Carolina
Exercise and Catecholamine-Induced Ventricular Arrhythmia

RAYMOND L. WOOSLEY, M.D., PH.D.

Professor and Chairman, Department of Pharmacology, Georgetown Unversity School of Medicine; Director, Division of Clinical Pharmacology, Georgetown University Medical Center, Washington, D.C.
Mexiletine

RAYMOND YEE, M.D.

Assistant Professor of Medicine, University of Western Ontario Faculty of Medicine; Director, Arrhythmia Monitoring Unit, University Hospital, London, Ontario, Canada
Atrial Fibrillation in the Wolff-Parkinson-White Syndrome
Antiarrhythmic Surgery: Supraventricular Arrhythmia in Patients with Preexcitation

PETER M. YURCHAK, M.D.

Associate Clinical Professor of Medicine, Harvard Medical School; Physician, Massachusetts General Hospital, Boston, Massachusetts
Multifocal Atrial Tachycardia

VICKI ZEIGLER, B.S.N.

Pediatric Pacemaker Clinic Coordinator, Division of Pediatric Cardiology, Medical University of South Carolina, Charleston, South Carolina
Cardiac Pacing in Children and Young Adults

PREFACE

The purpose of *Current Management of Arrhythmias* is to provide a summary of recent developments in the diagnosis and management of cardiac arrhythmias and to present management strategies for arrhythmias. Arrhythmias have been studied intensely over the past three decades. As a result, significant advances have been made yet vexing controversies have arisen. Since the introduction of such diagnostic techniques as invasive electrophysiologic studies and such therapies as implantable antitachycardia devices, many needs have been answered and many questions have been raised. "Old" questions, such as the ventricular premature complex (VPC) hypothesis, have received new attention. We have addressed the gamut of these issues in our volume.

Chapters are arranged within sections. Sections on basic concepts and diagnostic techniques are followed by discussions of individual arrhythmias, both tachyarrhythmias and bradyarrhythmias. Arrhythmias are then discussed in the context of the specific clinical situations in which they are encountered. Finally, sections on treatment address antiarrhythmic agents and nonpharmacologic therapies, emphasizing indications for specific therapies and the relative role of each drug or modality in the treatment of a specific arrhythmia and in a particular clinical situation. These issues are discussed in several contexts. Different points of view emerge in these discussions, and where controversy exists, I have endeavored to obtain disparate viewpoints. Because differing opinions are expressed by the contributing authors, the index has been meticulously constructed to allow ready reference to the individual discussions of specific arrhythmias and therapies.

This volume has been written by recognized experts in the many areas of arrhythmia management, and its chapters have been edited to read more as a consultation than as a textbook. Each chapter presents a personal point of view, a feature that characterizes books in the Current Therapy series.

I have attempted to make this a volume of value to medical students, internists, and cardiologists.

I am grateful to the contributors to this volume who have produced excellent and timely articles. I learned a great deal while editing this text. I should like particularly to express my appreciation to Ms. Mary E. Mansor and Ms. Kimberly A. LoDico of B. C. Decker for their support and editorial guidance. I am grateful to my secretary, Mrs. Kathleen Freeman, for her enthusiastic and meticulous secretarial assistance in the preparation of the manuscript and in coordinating the preparation of this work.

Leonard N. Horowitz, M.D.
Bryn Mawr, Pennsylvania

Dedicated to my wife, Dona, and our children, Adam, Joshua, and Aimee,
who are my inspiration.

CONTENTS

I BASIC CONCEPTS

MECHANISMS OF ARRHYTHMIAS AND BASIS OF ANTIARRHYTHMIC DRUG ACTION

ROBERT S. KIEVAL, V.M.D.
JOSEPH F. SPEAR, Ph.D.
E. NEIL MOORE, D.V.M., Ph.D.

Cardiac arrhythmias can result from a disruption of impulse generation, aberrant impulse conduction, or a combination of these conditions. Extensive laboratory research using both in vivo and in vitro animal models of myocardial disease has revealed several different mechanisms of arrhythmogenesis within each of these broad categories. Abnormalities of impulse initiation associated with cardiac arrhythmias include the abnormal manifestation of normal automaticity, abnormal automaticity, and triggered activity. Arrhythmogenic disturbances in the conduction of the cardiac impulse include conduction block, reentry, and reflection.

The multiplicity of anatomic and electrophysiologic substrates for cardiac arrhythmias has led to the development of a variety of antiarrhythmic drugs, each designed to prevent or eliminate specific arrhythmogenic conditions. Our increasing ability to characterize the cellular and subcellular pathophysiology of these conditions has enabled us to understand better the mechanism of action of established antiarrhythmic agents and to develop new drugs with increased efficacy. References for several recent reviews that offer in-depth descriptions of mechanisms of arrhythmogenesis and pharmacologic strategies in the treatment of cardiac arrhythmias are provided at the end of this chapter.

Traditionally, the study of the cellular mechanisms of cardiac arrhythmias has concentrated on aberrations of the active and passive electrical properties of the cell membrane. At present much attention is being focused on electrotonic cell coupling, or the transmission of electrical impulses from one cell to the next, and the potential role of altered cell coupling in cardiac rhythm disturbances. In this chapter we discuss the contribution of cell coupling to cardiac conduction patterns under normal and pathologic conditions. Our objectives are to highlight the role that cell coupling could play in the genesis of cardiac arrhythmias and to consider how the pharmacologic modulation of cell coupling could be an important mechanism of antiarrhythmic action. The role of cell-to-cell electrical coupling has been approached experimentally only recently. Consequently, much of the following discussion is based on relatively recent experimental findings; therefore many of the conclusions remain theoretical. Before beginning this discussion, a brief review of some classic concepts of arrhythmogenesis is presented.

CLASSIC MECHANISMS OF CARDIAC ARRHYTHMIAS

Abnormalities of Impulse Generation

In the normal heart, several different cell types possess the property of automaticity. These include the cells of the sinoatrial node, the specialized atrial conducting fibers, certain cells in the atrioventricular node, and cells within the His-Purkinje system. Working atrial and ventricular myocardial cells are not normally automatic. Abnormalities of impulse generation can be caused by an alteration of the spontaneous activity of heart cells that are normally automatic, the development of spontaneous activity in cells that are not normally automatic, or a combination of these events.

Abnormal Manifestation of Normal Automaticity

Under normal circumstances, the sinoatrial node is the dominant pacemaker of the heart with the fastest intrinsic rate of firing. The slower potential pacemakers do not capture the heart because they are depolarized by impulses from the sinoatrial node before they reach threshold themselves and because they are overdrive suppressed. A slowing or

1

suppression of depolarization of the sinoatrial node, owing to an increase in vagal tone for example, could permit a fiber with a lower intrinsic rate to capture the heart and produce an atrial or ventricular escape beat. Continued suppression of the sinus node would eventually lead to the emergence of a subsidiary automatic focus as the dominant pacemaker and a prolonged escape rhythm.

In addition to atrial or ventricular escape following suppression of the sinoatrial node, the augmentation of automaticity in latent pacemakers can also lead to their manifestation in the heart. An increase in sympathetic tone associated with high circulating levels of catecholamines, caffeine, or fatigue, for example, may accelerate the intrinsic rate of depolarization in normally quiescent automatic fibers. An increase in the firing rate of these fibers may appear as isolated extrasystoles or as persistent ectopic rhythms.

Abnormal Automaticity

Abnormal automaticity refers to the development of spontaneous activity in cells with a depolarized resting membrane potential. Working atrial and ventricular myocardial cells are not normally automatic. However, under conditions that cause a reduction of the resting membrane potential toward zero, these fibers can begin to depolarize spontaneously, to generate action potentials, and to become ectopic pacemakers.

The action potentials that are evoked at lower membrane potentials in these cells show characteristics similar to those of the slow response action potentials that are more characteristic of the natural pacemaker tissues of the sinoatrial and atrioventricular nodes. This depolarization-induced automaticity, also referred to as slow-response automaticity, is also seen in Purkinje fibers, which, although they are normally automatic, display an increased rate of firing and similarly abnormal action potentials at lower resting membrane potentials. Conditions that may cause a loss of resting membrane potential and thus may support the development of abnormal automaticity include electrolyte imbalances, ischemia, and certain drug toxicities.

Focal Excitation in Acute Ischemia

During acute ischemia, myocardial tissue in the ischemic zone becomes depolarized. Nonischemic cells adjacent to the ischemic zone maintain their resting membrane potential. As a result of the disparate membrane potentials of adjacent cells, current flows from the depolarized ischemic tissue into the nonischemic tissue. This flow of "injury current" is manifested at the body surface as an elevation or depression of the S-T segment in the electrocardiogram. If the electrical coupling between ischemic and nonischemic cells remains intact (see further on), a sufficient amount of current may flow across the ischemic border zone to cause focal excitation of the nonischemic tissue and aberrant impulse generation.

Triggered Activity

Triggered activity refers to the generation of action potentials resulting from afterdepolarizations. Afterdepolarizations of the cell membrane may occur either during or following action potential repolarization. An action potential that results from an afterdepolarization reaching threshold potential may be followed by another afterdepolarization, which in turn may stimulate further action potentials. Individual triggered action potentials appear as extrasystoles, whereas continuous triggered activity is seen as a sustained ectopic rhythm.

Early afterdepolarizations occur during the repolarization phase of the action potential. Experimentally, they can be evoked by interventions that cause an increase in depolarizing current flow or a decrease in repolarizing current flow during the action potential plateau. Action potentials resulting from early afterdepolarizations are typically slow-response action potentials, since, as in abnormal automaticity, the action potentials are evoked from a membrane potential at which the fast sodium channels of the sarcolemma are largely inactivated.

Delayed afterdepolarizations occur following action potential repolarization. This type of afterdepolarization can be demonstrated with interventions that raise the intracellular calcium concentration. One classic example of this effect is seen with cardiac glycoside toxicity. Inhibition of the membrane sodium-potassium-ATPase by cardiac glycosides results in a rise in cell calcium indirectly through modification of the sarcolemmal sodium-calcium exchange mechanism. The rise in intracellular calcium sparks an oscillatory uptake and release of calcium from the sarcoplasmic reticulum, which in turn leads to a transient flow of depolarizing current into the cell and a transient membrane depolarization. In a manner similar to the behavior of an early afterdepolarization, a delayed depolarization can be of sufficient amplitude to evoke an action potential, which in turn may be followed by additional afterdepolarizations and triggered action potentials.

Triggered rhythms are distinguished from true automatic rhythms because they are always associated with and caused by a preceding action potential. In the absence of external stimulation, fibers capable of generating triggered action potentials remain quiescent. However, once an action potential is evoked, afterdepolarizations and repetitive activity may result.

Abnormalities of Impulse Conduction

A uniform and constant sequence of activation in the heart is necessary for the synchronous contraction of the myocardium and the effective pumping of blood. A disruption of the normal sequence of activation compromises myocardial efficiency and could lead to malignant arrhythmias. The causes of conduction disturbances in the heart include altered myocardial anatomy, abnormal electrophysiology, and an interaction between both of these components.

Conduction Block

Conduction block may be described as the failure of an electrical impulse to propagate when it encounters a region of tissue that is temporarily or permanently inexcitable. Tissue that is encountered during its refractory period is temporarily inexcitable. For example, a premature impulse may fail to conduct because normal tissue along the conduction pathway has not had time to recover from preceding activation. Conversely, a normal impulse may fail to conduct if the refractory period in adjacent tissue is prolonged. An infarcted region of tissue that has been replaced by scar is permanently inexcitable. Tissue that is healthy but electrically uncoupled from adjacent tissue is functionally inexcitable and will also cause conduction to fail. The effects of electrical uncoupling on conduction are discussed in further detail later.

Conduction block may occur along the specialized conduction pathways of the heart, or it may occur within the myocardium. In either case, tissue distal to the site of block will be activated by electrical impulses arriving from other areas of the myocardium. In the special case of conduction block out of the sinoatrial node, no electrical impulse will excite the heart until the block is removed or until a subsidiary automatic focus becomes the dominant pacemaker. Likewise, conduction block at the atrioventricular node will result in a similar lack of excitation of the ventricles.

Reentry

Reentry refers to the reexcitation of a region of myocardium by one electrical impulse that returns to a given area after traveling over a circuitous route. This circuitous pathway may surround a fixed obstacle of inexcitable tissue, such as a myocardial scar from previous myocardial infarction. The presence of such an inexcitable segment of myocardium, however, is not a requirement for reentry to occur.

One necessary condition for establishing reentry is unidirectional conduction block in the reentrant circuit. When an impulse enters a potential reentrant circuit, conduction proceeds in both directions from the point of entry. The failure of conduction in one direction (antegrade) along this pathway permits conduction in the other direction (retrograde) to continue without being extinguished. A second condition for reentry to occur is that the tissue at the site of block must not still be refractory when the retrograde impulse arrives. This condition requires a short refractory period at the site of block, slow conduction of the oncoming impulse elsewhere in the circuit, a long reentrant circuit, or a combination of these factors. If this condition is satisfied, the retrograde impulse will excite this region of myocardium, travel around the circuit while stimulating adjacent myocardium to produce an ectopic beat, and return to the original site of unidirectional block to reexcite this tissue.

Continuous reentry along a short reentrant pathway can cause rapid reexcitation of the myocardium where the reentrant focus becomes the dominant pacemaker of the heart. Excessive heart rates caused by reentrant tachycardias often deteriorate into ventricular fibrillation. This may result from fractionation of the reentrant wavefront into multiple wavelets that desynchronize myocardial activation, or from myocardial ischemia that develops because of a compromise of the coronary circulation resulting from inadequate diastolic coronary perfusion.

Reflection

Reflection is a form of reentry in which reexcitation of previously active myocardium by one impulse occurs over a single linear conduction pathway instead of a reentrant circuit. Although reflection has only been seen in vitro, the conditions supporting it could arise in the intact heart. This topic is discussed further later.

ELECTROPHYSIOLOGY AND STRUCTURAL BASIS OF CELL COUPLING

The electrical coupling between myocardial cells provides for an ordered and constant sequence of activation of the heart. Until recently, the potential contribution of deficient cell coupling to cardiac arrhythmogenesis was poorly understood. At present, the delineation of the role of cell coupling as a determinant of cardiac impulse generation and conduction is actively being studied. The pharmacologic modification of cell coupling as an antiarrhythmic strategy, however, remains largely unexplored.

Local Circuit Theory

In order to adequately understand the role of cell coupling in the heart, it is necessary first to consider the local circuit theory of conduction and the function of intercellular junctions. Local circuit theory was first developed to describe electrical conduction in nervous tissue; however, it is applicable to conduction in cardiac muscle as well. The cardiac action potential conducts along the cell membrane because the active inward sodium current (responsible for the upstroke or depolarization phase of the action potential) generates a local electrotonic current that travels from the active membrane region through the intracellular space to depolarize an adjacent patch of resting membrane. To complete the local circuit, this current crosses the membrane and returns to the active site via the extracellular space. When the adjacent patch of membrane is depolarized to threshold potential, that region of membrane, in turn, generates an active sodium current to continue the progression of the action potential.

According to this model, current flow intracellularly, across the cell membrane, and through the extracellular space are all required for conduction to proceed. Alterations in the intracellular, extracellular, or membrane resistance markedly influence current flow and are manifested as changes in conduction velocity. Extreme increases in any of these resistances can disrupt the local circuit and cause complete conduction failure.

In order for action potentials to propagate from cell to cell, local circuit theory dictates that current must flow directly from the cytoplasm of one cell to that of the next. Although cardiac muscle is not an anatomic syncytium (that is, each myocardial cell or fiber is completely bound by a discrete cell membrane with a high resistance to current flow), specialized low-resistance junctions between myocardial cells facilitate the intercellular transmission of electrical impulses, thus allowing the tissue to behave as a *functional* syncytium. In this way, these low-resistance intercellular junctions serve to couple cells electrically by permitting intracellular currents from one cell to depolarize the membrane of a contiguous cell before returning extracellularly to complete the local circuit.

The Gap Junction

The low-resistance pathway for intercellular current flow is the gap junction or nexus. The gap junction is a specialized segment of sarcolemma containing numerous connexons, each of which consists of six identical protein subunits surrounding a central hydrophilic hemichannel. The connexons in the nexal membrane of two contiguous cells abut in a narrow (2 to 4 nm) intercellular "gap," thus forming complete transcellular aqueous channels. These channels permit the intercellular diffusion of ions and small molecules and thus provide the means for electrical current flow and the exchange of metabolites and possibly intracellular second messengers between cells.

Myocardial gap junctions are primarily located within intercalated disks and thus electrically couple cells aligned end-to-end. However, electrotonic coupling through gap junctions between cells that are situated side-to-side can also be demonstrated. The degree of electrotonic coupling between myocardial cells is dynamic and dependent on the variable electrical resistance (or conductance) of gap junctions. Changes in the gap junctional resistance can occur under a variety of physiologic and pathologic conditions and are mediated by the opening and closing of the junctional channels. The gap junctional resistance is a major determinant of the total intracellular resistance, and thus changes in this property can largely influence local circuit current flow and conduction velocity.

Although the exact nature of the gating of gap junctional channels is not known, a majority of the evidence obtained thus far suggests that channel closure is all or none and that the electrical conductance of each channel is either maximal or zero. Since each channel is either fully open or fully closed, the bulk electrical conductance of the gap junction at any given time is the sum of the unitary conductances of the open channels. Conditions that reduce the open-state probability of these channels thus uncouple cells and retard conduction by decreasing the total gap junctional conductance, and conversely, conditions that favor channel opening facilitate conduction by improving cell coupling.

Voltage clamp experiments in isolated cell pairs have shown that changes in the intracellular milieu profoundly affect gap junctional conductance. For example, pathologic elevation of the intracellular calcium ion concentration can completely uncouple myocardial cells. Intracellular acidification has also been shown to reduce gap junctional conductance, whereas increases in cytoplasmic cAMP levels augment it. (See DeMello, 1987 for review.)

Since the gap junctional conductance is sensitive to the intracellular environment, pharmacologic agents that affect the intracellular concentrations of ions and second messengers may also be expected to influence the degree of cell coupling. This expectation has proved to be well founded, as a variety of clinically used and experimental drugs have been found to alter gap junctional conductance.

IMPACT OF CELL COUPLING ON CONDUCTION OF THE CARDIAC IMPULSE

Anisotropy

The three-dimensional distribution of gap junctions within the myocardium and the high resistivity of the junctions relative to that of the myoplasm give rise to the anisotropy of conduction velocity observed in cardiac muscle. Experiments performed in isolated cells have shown that the electrotonic coupling between laterally connected cell pairs is equivalent to that of pairs joined end-to-end. However, since the myoplasm has a lower resistivity than the gap junction itself, and since more gap junctional resistances are encountered per unit distance transverse to myocardial fiber orientation by virtue of the fact that myocardial cells are longer than they are wide, the effective intracellular resistivity is less for a given distance along myocardial fibers than for the same distance transverse to the fibers. The effect of the increased resistivity transverse to fiber orientation is that conduction proceeds slower when moving in this direction than when moving along fiber orientation.

In addition to directional differences in conduction velocity, other electrophysiologic properties of cardiac muscle are affected by myocardial anisotropy. For example, there is evidence that the safety factor for conduction is lower for conduction longitudinal to fiber orientation (Spach et al, 1981). That is, slower conduction transverse to fiber orientation may be more resistant to disturbances in membrane properties than faster longitudinal conduction. One implication of this complex relationship is that longitudinal conduction of a premature impulse may fail, whereas transverse conduction is preserved. In a recent study of the characteristics of conduction in the epicardial border zone overlying a transmural infarct during premature stimulation, the combination of conduction block in the longitudinal direction of the fibers and slow but persistent transverse conduction was implicated in establishing the epicardial reentry and sustained ventricular tachycardia seen in this canine model (Diller et al, 1988).

Finally, it has been shown experimentally that the depolarization phase of the action potential is also influenced by the direction of conduction relative to myocardial fiber orientation. In anisotropic cardiac muscle, the amplitude and maximal rate of depolarization of action potentials are greater during transverse conduction of the cardiac impulse. This is explained by a directional difference in the net open time of active sodium channels. Consequently, the direction of conduction of the cardiac impulse may influence the binding of drugs to the sodium channel according to the "modulated receptor" theory (Hille, 1977).

Excitability and Refractoriness

Electrotonic interactions during repolarization of the action potential may modulate action potential duration and, as a result, refractoriness of cardiac tissue. Because of the electrotonic influence of adjacent tissue on a given region, the action potential duration is longer at the site of origin of a conducted wavefront than at a distance from the origin. In addition, at a site of collision of two approaching impulses, action potential duration is reduced.

In a recent study using a computer model of conduction in a two-dimensional grid of cells, we found that the degree of cell-to-cell coupling was also an important determinant of the heterogeneity of action potential duration. In regions with tight electrical coupling, action potential durations were uniform. However, when the modeled cells were progressively uncoupled, intrinsic differences in action potential duration between adjacent cells became manifest, because local current flow between regions that tended to repolarize early and those that remained depolarized longer was impeded. Moreover, this study suggested that a further reduction in the degree of cell coupling could exacerbate this tissue inhomogeneity to the point at which conduction block would occur in areas of prolonged action potential duration and refractoriness.

The importance of the electrotonic modulation of action potential duration in cardiac arrhythmogenesis has not been verified. However, a prerequisite for reentry to occur is the establishment of functional unidirectional block between adjacent regions of tissue. Attenuated cell coupling may facilitate such block by allowing the manifestation of intrinsic differences in action potential duration and refractoriness.

Membrane excitability, or the amount of current required to initiate a propagated action potential, is also influenced by cell coupling. According to Rushton's theory of liminal length, depolarization of tissue in a local region of stimulation will be resisted by hyperpolarizing current flow from adjacent resting myocardium. The amount of depolarizing current required to bring enough of the sarcolemma (the liminal length) to threshold in order to overcome this tendency is a function of the ease with which current can flow from the surrounding tissue. In this situation, electrical uncoupling of cells retards local current flow, reduces the liminal length, and increases local excitability (Joyner et al, 1989).

Electrotonus

A large increase in coupling resistance can curtail local current flow to the point at which active impulse propagation can no longer be supported and cell communication is reduced to electrotonic interaction. Such a consequence underlies the phenomenon of reflection, a form of reentry in which delayed, electrotonically mediated activation allows a cardiac impulse to reexcite previously active myocardium by retrograde conduction along a single pathway. Although reflection has only been seen in experimental preparations in vitro (Antzelevitch, 1988), it nevertheless highlights the dependence of active impulse transmission on cell coupling and the potential consequences of the electrotonic interactions that occur in its absence.

To demonstrate reflection, Purkinje fibers are placed in a partitioned, gapped chamber in which a sucrose solution fills the extracellular space in the gap between the proximal and distal segments of the fiber. The sucrose gap increases the extracellular resistance between proximal and distal segments and effectively electrically uncouples these regions by impeding local circuit current flow. Once this is achieved, the degree of electrical coupling between proximal and distal segments can be precisely controlled by placing various shunt resistors across the gap.

With high extracellular resistance, long delays between stimulation of the proximal segment and activation of the distal segment can be seen. Active membrane currents in the proximal segment are attenuated in the sucrose gap, and the distal segment of membrane is slowly charged to threshold electrotonically, producing an activation delay of up to several hundred milliseconds. This delay can be sufficient to allow the proximal segment to recover excitability. Activation of the distal segment can then similarly reexcite the proximal segment to produce a "reflected" action potential.

Even if the distal segment is not fully activated, large subthreshold depolarizations can occur beyond the site of block. These electrotonic responses can influence the membrane responsiveness of the distal region such that additional subthreshold stimulation will evoke a full action potential. Such electrotonic facilitation of excitability across a site of block was first demonstrated by Wedensky in nerve in 1903.

The contribution of these phenomena to clinical arrhythmias has not yet been documented. However, prepotentials and other electrotonic interactions are commonly observed in experimental models of myocardial infarction and other arrhythmogenic disease states. This suggests that reflection may play a role in certain cardiac conduction disturbances and is further evidence that altered cell coupling by any mechanism must be considered as a potential source of cardiac arrhythmias.

Atrioventricular Nodal Reentry

One final abnormality of cardiac conduction that may be attributable to poor cell coupling is atrioventricular (AV) nodal reciprocating tachycardia. Conceptually, for reentry to occur through the AV node, two functionally separate conduction pathways must be present: one to carry the impulse antegrade, the other to carry the retrograde reentrant beat (Mendez and Moe, 1966). Sufficient cellular uncoupling in this region could provide the necessary substrate for sustaining reentry by replacing the syncytial nature of this tissue with functionally separate conduction pathways.

CELL COUPLING AND CARDIAC IMPULSE INITIATION

Synchronization of Pacemaker Cells

The natural pacemaker tissues of the heart rely on cell-to-cell electrical continuity to synchronize their activity. If electrotonic coupling in the sinoatrial node is disrupted, usually inapparent differences in the intrinsic rates of depolarization of individual cells become manifest. Mutual modulation of automaticity as well as parasystolic behavior between functionally isolated adjacent pacemaker sites can develop and give rise to complex patterns of sinus node activity. This has been shown both experimentally and using computer models of pacemaker cells (Jalife and Michaels, 1985).

Suppression

At the edge of the sinoatrial node, spontaneous activity in pacemaker cells is suppressed by the adjacent nonautomatic atrial myocardium. This is because the resting membrane of working atrial myocytes effectively clamps the membrane potential of the contiguous pacemaker cells and prevents their diastolic depolarization. Uncoupling of the nonautomatic regions from the suppressed pacemaker sites allows the manifestation of pacemaker activity (Kirchhof et al, 1987). These subsidiary automatic foci can then compete with the dominant pacemaker sites for control of the sinoatrial node.

Age-Related Changes in Coupling

The combination of the expression of different intrinsic rates of automaticity, competition for dominance of the sinoatrial node, and complex patterns of sinus node activity discussed above is reminiscent of the sick sinus syndrome, which is characterized by paroxysms of bradycardia and tachycardia associated with electrocardiographic evidence of abnormal atrial conduction. In the human atrium, there is a progressive ingrowth of connective tissue with increasing age. In older atrial tissues studied in vitro, collagenous septa partition myocardial bundles, causing lateral cell-to-cell uncoupling. Transverse conduction in these older atrial tissues is characteristically discontinuous, producing multiple components in recorded extracellular electrograms and of nonuniform anisotropy (Spach, Dolber, and Heidlage, 1988). Since the bradycardia-tachycardia syndrome is more prevalent in older patients and is characterized in part by abnormal sinoatrial conduction, it is tempting to speculate that progressive cellular uncoupling with increasing age may be involved in the etiology of this disease.

CELL COUPLING IN MYOCARDIAL INJURY

Although its seemingly ubiquitous influence on cardiac impulse generation and conduction suggests an important role for cell coupling in cardiac arrhythmias, relatively little direct experimental evidence of this is available. However, the measurement of cell-to-cell current flow in isolated preparations has shown that cell coupling is responsible for certain characteristic electrophysiologic phenomena associated with acute ischemia. Additional evidence obtained in intact animals has implicated pathologic cell uncoupling in arrhythmias seen following chronic myocardial infarction.

Ischemia

Almost immediately after interruption of blood flow to the myocardium, individual cardiac cells undergo profound changes as a result of hypoxia, substrate deprivation, and the local accumulation of metabolites and electrolytes. The resting membrane potential becomes depolarized, and the intensity of the fast inward sodium current is decreased. Impulse conduction rapidly becomes slow and asynchronous.

The presence of coupling between the injured, depolarized ischemic region and adjacent nonischemic tissue allows for the difference in resting membrane potential to initiate a continuous flow of current between these two areas. This injury current is detected on the body surface as S-T segment elevation or depression. This flow of current between injured and border zone normal tissue may cause focal excitation of the normal tissue and induce arrhythmias.

As ischemia progresses, cell-to-cell uncoupling occurs as injured cells begin to die. Presumably the dying cells are calcium overloaded, and this functional isolation of injured tissue has been attributed to a calcium-induced increase in gap junctional resistance (see DeMello, 1987). As a result of this, current flow between healthy and depolarized regions decreases, reducing the magnitude of the injury potentials in the S-T segment.

Although the primary abnormality of conduction in the ischemic zone appears acutely to be due to depolarization of the membrane and a decrease in the magnitude of the fast inward current, the electrical uncoupling of ischemic cells also eventually contributes. Conduction in the ischemic zone is nonuniform and discontinuous, producing characteristic fractionation in recorded extracellular activity that is often associated with reentrant excitation (Kleber, Riegger, and Janse, 1987).

From these findings, cell coupling appears to contribute to the ventricular arrhythmias associated with acute ischemia in two ways. Initially, before uncoupling occurs, the flow of injury current between ischemic and normal tissue may allow focal excitation. Later, after the uncoupling of ischemic cells, the resulting dissociated conduction may support the continuous reentry from which ventricular tachyarrhythmias arise.

Infarction

Persistent myocardial ischemia leads to infarction, in which cardiac muscle dies and is replaced by scar tissue. Weeks or months after infarction, cardiac arrhythmias may still occur. Although the active membrane properties of surviving cells within an experimental infarct recover, conduction within the infarcted region remains bizarre. Experiments performed in our laboratory indicate that aberrant conduction in this region is caused by cell-to-cell electrical uncoupling. Additional evidence of this has been documented in a canine model of infarction in which permanent occlusion of the left anterior descending coronary artery leads to reentrant arrhythmias originating in the epicardium overlying the infarct. In one study using this model, the sluggish conduction seen during reentry consisted of abnormally slow conduction transverse to myocardial fiber orientation, apparently resulting from compromised cell coupling (Dillon et al, 1988).

In reperfused infarcts in which the surviving myocardium is dispersed transmurally within a matrix of scar, the reentrant pathway is anatomically circuitous, indicating that cell-to-cell coupling must be disrupted. In animals with this type of experimental infarction, arrhythmias may be inducible for years. The unique substrate in these myocardial infarcts, in which the active membrane properties are normal and the basis for the abnormal conduction leading to reentry is anatomic, may be responsible for the notorious difficulty in controlling these types of arrhythmias with conventional pharmacologic therapy.

PHARMACOLOGIC MODIFICATION OF CELL COUPLING: A POSSIBLE ROLE IN ANTIARRHYTHMIC ACTION

The sensitivity of gap junctional conductance to the intracellular milieu has led to the expectation that drugs that modify the intracellular ionic environment or lead to the production of intracellular second messengers affect the magnitude of cell coupling. This hypothesis has been confirmed using in vitro techniques to measure intercellular current flow before and after drug administration. Several classes of drugs, including general anesthetics, positive inotropic agents, and antiarrhythmic agents have been found to influence cell-to-cell coupling directly.

For example, digitalis-like agents uncouple myocardial cells (Weingart, 1977). This effect is most probably caused by blockade of the sodium-potassium ATPase system and a resultant increase in intracellular sodium concentration. The latter mediates an increase in cell calcium via altered sodium-calcium exchange. The direct effect of increased intracellular calcium is a closure of gap junctional channels and increased intercellular resistance to current flow.

Halothane, a widely used general anesthetic, has also been shown to cause cellular uncoupling. This is of particular interest because halothane is known to be arrhythmogenic. Cellular uncoupling by halothane was first shown as a decreased space constant in Purkinje fibers (Hauswirth, 1967), but this was later confirmed as an increase in the internal longitudinal resistance in papillary muscles (Wojtczak, 1984), and most recently it was demonstrated as an increase in the gap junctional resistance between isolated cell pairs (Niggli et al, 1989). Unlike the effects of cardiac glycosides, the mechanism of uncoupling by halothane may be unrelated to cell calcium, since inhibition of calmodulin, a primary mediator of intracellular calcium action, does not inhibit halothane-induced electrical dissociation.

Isoproterenol, a positive inotropic agent, has been shown to increase gap junctional conductance (DeMello, 1988). This improvement in cell coupling may facilitate enhanced inotropy by maximally synchronizing cardiac contraction. The effects of isoproterenol are thought to be mediated by increased intracellular cAMP production, since inhibition of cAMP-dependent protein kinase abolishes the effects of this drug.

Procainamide, a class I antiarrhythmic agent, has also been shown to augment cell coupling by increasing the space constant of Purkinje fibers (Arnsdorf and Bigger, 1976). This effect appears primarily attributable to an increase in membrane resistance, but it may also involve a direct effect of these agents on gap junctional conductance. As a sodium channel blocking agent, procainamide causes a fall in the intracellular sodium concentration and, through the sodium-calcium exchange mechanism, should lead to a decrease in the intracellular calcium concentration. This postulated fall in cell calcium may be responsible for the negative inotropic effects of this and other class I agents and could also mediate an increase in gap junctional conductance.

Matrix Concept of Antiarrhythmic Drug Action

Although it has been known for some time that antiarrhythmic drugs modify cell coupling, there has been relatively little theoretical or experimental analysis of this as an antiarrhythmic mechanism of action. Recently, Arnsdorf 1984 presented a concep-

tual technique for evaluating drug action. His matrix concept involves a mutual interaction among active and passive electrophysiologic properties, including cell coupling as manifested by the space constant. Different drugs affect these properties to varying degrees. However, regardless of its primary mechanism of action, any agent that affects one of these properties will, because of the interrelationships among them, influence all other parameters to some degree. This fact emphasizes the need to consider a change in cell coupling as a potentially significant antiarrhythmic mechanism and possibly to reexamine what are considered the "primary" mechanisms of action of antiarrhythmic agents in this light.

Influence of the Anisotropic Nature of Cardiac Muscle

The anisotropic properties of myocardial tissue can greatly influence the effects of drugs on the cardiac cell membrane. For example, the open time of the sodium channels in the sarcolemma is longer during impulse propagation longitudinal to myocardial fiber orientation. Because of this, drugs that preferentially bind to sodium channels in the active state will bind to a greater degree in areas where conduction is proceeding primarily longitudinally. Accordingly, certain class I antiarrhythmic agents that block the fast inward current have a greater effect on depressing conduction velocity in the longitudinal direction. Furthermore, the electrotonic modulation of action potential duration may also contribute to differences in drug binding. Drugs that bind to the inactive state of the sodium channel have a greater effect in those areas that have action potentials of longer duration.

The directional difference in internal axial resistance that results from the greater number of gap junctions encountered per unit distance transverse to fiber orientation is also a determinant of the magnitude of a drug effect on conduction. Drugs that change gap junctional resistance have a greater effect on propagation in the transverse direction. The most definitive example of this can be seen with heptanol, an aliphatic alcohol that increases gap junctional resistance without significant effects on the fast inward current. After exposure to heptanol, conduction traveling transverse to myocardial fiber orientation is markedly depressed, whereas longitudinal conduction is less severely affected.

In contrast to heptanol, procainamide has been found to slow conduction to a greater degree longitudinal to fiber orientation. This effect could be due to the aforementioned greater degree of binding to activated sodium channels. However, an alternative explanation is that procainamide, while decreasing the fast inward current and slowing conduction by this mechanism, also decreases gap junctional resistance through its modulation of intracellular calcium concentration. The latter action would have a greater effect on conduction transverse to fiber orientation such that although conduction would be retarded in both directions, transverse conduction would be preferentially preserved.

The implications of the dependence of drug action on anisotropy for an antiarrhythmic effect have yet to be elucidated. However, it is possible to speculate that if anisotropy plays a role in the unidirectional block and slow conduction initiating and sustaining reentry, any drug that preferentially depresses conduction longitudinal and not transverse to fibers may have an antiarrhythmic advantage. For example, with a drug of this type the unidirectional block occurring longitudinally in canine models of myocardial infarction could be converted to bidirectional block without substantially further retarding transverse conduction (Dillon et al, 1988).

Moreover, drugs that alter cell-to-cell coupling by changing the gap junctional conductance could also contribute to the elimination of aberrant conduction pathways. This is because regions of the heart having greater gap juntional resistance as a result of a pathologic condition are more sensitive to the effect of an agent that modifies gap junctional resistance. In the surviving tissue of the healed infarct, the slow conduction and block that provide the probable substrate for reentrant ventricular tachycardia occur in regions having the highest junctional resistance. This raises the possibility that such abnormal regions could be pharmacologically "ablated" using an agent that further increased gap junctional resistance, thus selectively eliminating them from the conduction path. Pharmacologically enhancing junctional conductance in areas where it is depressed represents an alternative method of abolishing the abnormal pathway (Spear et al, 1989).

Although the modification of cell coupling could be a significant antiarrhythmic mechanism, the possibility remains that it could also contribute to the genesis of cardiac arrhythmias. We have just discussed many instances in which electrical dissocation in myocardial tissue may be responsible for conduction disturbances. A pharmacologic agent, then, by its tendency to uncouple myocardial cells, could theoretically enhance the likelihood that an arrhythmia will occur. The fact that the toxic effects of digitalis, procainamide, and many other antiarrhythmic drugs include cardiac arrhythmias supports this possibility.

Several antiarrhythmic agents have been shown to influence cell-to-cell electrical coupling. However, little is known about how such modulation contributes to their antiarrhythmic or proarrhythmic action. Recent studies have demonstrated the likely role of abberant cell coupling in cardiac rhythm disturbances. The potential for eliminating these abnormalities using pharmacologic methods deserves further investigation.

SUGGESTED READING

Antzelevitch C. Reflection as a mechanism of reentrant cardiac arrhythmias. In: Zipes DP, Rowlands DJ, eds. Progress in cardiology. Philadelphia: Lea & Febiger, 1988: 3–16.

Arnsdorf MF. Basic understanding of the electrophysiologic actions of antiarrhythmic drugs: Sources, sinks and matrices of information. Med Clin North Am 1984; 68:1247–1280.

Arnsdorf MF, Bigger JT Jr. The effect of procaine amide on components of excitability in long mammalian cardiac Purkinje fibers. Circ Res 1976; 38:115–122.

Bailey JC, Spear JF, Moore EN. Microelectrode demonstration of Wedensky facilitation in canine cardiac Purkinje fibers. Circ Res 1973; 33:48–53.

Bajaj AK, Kopelman HA, Wikswo JP Jr, et al. Frequency- and orientation-dependent effects of mexiletine and quinidine on conduction in the intact dog heart. Circulation 1987; 75:1065–1073.

Balke CW, Lesh MD, Spear JF, et al. Effects of cellular uncoupling on conduction in anisotropic canine ventricular myocardium. Circ Res 1988; 63:879–892.

Boineau JP, Cox JL. Slow ventricular activation in acute myocardial infarction: A source of reentrant premature ventricular contraction. Circulation 1973; 48:702–713.

De Felice LJ, Challice CE. Anatomical and ultrastructural study of the electrophysiological atrioventricular node of the rabbit. Circ Res 1969; 24:457–474.

De Mello WC. Effect of intracellular injection of calcium and strontium on cell communication in heart. J Physiol 1975; 250:231–245.

De Mello WC. Modulation of junctional permeability. In: De Mello WC, ed. Cell-to-cell communication. New York: Plenum Press, 1987:29–64.

De Mello WC. Increase in junctional conductance caused by isoproterenol in heart cell pairs is suppressed by cAMP-dependent protein-kinase inhibitor. Biochem Biophys Res Commun 1988; 154:509–514.

Dillon SM, Allessie MA, Ursell PC, Wit AL. Influences of anisotropic tissue structure on reentrant circuits in the epicardial border zone of subacute canine infarcts. Circ Res 1988; 63:182–206.

Guevara MR, Glass L. Phase locking, period-doubling bifurcations and chaos in a mathematical model of a periodically driven oscillator: A theory for the entrainment of biological oscillators and the generation of cardiac dysrhythmias. J Math Biol 1982; 14:1–23.

Hanich RF, De Langen CDJ, Kadish AH, et al. Inducible sustained ventricular tachycardia 4 years after experimental canine myocardial infarction: Electrophysiologic and anatomic comparisons with early healed infarcts. Circulation 1988; 77:445–456.

Hauswirth O. The influence of halothane on the electrical properties of cardiac Purkinje fibers. J Physiol 1969; 201:42P–43P.

Hille B. Local anesthetics: Hydrophilic and hydrophobic pathways for the drug-receptor reaction. J Gen Physiol 1977; 69:497–515.

Hodgkin AL. Evidence for electrical transmission in nerve. J Physiol 1937; 90:183–232.

Hoffman BF, Dangman KH. Mechanisms for cardiac arrhythmias. Experientia 1987; 43:1049–1056.

Hoyt TH, Cohen ML, Saffitz JE. Distribution and three-dimensional structure of intercellular junctions in canine myocardium. Circ Res 1989; 64:563–574.

Jalife J, Michaels DC. Phase-dependent interactions of cardiac pacemakers as mechanisms of control and synchronization in the heart. In: Zipes DP, Jalife J, eds. Cardiac electrophysiology and arrhythmias. Orlando:Grune & Stratton, 1985:109–119.

Jalife J, Moe GK. Effect of electrotonic potentials on pacemaker activity of canine Purkinje fibers in relation to parasystole. Circ Res 1976; 39:801–808.

Janse MJ, Van Capelle FJL. Electrotonic interactions across an inexcitable region as a cause of ectopic activity in acute regional myocardial ischemia: A study in intact porcine and canine hearts and computer models. Circ Res 1982; 50:527–537.

Janse MJ, Van Capelle FJL, Morsink H, et al. Flow of "injury" current and patterns of excitation during early ventricular arrhythmias in acute regional myocardial ischemia in isolated porcine and canine hearts. Circ Res 1980; 47:151–165.

Joyner RW, Ramza BM, Tan RC, et al. Effects of tissue geometry on initiation of a cardiac action potential. Am J Physiol 1989; 256:H391–H403.

Kadish AH, Spear JF, Levine JH, Moore EN. The effects of procainamide on conduction in anisotropic canine ventricular myocardium. Circulation 1986; 74:616–625.

Kirchhof CJHJ, Bonke FIM, Allessie MA, Lammers WJEP. The influence of the atrial myocardium on impulse formation in the rabbit sinus node. Pflugers Arch 1987; 410:198–203.

Kleber AG, Riegger CB, Janse MJ. Electrical uncoupling and increase of extracellular resistance after induction of ischemia in isolated, arterially perfused rabbit papillary muscle. Circ Res 1987; 61:271–279.

Lesh MD, Pring M, Spear JF. Cellular uncoupling can unmask dispersion of action potential duration in ventricular myocardium—a computer modeling study. Circ Res 1989; 65:1426–1440.

Mendez C, Moe GK. Demonstration of a dual AV nodal conduction system in the isolated rabbit heart. Circ Res 1966; 19:378–393.

Niggli E, Rudisuli A, Maurer P, Weingart R. Effects of general anesthetics on current flow across membranes in guinea pig myocytes. Am J Physiol 1989; 256:C273–C281.

Rosen MRR. Mechanisms for arrhythmias. Am J Cardiol 1988; 61:2A–8A.

Rosen MR, Danilo P Jr: Cellular electrophysiologic mechanisms of antiarrhythmic drug action. In: Reiser HJ, Horowitz LN, eds. Mechanisms and treatment of cardiac arrhythmias: Relevance of basic studies to clinical management. Baltimore:Urban & Schwarzenberg, 1985:71–88.

Rushton WAH. Initiation of the propagated disturbance. Proc R Soc Lond 1937; B124:210–243.

Spach MS, Dolber PC. Relating extracellular potentials and their derivatives to anisotropic propagation at a microscopic level in human cardiac muscle. Evidence for electrical uncoupling of side-to-side fiber connections with increasing age. Circ Res 1986; 58:356–371.

Spach MS, Dolber PC, Heidlage JF, et al. Propagating depolarization in anisotropic human and canine cardiac muscle: Apparent directional differences in membrane capacitance. Circ Res 1987; 60:206–219.

Spach MS, Dolber PC, Heidlage JF. Influence of the passive anisotropic properties on directional differences in propagation following modification of the sodium conductance in human atrial muscle. A model of reentry based on anisotropic discontinuous propagation. Circ Res 1988; 62:811–832.

Spach MS, Kootsey JM. Relating the sodium current and conductance to the shape of transmembrane and extracellular potentials by simulation: Effects of propagation boundaries. IEEE Transactions on Biomedical Engineering 1985; BME32: 743–755.

Spach MS, Kootsey JM, Sloan JD. Active modulation of electrical coupling between cardiac cells of the dog. A mechanism for transient and steady state variations in conduction velocity. Circ Res 1982; 51:347–362.

Spach MS, Miller WT III, Geselowitz DB, et al: The discontinuous nature of propagation in normal canine cardiac muscle. Evidence for recurrent discontinuities of intracellular resistance that affect the membrane currents. Circ Res 1981; 48:39–54.

Spear JF, Balke CW, Lesh MD, et al. The effect of cellular uncoupling by heptanol on conduction in infarcted myocardium. Circ Res 1990; 66:202–217.

Spear JF, Michelson EL, Moore EN. Cellular electrophysiologic characteristics of chronically infarcted myocardium in dogs susceptible to sustained ventricular tachyarrhythmias. J Am Coll Cardiol 1983; 1:1099–1110.

Spear JF, Michelson EL, Moore EN. Reduced space constant in slowly conducting regions of chronically infarcted canine myocardium. Circ Res 1983; 53:176–185.

Steinbeck G, Bonke FIM, Allessie MA, Lammers WJEP. Cardiac glycosides and pacemaker activity of the sinus node—A microelectrode study on the isolated right atrium of the rabbit. In: Bonke FIM, ed. The sinus node: Structure, function, and clinical relevance. The Hague:Martinus Nijhoff Medical Division, 1978:258–269.

Toyoshima H, Burgess MJ. Electrotonic interaction during canine ventricular repolarization. Circ Res 1978; 43:348–356.

Ursell PC, Gardner PI, Albela A, et al. Structural and electrophysiological changes in the epicardial border zone of canine myocardial infarcts during infarct healing. Circ Res 1985; 56:436–451.

Van Capelle FJL, Durrer D. Computer simulation of arrhythmias in a network of coupled excitable cells. Circ Res 1980; 47:454–466.

Wedensky NE: Die erregung, hemmung und narkose. Pfluegers Arch 1903; 100:1–144.

Weingart R. The actions of ouabain on intercellular coupling and conduction velocity in mammalian ventricular muscle. J Physiol 1977; 264:341–365.

Wit AL. Cardiac arrhythmias: Electrophysiologic mechanisms. In: Reiser HJ, Horowitz LN, eds. Mechanisms and treatment of cardiac arrhythmias: Relevance of basic studies to clinical management. Baltimore: Urban & Schwarzenberg, 1985:11–37.

Wojtczak JA. Effects of general and local anesthetics on intercellular coupling in the heart muscle. Biophys J 1984; 45:22a.

AUTONOMIC INFLUENCES AND CARDIAC ARRHYTHMIAS

RICHARD L. VERRIER, Ph.D.

Remarkable progress has been made in recent years in defining the influence of neural and behavioral factors in the genesis of cardiac arrhythmias. This has been attributable to the development of clinically relevant experimental models and to the innovation of quantitative methods for assessing cardiac electrical stability. The availability of improved pharmacologic probes and the refinement of cardiac denervation procedures have also contributed significantly to the advancement of the field.

ADRENERGIC INFLUENCES

It is well established that enhanced adrenergic activity is conducive to cardiac arrhythmias. For example, it has been demonstrated that electrical stimulation of neural structures, such as the posterior hypothalamus or the stellate ganglia, increases susceptibility to ventricular fibrillation. Infusion of catecholamines, including norepinephrine and epinephrine, has also been shown to increase the incidence of ventricular fibrillation during coronary artery occlusion.

A close temporal relationship has been shown to exist between the sympathetic neural discharge rate and vulnerability to ventricular fibrillation during acute myocardial ischemia (Fig. 1). Within 2 minutes of coronary artery occlusion, there was maximal activation of cardiac sympathetic preganglionic fibers, which coincided with the time during which ventricular fibrillation threshold was at its lowest level. The period of enhanced vulnerability lasted for 5 to 6 minutes, after which time nerve discharge rate and vulnerability returned to the preocclusion level despite continued obstruction of the coronary vessel. A short-lived but significant decrease in fibrillation threshold occurred during release reperfusion, but this was not accompanied by an enhancement of sympathetic neural activity.

Bilateral stellectomy prevented the changes in ventricular fibrillation threshold observed during coronary artery occlusion, thus indicating that increased cardiac sympathetic neural activity is a primary factor contributing to ventricular vulnerability during acute myocardial ischemia. During the reperfusion phase, however, stellectomy did not confer protection and may have actually augmented susceptibility to fibrillation. The basis for this action is

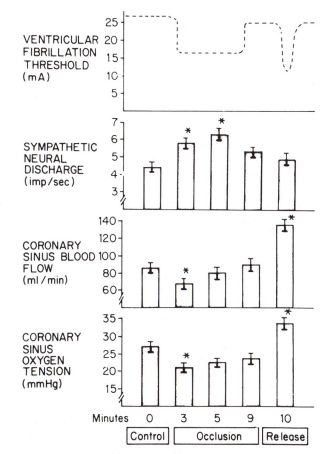

Figure 1 Effects of a 10-minute period of left anterior descending coronary artery occlusion and release on sympathetic neural activity, coronary sinus blood flow, and oxygen tension. A schematic representation of the time course of changes in ventricular fibrillation threshold is also displayed. Left anterior descending coronary artery occlusion results in a consistent activation of sympathetic preganglionic fibers that corresponds with the period of maximal increase in vulnerability to ventricular fibrillation. The concomitant changes in coronary sinus blood flow and reperfusion are also displayed. *P <0.05 compared with control period. (Reprinted from Lombardi F, Verrier RL, and Lown B. Relationship between sympathetic neural activity, coronary dynamics, and vulnerability to ventricular fibrillation during myocardial ischemia and reperfusion. Am Heart J 1983; 105:958; with permission.)

unclear. A reasonable possibility is that the loss of sympathetic tone to the coronary vasculature increased the reactive hyperemic response. This, in turn, resulted in an enhanced release of ischemic byproducts, thought to be the triggers for reperfusion arrhythmias.

Role of Beta-1- and Beta-2-Adrenergic Receptors

Several beta-adrenergic receptor blocking drugs, including propranolol, practolol, and metoprolol, have been shown to exert a significant antifibrillatory effect during coronary artery occlusion in experimental animals. The beneficial effects of these drugs appear to be due mainly to their adrenergic receptor blocking properties rather than to their nonspecific membrane stabilizing influences. Pindolol exerted the weakest antifibrillatory effect of all beta blockers tested, a result that was found to be related to its intrinsic sympathomimetic activity. Practolol was found to be superior to propranolol in protecting against ventricular fibrillation during coronary artery occlusion. It has been suggested that cardioselectivity circumvents the potential for deleterious coronary vasoconstrictor effects associated with nonselective agents such as propranolol.

None of the beta-adrenergic receptor blocking agents tested so far has exerted protection against reperfusion-induced ventricular fibrillation. This observation is consistent with the fact that adrenergic factors did not appear to play a role during reperfusion after a period of occlusion of 10 minutes or less. With longer periods of occlusion, changes can occur in receptor responsivity that alter the response to adrenergic drugs, as discussed below.

Beta-2-adrenergic receptor blocking agents do not appear to influence electrophysiologic properties in the canine myocardium. This conclusion is based on the observation that selective beta-2-adrenergic receptor stimulation or blockade with salbutamol and ICI 118,551, respectively, were completely without effect on cardiac excitable properties.

Role of Alpha-Adrenergic Receptors

In the normal heart, alpha-adrenergic receptor stimulation or blockade does not appear to alter ventricular electrical stability. Intravenous injection of alpha-adrenergic agonists, including phenylephrine and methoxamine, did not alter the vulnerable period threshold when the pressor responses to the drugs were controlled to prevent the baroreflex changes in autonomic tone. Injection of the alpha-adrenergic receptor blocking agent phenoxybenzamine likewise did not alter ventricular vulnerability.

In the setting of protracted myocardial ischemia, a different picture has emerged. Corr and colleagues demonstrated that the idioventricular rate was enhanced during reflow by localized infusion of methoxamine, an alpha-agonist, into the reperfused zone. This finding is in contrast with the effects mediated by beta-adrenergic receptors on idioventricular rate in nonischemic animals. Thus it appears that alpha-1-adrenergic stimulation may result in electrophysiologic derangements peculiar to ischemia and reperfusion and not evident in normal tissue. Recent work using x-ray microprobe analysis has also suggested that alpha-adrenergic mechanisms may mediate a large portion of the increase in intracellular calcium during reperfusion.

SYMPATHETIC-PARASYMPATHETIC INTERACTIONS

The contemporary view is that the effects of vagus nerve activity on ventricular vulnerability are contingent on the level of preexisting cardiac sympathetic tone. This conclusion is based on the observation that when sympathetic tone to the heart was augmented by thoracotomy, sympathetic nerve stimulation, or catecholamine infusion, simultaneous vagal activation exerted a protective effect on ventricular vulnerability. Vagus nerve stimulation was without effect on ventricular vulnerability when adrenergic input to the heart was ablated by beta-adrenergic receptor blockade.

The influence of the vagus nerve on ventricular vulnerability appears to be due to activation of muscarinic receptors, because vagally mediated changes in vulnerability were prevented by atropine administration. The diminution of adrenergic effects by muscarinic activation has a physiologic and cellular basis. Muscarinic agents inhibit the release of norepinephrine from sympathetic nerve endings as well as attenuate the response to norepinephrine at receptor sites by cyclic nucleotide interactions.

Vagus nerve stimulation also exerts an antifibrillatory action during acute coronary artery occlusion. We showed that cholinergic stimulation by electrical stimulation of the decentralized vagus nerves or by direct muscarinic receptor stimulation with methacholine afforded substantial protection during myocardial ischemia in dogs. This effect was independent of heart rate, as this variable was maintained constant by pacing. No protective influence of vagus nerve stimulation was observed, however, during the reperfusion phase (Fig. 2). These observations are consistent with the concept that the antifibrillatory effect of vagus nerve activation is due to accentuated antagonism of adrenergic activity.

The role of vagal influences in the context of myocardial ischemia is a subject of current investigation. In an elegant series of experiments, Zipes and coworkers described the functional neuroanatomy of the heart and the manner in which it is influenced by myocardial ischemia and infarction. Particularly significant is their observation that damage to the epicardium or endocardium may preferentially interrupt one or another limb of the autonomic nervous system and this could, in turn, augment the arrhythmogenic effect of neural activation. Our current view of vagal influences on ventricular electrical stability is summarized in Table 1.

EXPERIMENTAL STUDIES OF BEHAVIORALLY INDUCED ISCHEMIA AND ARRHYTHMIAS

A few years ago we undertook to develop an experimental counterpart to anger. This was prompted by clinical reports linking this emotional

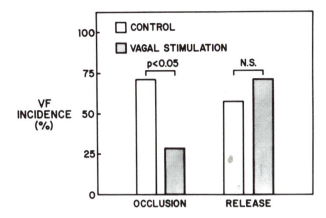

Figure 2 Influence of vagal stimulation on the incidence of ventricular fibrillation during a 10-minute period of left anterior descending coronary artery occlusion followed by abrupt release. Stimulation of the vagus nerve conferred significant protection against ventricular fibrillation during occlusion. No protection was noted during reperfusion, however. Heart rate was maintained constant by ventricular pacing at 200 beats per minute. Open columns, control; stippled columns, vagal stimulation. (Reprinted from Verrier RL, Hohnloser SH. How is the nervous system implicated in the genesis of cardiac arrhythmias? In: Hearse DJ, Manning AS, Janse MJ, eds. Life-threatening arrhythmias during ischemia and infarction. New York: Raven Press, 1987; with permission.)

state with cardiovascular disorders, including angina pectoris and cardiac arrhythmias. The experimental paradigm consisted of inducing an anger-like state in dogs by denial of access to food. After an overnight fast, the instrumented dog was brought to the experimental laboratory and allowed to acclimate for 20 to 30 minutes. While secured by a leash, the animal was presented with a dish of food. At this point, the food was moved just out of reach and a second leashed dog was permitted to consume the food. Upon observing this, the first dog almost invariably exhibited an anger-like behavioral state, as evidenced by growling and exposing its teeth. The animals were not allowed to come into contact. The

Table 1 Sympathetic-Parasympathetic Interactions and Cardiac Arrhythmogenesis

Vagal tone increases myocardial electrical stability and protects against ventricular fibrillation during myocardial ischemia. This indirect effect results from antagonism of adrenergic influences.

The basis for parasympathetic-sympathetic interactions is inhibition of norepinephrine release from nerve endings and attenuation of response to catecholamines at receptor sites.

Beneficial effects of vagal activity may be annulled if profound bradycardia and hypotension ensue.

Myocardial infarction may alter autonomic influences by damaging neural pathways.

Reprinted from Verrier RL Autonomic substrates for arrhythmias. Prog Cardiol 1988; 1:74, with permission.

anger response persisted as long as the animals remained within sight of each other. The behavioral response was associated with consistent increases in heart rate, mean arterial blood pressure, and plasma catecholamine levels and a significant decrease in the repetitive extrasystole threshold. The latter effect indicates that induction of anger is capable of substantially decreasing the electrical stability of even the normal myocardium. It is reasonable to assume, although it has not yet been established, that major arrhythmias would be precipitated in the damaged myocardium.

Delayed Myocardial Ischemia

Employing the anger model, we made a serendipitous observation regarding the effects of the post-stress state on myocardial perfusion. Specifically, we observed that after induction of the anger-like state, a progressive increase in coronary vascular resistance ensued within 2 to 3 minutes and persisted for 10 to 15 minutes after the anger episode. The vasoconstrictor state lasted well after heart rate and arterial blood pressure had returned to control levels, indicating primary coronary vasoconstriction. In some animals the response was so intense as to obstruct flow in the affected vessel completely. The presence of myocardial ischemia was indicated by significant S-T segment changes (Fig. 3). Although the delayed myocardial ischemia phenomenon is not fully understood, some important insights have emerged from recent studies. Specifically, it appears that activation of the sympathetic nervous system is a critical factor. This is based on two lines of evidence. The first is that the phenomenon can be induced by direct electrical stimulation of the left stellate ganglion and that the vasoconstrictor response can be averted by alpha-adrenergic receptor blockade with prazosin. The second line of evidence is based on the recent observation that bilateral stellectomy prevents delayed ischemia induced by anger.

The delayed nature of the response remained an enigma, however. A clue was provided by the finding that there is a close temporal association between the onset of ischemia and the return of coronary arterial blood pressure to the control level following anger or sympathetic stimulation. Experimental interventions were carried out in order to define the role of pressure in delayed ischemia. The first involved preventing the hypertensive response to stellate stimulation by controlled exsanguination. When this procedure was carried out, the coronary vasoconstrictor response was not delayed but occurred during stimulation. A series of interventions designed to raise arterial blood pressure was performed next. These entailed stimulating the left stellate ganglion without blood pressure regulation and allowing the delayed coronary vasoconstriction to occur. Thereafter, systemic blood pressure was raised to the stimulation level by occluding the aorta with a snare. Increasing

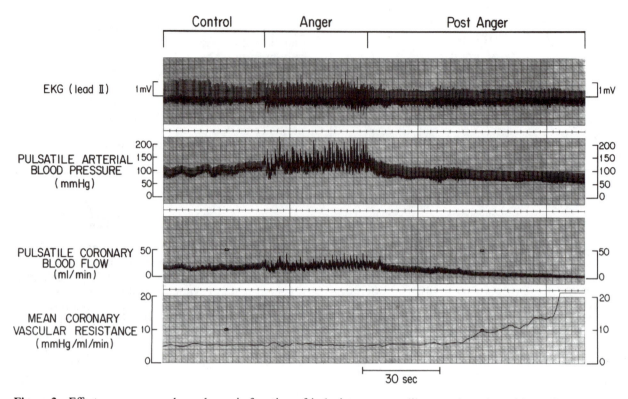

Figure 3 Effects on coronary hemodynamic function of inducing an anger-like state in a dog with a coronary artery stenosis. During the stress state, coronary arterial blood flow increased and coronary vascular resistance decreased. During the poststress recovery period, pronounced coronary vasoconstriction was evidenced by a fall in coronary arterial blood flow and an increase in coronary vascular resistance. These changes occurred when heart rate and arterial blood pressure returned to the prestress levels, a response suggesting primary coronary vasoconstriction. (Reprinted from Verrier RL, Hagestad EL, and Lown B. Delayed myocardial ischemia induced by anger. Circulation 1987; 75:249. Reprinted by permission of the American Heart Association.)

arterial blood pressure in this manner consistently returned coronary arterial flow and intracoronary pressure to the control values. By contrast, elevating systemic pressure by restimulating the stellate ganglion failed to restore flow through the coronary artery.

SLEEP AND CARDIAC DISORDERS

Arrhythmias

Clinical studies indicate that sleep suppresses ventricular arrhythmias. In particular, Lown and co-workers found that 45 of 54 subjects undergoing 24-hour ambulatory monitoring exhibited significant reduction in ventricular ectopic activity during sleep. When sleep stages were monitored, these investigators noted reduction of ventricular premature complexes during all stages except rapid eye movement (REM) sleep. The frequency of ventricular premature complexes during REM was similar to that during awake periods. The most marked lessening of arrhythmias was recorded during slow wave sleep

(stages 3 and 4). The change in ventricular ectopic activity was not correlated with changes in heart rate because heart rate remained relatively stable during the various sleep stages. A beneficial effect of sleep on myocardial electrical stability is also suggested by the infrequency of sudden cardiac death during sleep, although sleep occupies about one-third of the diurnal cycle. Ventricular tachycardia and fibrillation, however, have been noted to occur in association with violent or frightening dreams. Notwithstanding these observations, it remains highly inferential that when sudden death does occur nocturnally, it is during REM sleep.

Recently, we obtained evidence suggesting that alterations in vagal tone may modulate cardiac electrophysiologic properties during sleep. Specifically, the effects of REM and slow wave sleep on ventricular refractoriness were studied in chronically instrumented cats. Electrodes were implanted to record electrooculograms, electromyograms, and electroencephalograms for sleep stage determination. A right ventricular catheter was employed for cardiac electrical testing using the single stimulus technique. Both REM and slow wave sleep significantly increased the effective refractory period. This effect was independent of alterations in heart rate, as this variable was maintained constant by pacing. These alterations were not prevented by bilateral stellectomy. However, when the muscarinic receptor blocking agent atropine methylnitrate was administered, the sleep-induced changes were completely abolished. These results suggest that the electrophysiologic changes associated with sleep are mediated through fluctuations in cardiac vagal tone.

Myocardial Ischemia

There may be hemodynamic concomitants as well as coronary artery flow changes linked to neural alterations during sleep stages that influence the electrically unstable ischemic heart. Clinical studies indicate that phasic changes in coronary blood flow occur throughout the diurnal cycle. In particular, Deanfield and coworkers found during 24-hour Holter monitoring in patients with stable angina that S-T segments fluctuate substantially during day and night. King and associates studied the effects of sleep on the occurrence of Prinzmetal's variant angina. In an individual with angiographically documented coronary artery spasm, they found that the episodes of nocturnal chest pain accompanied by S-T segment elevation occurred primarily during the REM stage of sleep. The factors responsible for the episodes of nocturnal angina, however, were not defined.

We addressed the issue of sleep-induced coronary blood flow changes in a recent series of experiments carried out in chronically instrumented dogs. The animals were prepared for recording sleep stage and systemic and coronary hemodynamic function. The animals were studied during natural sleep and the cycles were divided into 1-minute periods of quiet wakefulness, slow wave sleep, or REM sleep. The findings indicate that during slow wave sleep there were moderate but significant reductions in heart rate and coronary blood flow and increases in coronary vascular resistance. In REM, the coronary blood flow baseline was moderately elevated compared with during slow wave sleep, and there were striking episodic surges in flow. Coronary vascular resistance was reduced correspondingly. Heart rate and mean arterial pressure were also elevated during the flow surges, indicating that an increase in cardiac metabolic activity may be the basis for the coronary

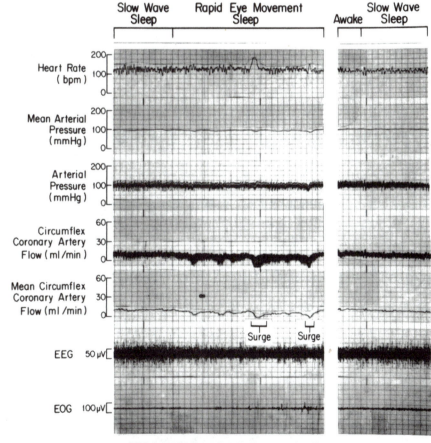

Figure 4 The effects of sleep stage on heart rate, mean and phasic arterial blood pressure, and mean and phasic circumflex coronary artery flow are shown in a typical dog during stenosis. Note the phasic decreases in coronary artery blood flow that occur during heart rate surges when the dog is in REM sleep. (Reprinted from Kirby DA, Verrier RL. Differential effects of sleep stage on coronary hemodynamic function during stenosis. Physiol Behav 1989; 45:1018. Copyright 1989, Pergamon Press, with permission.)

vasodilation. Since bilateral stellectomy prevented the surges in coronary blood flow, this response does not appear to be caused by nonspecific effects of somatic activity or respiratory fluctuations. Rather, the changes appear to be the direct result of enhanced adrenergic discharge. We also examined the influence of sleep on coronary hemodynamic function during coronary stenosis. The results indicate that in the presence of coronary stenosis, the phasic increases in sympathetic discharge during REM sleep result in a decrease rather than an increase in coronary arterial blood flow (Fig. 4). These observations carry important implications, as a heuristic laboratory model may thus be available to investigate the prevalent but poorly understood phenomenon of nocturnal angina.

Supported by Grants HL-32905, HL-33567, and HL-35138 from the National Institutes of Health, Bethesda, Maryland.

SUGGESTED READING

Corr PB, Yamada KA, Witkowski FX. Mechanisms controlling cardiac autonomic function and their relation to arrhythmogenesis. In: Fozzard HA, et al, eds. The heart and cardiovascular system. New York: Raven Press, 1986:1343.

Lown B. Sudden cardiac death: Biobehavioral perspective. Circulation 1987; 76(Suppl I):I186–I196.

Schwartz PJ, Stone HJ. The analysis and modulation of autonomic reflexes in the prediction and prevention of sudden death. In: Zipes DP, Jalife J, eds. Cardiac electrophysiology and arrhythmias. Orlando: Grune & Stratton, 1985:165.

Verrier RL. Autonomic substrates for arrhythmias. Prog Cardiol 1988; 1:65–85.

Verrier RL. Behavioral stress, myocardial ischemia, and arrhythmias. In: Zipes DP, Jalife J, eds. Cardiac electrophysiology and arrhythmias: From cell to bedside. Philadelphia: WB Saunders, 1990.

Zipes DP, Barber MJ, Takahashi N, Gilmour RF Jr. Recent observations on autonomic innervation of the heart. In: Zipes DP, Jalife J, eds. Cardiac electrophysiology and arrhythmias. Orlando: Grune & Stratton, 1985:181.

II DIAGNOSTIC TECHNIQUES

HISTORY AND PHYSICAL EXAMINATION OF PATIENTS WITH ARRHYTHMIA

BERNARD L. SEGAL, M.D.

There is a tendency in modern medicine to educate and graduate technologists rather than practicing cardiologists. As in many other fields of medicine, there is a temptation to order expensive, highly technical, and sophisticated procedures that are uncomfortable and sometimes hazardous for the patient. Frequently, a precise pathophysiologic diagnosis can be established on the basis of a detailed patient history and physical examination. A compassionate, thoughtful physician will not order unnecessary procedures. Accurate decision making is often difficult, requiring experience and a comprehensive knowledge of the available technologic equipment. With the ever-increasing array of specialized procedures, the physician must make the appropriate choice.

HISTORY TAKING

Use of a questionnaire or delegating responsibility for the history to a nurse or a physician's assistant is inadvisable. Skillful history taking provides a rich source of information concerning the patient's illness. The physician should establish a bond with the patient that will prove valuable in securing his or her compliance. Establishing this rapport engenders confidence and encourages the patient to accept decisions with regard to laboratory procedures, hospitalization, and medical and even surgical management.

A careful history allows the physician to evaluate the accuracy of the patient's complaints and to recognize the importance of certain symptoms, the effects of the disease, and the patient's fears and anxieties. This is an opportunity to understand the patient's personality and lifestyle and the role of the family. The patient should be put as much at ease as possible. If the presence of the spouse can lessen the anxiety, the examination should be so conducted. Often the spouse can augment the history, especially when the patient is forgetful or confused or underestimates the significance of symptoms or the importance of habits.

Patients should first be given the opportunity to present their experiences and complaints in their own way, without interruption. Although it is time-consuming and may include much irrelevant information, this technique has the advantage of providing considerable information about the patient's intelligence and emotional state and assures the patient the satisfaction of knowing that he or she has been listened to. After the patient has given an account of the symptoms, the physician should obtain information concerning their onset and chronology, location, quality, and intensity, the precipitating, aggravating, and relieving circumstances, and the response to any past therapy.

The detailed medical history, including a personal history, previous hospitalizations, and occupational and nutritional histories, should be recorded. Personal habits such as exercise, smoking, alcohol intake, and use of drugs should be investigated further. All medications should be reviewed. The genetic factor in many forms of heart disease emphasizes the importance of taking a family history, which should include risk factors for coronary heart disease: a similar history in other members of the family, smoking, hypertension, lipid abnormalities, diabetes mellitus, or onset of menopause (natural or induced).

As the patient relates the history, important nonverbal clues are often given. The doctor should observe the patient's attitude, responses, gestures, body motion, choice of words, and emotional state.

Palpitation

This common symptom is defined as an unpleasant awareness of rapid or forceful beating of the heart. It may be brought about by changes in rhythm or rate, including premature beats, compensatory pauses, augmented stroke volume owing to valvular regurgitation, high output states, and sudden conduction problems with slowing of the heartbeat and advanced heart block. In cases of premature contractions, the patient is more commonly aware of the postextrasystolic contraction than of the premature contraction itself. The increased motion of the heart within the chest is perceived rather than the increase in cardiac contractility.

When palpitations are confined to one or two beats, patients describe them as "skipped beats" or a "flopping sensation" in the chest; these are most commonly due to atrial and ventricular premature contractions. On the other hand, the sensation that the heart has "stopped beating" often correlates with the long compensatory pause following a premature contraction. Palpitations caused by slowing of the heartbeat may be due to sinus node or atrioventricular conduction system disease with advanced block. When palpitation begins and ends abruptly, the patient describes a rapid throbbing in the chest that is often attributable to paroxysmal tachycardia, such as paroxysmal atrial or junctional tachycardia or atrial flutter or fibrillation. During spontaneous conversion to sinus rhythm, the patient experiences a sudden throbbing or a jolt in the chest. In patients with sinus tachycardia, the palpitations are described as a gradual onset and cessation of the attack and are often accompanied by anxiety and apprehension. Patients with paroxysmal atrial flutter and fibrillation often describe a rapid heart action that is frequent and repetitious. When patients take their pulse during the palpitation, they usually describe a particular rhythm or cadence, slow or rapid, regular or irregular, weak or strong. A rate between 100 and 140 beats per minute suggests sinus tachycardia; a rate of 150 beats per minute suggests atrial flutter; and rates exceeding 160 beats per minute suggest paroxysmal supraventricular tachycardia.

The complaint of palpitation during or after strenuous physical activity is normal, whereas palpitations during mild exercise may suggest cardiac disease or may indicate that the individual is not in good physical condition. The feeling of a forceful heart action accompanied by a neck throb may indicate increased stroke volume, as in aortic regurgitation, or right atrial contraction against a closed tricuspid valve, as in premature ventricular beats or in junctional rhythm. When palpitations are relieved abruptly by stooping, the patient's holding his or her breath, gagging, vomiting, or straining at stool (vagal maneuvers), the diagnosis of paroxysmal supraventricular tachycardia is suggested. A history of palpitation associated with emotional symptoms (a lump in the throat, lightheadedness, face or hand paresthesia) suggests sinus tachycardia with hyperventilation.

The patient should be asked to simulate the cadence and the rhythm of the palpitation by a tapping of the finger or hand. In this way, the physician is able to learn more about the rate, rhythm, and pattern of the arrhythmia.

Syncope

Syncope, the loss of consciousness, results most commonly from reduced perfusion of the brain. The history is important in differentiating its precise causes. Cardiac syncope is usually of rapid onset, without aura, and is not usually associated with convulsive movements, urinary incontinence, or confusion states. When a state of unconsciousness develops gradually and lasts for a few seconds, this may suggest vasodepressor syncope or syncope due to orthostatic hypotension. When syncope is not accompanied by any change in pulse or blood pressure, the diagnosis of hysterical syncope is suggested. This condition is often associated with paresthesia of the hands or face, hyperventilation, shortness of breath, chest pain, and feelings of acute anxiety.

Syncope occurring with change in posture and position may also be caused by a ball-valve thrombus or a left atrial myxoma. Syncope brought on by severe exertion may suggest aortic stenosis, hypertrophic obstructive cardiomyopathy, or primary pulmonary hypertension.

Vasodepressor syncope is often the result of emotional stress or painful stimuli and may be precipitated by the sight or loss of blood or by severe emotional stress. It is often preceded by sweating, nausea, and vomiting. Carotid sinus hypersensitivity may be diagnosed when the patient has a history of sudden syncope in association with sudden movements of the head, shaving the neck, or wearing a tight collar.

Syncope is most unusual in patients with coronary heart disease and angina pectoris unless advanced heart block or ischemia-induced tachyarrhythmia is present. Syncope in patients with hypertrophic obstructive cardiomyopathy may be precipitated by a sudden Valsalva maneuver or positional changes. Orthostatic or drug-induced hypotension may also be responsible for syncope. Syncope that is associated with severe angina pectoris is usually caused by advanced heart block or a tachyarrhythmia produced by ischemia.

A family history of syncope suggests the possibility of hypertrophic obstructive cardiomyopathy or ventricular tachyarrhythmia associated with a prolonged Q-T interval. Syncope and cyanosis, which are likely to occur in cyanotic congenital heart disease, are attributable to cerebral anoxia that results in an increase in the right-to-left shunting (because of an obstruction in the right ventricular outflow track) or to a reduction in the systemic vascular resistance. Syncope during childhood suggests subvalvular or supravalvular or aortic valvular disease. Syncope associated with cerebral vascular insufficiency is usually accompanied by localizing neurologic features.

PHYSICAL EXAMINATION

The patient should be examined in a quiet room with closed doors. The patient should be placed on a bed or an examining table having a head section that can be raised or lowered so that the patient's trunk is at a 30- to 45-degree elevation from the horizontal. Posture changes help in the evaluation of jugular venous pressure. Good lighting is also important, and daylight is preferable.

The patient's temperature should be taken, since a fever may be responsible for sinus tachycardia and supraventricular arrhythmia. A very husky voice of low pitch suggests myxedema with sinus bradycardia. A puffy face, an enlarged tongue, somnolence, and the loss of eyebrow and scalp hair may also suggest hypothyroidism. Examination of the thyroid gland is important. A moderately firm enlarged gland may be found in patients with hyperthyroidism. Sinus tachycardia is the most common arrhythmia in these patients, and bruits over the thyroid gland are usually systolic in timing and arterial in origin. Exophthalmos combined with eyelid lag may suggest hyperthyroidism.

Arterial and Venous Pulses

Examination of the neck veins enables the physician to estimate the venous pressure and thus confirm or rule out right-sided heart failure or cardiac tamponade. Proper interpretation of the patient's venous pulse wave may aid in the diagnosis of complete atrioventricular block. The peripheral pulse may lead to the diagnosis of many cardiac arrhythmias.

The venous pulse is most readily evaluated by inspecting the external and internal jugular veins. As a rule, the right internal jugular vein is best for this purpose. In patients with normal sinus rhythm, an A wave precedes the first sound and a V wave follows the first sound. The A wave, produced by atrial contraction, is absent in atrial fibrillation, and in atrial flutter it is replaced by rapid smaller oscillations occurring approximately 300 times per minute. The interval between the A wave and the carotid pulse is an estimation of atrioventricular (AV) conduction time. With practice, the AV conduction time may be estimated.

When there is AV junctional rhythm or a very long AV conduction time, the atrium may contract at a time when the tricuspid valve is closed, resulting in prominent A waves. Giant A waves or cannon waves occur in patients with complete AV block. This phenomenon is one of the most common and

reliable physical signs of complete AV block. The giant A waves are irregular. In complete AV block, one may be able to time the atrial rhythm, which is usually normal at 60 to 100 beats per minute. These A waves are mostly normal in size, but at irregular intervals they become large when the atrium contracts while the tricuspid valve is closed. By a similar mechanism, irregular large A waves may occur with atrial, junctional, or ventricular premature contractions, when right atrial systole coincides with ventricular systole. Irregular large A waves do not appear when there is atrial fibrillation.

In adults with complete AV block, the ventricular rate as determined by the carotid pulse is usually about 40 beats per minute. One must be cautious in estimating the heart rate from the arterial pulse rate when there is an arrhythmia. An arterial rate of 40 beats per minute may be found here when the true ventricular rate is 80 beats per minute. This is observed when there is bigeminal rhythm caused by premature beats, if the premature contractions are too feeble to produce an arterial pulse (pulse deficit). In patients with tricuspid valve regurgitation, a large positive wave, the V wave, is conspicuous. In patients with atrial fibrillation, the only visible wave is the V wave in the jugular venous pulse. The variation in these waves with change of posture or their obliteration by light pressure over the base of the neck demonstrates that the carotid artery is not the source of these pulses and that the wave is venous in origin.

The carotid arterial pulse normally has a single positive wave. An exaggerated carotid pulse may be seen in patients with sinus tachycardia or those who are anxious or apprehensive. With complete AV block in adults, the heart rate is usually near 40 beats per minute; the diastolic pressure is low and the cardiac stroke volume is increased, thus causing a prominent arterial pulse. For the same reason, 2:1 AV block or sinus bradycardia may also cause an exaggerated arterial pulse.

Under certain circumstances in which atrial activation is not transmitted to the ventricles, the peripheral pulses wax and wane in relation to varying time intervals between atrial and ventricular systole. This variation of pulse magnitude occurs most commonly in patients with ventricular tachycardia and in those with AV block or dissociation. The pulse is strong when atrial systole precedes ventricular systole by short intervals. When there is a long interval or no preceding atrial contraction, the pulse is weak. This finding may be a valuable physical clue in the diagnosis of ventricular tachycardia in patients who have paroxysmal tachycardia. Variations of the blood pressure cuff may aid in demonstrating or confirming this mechanism. This finding is absent in ventricular tachycardia when there is retrograde conduction from ventricles to atria.

Palpation of the radial or other arteries may disclose alternate strong and weak pulses, usually a result of bigeminal rhythm caused by premature contractions. In alternating pulses, the premature contractions are usually weaker and can be confirmed with a blood pressure cuff.

Auscultation

Specific auscultatory findings are not typically helpful in assessing the presence or type of arrhythmia.

Carotid Sinus Pressure

When the heart rate is 150 beats per minute or more and the rhythm is regular, it may be necessary to distinguish between sinus tachycardia and one of the paroxysmal tachycardias, such as atrial tachycardia, AV junctional tachycardia, ventricular tachycardia, or atrial flutter with 2:1 AV block.

It may be helpful to observe the response of the arrhythmia to carotid sinus pressure. With sinus tachycardia there is usually no response or a slight slowing of the heart rate, usually by no more than 10 to 20 beats per minute; with release of the carotid sinus pressure there is a gradual return to the previous rate. With ventricular tachycardia there is virtually no response to carotid sinus pressure; with atrial or AV junctional tachycardia, either there is no response or the heart rate suddenly decreases to a normal rate and remains there upon release of the pressure. With paroxysmal atrial flutter with 2:1 AV block, the ventricular rate is usually near 150 beats per minute, since the atrial flutter rate is usually close to 300 beats per minute. There may be either no response to carotid sinus pressure or a sudden slowing of the ventricular response from about 150 to perhaps 75 to 50 beats per minute. This is the result of increasing the AV block to 2:1 or 3:1 or 4:1. Upon release of the carotid sinus pressure, there is a sudden return of the ventricular rate to the original value of about 150 beats per minute.

In general, carotid sinus pressure is somewhat hazardous and probably should not be used in patients over 75 years old. The carotid sinus pressure is best applied with the patient lying supine in a comfortable position, and only on one side at a time, not bilaterally and simultaneously. The patient's head should be supported comfortably on a pillow and turned slightly away from the examiner. The pressure should be exerted firmly over the carotid artery just above the bifurcation with a slight massaging motion for about 5 seconds but no more. Ideally, the procedure should be carried out with an electrocardiograph recording any changes in rhythm.

SPECIFIC ARRHYTHMIAS

Premature Complexes

Premature complexes, supraventricular and ventricular, are the commonest of the disorders of the heartbeat. Generally they cause no symptoms, but in some patients they are disturbing. When appreciated they are usually felt particularly at night just before falling asleep. As the heart rate slows, the premature contractions tend to appear more readily and may cause or aggravate insomnia. The patient is most commonly aware of the pause following the premature contraction or of the forceful contraction that follows the pause. The patient may complain of a flip-flop or a skipped beat. The carotid or radial pulse is irregular, with a possible pulse deficit. Occasionally the premature complex is so early, with very little cardiac output, that only a first heart sound is heard and no second sound is audible.

It is difficult to distinguish between atrial and junctional premature complexes on the one hand and ventricular premature complexes on the other without the help of an electrocardiogram. Ventricular premature complexes do not ordinarily interfere with the sinus discharge of the atrium, and thus the next complex following the pause occurs on time. With atrial and AV junctional premature complexes, the basic atrial rhythm is usually disturbed, and the pause following an atrial or AV junctural complex is shorter than that following a ventricular complex; hence the pause is not compensatory.

Tachyarrhythmias

Patients with paroxysmal tachycardia may have difficulty maintaining the upright posture and near-syncope or syncope may ensue. The patient may complain of sweating, nausea, and tightness, discomfort, or a squeezing sensation over the precordium.

With ventricular tachycardia there is often variation in the intensity of the first heart sound because of the dissociation between the atrial and ventricular rhythms. This mechanism is similar to that in complete AV block. This variation is not detected in paroxysmal or AV junctional tachycardia. The most useful clue to the diagnosis of ventricular tachycardia is the beat-to-beat variation in blood pressure, which occurs because of the varying contribution of atrial systole to ventricular filling. The blood pressure may vary as much as 25 to 30 mm Hg between the lowest and the highest systolic values. Auscultation during ventricular tachycardia can reveal a third (S3) and fourth (S4) heart sound, a summation gallop (S3 + S4) in shorter diastolic intervals, and the murmur of papillary muscle dysfunction.

Ventricular fibrillation, cardiac standstill, and, on occasion, extremely rapid ventricular tachycardia may be responsible for the syndrome of cardiac or circulatory arrest. With circulatory arrest there is no measurable blood pressure, no arterial pulse, and no audible heart sounds. The patient appears to be dead. The differential diagnosis between ventricular fibrillation and cardiac asystole cannot be made without an electrocardiogram, since there are no heart sounds with either disorder.

Suggested Reading

Braunwald E. Heart disease: A textbook of cardiovascular medicine. 3rd Ed. Philadelphia: W.B. Saunders, 1988:1.
Constant J. The evolving checklist of history-taking. In: Bedside cardiology. 3rd Ed. Boston: Little, Brown & Co., 1985:1.
Fowler NO. The history in cardiac diagnosis. In: Fowler NO, ed. Cardiac diagnosis and treatment. 3rd Ed. Hagerstown, MD: Harper & Row, 1980:23.

AMBULATORY ELECTROCARDIOGRAPHIC MONITORING

WALTER R. HEPP, M.D.
LEONARD N. HOROWITZ, M.D.

Electrocardiography and long-term ambulatory monitoring have become indispensable modalities for both the diagnosis and management of cardiac arrhythmias. For many years, standard resting electrocardiographic rhythm strips were the only format available for studying rhythm disturbances. The limitations of this technology were obvious. Rhythm disturbances are often sporadic, with a high rate of spontaneous variability, and their presence may go undetected by the patient. However, in the 1950s advances were made in the recordings of long-term electrocardiograms (ECGs) in ambulatory patients. These developments enabled us to study patients under normal ambulatory conditions and enhanced our ability to detect and study the nature of cardiac arrhythmias. These devices, which initially lacked sophistication, were cumbersome and heavy. They provided limited information because of lack of fidelity of their recording signal, and they were not able to quantitate arrhythmia detection. Over the years, with eventual commercialization of ambulatory monitors, refinements greatly advanced our technical capabilities regarding monitor size, recording modes, analysis systems, data storage, and data formatting capabilities.

INSTRUMENTATION

Recording from an ambulatory monitor requires three to five disposable, self-adhesive, skin electrodes that are placed on the patient's chest. The three-lead system records single-channel electrocardiographic data, whereas the five-lead system records two channels of electrocardiographic data, often monitoring from V_1 and V_5 of the standard 12-lead ECG. The skin electrodes are connected to a small, lightweight, battery-operated recorder by electrical cables. Recorders differ dramatically in regard to their recording modes, data analysis, and data formatting capabilities.

Recorders are available in two distinct formats —solid-state digital memory recorders and conventional analog tape recorders. Solid-state recorders record 24 hours of electrocardiographic data into digital memory. This method eliminates the possibility of tape jamming found in conventional analog systems. Additionally, there is no signal distortion, which is also found in the analog systems. However, because this format records all of its electrocardiographic data into digital memory, some form of data compression is necessary. Data compression optimizes limited memory space by using algorithms devised to recognize electrocardiographic morphologies similar to previously established templates and store into memory abnormal waveforms that differ from the established templates. Subtle electrocardiographic changes may, however, not be recognized, and artifacts tend to saturate memory stores rapidly. This may allow genuine electrocardiographic changes to go unnoticed or unstored because memory storage space is saturated. Digital memory systems also tend to have poor high-frequency recording capabilities and therefore high QRS frequencies, and pacemaker spikes may not be recorded.

The most commonly used recorder format is that of the conventional analog tape recorder. These systems record electrocardiographic data directly onto magnetic tape, which is either a cassette or reel-to-reel. The tape is motor-driven and records electrical signals between the frequencies of 0.05 and 100 Hz. Cassette tapes are used more often in clinical settings because of their lighter weight and compact size. These systems are therefore more convenient and less conspicuous for the patient wearing the device. Reel-to-reel tape systems, however, have a better signal-to-noise ratio, speed stability, and dynamic range than cassette recorders. They also have a lower incidence of recording failures and are more commonly used for research and experimental studies. Both of these recorder formats are usually equipped with internal calibration systems, especially if S-T segment analysis is considered. Most recorders also have event markers that are activated by the patient and allow for a direct comparison of the patient's symptoms with the rhythm present at that time.

There are three basic recording modes in ambulatory monitoring that utilize different data analysis systems. Continuous recordings are the standard mode for electrocardiographic recordings. Here a 24-hour electrocardiographic recording is completed without interruption. At the end of the study, the tape and battery are replaced. The tape is retrospectively analyzed by a variety of interactive and noninteractive methods. Interactive systems utilize a technician to assist with computer analysis. The tapes are computer scanned at 60 to 240 times that of the normal recording speed. All electrocardiographic data found to be abnormal in the rate, rhythm, QRS morphology, or S-T segment analysis by the accelerated analysis program are visibly inspected, reviewed, and verified by the technician. These are the most popular analysis systems, since all electrographic data is available for review.

Real-time data analysis recorders examine continuous ambulatory electrocardiographic data by microcomputer on a beat-by-beat basis while the patient is wearing the device. The microcomputer is programmed to analyze and record long-term electrocardiographic data in a noncontinuous excerpt fashion after editing and generating an analog and graphic hard copy. The decision analysis summary, or compressed data format, is then recorded in solid-state memory or tape storage. These systems lack any standardization and do not allow for interactive confirmation of the electrocardiographic findings, but they are a low-cost method for acquiring and processing ambulatory electrocardiographic data.

Patient-activated or intermittent recorders are the third recording mode available today. Recording formats for these devices are either solid-state memory or tape recordings. These devices are used in patients with unpredictable or infrequent symptoms in whom continuous recordings would be impractical. These devices are not continuous recorders, and they may be either patient-activated or activated automatically at predetermined intervals or by specific signals, e.g., a cardioversion artifact.

After completion of the 24-hour recording and analysis of the data, information regarding the study should be presented in a format that is both clear and concise. The duration of the recording period that is analyzed should be noted at the beginning of the report. Traditional parameters analyzed by Holter recordings include analysis of heart rate, presence of supraventricular and ventricular complexes, and ventricular couplets and ventricular tachycardia. These parameters should be reported and presented with low, high, and mean frequencies on an hourly basis as well as an overall 24-hour basis. Details regarding any form of conduction abnormalities, bradyarrhythmias, and tachyarrhythmias should also be recorded and noted if present. In patients with permanent pacemakers, a summary of the pacemaker's functional status should be included in the report. Analysis of S-T segment shifts should be summarized in the Holter report and correlated with any patient's symptoms. Other parameters that are reported in the ambulatory report include any changes in the native rhythm, P-R interval, QRS complex, or Q-T interval as well as any R on T phenomenon. Finally, it should be noted whether any of the reported symptoms the patient may have had during the study correlated with any observed arrhythmia, S-T segment shift, or conduction abnormality.

It is worth noting that in the past ventricular arrhythmias were reported according to a variety of classification schemes. The most popular scheme for classifying ventricular arrhythmias was proposed by Lown and coworkers, who graded ventricular arrhythmias in terms of their prognostic significance in order of ascending gravity. This system was initially widely accepted and used in both the research and clinical settings because of its pragmatic simplicity. Problems eventually arose with this grading system, however, and subsequently this classification has fallen out of favor. By and large, currently ventricular arrhythmias are reported quantitatively in terms of frequency and forms observed.

In general, manufacturers claim a high accuracy for the diagnostic and quantitative capabilities of their analyzing systems in determining premature complexes. Published information on the accuracy of these analyzing systems is extremely limited, however. Firms generally test the accuracy of their system against hand-counted 1- to 24-hour recordings. Criticism of these accuracy testing practices in the past has been that details regarding arrhythmia frequency, recording quality, and selection processes have not been routinely disclosed. Standardized tapes are now available for such testing.

VARIABILITY AND REPRODUCIBILITY OF AMBULATORY MONITORING

In the past, ambulatory ECGs were recorded for variable periods of time. During this period, great uncertainty existed regarding the proper length of monitoring time required to detect cardiac arrhythmias optimally. Shorter monitoring intervals were clearly less effective in detecting the maximum frequency of ventricular arrhythmias and complex forms, such as couplets and ventricular tachycardia. Studies compared increasing hourly monitoring periods and demonstrated a greater frequency of ventricular arrhythmias and complex forms with longer monitoring periods. With these findings also came the observation that there was marked spontaneous variability of ventricular arrhythmias on an hourly and daily basis in stable patients. This variability might therefore mimic drug efficacy if a high single dose of antiarrhythmic drug was administered, since drug efficacy was generally defined at that time as a 50 to 75 percent reduction in the frequency of ventricular arrhythmias. This posed a serious dilemma in evaluating antiarrhythmic drug efficacy, which compared baseline ambulatory electrocardiographic monitoring with that obtained while the patient was receiving drug therapy.

Eventually, statistical analysis was applied to the frequency of ventricular arrhythmias and complex forms, which demonstrated the limitations of 24-hour ambulatory electrocardiographic monitoring as a diagnostic modality. Spontaneous variability was evaluated in consecutive 24-hour ambulatory monitoring of stable patients with ventricular arrhythmias and complex forms. The analysis data determined the required reduction in the frequency of ventricular arrhythmias and complex forms necessary to constitute a therapeutic response rather than a biologic or spontaneous variability in arrhythmia frequency. Statistical data established that for two 24-hour ambulatory electrocardiographic monitors, an 83 percent greater reduction in ventricular premature complexes was required to demonstrate a therapeutic efficacy rather than spontaneous variability. Likewise, a 65 percent decrease in mean hourly frequency of ventricular tachycardia and a 75 percent reduction in the frequency of couplets are required to demonstrate therapeutic efficacy rather than spontaneous variability alone.

The efficacy of an antiarrhythmic agent in demonstrating abolition or a statistically significant reduction in ventricular arrhythmias and complex forms is interpreted, therefore, as a beneficial effect and may improve survival. It must be remembered, however, that efficacy does not imply that such a reduction prevents sudden death, since the frequency of ventricular arrhythmias does not always correlate with the risk of sudden death.

In clinical studies and in practice, once efficacy is established for a particular drug, we assume that the frequency and variability of the arrhythmias remain constant for long periods of time. This may not be the case, and there are data to suggest that for non–life-threatening ventricular arrhythmias, patients should be periodically restudied when off drug treatment to assess whether long-term antiarrhythmic therapy continues to be necessary.

CLINICAL USES OF AMBULATORY MONITORING

Numerous studies of normal subjects without apparent heart disease have examined the association of premature supraventricular and ventricular arrhythmias and their significance. These have shown that supraventricular arrhythmias occur in both men and women but are generally more common in men. They occur in both young and old subjects and appear to increase in prevalence with increasing age. Supraventricular complexes are not associated with any increased prevalence of coronary artery disease or sudden death. Premature ventricular complexes have also been noted in patients with no evidence of structural heart disease. They, too, are more common in men, although they are found in both men and women and also appear to increase in prevalence with increasing age. Patients over age 30 with ventricular arrhythmias appear to have an increased prevalence of coronary artery disease as well as risk of sudden death.

Prolonged electrocardiographic recordings provide clinicians with a noninvasive and practical method of monitoring a patient's cardiac status under normal physiologic conditions. In general, there are three basic indications for ambulatory electrocardiographic monitoring: (1) to evaluate patients' symptoms suspected of being cardiac in origin, (2) to evaluate patients at high risk for cardiac arrhythmias, and (3) to evaluate therapeutic efficacy.

Patients with symptoms thought to be of cardiac origin often complain of an awareness of their heart pounding or of palpitations. They often describe "skipped beats," "jumping" in their chests, or "a rushing sensation in their ears." These perceptions of abnormal cardiac function may be attributable to ectopic beats, tachyarrhythmias, pacemaker malfunction, or disturbances of cardiac conduction. In general, patients are not usually aware of the majority of the ectopic beats they experience, and often symptoms do not correlate with detected arrhythmias. This emphasizes the need to demonstrate clearly a valid correlation between symptoms and cardiac arrhythmias if treatment of non–life-threatening arrhythmias is considered.

Some symptoms, such as lightheadedness or syncope, are suggestive of more serious cardiac disease. In these cases, ambulatory electrocardiographic monitoring is helpful in evaluating the etiology, which may be due to sinus arrest, conduction disturbances, pacemaker malfunction, or supraventricular and ventricular arrhythmias.

Chest pain is another symptom that may be evaluated by ambulatory ECG monitoring. Typical angina pectoris is best evaluated noninvasively by stress testing. But in those patients with "atypical chest pain," which is unpredictable or nonreproducible, prolonged electrocardiographic recordings or event recorders may be advantageous. These symptoms, if of cardiac origin, may be due to Prinzmetal's angina, ischemic heart disease, or noncardiac causes.

Prolonged electrocardiographic recordings are also used to assist in the evaluation of "high-risk" cardiac patients. These patients generally suffer from coronary artery disease, cardiomyopathy, or valvular heart disease. Frequent and repetitive ventricular premature complexes and unsustained ventricular tachycardia increase the risk of mortality.

Ambulatory electrocardiographic monitoring is also commonly used to assess therapeutic efficacy. This may be to evaluate supraventricular or ventricular arrhythmia suppression, to evaluate pacemaker function, or to detect ischemic events over a 24-hour period. Additionally, treatment may have an adverse effect, such as a "proarrhythmic response" to a particular antiarrhythmic agent. In this case, the antiarrhythmic agent would need to be discontinued and an alternative drug administered.

SUGGESTED READING

Harrison DC, Fitzgerald JW, Winkle RA. Ambulatory electrocardiography for diagnosis and treatment of cardiac arrhythmias. N Engl J Med 1976; 294:373–380.

Holter NJ. Radioelectrocardiography: A new technique for cardiovascular study. Ann NY Acad Sci 1959; 65:913–923.

Kennedy HL, Caralis DG. Ambulatory electrocardiography: A clinical perspective. Ann Intern Med 1977; 87:729–739.

Lown B, Graboys TB. Management of patients with malignant ventricular arrhythmias. Am J Cardiol 1977; 39:910–919.

Michelson EL, Morganroth J. Spontaneous variability of complex ventricular arrhythmias detected by long-term electrocardiographic recording. Circulation 1980; 64:690–695.

Morganroth J. Ambulatory Holter electrocardiography: Choice of technologies and clinical uses. Ann Intern Med 1985; 102:73–81.

Morganroth J, Michelson E, Horowitz LN, et al. Limitations of routine long-term electrocardiographic monitoring to access ventricular ectopic frequency. Circulation 1978; 58:408–414.

EXERCISE TESTING

PHILIP J. PODRID, M.D.

Exercise testing has assumed an important role in cardiology and is a valuable tool for the evaluation and management of patients with coronary artery disease and other cardiovascular problems, such as congestive heart failure, hypertension, and arrhythmia. Although ambulatory monitoring and electrophysiologic testing are the principal techniques most often used for the management of patients with arrhythmias, exercise testing is an important adjunctive method that provides information complementary to that derived from ambulatory monitoring or invasive studies. In a subset of patients, exercise testing may be the only reliable method for arrhythmia management. This noninvasive technique is not only useful for the exposure of arrhythmia but also has an important role in evaluation of the beneficial and toxic effects of antiarrhythmic drugs.

The usefulness of exercise testing for arrhythmia management is based on the same physiologic changes that are important for evaluating patients with coronary artery disease. In response to exercise, there is withdrawal of vagal tone and a marked increase in sympathetic neural activity and the level of circulating catecholamines (Fig. 1). Sympathetic stimulation plays a major role in the genesis or maintenance of many arrhythmias, regardless of the

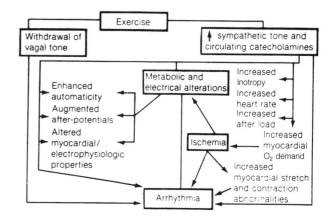

Figure 1 Schema of physiologic changes occurring during exercise and relationship to arrhythmogenesis.

underlying mechanism responsible for their occurrence.

Three etiologic mechanisms have been proposed to explain arrhythmogenesis. The first mechanism, which is considered to be the most important and is responsible for the majority of clinical arrhythmias, is reentry. This results from a disparity of electrophysiologic properties that exist between damaged and normal myocardial tissues that are anatomically adjacent to each other or are linked to each other proximally and distally, thereby forming a circuit. As a result of a nonuniformity of membrane conduction velocities and refractory periods that may exist within these pathways, an appropriately timed premature impulse may "activate" this circuit and initiate continuous electrical activity, which circulates around the reentrant loop, resulting in a sustained tachyarrhythmia. The sympathetic nervous system and circulating catecholamines also alter membrane conductivity and refractoriness, and when underlying differences in these properties already exist, inhomogeneity and the propensity for arrhythmia are further increased.

The second proposed mechanism for arrhythmogenesis is enhanced automaticity of ectopic foci that are located within abnormal or damaged tissue, which is the result of underlying cardiac disease. These automatic foci are capable of exhibiting spontaneous depolarizations. If the automaticity of these foci is enhanced by other factors, such as circulating catecholamines, their rate of spontaneous depolarization increases. If the firing rate of this ectopic focus exceeds that of the normal pacemaker, an ectopic or automatic rhythm is generated.

The third arrhythmogenic mechanism is triggered automaticity or delayed afterdepolarizations, which are low-amplitude oscillations occurring at the end of the action potential. These oscillations are triggered by the preceding action potential and are the result of calcium ion fluxes into the myocardium. If these oscillations are of sufficient amplitude, reaching threshold potential, a spontaneous action potential is produced. If this process continues, a sustained tachyarrhythmia may be generated. Any factor that increases the influx of calcium ions into the myocardial cell increases the amplitude of these after potentials and may result in the induction of arrhythmia owing to triggered automaticity. Among the most important of these factors are digitalis and circulating catecholamines.

Therefore, regardless of the mechanism, the sympathetic nervous system and circulating catecholamines play an important role in arrhythmogenesis. Sympathetic stimulation causes a number of other changes that are important for the induction of arrhythmia. Catecholamines can produce metabolic changes, for example, hypokalemia or pH shifts, which may directly provoke arrhythmias or may alter the underlying electrophysiologic properties of the myocardium, enhancing the preconditions for arrhythmia generation. As a result of a sympathetically mediated increase in myocardial inotropy, heart rate, blood pressure, or afterload, myocardial ischemia may result. Hypoxia can directly provoke arrhythmia, or it may produce metabolic and electrophysiologic alterations that are important for generation of arrhythmia. Additionally, ischemia may produce ventricular contraction abnormalities and an increase in myocardial stretch, which may enhance arrhythmogenesis.

It appears that exercise testing, which is a clinically important and frequently used method for activating the sympathetic nervous system and increasing the level of circulating catecholamines, can induce arrhythmia as the result of a number of interrelated physiologic changes. These factors are not only associated with the provocation of arrhythmia but are also of importance in the evaluation of beneficial and adverse antiarrhythmic drug effects.

INCIDENCE OF ARRHYTHMIA DURING EXERCISE TESTING

Although atrial and ventricular arrhythmias are often observed during exercise testing, their presence, frequency, and complexity can be established accurately only when continuous electrocardiographic recording is used. Additionally, it is known that the prevalence, frequency, and complexity of arrhythmias are directly related to the presence, type, and extent of underlying heart disease.

Supraventricular Arrhythmia

Supraventricular arrhythmia is often induced by exercise testing, although the actual prevalence is uncertain, since such arrhythmia is usually overlooked or unrecognized. Atrial or junctional premature complexes are the most frequent form of supraventricular arrhythmia, reported in 10 to 20 percent of normal subjects, whereas they are observed in 40 percent of those with underlying cardiac disease (Table 1). There is also a relationship between age and frequency of supraventricular premature complexes observed during exercise.

In contrast to premature complexes, the provocation of a sustained supraventricular tachyarrhythmia is infrequent, but its prevalence is related to the patient group studied. In a general population of patients with and without heart disease, 2 to 3 percent have supraventricular tachycardia induced by exercise, whereas atrial fibrillation occurs in 1 to 2 percent. In contrast, the incidence of supraventricular tachyarrhythmias during exercise is 15 percent in a group of patients with a history of such arrhythmia.

Table 1 Prevalence of Supraventricular Arrhythmia During Exercise

	Without Heart Disease	With Heart Disease
SVPC	3–18%	10–40%
SVT	0.1–3%	12%*
AF	0.1–1%	2–4%*

*With a history of SVT or AF.
SVPC = supraventricular premature complexes, SVT = supraventricular tachycardia, AF = atrial fibrillation.

Ventricular Arrhythmia

As in supraventricular arrhythmia, the prevalence of all forms of ventricular arrhythmia during exercise testing is related to the presence and extent of underlying heart disease and to age (Table 2). Continuous electrocardiographic recording is essential for the documentation and quantification of ventricular arrhythmia. This is especially important for the recognition of complex or repetitive forms, and their observed frequency is increased by six-fold when continuous recording is utilized. Single ventricular premature complexes (VPCs) are observed during exercise in 20 to 40 percent of normal subjects, whereas they are documented in 50 to 60 percent of patients with underlying heart disease. In contrast to simple VPCs, repetitive ventricular arrhythmia (couplets and runs of ventricular tachycardia) provoked by exercise testing is related to the presence of underlying heart disease. In a number of studies, the prevalence of repetitive arrhythmia in a normal population ranges from 0 to 6 percent, whereas this arrhythmia is documented in 10 to 30 percent among those with underlying heart disease. The incidence of ventricular arrhythmia during exercise testing is highest among those patients who have experienced a sustained ventricular tachyarrhythmia, that is, ventricular tachycardia or ventricular fibrillation. All these patients have VPCs, whereas in 50 to 75 percent repetitive arrhythmia is induced.

The induction of sustained ventricular tachycardia or ventricular fibrillation during exercise is rare (0.2%) and occurs primarily in those with heart disease. As with sustained supraventricular tachycardia, the incidence of a sustained ventricular tachyarrhythmia is higher (9 percent) among patients with a history of such arrhythmia.

PROGNOSTIC SIGNIFICANCE OF EXERCISE-INDUCED ARRHYTHMIA

There have been a number of studies reporting a significant association between repetitive arrhythmia documented during 24-hour ambulatory monitoring and an increased risk of sudden cardiac death. These studies have primarily involved patients with a recent myocardial infarction or those with congestive cardiomyopathy. Only a few studies have examined the prognostic importance of exercise-induced arrhythmia, and these have principally involved patients with coronary artery disease, especially in association with an acute myocardial infarction (Table 3). Unfortunately, there is a lack of agreement about the prognostic significance of exercise-induced ventricular arrhythmia. In most of these studies, which have involved postinfarction patients, the presence of repetitive ventricular arrhythmia increased the risk of sudden death by approximately two-fold. Ventricular arrhythmia during exercise is of less significance among the population of patients with coronary artery disease who have not had a recent infarction, and studies involving this group are contradictory. Exercise-induced ventricular arrhythmia has no prognostic significance in normal subjects.

ROLE OF EXERCISE TESTING IN ARRHYTHMIA MANAGEMENT

Although ambulatory monitoring is a more useful technique for exposure of arrhythmia and risk stratification, especially of postinfarction patients, exercise testing has an important role in the evaluation of antiarrhythmic drug effect and serves as an adjunctive tool, used along with ambulatory monitoring or electrophysiologic testing. In approximately 10 to 15 percent of patients with a history of a sustained ventricular tachyarrhythmia, exercise testing may be the only method for exposing spontaneously occurring ectopy, and for such patients it is the principal, perhaps only, technique for drug evaluation and selection.

Table 2 Prevalence of Ventricular Arrhythmia During Exercise Testing

	Normals	Heart Disease	History of VT/VF
Simple VPCs	3–34%	15–60%	80–100%
Repetitive VPCs	0–6%	15–30%	50–75%
VT/VF	0.02%	0.05–0.5%	9%

VPC = ventricular premature complexes, VT = ventricular tachycardia, VF = ventricular fibrillation.

Table 3 Prognostic Significance of Exercise-Induced Ventricular Arrhythmia

		Percent Mortality			
Study	Population	No VPCs	Simple VPCs	Complex VPCs	Significance
Weld	After MI	4	12	?	Yes
Krone	After MI	3	7	13	Yes
Henry	After MI	8	25	?	Yes
Udall	CAD + ST	10	33	42	Yes
	CAD − ST	2	15	29	Yes
Califf	CAD	10	17	25	Yes
	Normals	0	0	0	No
Weiner	Significant CAD	11	13	?	No
	Minimal CAD	2	9	?	No

VPCs = ventricular premature complexes, MI = myocardial infarction, CAD = coronary artery disease, + ST = S-T segment depression, − ST = no S-T segment depression.

For the majority of patients requiring treatment with antiarrhythmic agents, exercise testing provides important information that is complementary to that derived from either ambulatory monitoring or electrophysiologic testing (Fig. 2). This is based on the physiologic changes that occur during exercise testing that can interact with and perhaps modify antiarrhythmic drug activity. As previously indicated, exercise testing enhances sympathetic neural tone and increases the level of circulating catecholamines. The heightened sympathetic stimulation increases membrane automaticity and impulse conduction velocity and shortens the membrane refractory period, resulting in an enhancement of membrane excitability. These changes are in contrast to the electrophysiologic effects of the membrane-active antiarrhythmic drugs, which reduce membrane automaticity, excitability, and conductivity. Theoretically, catecholamines may negate the beneficial antiarrhythmic effects of these drugs, and there is now growing evidence that this is a clinically important concern. Indeed, in approximately 15 percent of patients, potentially serious repetitive arrhythmia continues to be provoked during exercise stress testing despite its suppression as observed during 24 hours of ambulatory monitoring. The continued presence of such arrhythmia either during exercise testing or on ambulatory monitoring correlates with a poorer prognosis as a result of a higher incidence of recurrent arrhythmia and sudden cardiac death, whereas its suppression predicts a favorable outcome.

Exercise testing is also useful for the selection of an effective drug to prevent supraventricular tachycardia when this arrhythmia is reproducibly provoked by exercise (Fig. 3). Exercise testing is an important technique for judging the adequacy of drugs for ventricular response rate control in patients with chronic atrial fibrillation. Although the ventricular rate may be well controlled, with or without digitalis therapy while the patient is at rest, it is usually poorly controlled during exercise, at a time when catecholamine levels are increased and conduction through the atrioventricular node is enhanced (Fig. 4). In this situation the addition of a beta blocker or calcium channel blocker along with digitalis provides optimal rate control during times of sympathetic stimulation, and this effect is best evaluated with exercise testing (see the chapter *Atrial Fibrillation*).

In addition to the important role of exercise testing for evaluating the beneficial effects of antiarrhythmic drugs, this technique is also important for the exposure of potentially serious drug-induced cardiac toxicity. Each of the antiarrhythmic drugs is negatively inotropic and has the potential for reducing left ventricular function and inducing congestive heart failure. Often this depressive effect on myocardial contractility is not obvious while the patient is at rest but becomes manifest during physical activity.

Figure 2 Exercise testing for management of ventricular arrhythmia. During the control exercise, test runs of unsustained ventricular tachycardia were induced. A high density of ventricular arrhythmia was also observed on monitoring. There were frequent ventricular premature complexes (VPCs) for 23 hours (2^{23}), couplets during 23 hours with up to 38 episodes per hour ($4A^{23}_{38}$), and runs of unsustained ventricular tachycardia 4B for 23 hours with as many as 40 episodes per hour, up to 38 beats in length and at a rate of 160 ($4B^{23}_{40,36(160)}$). With quinidine, arrhythmia is abolished during exercise. Monitoring demonstrates no VPC for 1 hour (0^1), infrequent VPCs (>30/hour) for 8 hours (1^8), frequent VPCs (>30/hour) for 13 hours (2^{13}), and 9 hours during which 3 couplets per hour occurred ($4A^9_3$).

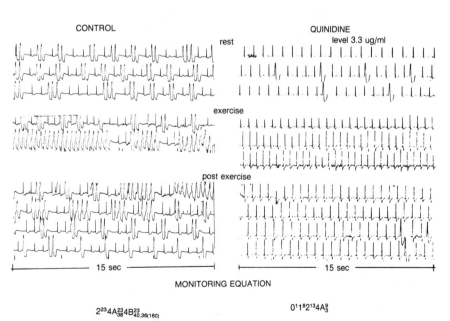

CONTROL

QUINIDINE

rest

level 3.3 ug/ml

exercise

post exercise

|— 15 sec —|

|— 15 sec —|

MONITORING EQUATION

$2^{23}4A^{23}_{38}4B^{23}_{40,36(160)}$

$0^11^82^{13}4A^9_3$

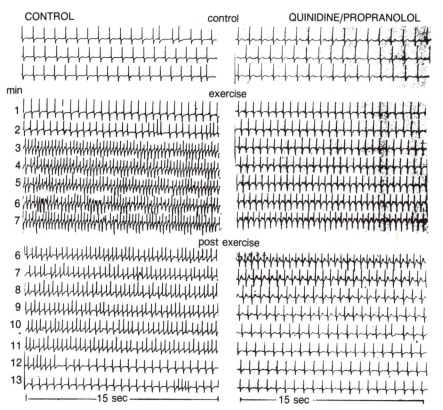

CONTROL control QUINIDINE/PROPRANOLOL

min exercise

post exercise

Figure 3 Use of exercise testing for management of exercise-induced atrial fibrillation. During the baseline study, the patient went into atrial fibrillation after 3 minutes of exercise. This terminated spontaneously 12 minutes into recovery. During therapy with quinidine and propranolol, no atrial fibrillation is provoked by exercise.

Exercise testing is therefore an important tool for exposing this negative inotropic effect, which may result in a reduction in exercise tolerance, a decrease in peak blood pressure, or a decrease in left ventricular ejection fraction measured during exercise.

Another adverse cardiac reaction is related to the slowing of impulse conduction through the myocardium caused by some of the antiarrhythmic drugs. This may result in the occurrence of significant atrioventricular nodal or intraventricular conduction abnormalities that may not be observed while the patient is at rest but that are rate-related and become apparent during exercise (Fig. 5). Such conduction abnormalities may produce symptoms suggestive of arrhythmia recurrence or cause confusion because of an electrocardiographic pattern resembling a ventricular tachyarrhythmia.

Last, all antiarrhythmic drugs have the potential to aggravate the very arrhythmia being treated or to provoke an arrhythmia that is new for the patient. Aggravation of arrhythmia by antiarrhythmic drugs is one of the most serious adverse reactions associated with this class of agents and has been reported to occur in 9 percent of noninvasively guided drug studies and in over 30 percent of patients undergoing multiple drug tests. Although it is difficult to identify the patient at risk for developing this toxic side effect, exercise testing is an extremely important method for exposing this complication. The physiologic effects caused by exercise play an important role by modifying antiarrhythmic drug activity as well as the properties of the underlying myocardial substrate, thereby possibly enhancing arrhythmogenesis in the vulnerable patient. Indeed, it has been

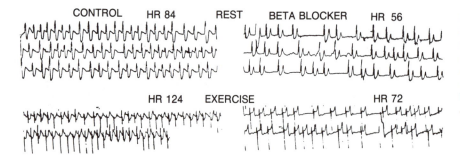

CONTROL HR 84 REST BETA BLOCKER HR 56

HR 124 EXERCISE HR 72

Figure 4 Role of exercise testing for rate control of atrial fibrillation. Prior to therapy, exercise produced a marked acceleration of the ventricular response rate. After treatment with a beta blocker, this exercise-induced increase in heart rate is blunted.

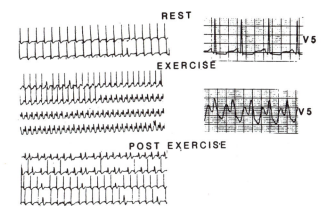

REST

EXERCISE

V5

V5

POST EXERCISE

Figure 5 Conduction abnormality exposed by exercise testing. During therapy with an antiarrhythmic agent, the QRS is normal at rest. However, exercise testing exposes a rate-related left bundle branch block, which resolves during recovery. This was initially interpreted as ventricular tachycardia.

reported that one-third of all episodes of drug-induced arrhythmia aggravation occurred during exercise testing, usually at a time when ambulatory monitoring demonstrated arrhythmia suppression (Fig. 6).

REPRODUCIBILITY OF ARRHYTHMIA DURING EXERCISE TESTING

One of the major limitations of the use of noninvasive techniques for assessing antiarrhythmic drug effect is the random variability of spontaneously occurring ventricular arrhythmia. Although most of the studies reporting wide variability of arrhythmia frequency have involved analysis of ambulatory monitoring data, there have been a few studies that have examined variability of arrhythmia during exercise testing. In patients with and without coronary artery disease but no history of serious or symptomatic arrhythmia, two sequential exercise tests performed within 45 minutes of each other result in a significant difference in the frequency of VPCs. In contrast, reproducibility is greater when the two exercise tests are separated by a longer period of time. Moreover, the reproducibility is directly related to age and more significantly to the presence and severity of underlying cardiac disease.

In the patient with a history of a sustained ventricular tachyarrhythmia who has repetitive ventricular arrhythmia provoked by exercise testing, reproducibility is good. Similar results have been reported when ambulatory monitoring data in this population are analyzed. Therefore noninvasive methods, including exercise testing and ambulatory monitoring, are reliable for evaluation of drug efficacy and

Figure 6 Aggravation of arrhythmia during exercise testing. During the control period exercise provokes frequent ventricular premature complexes (VPCs) and rare repetitive forms. During therapy with morcizine, arrhythmia documented with monitoring was suppressed, but exercise provoked ventricular fibrillation, not previously experienced by the patient. After multiple attempts at defibrillation, sinus rhythm is restored.

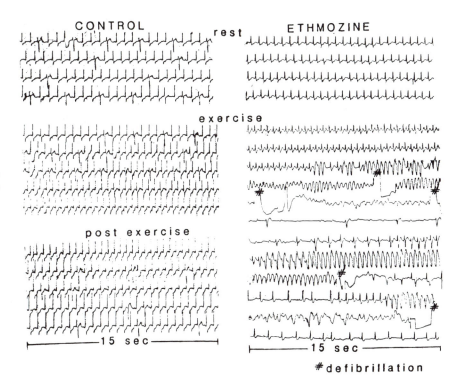

CONTROL   rest   ETHMOZINE

exercise

post exercise

├─── 15 sec ───┤   ├─── 15 sec ───┤

#defibrillation

for drug selection in the patient who manifests a high density of spontaneously occurring repetitive ventricular arrhythmia, primarily runs of nonsustained ventricular tachycardia, which is reproducibly present from day to day.

SAFETY OF EXERCISE TESTING

Although exercise testing is an important and reliable method for assessing drug effect and selecting an effective agent, an important concern is its safety. In a number of large surveys, mortality or the provocation of a serious arrhythmia during an exercise test has been reported to be from 0.2 to 0.5 percent, although most of these studies excluded patients with a history of a serious ventricular tachyarrhythmia. However, one study has reported that in such a group of patients exercise testing provoked a serious arrhythmic complication requiring an emergency intervention in 2.3 percent of tests and in 9 percent of patients. It is important to note,

however, that many of these events occurred during the course of drug evaluation and represented arrhythmia aggravation.

SUGGESTED READING

Califf RM, McKinnis RA, McNeer F, et al. Prognostic value of ventricular arrhythmias associated with treadmill exercise testing in patients studied with cardiac catheterization for suspected ischemic heart disease. J Am Coll Cardiol 1983; 2:1060–1067.

Podrid PJ. Treatment of ventricular arrhythmias: Noninvasive versus invasive approach—application and limitations. Chest 1985; 88:121–128.

Ryan M, Lown B, Horn H. Comparison of ventricular ectopic activity during 24 hour monitoring and exercise testing in patients with coronary heart disease. N Engl J Med 1975; 292:224–229.

Slater W, Lampert S, Podrid PJ, Lown B. Clinical predictors of arrhythmia worsening by antiarrhythmic drugs. Am J Cardiol 1988; 61:349–353.

Young D, Lampert S, Graboys TB, Lown B. Safety of maximal exercise testing in patients at high risk for ventricular arrhythmia. Circulation 1984; 70:184–189.

SIGNAL-AVERAGED ELECTROCARDIOGRAPHY

MICHAEL B. SIMSON, M.D.

Since 1978, investigators have detected small, high-frequency waveforms on signal-averaged electrocardiograms (ECGs) in patients with ventricular tachycardia (VT) after myocardial infarction. The microvolt (μV) level signals, termed late potentials, are continuous with the QRS complex and persist for tens of milliseconds into the S-T segment. Late potentials correspond to delayed and fragmented ventricular activation that has been observed in epicardial and endocardial electrograms recorded from patients with VT. The delayed electrograms are low in amplitude and occur in only a few areas of the heart. A standard ECG cannot reliably detect late potentials on the body surface because they are masked by noise.

Examples of signal-averaged ECGs obtained during sinus rhythm from patients without VT after myocardial infarction are shown in Figure 1. The unfiltered, signal-averaged leads (top) are displayed at high gain. On the bottom is the filtered QRS complex, a measure that depicts high-frequency information (greater than 25 Hz) contained in all three

leads. The filtered QRS complex in patients without VT is symmetric and abruptly declines to noise level at the end of the QRS complex. There is no signal above noise level (less than 1 μV) in the S-T segment. the Peak of the T wave has a small amount of high frequency content.

The initial portion of the filtered QRS complex recorded from patients with VT after myocardial infarction (Fig. 2) is generally similar to that of patients without VT. At the end of the filtered QRS complex, however, there is a late potential that is not present in patients without VT. The late potential corresponds to fine ripples in the QRS complexes of the signal-averaged unfiltered leads. The amplitude of the late potential varies from 1 to 25 μV with 25-Hz high-pass filtering.

This chapter briefly reviews signal-averaging methods and discusses the clinical significance of ventricular late potentials after myocardial infarction.

SIGNAL AVERAGING

The purpose of signal averaging is to decrease the amplitude of noise that contaminates the ECG. The primary source of noise is skeletal muscle activity, which is typically 5 to 25 μV under optimal conditions before averaging. The muscle noise cannot be eliminated by filtering.

Figure 1 Signal-averaged ECGs in two patients who did not have VT. The signal-averaged leads are shown at high gain (*top*). The filtered QRS complex is on the bottom. The filtered QRS complex is less than 100 msec in duration in both, and there is a large amplitude of signal in the last 40 msec (100 and 53 μV, respectively). The patients had an inferior (*left*) and an anterior (*right*) myocardial infarction. (From Simson MB. Signal-averaged electrocardiography: Methods and clinical application. In: Braunwald E, ed. Heart disease update. Philadelphia: WB Saunders, 1989:145; with permission.)

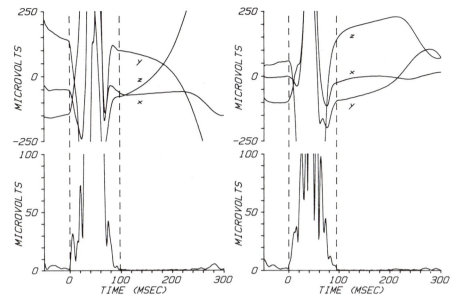

Signal averaging is a computer process that averages multiple samples of a repetitive waveform, such as the QRS complex. Random noise cancels and is reduced. Averaging 100 to 400 cycles decreases noise by a factor of 10 to 20. The technique allows a low-level signal that is hidden by noise to be readily detected. The noise content in most studies after averaging is under 1 μV or 1/100 of a millimeter at standard ECG scale.

Once the ECG is signal averaged, it is high-pass filtered to reduce large-amplitude, low-frequency signal content. The high-pass filter allows high-frequency waveforms to pass without attenuation but minimizes low-frequency waveforms. The rationale for filtering is that depolarization of cells and the movement of wavefronts of activation generate high frequencies on the body surface. The plateau or repolarization phases of the action potential produce slowly changing, lower frequency signals. The S-T segment, for example, may contain slowly changing potentials of 100 μV or more. If displayed at high gain without high-pass filtering, microvolt signals corresponding to depolarization of small areas of the myocardium would be difficult to perceive. Filter frequencies of 25 to 40 Hz are used in most studies.

Figure 2 Signal-averaged ECGs in patients with VT. For each patient the filtered QRS complex shows a longer duration and a late potential (*arrow*), which is not present in the filtered QRS complexes from control patients (see Fig. 1). The voltage in the last 40 msec of the filtered QRS complex measured 3.1 and 4.3 μV, respectively. The patients had an inferior (*left*) and an anterior (*right*) myocardial infarction. (From Simson MB. Signal-averaged electrocardiography: Methods and clinical application. In: Braunwald E, ed. Heart disease update. Philadelphia: WB Saunders, 1989:145; with permission.)

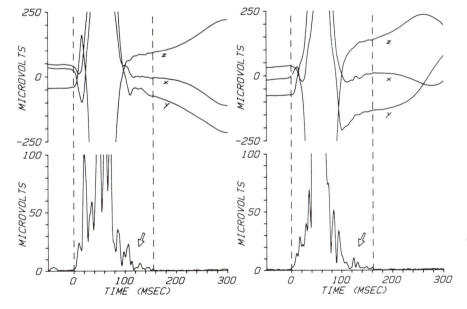

A problem with conventional high-pass filters is that they create an artifact (ringing or overshoot) after a large signal abruptly ends. This property impedes the detection of low-level late potentials that exist for only a few tens of milliseconds after the QRS complex. A bidirectional digital filter free of ringing artifact was developed to study late potentials.

High-pass filtering is called time domain analysis; the filter output corresponds in time with the input signal. Another means of extracting high-frequency content from a signal-averaged ECG is frequency domain analysis, performed by the Fourier transform. The input signal is mathematically decomposed into fundamental and harmonic frequencies, such as 8, 16, or 24 Hz, and a spectrum is formed that displays amplitude versus frequency. Most studies use time domain analysis (high-pass filtering).

Orthogonal XYZ leads are used in most investigations of late potentials. After signal averaging and high-pass filtering, the leads are often combined into a vector magnitude, a measure that sums the high-frequency information contained in all leads. The vector magnitude is termed the "filtered QRS complex." Clinical signal-averaging ECG equipment is available from several manufacturers. The entire process is automated and takes 10 to 20 minutes to perform.

Ventricular Late Potentials

Various measurements are made by the computer on the filtered QRS complex in order to detect the presence of a late potential. The late potential extends the duration of the filtered QRS complex in patients with VT after myocardial infarction by an average of 45 msec. The late potential has low amplitude. The voltage in the last 40 msec of the filtered QRS complex has been found to distinguish well between patients with and without VT after myocardial infarction. Those with VT had a means of 15 μV of signal at the end of the filtered QRS complex. Patients without the arrhythmia, in contrast, had an average of 74 μV. Another good criterion used to identify the late potential is the duration that the terminal portion of the filtered QRS complex remains below a 40-μV threshold. Late potentials are relatively high-frequency waveforms that extend into the S-T segment. When this region is analyzed by the Fourier transform, an increase in high-frequency signal content is detected.

Since late potentials were first described in 1978, many groups have recorded them with a signal-averaged ECG from patients with VT after myocardial infarction. Patients with sustained and inducible VT after myocardial infarction have abnormal signal-averaged ECGs in 79 to 92 percent of cases; in contrast, 7 to 15 percent of patients without VT after myocardial infarction and Lown class 0–1 ectopy have abnormal signal-averaged ECGs. Only 0 to 2 percent of healthy volunteers have abnormal signal-averaged ECGs; most studies report that no late potentials are detected in normal subjects.

The definition of a late potential and the scoring of a signal-averaged ECG as normal or abnormal are highly technique-specific, and standards vary. Representative criteria are that a late potential exists when the filtered QRS complex is longer than 114 to 120 msec, or there is less than 20 μV of signal in the last 40 msec of the filtered QRS complex, or the terminal filtered QRS complex remains below 40 μV for longer than 38 msec (40 Hz bidirectional filtering). The European Society of Cardiology and the American Heart Association have convened a committee to establish standards for the recording and analysis of signal-averaged ECGs.

Late potentials appear to originate from small areas of delayed and disorganized ventricular activation. Patients with VT after myocardial infarction have prolonged fragmented electrograms during sinus rhythm that often outlast the end of the QRS complex as conventionally recorded. Studies in experimental myocardial infarction have shown that delayed ventricular activation, recorded directly from ischemic or infarcted myocardium, can span diastole and that VT depends on a wavefront that slowly conducts over a reentrant pathway. Endocardial recordings in humans have demonstrated that delayed fragmented activity can outlast the surface QRS complex, that it prolongs under the stress of premature beats, and that the onset and maintenance of VT depend on continuous diastolic activity. After experimental myocardial infarction, the fragmented electrograms occurred in areas of infarction where interstitial fibrosis caused wide separation of individual myocardial fibers. A similar anatomic substrate has been found in endocardium resected from patients undergoing surgery for control of VT.

The time relationship between the body surface late potentials and delayed ventricular activation has been studied in patients with VT after myocardial infarction. The late potentials correlated with delayed fragmented electrogram activity, recorded primarily from endocardial sites. Studies in animals with experimental myocardial infarctions have shown a similar relationship between delayed ventricular activation and late potentials.

Prognostic Significance of Late Potentials After Acute Myocardial Infarction

The prognostic value of late potentials or an abnormal signal-average ECG in patients after an acute myocardial infarction has been evaluated in multiple studies sing 1983. Table 1 presents four peer-reviewed prospective studies on a total of 778

Table 1 Prognostic Significance of the Signal-Averaged ECG in Patients After Myocardial Infarction

	N	Day of Study After Myocardial Infarction	Follow-Up Duration (mo)	Incidence of Arrhythmia or Sudden Death		
					Sudden Death	Sustained VT
Breithardt et al (1983)	160	25.5 (median)	7.5 ± 3.3 mean ± SD	No LP LP > 40 msec LP < 40 msec	3.8% 3.2% 11.1%	0% 4.8% 16.6%
					Sudden death	Sustained VT or VF
Denniss et al (1986)	306	7–28	24 mean 12	Normal Abnormal	2% 15% (1 yr)	4% 19% (2 yr)
Gomes et al (1987)	102	10 ± 6	12 ± 6	Normal Abnormal		3.5% 28.9%
Kuchar et al (1987)	210	11 (mean)	6–24 mean 14	Normal Abnormal		0.8% 16.7%

Key: VT = ventricular tachycardia, N = number of patients, LP = late potentials, VF = ventricular fibrillation.
Normal or abnormal refers to a normal or abnormal signal-averaged ECG.

patients. The signal-averaged ECG was performed less than 1 month after an acute myocardial infarction, and the mean duration of follow-up was 7.5 to 14 months. Late potentials or an abnormal signal-averaged ECG was found in 24 to 44 percent of patients. Patients with a normal signal-averaged ECG or no late potentials had a 0.8 to 3.5 percent incidence of sudden cardiac death or sustained VT during follow-up. In contrast, patients with an abnormal signal-averaged ECG or definite late potentials (greater than 40 msec) had an incidence of sudden death or sustained VT of 16.7 to 28.9 percent. One study showed a higher incidence of sudden death and sustained VT in patients with anterior wall myocardial infarction as compared with those with inferior wall myocardial infarction, but the other three studies showed no difference. An abnormal signal-averaged ECG appears to predict an increase in overall cardiac mortality as well as serious arrhythmic events following an acute myocardial infarction; Denniss reported that patients with an abnormal signal-averaged ECG had a 10 percent mortality in the first year following a myocardial infarction as compared with 2 percent for patients with a normal signal-averaged ECG.

Studies performed in the 1980s demonstrated that ventricular arrhythmias and left ventricular dysfunction are independently related to the risk of mortality and sudden cardiac death following an acute myocardial infarction. Two large multicenter studies showed, for example, that patients with repetitive ventricular premature complexes were 2.3 to 5.6 times more likely to die during follow-up than patients without the arrhythmias. Similarly, those patients with a left ventricular ejection fraction of less than 40 percent showed an odds ratio of dying during follow-up of 3.4 to 5.1 as compared with patients with a higher ejection fraction. The risk of sudden death following myocardial infarction was also increased by left ventricular dysfunction and, independently, by ventricular arrhythmias.

An important question to be answered was whether the signal-averaged ECG provided information that was independent of left ventricular dysfunction or ventricular ectopy, and that was useful in identifying patients with lethal tachyarrhythmias. A partial answer was provided by a retrospective study that compared the findings on a signal-averaged ECG, Holter monitoring, and cardiac catheterization in 98 patients who had recurrent sustained VT and 76 patients without VT after myocardial infarction. Multivariant analysis showed that only three variables provided significant independent information to identify patients with VT: an abnormal signal-averaged ECG, a peak ventricular premature complex rate of more than 100 per minute, and the presence of a left ventricular aneurysm. When aneurysm was excluded as a variable in the analysis, a left ventricular ejection fraction of less than 40 percent replaced aneurysm as a third independent variable. The study suggested that the signal-averaged ECG could be combined with other clinical information to provide a more accurate identification of patients with VT after myocardial infarction. Multiple investigations have demonstrated that the signal-averaged ECG provides data independent of left ventricular ejection fraction or ventricular ectopy in identifying patients with VT.

Recent prospective studies by Gomes and co-workers, and Kuchar and colleagues have evaluated the signal-averaged ECG, prolonged ECG monitoring, and radionuclide ventriculography as a means of predicting sustained VT or sudden death after myocardial infarction. A total of 312 patients were studied for a mean of 12 to 14 months after an acute myocardial infarction. The median time to development of life-threatening arrhythmias was less than 2 months. Multivariant analysis in both studies showed that the signal-averaged ECG, an ejection fraction of less than 40 percent, or complex ventricular ectopic activity each had independent value to predict serious arrhythmic events after myocardial infarction. The tests could be combined to identify high-risk patients more accurately. The combination of a signal-averaged ECG and a low ejection fraction had the highest sensitivity and specificity in both studies. No patient in either study with a normal signal-averaged ECG and ejection fraction greater than 40 percent had sustained VT or sudden death during follow-up. In contrast, patients with an abnormal signal-averaged ECG and an ejection fraction of less than 40 percent had a 34 to 36 percent incidence of sustained VT or sudden death during follow-up. A combination of an abnormal signal-averaged ECG and a low ejection fraction provided a sensitivity of 80 percent and 100 percent and a specificity of 89 percent and 59 percent to identify patients in whom sudden death or sustained VT would occur in the studies by Kuchar and coworkers and Gomes and associates, respectively.

The two studies argue that a combination of noninvasive tests, including the signal-averaged ECG, can be used to stratify patients according to risk of serious arrhythmic events after an acute myocardial infarction. Patients with normal tests are at low risk for arrhythmic events and need no further therapy. Patients with a combination of abnormal tests are at high risk for developing sustained VT or sudden death. The most effective therapy for high-risk patients is unknown and requires further investigation. The roles of new antiarrhythmic agents, antitachycardia devices, implantable defibrillators, and therapy guided by electrophysiologic stimulation tests need to be defined. A recent prospective study by Breithardt and coworkers suggests that programmed ventricular stimulation, along with the signal-averaged ECG, may be used to define the patients at highest risk for sustained VT after an acute myocardial infarction; in their study, the patients at highest risk were characterized by the presence of a ventricular late potential and an inducible sustained VT at a rate of less than 270 beats per minute.

The signal-averaged ECG may be useful in de-fining a patient group at high risk of developing ventricular fibrillation or sustained VT in the acute stage of a myocardial infarction. McGuire and associates found that a signal-averaged ECG recorded a mean of 12 hours after onset of chest pain identified patients with sustained VT or ventricular fibrillation within the first day after myocardial infarction with a sensitivity of 80 percent and a specificity of 72 percent. Another study of Gomes and coworkers reported that a signal-averaged ECG performed 3 days after a myocardial infarction predicted sustained VT or ventricular fibrillation within 13 to 15 days after an acute myocardial infarction, with a sensitivity of 80 to 100 percent. The signal-averaged ECG may prove useful in selecting patients who could benefit from more intense or prolonged monitoring after an acute myocardial infarction.

SUGGESTED READING

Breithardt G, Borggrefe M. Recent advances in the identification of patients at risk of ventricular tachyarrhythmias: Role of ventricular late potentials. Circulation 1987; 75:1091–1096.

Breithardt G, Schwarzmaier M, Borggrefe M, et al. Prognostic significance of late ventricular potentials after acute myocardial infarction. Eur Heart J 1983; 4:487–495.

Denniss AR, Richards DA, Cody DV, et al. Prognostic significance of ventricular tachycardia and fibrillation induced at programmed stimulation and delayed potentials detected on the signal-averaged electrocardiograms of survivors of acute myocardial infarction. Circulation 1986; 74:731–745.

Gomes JA, Mehra R, Barreca P, et al. Quantitative analysis of the high-frequency components of the signal-averaged QRS complex in patients with acute myocardial infarction: A prospective study. Circulation 1985; 72:105–111.

Gomes JA, Winters SL, Stewart D, et al. A new noninvasive index to predict sustained ventricular tachycardia and sudden death in the first year after myocardial infarction: Based on signal-averaged electrocardiogram, radionuclide ejection fraction and Holter monitoring. J Am Coll Cardiol 1987; 10:349–357.

Kanovsky MS, Falcone RA, Dresden CA, et al. Identification of patients with ventricular tachycardia after myocardial infarction: Signal-averaged electrocardiogram, Holter monitoring, and cardiac catheterization. Circulation 1984; 70:264–270.

Kuchar DL, Thorburn CW, Sammel NL. Prediction of serious arrhythmic events after myocardial infarction: Signal-averaged electrocardiogram, Holter monitoring and radionuclide ventriculography. J Am Coll Cardiol 1987; 9:531–538.

McGuire M, Kuchar D, Ganis J, et al. Natural history of late potentials in the first ten days after acute myocardial infarction and relation to early ventricular arrhythmias. Am J Cardiol 1988; 61:1187–1190.

Simson MB. Signal-averaged electrocardiography: Methods and clinical applications. In: Braunwald E, ed. Heart disease update. Philadelphia: WB Saunders, 1989:145.

ELECTROPHYSIOLOGIC TECHNIQUES

STEVEN J. NIERENBERG, M.D.

The recording and validation of the His potential in humans by Scherlag and Helfant in 1969, followed by further confirmation and extensive study in the 1970s, catapulted cardiac electrophysiology to its position in the 1980s as a well accepted and widely used technique in diagnosing and treating cardiac arrhythmias. The catheter recording of a His potential has enabled us to verify directly what many of the expert electrocardiographers of the middle part of this century deduced from the surface electrocardiogram concerning atrioventricular (AV) block and concealed conduction.

In many cases, however, the level of AV block cannot be deduced with certainty from the surface electrocardiogram, and because supra-Hisian block carries with it a different prognosis than intra- or infra-Hisian block, it may be necessary to record a His bundle electrogram to make an accurate diagnosis concerning the mechanism of AV block. Additionally, when the presenting rhythm is a wide complex tachycardia, the recording of a His potential enables us to differentiate clearly supraventricular from ventricular tachycardia as well as to further elucidate the mechanisms of these tachycardias. Antiarrhythmic drug testing also is facilitated by electrophysiologic studies.

EQUIPMENT

The principles of recording electrical potentials from inside the heart are basic to those of electrocardiography in general. In the electrophysiology laboratory, we use a multichannel recorder that amplifies and filters the intracardiac signals. The filters must be able to filter both low and high frequencies. The signals are usually transmitted by electrode catheters made of woven dacron and having at least two electrode poles and diameters of Nos. 5 to 7 French. Recordings made between two poles of the electrode catheter are termed bipolar. A unipolar recording can be obtained from any single electrode on the catheter and a common central terminal, often called the Wilson central terminal at the electrical center of the heart (a principle similar to recording the unipolar precordial V leads developed by Wilson in 1934). Intraelectrode distances may vary, but they are generally 0.5 to 1.0 cm for most studies. To record and stimulate simultaneously in a bipolar fashion, two pairs (quadripolar) of electrodes are needed (Fig. 1).

The electrode catheters are usually connected to a junction box. This enables recording from any single pole or pair of poles of the catheter to be done easily by the flip of a switch or utilizing a computer program to select recording sites. Electrically isolated cables that ideally run under the floor are connected to an electrically isolated amplifier system. The intracardiac and surface electrograms are amplified to approximately 1 cm amplitude per millivolt, which is similar to a standard electrocardiographic recorder. We generally filter our intracardiac signals below 40 and above 400 Hz.

Surface electrocardiographic leads I, aVF, and V_1, along with intracardiac electrograms from the atrium, His bundle area, and ventricle, are typically displayed on an oscilloscope for viewing as well as printed for hard copy (Fig. 2). We use an ink jet printer with the capability of high-speed recording of signals up to 250 mm per second with a frequency response of greater than 500 Hz. Photographic recorders with these capabilities would also be adequate. We also record the entire study on magnetic tape as a permanent record.

A stimulator is necessary both for pacing the heart and to deliver extrastimuli. This stimulator should have the minimal capability to pace the heart at cycle lengths of 2,000 msec down to 50 msec (30 to 1,200 pulses per minute) with minimal incremental changes of no more than 10 msec. The current or voltage output should be adjustable on at least two separate channels that have the capability of simultaneously or sequentially delivering pulses at two separate sites. Additionally, synchronization of these pulses to the intrinsic heart rhythm and the ability to deliver at least three timed extrastimuli after a train of paced beats are necessary for most stimulation protocols.

During an electrophysiologic study, we continuously record surface electrograms from two stan-

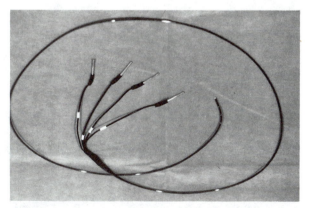

Figure 1 A typical quadripolar electrode catheter made of woven Dacron. Note the four separate poles that exit the proximal end of the catheters separately for ease of connection to a junction box.

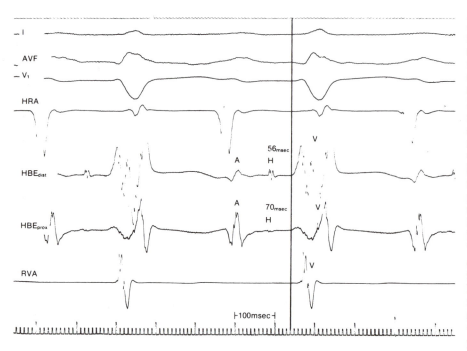

Figure 2 Ink jet recording of surface leads 1, AVF, and V_1 at the top of the tracing. Note the small far field ventricular electrogram in the high right atrial (HRA) recording. In the His bundle electrogram (HBE) recording, note the smaller atrial electrogram recorded from the distal electrode pair when compared with the proximal His bundle electrogram recorded from the proximal pair of electrodes. When measured from the most proximal His bundle recording, the H-V interval is mildly prolonged at 70 msec. If the distal His bundle recording had been used, the H-V interval would have been erroneously measured as normal. The right ventricular apex (RVA) electrogram reveals a narrow, discrete, multiphasic potential.

dard anterior/posterior electrode pads and display this recording on the oscilloscope of a standard cardioverter-defibrillator. Additionally, we keep precordial and limb lead electrodes attached to an electrocardiographic recorder to record a full 12-lead electrocardiogram after induction of arrhythmias. With this system, hemodynamically poorly tolerated arrhythmias can be recorded and terminated with direct current cardioversion, quickly and with minimal activity from staff.

TECHNIQUE

Cardiac electrophysiologic studies involve the insertion of electrode catheters at various intracardiac sites, usually via the venous system using a fluoroscopic tube to guide catheter placement. It is preferable, although not absolutely necessary, to have a laboratory dedicated to electrophysiologic studies so as to minimize technical problems (Fig. 3). The most commonly used veins for electrophysiolo-

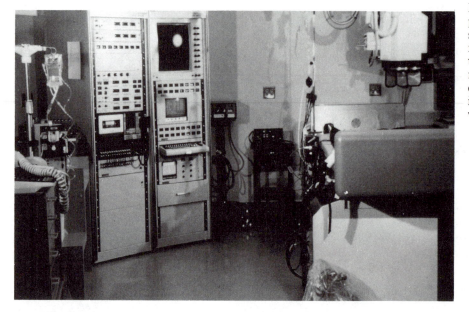

Figure 3 A dedicated electrophysiology laboratory demonstrating (from right to left) a fluoroscopic table and x-ray tube, pulse oximetry equipment, electrophysiologic recording and stimulator unit, ink jet printer, and code cart with defibrillating equipment.

gic studies are the femoral veins, from which catheter positioning in various right atrial and right ventricular sites can be accomplished with catheter manipulation. Entrance into the venous system is performed via percutaneous needle puncture under local anesthesia. Techniques vary from laboratory to laboratory, but generally they involve some variation of the Seldinger technique, in which a flexible wire is passed through the needle into the vein. The needle is then removed with the placement of a dilator and sheath over the wire into the vein through which the catheter will pass. It has been my experience that palpation of the femoral artery with two or three fingers along its course delineates the anatomy of the artery, facilitating arterial and venous punctures. The femoral venipuncture is then done 1 cm medial to the artery and 1 cm inferior to the inguinal ligament. A second puncture can be made 1 to 2 cm inferior to the first for placement of a second venous catheter (Fig. 4). For most ventricular tachycardia cases, we position catheters in the high right atrium, His bundle area, and right ventricular apex. A coronary sinus catheter is often placed for cases of supraventricular tachycardia to record left atrial potentials (Fig. 5). One of these catheters is later moved to the right ventricular outflow tract for recording and stimulation. We generally place a No. 5 French sheath in the right femoral artery for hemodynamic monitoring, unless there is a contraindication such as severe peripheral vascular disease.

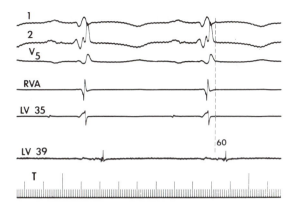

Figure 5 Recording during sinus rhythm demonstrating a narrow discrete electrogram recorded from a catheter in the right ventricular apex (RVA). By comparison, note the fractionated, low-amplitude potentials recorded from the left ventricular posteroapical epicardium (LV 39). These fractionated potentials represent slow conduction in the region of a left ventricular aneurysm.

Once a catheter is positioned in the right atrium or right ventricle, the electrogram recorded should be observed. The electrogram should be discrete and relatively narrow (less than 70 msec) (see Fig. 2). It should not be broad or fractionated, with low-amplitude potentials (Fig. 5). Fractionated electrograms may indicate positioning of the catheter in an area of electrically inert tissue such as scar or fibrous tissue. This is less desirable during the stimulation protocol, because it requires higher energies to pace these areas and may make tachycardia induction more difficult. If the appearance of the electrograms is acceptable, the threshold to capture is determined by a fixed rate pacing technique. At a pulse duration of 0.2 msec, a current of 1.0 mA or less should cause depolarization of the myocardium. In our laboratory, as in most others, the remainder of the study is done at twice the diastolic threshold. Higher currents are reserved for tachycardia induction in some laboratories when the lower current has failed.

One main exception to the femoral vein approach is when cannulation of the coronary sinus is desired. Because of the posterior location of the coronary sinus, it is frequently easier to cannulate via the superior vena cava. We usually utilize the left median basilic vein for this cannulation; however, the subclavian or internal jugular veins (preferably the left) can be used as well. In this technique a multipolar catheter (hexapolar in our laboratory) with a gentle curve at the tip is advanced into the right atrium. The region of the right atrium, inferoposterior to the tricuspid valve, is then investigated with the catheter until cannulation of the os of the coronary sinus occurs. Sometimes a deep breath or

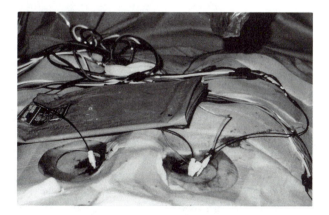

Figure 4 A view of the right and left sides of the groin from the head of the bed demonstrating two venous sheaths in the right femoral artery approximately 1 cm apart and one arterial sheath in the right femoral artery and one venous sheath in the left femoral vein. Through these sheaths are the electrode catheters, which are then connected via cables to our junction box located at the foot of the table.

coughing facilitates this process. In some situations it may be helpful to turn the patient to the 30-degree right anterior oblique position. The AV fat pad is well visualized in this view. The os of the coronary sinus lies at the base of the fat pad. The catheter should be advanced gently to its most lateral position at the border of the left side of the heart and should make a curve toward the patient's left shoulder (Fig. 6). Verification of catheter position within the coronary sinus is usually done by inspection of the electrograms recorded from the distal electrode pair. This should demonstrate large atrial and ventricular potentials. Pacing at low current (less than 5 mA) from the middle or distal electrode pair should result in depolarization of the left atrium with conduction to the ventricle. Additionally, we usually rotate the table into the left anterior oblique position to demonstrate the posterior location of the catheter. Final verification (rarely necessary) could be accomplished by demonstrating desaturated blood withdrawn through a lumen catheter.

The His bundle electrogram is easily recorded when approached with a catheter via the inferior vena cava. A No. 6 or 7 French tripolar or quadripolar catheter, with varying curves at the tip, is frequently used for this purpose. Electrograms can be recorded from the distal electrode pair and from the proximal electrode pair of a quadripolar catheter simultaneously. The usual technique is to cross the tricuspid valve with the catheter so that a large ventricular electrogram and a small atrial electrogram

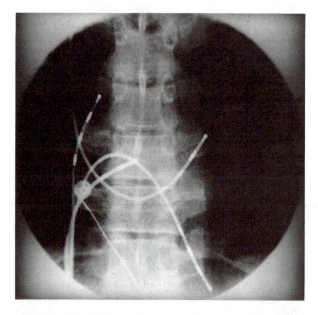

Figure 6 Fluoroscopic image of the heart with catheter positions as follows. Clockwise from the top, there is a high right atrial catheter, His bundle electrogram catheter, right ventricular apex, and coronary sinus catheter. Note the typical curve of the coronary sinus catheter toward the left shoulder.

are recorded from the distal electrode pair. The catheter is then gently withdrawn, usually with clockwise torque turning the catheter more posteriorly against the septum and tricuspid valve. As the catheter is withdrawn, a narrow potential is sometimes observed just in front of the large ventricular potential at a time when the atrial electrogram is small. This usually represents the right bundle branch recording. The catheter should be further withdrawn until the largest atrial electrogram is recorded while still recording a His potential. It is at this point that the recording electrodes are near the most proximal portion of the His bundle, and measurement of the H-V interval should be obtained (Figs. 2 and 7). Verification of the catheter position at the proximal His bundle can be obtained by pacing from the same electrode pair, in which case a narrow QRS complex should be obtained that is identical to the QRS complex during sinus rhythm in all leads. The stimulus to activation of the ventricle time (S-V) should be the same as the H-V interval time, indicating no latency from stimulus artifact to His bundle activation. This pacing should be done at less than 1.0 mA so as not to activate surrounding tissue. Additionally, the atrial electrogram should follow the His potential during His bundle pacing. Once the His potential is recorded, an additional 90 or 180 degrees of clockwise torque is sometimes applied to secure the catheter against the septum for stability. Sometimes we make a small loop in the catheter outside the body and lay a sterile towel across it to maintain position.

Utilizing the femoral venous approach, a His bundle recording can be made in almost all patients. Rarely, because of contraindications against using the femoral venous system, such as deep vein thrombosis, active phlebitis, infection, or other anatomic reasons, a superior vena cava approach may be utilized to record a His bundle. Recording of the His potential from the superior vena cava approach is difficult with a standard quadripolar catheter. It is usually necessary to prolapse the catheter across the tricuspid valve into the right ventricle and gently withdraw the catheter so that its tip comes into proximity with the tricuspid valve while the catheter is still looped in the right ventricle. Looping the catheter in the right atrium so the tip contacts the tricuspid area has also been done. A retrograde arterial approach can also be used but is rarely employed. In this technique, the catheter is introduced into the arterial system and advanced retrogradely to the aortic valve to lie in the noncoronary or posterior sinus of Valsalva. In this position, accurate and comparable recordings of the His potential may be obtained.

Once the electrode catheters are placed, the electrogram recorded should be inspected, as should the sequence of atrial activation during normal sinus rhythm. Generally, the catheter recording high right

Figure 7 An ink jet recording, again from the distal and proximal pairs of a His bundle electrogram (HBE) catheter, demonstrating the importance of pulling the catheter back until a large atrial electrogram is obtained prior to measuring the H-V interval. These measurements may differ by 5 to 10 msec in normal individuals, reflecting His bundle conduction time. However, in patients with His-Purkinje dysfunction, the differences between proximal and distal H-V intervals can be greater. RVA = right ventricular apex; RFA = right femoral artery.

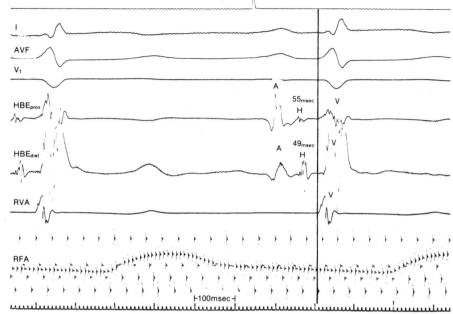

Figure 8 Typical atrial activation pattern in sinus rhythm demonstrating the earliest atrial activation in the high right atrium (HRA). This is usually rapidly followed by activation of the atrium in the tricuspid area near the His bundle (HBE). The rapid activation of this area 30 to 40 msec prior to low right atrial or proximal coronary sinus activation suggests the presence of rapidly conducting internodal tissue. Note the late activation of the distal coronary sinus (CS$_d$) when compared with the proximal coronary sinus area (CS$_p$). RVA = right ventricular apex.

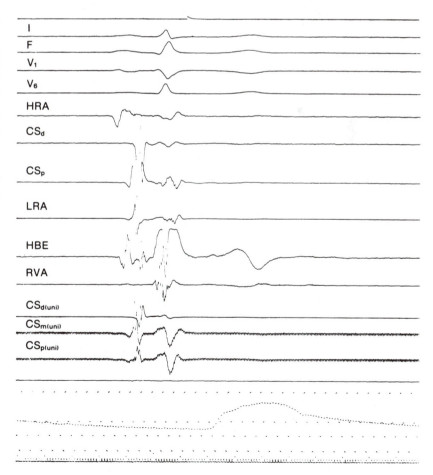

atrial electrograms is activated earliest and is usually followed by the His bundle catheter recording approximately 30 to 40 msec later. Activation of the region surrounding the coronary sinus (left atrium) is last and is usually activated from medial to lateral (Fig. 8). Occasionally, the distal coronary sinus electrode recording the posterolateral left atrium is activated prior to the proximal coronary sinus electrode (Fig. 9). Some electrophysiologists interpret this as evidence of a specialized interatrial conduction system (Bachmann's bundle). Additionally, the rapid activation of the His bundle area prior to the os of the coronary sinus or low right atrium has been felt to be attributable to specialized conducting tissue connecting the sinus and AV nodes.

ELECTROPHYSIOLOGIC PROTOCOLS

Electrophysiologic protocols vary from laboratory to laboratory as well as from case to case. Generally, measurements of the P-R, R-R, QRS, and QTc intervals are made at the beginning of the study. Following that, measurement of the A-H interval, which approximates conduction through the AV node, is made. This measurement is made in the His bundle recording from the earliest rapid atrial deflection to the initial deflection of the His potential at a paper speed of at least 100 mm per second

(see Fig. 7). The normal A-H interval ranges from 60 to 125 msec.

The H-V interval is also measured in the His bundle recording and approximates conduction down the His-Purkinje system to the activation of the ventricles. This measurement is also done at least 100 mm per second paper speed, although we make this measurement at 250 mm per second paper speed for greater accuracy. Accurate measurement of the H-V interval is frequently crucial for decision making, since 20-msec differences in this measurement can separate normal His-Purkinje conduction from moderately prolonged His-Purkinje conduction. Again, it is important that the His electrogram with the largest possible atrial electrogram is selected for measurement of the H-V interval so as to record the most proximal portion of the His potential. If a distal His bundle electrogram recording is used, erroneously "normal" H-V interval measurements may be made in patients with abnormal His-Purkinje function (see Fig. 2). Measurement of the H-V interval is made from the initial deflection of the His electrogram from the isoelectric baseline to the earliest activation of the ventricle, whether on the surface or on an intracardiac recording (see Fig. 7). Generally, the earliest activation of the ventricle is seen on one of the surface ECG leads (often V_1), because activation of the septum, which is seen well on a surface electrocardiogram, occurs before activation

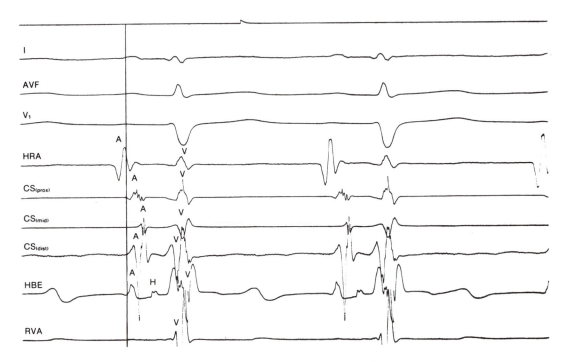

Figure 9 In this tracing of a patient also in sinus rhythm, there is rapid activation of the distal coronary sinus (CS). This activation is nearly simultaneous with the proximal coronary sinus area and His bundle electrogram (HBE). This may indicate specialized conducting tissue connecting the right and left atria (Bachmann's bundle).

of the right ventricular apex. The normal H-V interval is 35 to 60 msec. The normal His potential duration is no more than 25 msec. With careful attention to detail, accurate measurement of the H-V interval can be made with a margin of error of less than 5 msec.

After baseline electrocardiographic and electrophysiologic measurements are made, we begin programmed electrical stimulation in the atria, first to assess sinus node function. This includes measurement of the sinoatrial conduction time by the method of Narula, followed by measurement of the sinus node recovery time after 30 seconds of constant rate atrial pacing at varying cycle lengths.

Following the sinus node evaluation, evaluation of AV conduction is made. First the point at which AV nodal block occurs during incremental atrial pacing is assessed. Following this, atrial and AV conduction and refractoriness are assessed by the extrastimulus method. This generally involves delivering a train of eight paced complexes in the atria followed by an extrastimulus. The coupling interval of the extrastimulus is gradually tightened as one assesses the refractoriness and conduction in the

atria and AV node-His-Purkinje system (Fig. 10). We generally do this during sinus rhythm as well as during an atrial paced rhythm of 600 msec. Assessment of AV nodal and His-Purkinje function is made during these extrastimulus scans, including assessment of dual AV nodal pathways and supra- versus infra-Hisian block during extrastimulus. The ability to induce varying atrial, AV nodal, and, atrioventricular rhythms is also assessed.

Following the assessment of sinus node and AV nodal and His-Purkinje function, the assessment of ventricular function and of the ability to induce ventricular arrhythmias is carried out. Initially we perform straight ventricular pacing at varying cycle lengths to assess the presence and pattern of ventriculoatrial conduction as well as the cycle length at which ventriculoatrial block occurs during incremental ventricular pacing. Ventricular refractoriness is then assessed by the extrastimulus method similar to that described in the atria and involves a train of eight paced beats in the ventricle followed by a single extrastimulus. Ventricular extrastimulus scans are generally done during at least two different ventricular drives. In our laboratory we use 600 msec and

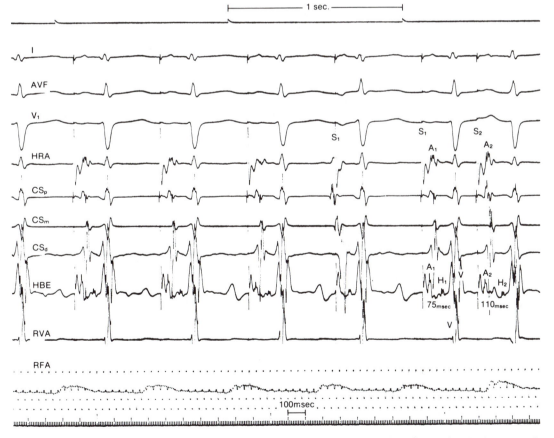

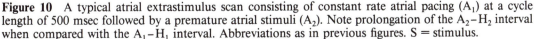

Figure 10 A typical atrial extrastimulus scan consisting of constant rate atrial pacing (A_1) at a cycle length of 500 msec followed by a premature atrial stimuli (A_2). Note prolongation of the A_2-H_2 interval when compared with the A_1-H_1 interval. Abbreviations as in previous figures. S = stimulus.

400 msec drives routinely and occasionally a 500 msec drive as well. Following the determination of ventricular refractoriness by single extrastimuli, double and in most laboratories triple extrastimuli are employed in an attempt to induce ventricular arrhythmias. We start our extrastimulus scan at 40 msec beyond refractoriness and gradually shorten the coupling interval by 10-msec increments until refractoriness occurs in our last extrastimulus. At this point we shorten the next to last extrastimulus by 10 msec. If that combination of coupling intervals captures the ventricle, we then try to tighten the last extrastimulus again by 10 msec. We follow this routine in an effort to hit all possible combinations of coupling intervals and therefore to maximize our chances of inducing an arrhythmia.

If a sustained ventricular arrhythmia is induced, we quickly measure the cycle length at 100 mm per second paper speed and obtain a 12-lead electrocardiogram for morphologic comparison. The mean arterial pressure recorded by an intraarterial catheter is observed, as is the patient's response to the arrhythmia. If the patient and his or her blood pressure appear stable, we observe the patient for 30 seconds before intervening to terminate the tachycardia. If the patient is hypotensive and symptomatic, we frequently intervene with ventricular burst pacing prior to 30 sec in an effort to terminate a tachycardia before loss of consciousness occurs. Should loss of consciousness occur, direct current external cardioversion is performed. The initial energy used varies from laboratory to laboratory but is generally in the 100 to 200 J range. If this fails, rescue shocks with greater energy are employed. Following the initiation and termination of a hemodynamically poorly tolerated arrhythmia, we usually wait at least 10 to 15 minutes for hemodynamic stabilization of the patient before resuming the study. Generally we try to reproduce all induced arrhythmias at least once unless the patient is unstable. Following the initiation and reproduction of a sustained ventricular arrhythmia, we generally administer intravenous procainamide in a dose of 15 mg per kilogram. Baseline electrocardiographic and electrophysiologic measurements are then made. This is followed by programmed electrical stimulation identical to the initial ventricular protocol. The response of the patient to intravenous procainamide gives us important information concerning management of the patient's ventricular arrhythmias.

RISKS AND COMPLICATIONS

Cardiac electrophysiologic study carries an acceptably low incidence of serious complications. The risk of a significant complication or death is approximately 1 per cent of cases. This is similar to the major complication rate of cardiac catheterization.

Table 1 Significant Complications of Electrophysiologic Studies in 1,000 Patients

Complication	Incidence/1,000 Patients Exposed (%)	Incidence/ Procedure (%)
Death	1 (0.1)	1/2,210 (0.05)
Vascular	12 (1.2)	12/1,782* (0.7)
Arterial injury	4 (0.4)	4/1,782 (0.2)
Thrombophlebitis	6 (0.6))	6/1,782 (0.3)
Severe hematoma	2 (0.2)	2/1,782 (0.1)
Embolic	4 (0.4)	4/2,210 (0.2)
Systemic arterial embolus	1 (0.1)	1/2,210 (0.5)
Pulmonary embolus	3 (0.3)	3/2,210 (0.15)
Cardiac perforation	2 (0.2)	2/1,782 (0.1)
Hypotension	20 (2.0)	20/2,210 (1.0)

*The number of studies in which catheter insertion occurred

In a series of 1,000 consecutive patients, Horowitz reported one death (Table 1). Arterial complications occurred in four patients. Venous complications, mainly thrombophlebitis, were more common and occurred in six patients. Three of these patients developed pulmonary emboli and were treated successfully with anticoagulation. (We routinely aspirate the venous sheaths during their removal to reduce the risk of venous thrombosis.) Cardiac perforation occurred in two patients, one of whom became profoundly hypotensive and required emergency pericardiocentesis. Blood pressure was restored with fluids, and the patient recovered.

The induction of incessant ventricular tachycardia is the one arrhythmia that even experienced electrophysiologists fear. This occurred in 14 of 1,000 patients in the Horowitz series. Only two such arrhythmias occurred at baseline when the patient was off antiarrhythmic drugs. In the other 12 patients, incessant ventricular tachycardia occurred while the patient was taking an antiarrhythmic agent. These drugs included oral flecainide (three patients), intravenous procainamide (three patients), intravenous indecainide (one patient), intravenous pirmenol (one patient), intravenous amiodarone (one patient), oral disopyramide with intravenous mexiletine (one patient), oral amiodarone (one patient), oral amiodarone with oral procainamide (one patient). This complication occurred in 3 percent of 397 patients undergoing serial electrophysiologic drug evaluation who had a sustained tachyarrhythmia.

SUGGESTED READING

Horowitz LN, Josephson ME, Farshidi A, et al. Recurrent sustained ventricular tachycardia. Role of the electrophysiologic study in selection of antiarrhythmic regimens. Circulation 1978; 58:987–997.

Horowitz LN, Kay HR, Kutalek SP, et al. Risk and complications of clinical cardiac electrophysiologic studies: A perspective analysis of 1000 consecutive patients. J Am Coll Cardiol 1987; 9:1261–1268.

Narula OS. Validation of His bundle recordings: Limitations of the catheter technique. In: Narula OS, ed. His bundle electrocardiography and clinical electrophysiology. Philadelphia: FA Davis Co, 1975:pp 65–93.

Rosen KM. The contribution of His bundle recording to the understanding of cardiac conduction in man. Circulation 1971; 43:961–966.

Scherlag BJ, Berbari EJ. Techniques for His bundle recordings. In: Narula OS, ed. His bundle electrocardiography and clinical electrophysiology. Philadelphia: FA Davis Co., 1975:pp 51–63.

Scherlag BJ, Lau SH, Helfant RH, et al. Catheter technique for recording His bundle activity in man. Circulation 1969; 29:13–18.

Ward DE, Camm AJ. Clinical electrophysiologic methods. In: Clinical electrophysiology of the heart. London: Edward Arnold Publishers, 1987:pp 9–31.

III SUPRAVENTRICULAR TACHYARRHYTHMIAS

SUPRAVENTRICULAR TACHYARRHYTHMIAS: CLASSIFICATION AND GENERAL PRINCIPLES OF THERAPY

JOHN A. KASTOR, M.D.

Supraventricular tachyarrhythmias can be defined by what they are not. Ventricular tachyarrhythmias (see Section V, Ventricular Arrhythmias) start in the ventricles. Most supraventricular tachyarrhythmias originate elsewhere.

IDENTIFICATION

Although there are several methods of identifying supraventricular tachyarrhythmias, I have always found it helpful to describe them first as regular or irregular. This is one of the first features usually observed when examining the electrocardiogram of a patient with a tachycardia.

Regularity

Atrial fibrillation, atrial flutter, and multifocal atrial tachycardia (MAT) are three supraventricular tachyarrhythmias that can be irregular. Fibrillation and MAT usually, flutter some of the time. Other supraventricular tachyarrhythmias are generally regular with only slight variations in the duration of the R-R intervals.

Electrocardiographic Morphology

Having determined whether the ventricular rate is regular or irregular, most observers then pay attention to the form or morphology of the various elements in the electrocardiogram, including the baseline, the atrial activity, the QRS complexes, and the relationship between the atrial activity and the QRS complexes.

Baseline. The portion of the electrocardiographic signal between the end of the T wave and the beginning of either formed atrial activity or the QRS complex should be examined for the presence of continuous atrial activity, which usually indicates the presence of atrial flutter or fibrillation. If the electrocardiographic signal appears flat during this period, one can usually assume that the atria are quiescent or that their activation is hidden in the QRS complex or S-T segment or T wave.

QRS Complexes. One usually examines the morphology of the QRS complexes next, noting in each lead their width, height, and depth and other special characteristics.

Most of us have been taught that the QRS complexes of ventricular arrhythmias are wide and those of supraventricular tachyarrhythmias are narrow; this is often correct but all too frequently untrue. Some ventricular arrhythmias, fascicular rhythms for example, have narrow, almost normal QRS widths. Many supraventricular tachyarrhythmias have wide QRS complexes, such as those associated with bundle branch block or antegrade conduction through accessory pathways.

The specific form of the QRS complex can also help one distinguish supraventricular tachycardia (SVT) from ventricular tachycardia. These details are discussed elsewhere in this text.

P Waves. The form of the P waves—if any are present—should be carefully examined in each of the electrocardiographic leads. Are they identical to those in sinus rhythm? If not, what is their vector? If it is markedly to the left, retrograde activation of the atria from the atrioventricular junction is suggested. This finding suggests that the tachyarrhythmia is sustained by a mechanism that incorporates the atrioventricular node. The rhythm itself may be either supraventricular or ventricular.

Is the form of the P waves constant or changing? Varying morphology of P waves is characteristic of multifocal atrial tachycardia.

P Wave–QRS Complex Relationships. The important question to be answered here is whether or not the P waves and QRS complexes depend upon one or the other. A constant relationship between P waves and QRS complexes is the rule in the regular SVTs. In most cases one P wave is associated with one QRS complex. In true atrial tachycardias, such as multifocal, sinus nodal, and ectopic atrial tachycardias, some atrioventricular block may be present so that not all of the abnormal P waves are conducted to the ventricles.

Does the P wave precede or follow the QRS complex? The location of the P wave with respect to the QRS complex can help define the mechanism of the tachycardia.

MECHANISMS AND THEIR RELATION TO THERAPY

We may classify supraventricular tachyarrhythmias by the mechanisms that sustain them (Table 1).

Atrial Fibrillation

Fibrillation in the atria develops when these chambers can no longer sustain a regular coordinated rhythm. Many individual electrical circuits in one or both atria now begin to discharge hundreds of times per minute. The atrioventricular (AV) node prevents each of these impulses from reaching the ventricles so that the ventricular response, although relatively rapid, is not so fast as to induce ventricular fibrillation. Since the AV node blocks an inconstant number of impulses, the ventricular response is characteristically irregular.

Treatment is initially directed toward slowing the ventricular rate by increasing the number of signals that are blocked in the AV node with digitalis or beta blocking or calcium channel blocking drugs. After the ventricular rate has been reduced to a clinically satisfactory level, restoration of normal, regu-

Table 1 Supraventricular Tachyarrhythmias Classified by Mechanisms

Atrial fibrillation
Atrial flutter
Reentrant supraventricular tachycardias, sustained within
  Atrioventricular node
  Accessory pathway
  Atrium
  Sinus node
Automatic supraventricular tachycardias
  Automatic atrial tachycardia
    Paroxysmal atrial tachycardia with block
  Automatic junctional tachycardia
    Nonparoxysmal junctional tachycardia
Supraventricular tachycardia of uncertain mechanism
  Multifocal atrial tachycardia

lar atrial electrical activity may be attempted with any of several antiarrhythmic drugs or with electrical cardioversion. Selecting which patients with atrial fibrillation should be restored to sinus rhythm is discussed in the chapter *Atrial Fibrillation*.

Atrial Flutter

Flutter in the atria is almost certainly produced by reentry within an electrophysiologically abnormal portion of atrial myocardium. The pathway of reentry may be relatively large and located in different regions of either atria, although more commonly it is found in the right atrium. The rate of repetitive reentry is relatively rapid, usually 250 to 400 beats per minute. The AV node can rarely accept each of the impulses, and consequently the ventricular rate is usually a fraction of the atrial rate, often 50 percent in untreated patients. However, if the AV node conducts relatively slowly or if AV nodal blocking drugs have been administered, the ventricular response will occur at a lesser or changing ratio, producing an irregular ventricular response.

Atrial flutter is best converted to sinus rhythm with electrical cardioversion or rapid atrial pacing rather than with drugs. The ventricular response to atrial flutter may be decreased by agents that slow AV nodal conduction, such as digitalis or beta or calcium channel blockers (see the chapter *Atrial Flutter* for further details).

Reentrant Supraventricular Tachycardia

The term SVT is used to describe two groups of arrhythmias: (1) all nonventricular tachyarrhythmias except fibrillation and flutter, and (2) those reentrant tachycardias that are sustained, for the most part, within atrial or AV junctional tissue. (The phrase paroxysmal supraventricular tachycardia (PSVT) is frequently employed for this group of arrhythmias.) In this discussion, SVT will be used in the second context.

Reentry, the mechanism of most regular tachycardias, produces arrhythmias when electrophysiologic continuity develops between tissues with different degrees of refractoriness and/or rates of conduction. In SVT, these circuits operate within the AV node, the atrial myocardium, the sinus node, or accessory pathways.

Reentry within fast and slow pathways in the *AV node* is the most common mechanism of SVT.

Next most frequently encountered is reentry utilizing an *accessory pathway* for one (usually the retrograde or caudad-to-cephalic) limb of the circuit. The reentrant wavefront in such cases usually courses through the atrium and down the AV node, bundle of His, bundle branches, Purkinje tissues, and ventricular myocardium. In sinus rhythm, antegrade conduction through the accessory pathway can produce the electrocardiographic features of ventricular preexcitation, as seen in patients with the Wolff-Parkinson-White syndrome.

Reentrant SVT also occurs, although infrequently, within *atrial tissues* themselves or in the *sinus node.*

Treatment. For decades, clinicians have converted SVT to sinus rhythm by carotid sinus massage, the Valsalva maneuver, and even by submerging the face of the patient in cold water. Digitalis, beta blocking drugs, calcium channel blocking drugs, vasopressors, and parasympathomimetic agents have also been administered for conversion.

Why is such a large group of drugs and maneuvers, with apparently disparate properties, effective in converting many patients with SVT? It is because each of them decreases conduction in the AV node and thereby interrupts the balance of conduction and refractoriness required within the reentrant circuit to sustain the tachycardia.

In the case of AV nodal reentry, these maneuvers and drugs act on the more slowly conducting of the two pathways in the AV node. In patients with accessory pathway reentry, they decrease the rate of conduction in the antegrade limb also within the AV node. Such drugs and maneuvers can convert reentrant SVT similarly in the sinus node and in atrial tissue. They act directly by AV nodal and parasympathetic stimulation or indirectly through autonomic responses following baroreceptor activation produced, for example, by raising the blood pressure with alpha-adrenergic drugs.

Reentry in SVT may also be disrupted by giving drugs that slow conduction within the more rapidly conducting pathway, usually the retrograde limb in AV nodal reentry or the accessory pathway when SVT is sustained through bypass tracts. The type I agents quinidine, procainamide, and disopyramide, exert their action in this manner. In converting patients from reentrant SVT to sinus rhythm acutely, however, we usually choose an agent such as verapamil, which decreases conduction in the slow pathway.

Cardioversion. Of course paroxysmal SVT can almost always be converted by electric shock, which quite effectively interrupts the reentry. Such treatment is seldom required, however, except when the arrhythmia has produced severe cardiovascular decompensation and the patient shows signs of congestive heart failure, hypotension, angina, or cerebral hyperperfusion, or if the drugs have been ineffective or have produced intolerable side effects.

Pacing. Reentrant SVT can often be converted with atrial pacing, either with properly timed individual beats or with bursts at fairly rapid speed. Like drugs, such impulses interrupt the reentrant signal and restore sinus rhythm.

Chronic Suppression. Sustaining sinus rhythm and preventing SVT are more difficult to accomplish than converting a paroxysm to normal rhythm. All the drugs already mentioned plus others are employed, either alone or in combinations. This topic is developed more fully in the chapters that follow.

Surgery. For more than 20 years, cardiac surgeons have been able to sever accessory pathways in patients with reentrant SVT sustained through bypass tracts. Such treatment cures patients of the arrhythmia, and in those with the Wolff-Parkinson-White syndrome, it eliminates the delta waves and short P-R intervals that their electrocardiograms in sinus rhythm may show. More recently, an operation has been developed that interrupts part of the circuit sustaining reentry within the AV node. These operations should only be performed at centers with highly trained medical and surgical teams experienced in clinical electrophysiology and the specialized diagnosis and treatment of arrhythmias.

Automatic Supraventricular Tachycardias

A few SVTs develop because of abnormal, enhanced automaticity in the atrium or bundle of His. The mechanism in these cases depends on the acquisition by diseased tissue of rapid diastolic depolarization in phase 4 of the action potential. Tissues that do not normally function as pacemakers can then assume control of the heart rate.

Automatic Atrial Tachycardia. This tachycardia can be produced by drugs such as digitalis or catecholamines, by infarction or inflammation of atrial tissue, or, rarely, by tumors.

Paroxysmal Atrial Tachycardia (PAT) With Block. Enhanced automaticity is probably the mechanism for the familiar variety of automatic atrial tachycardia known as PAT with block; which is often produced by digitalis intoxication. The drug, acting on abnormal atrial tissue and sometimes augmented by hypokalemia, produces a rapidly discharging automatic focus. The AV node, whose antegrade conduction has been partially suppressed by the digitalis, blocks some of the beats, producing the typical pattern of the arrhythmia.

Automatic Junctional Tachycardia. Rapid automatic junctional tachycardias are seldom seen in adults, but they have been reported with some frequency in children.

Nonparoxysmal Junctional Tachycardia. This is a relatively slow and far from rare arrhythmia in adults, probably the result of enhanced automaticity. It is seen in patients with (1) digitalis intoxication, particularly those who have atrial fibrillation; (2) myocarditis, including that now rare disease acute rheumatic fever; (3) recent cardiac surgery, and (4) acute, often inferior, myocardial infarction.

In this arrhythmia, narrow QRS complexes appear at a rate usually slightly faster than the fundamental rate, producing atrioventricular dissociation and the characteristic appearance of the arrhythmia.

In atrial fibrillation, nonparoxysmal junctional tachycardia is recognized by regularization of the ventricular response. This arrhythmia, which seldom produces serious hemodynamic difficulties, usually disappears when the acute disease process resolves.

Treatment. The automatic atrial and junctional tachycardias do not ordinarily convert to sinus rhythm with the maneuvers or drugs that interrupt reentrant SVT. Cardioversion or pacing usually has only a transient effect. These tachycardias are best treated by reducing the amount of such agents as digitalis or giving drugs that decrease the rate of diastolic depolarization, such as quinidine, procainamide, disopyramide, flecainide, or amiodarone. Electrical ablation or excision of the automatic foci, located by mapping techniques, has cured a few patients.

Supraventricular Tachycardia of Uncertain Mechanism

Multifocal Atrial Tachycardia. The mechanism of MAT has not yet been definitely established.

We do know that the arrhythmia seems to appear because of the presence of several automatic and/or reentrant foci within the atria. These centers are aroused in abnormal cardiac tissues by certain drugs such as theophylline or catecholamines, and by hypercapnia, hypoxia, electrolyte abnormalities, infections, or other systemic disorders. Since not all the atrial impulses in MAT can traverse the AV node, some block is usually present. Digitalis often causes paroxysmal atrial tachycardia with block but seldom, if ever, produces MAT.

Treatment. MAT should first be treated by improving the systemic abnormalities that exacerbate the tachycardia. Treatment of chronic obstructive pulmonary disease, reduction in the doses of certain excitatory drugs, and correction of electrolyte disturbances and infections can produce sinus rhythm. In some cases, however, MAT persists despite these efforts. Verapamil and the cardioselective beta blocker metoprolol can reduce the atrial and ventricular rates and sometimes suppress the arrhythmia entirely. Type I agents are occasionally helpful.

SUPRAVENTRICULAR (ATRIAL AND JUNCTIONAL) PREMATURE COMPLEXES

DANIEL V. WILKINSON JR., M.D.

Table 1 Agents and Factors Predisposing to Atrial Premature Complexes

Caffeine	Atrial distention
Nicotine	Gastrointestinal reflexes
Alcohol	Toxic states
Digoxin	Fatigue
Monoamine oxidase	Pregnancy
inhibitors	Hyperthyroidism
Anesthetic agents	Mitral valve disease
Sympathomimetics	Occlusion of sinoatrial
	nodal artery
	Hypokalemia

ATRIAL PREMATURE COMPLEXES

Supraventricular ectopic complexes are, by definition, those that differ from the prevailing, usually sinus, rhythm. They reflect electrical depolarizations that are abnormal by virtue of site of genesis, timing, or both.

Atrial premature complexes (APCs) are notable more for their frequency and variety of presentation than for their gravity. It is estimated that 10 percent of a normal population will demonstrate atrial ectopic activity with prolonged monitoring. The likelihood rises to 80 percent in those with evidence of structural atrial abnormalities (e.g., dilatation, conduction disease).

A multitude of precipitating or causative factors have been identified relative to APCs (Table 1).

ELECTROCARDIOGRAPHIC DIAGNOSIS

Premature appearance and altered morphology of a P wave are the hallmarks of APCs in surface electrocardiography. They may be taller, shorter, notched or widened, or superimposed on the preceding T wave (Figs. 1 and 2). The polarity of the P wave has been used to suggest the location of impulse generation (Table 2). Such designations should be accepted with caution, as mapping studies of atrial tachycardias have not confirmed their accuracy. The general descriptive term of ectopic atrial complex is preferred to "left atrial" or "coronary sinus" complex or rhythm.

Recovery of the ensuing sinus complex after an APC can follow one of three patterns. An APC may

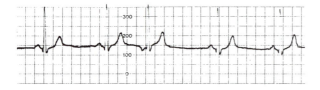

Figure 1 An atrial premature complex with an inverted P wave.

Table 2 Morphology of Premature Atrial Complexes

P Wave Morphology on Surface Electrocardiogram	Presumed Anatomic Focus
Inverted in leads II, III, F	Inferior, usually right atrial or coronary sinus
Inverted in leads I, aVL	Left atrium
Similar to sinus complex	Perisinoatrial nodal

be sufficiently premature that it can penetrate the sinus node and cause it to "reset." This will result in a pause that is more than compensatory. Collision of a sinus complex with an APC will prevent sinus node reset, and the pause will be fully compensatory. Interpolation of an APC within the sinus cycle may leave the latter undisturbed.

Atrioventricular Nodal and His-Purkinje Conduction

Prematurity normally elicits conduction delay in the atrioventricular (AV) node. Hence, an APC typically conducts with a longer P-R interval than a sinus complex. Blocked (or nonconducted) APCs result when the ectopic impulse encroaches on the effective refractory period of the AV node. This occurs either when the APC is very early or when there is intrinsic AV nodal conduction disease with a relatively long refractory period.

Further conduction to the ventricle along the His-Purkinje system is also frequently manifested by delay. Relative refractoriness in the bundle branches causes surface electrocardiographic appearance of aberrant conduction. When aberration is present, it is usually of a right bundle branch block morphology (Fig. 3).

Mechanisms

APCs may represent reentry within the atrium. This is postulated to occur at anatomic junctions such as that of atrial muscle with the sinus or AV node, venae cavae, or foramina, where conduction velocities slow and allow the requisite conditions for reentry. Impaired conduction in diseased atrial muscle is also a possible substrate.

Enhanced automaticity results from a reduction in the excitation threshold, allowing expression of depolarizations that would normally remain subthreshold. This may be a response to ambient conditions such as hypoxia, hypokalemia, or ischemia as well as to the use of stimulants and sympathomimetic agents.

Triggered activity due to delayed afterdepolarizations may produce single ectopic complexes or sustained arrhythmias.

Treatment

APCs in healthy individuals pose little risk and should be treated accordingly. Patients typically complain of the irregularity of their heart rhythm, disturbing pauses, and occasionally unusually forceful contractions.

Holter monitoring or an office rhythm strip is all that is needed to identify the arrhythmia, but a great deal of patient reassurance is often required to keep it in its proper perspective. The more severe the complaints—including those of dizziness, lightheadedness, and near-syncope—the more discussion is usually required to reconcile the perceived abnormality with the physiologic event.

By showing the patient graphically what occurred at the time symptoms were experienced, the irregular beats and anxiety-provoking pauses can be visualized and reduced to concrete and more manageable images.

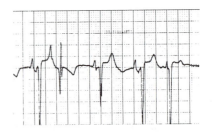

Figure 3 The first APC in this sequence deforms the previous T wave and conducts with the right bundle branch block.

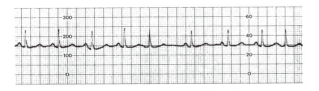

Figure 2 The atrial premature complex deforms the previous T wave.

If the APCs are highly symptomatic, reassurance alone may fail. When a decision to treat APCs has been made, it is important that the therapy not constitute a greater danger than the arrhythmia itself. Beta blockers are useful in this situation. They both depress automaticity and increase refractoriness in the AV node. Toxic effects are infrequent, and the blunting of the cathecholamine response may be anxiolytic.

Suppression of the APCs with type IA antiarrhythmic drugs is another possibility. Unfortunately, these drugs have a high incidence of side effects as well as the potential for producing more severe arrhythmias (e.g., long QT syndrome). Toxic effects with long-term use are also a potential hazard (e.g., lupus erythematosus and agranulocytosis with procainamide), and the need for such therapy has to be carefully deliberated in this setting (compare the chapters entitled *Disopyramide, Procainamide,* and *Quinidine*).

When supraventricular tachycardias are triggered by the APCs, the need to treat the ectopy becomes more acute. Aggressive suppression of these ectopic complexes would warrant the use of therapeutic doses of type IA antiarrhythmics (quinidine, procainamide, disopyramide). Because of the controversy surrounding type IC drugs, they cannot be recommended at this time. The addition of beta blockers, digoxin, or verapamil is sometimes required to increase AV nodal refractoriness and prevent a rapid ventricular response. In patients who are at risk from these tachyarrhythmias, therapy should be administered prophylactically to prevent clinical compromise.

JUNCTIONAL PREMATURE COMPLEXES

The AV node is actually three electrophysiologically distinct regions (AN, N, and NH), along with the bundle of His. However, since the surface electrocardiogram is unable to discriminate between a coronary sinus rhythm and one emanating from the NH region or His bundle, a broader concept is more practical.

AV junctional rhythms are, therefore, described electrocardiographically as complexes whose QRS morphology is identical to that of sinus complexes but whose P wave either is absent, is inverted, or follows the QRS complex. Outside of the sinus node, the coronary sinus, low atrium, and NH regions have the greatest automaticity.

With junctional premature complexes (JPCs), the presence and location of associated P waves reflect one of three possibilities. Atrial activation may precede ventricular, in which case the P-R interval is short and the P wave is typically inverted with an axis of −60 to −120 degrees, indicative of retrograde activation of the atria. There may be simulta-

Table 3   Causes of Junctional Premature Complexes

Hypokalemia
Digitalis toxicity
Chronic lung disease
Sinus node dysfunction
Parasystolic rhythm

neous atrial and ventricular depolarizations, with the P waves buried in the QRS complex and unrecognizable on the surface electrocardiogram; or, ventricular activation may precede atrial depolarization, in which case the P waves follow the QRS complex.

More accurately, the position of the P wave relative to the QRS depends on the respective antegrade and retrograde conduction velocities rather than the precise site of origin of the impulse. Although a low atrial impulse would more likely depolarize the atria first and a His impulse would depolarize the ventricle first, they cannot be reliably distinguished on that basis. Inter- and intra-atrial conduction time, AV nodal pathways, and accessory pathways all influence the P-QRS relationship on the electrocardiogram.

JPCs are much less common than either APCs or premature ventricular complexes. They occur in the setting of hypokalemia, digitalis toxicity, acute myocardial infarction, chronic lung disease, and sinus node dysfunction (Table 3). Although aberrant conduction may occur, a wide QRS complex cannot be easily distinguished from a premature ventricular complex.

JPCs can occur as a parasystolic rhythm (Fig. 4), which may be concealed or manifest. However, the presence of frequent single junctional complexes

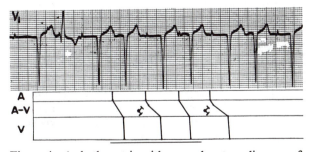

Figure 4   A rhythm strip with an explanatory diagram of a concealed junctional parasystole. The concealed junctional premature complexes effect a prolongation in the P-R interval, which is otherwise unexplained. (From Langendorf R, Mehlman JS. Blocked (nonconducted) A-V nodal premature systoles imitating first and second degree A-V block. Am Heart J 1947;34:500, with permission.)

should alert one to the possibility of a concealed junctional parasystole. Extended rhythm analysis may show the influence of concealed junctional complexes on the AV node, causing P-R interval prolongation in the next sinus cycle. Pseudo-AV block caused by concealed junctional complexes may also occur.

Treatment of JPCs is directed at the underlying disease process, with appropriate correction of electrolyte imbalance and digitalis levels. Antiarrhythmic therapy is usually not indicated.

SUGGESTED READING

Langendorf R, Mehlman, JS. Blocked (nonconducted) A-V nodal premature systoles imitating first and second degree A-V block. Am Heart J 1947; 34:500.
Scherf D, Schott A. Extrasystoles and allied arrythmias. 2nd ed. Chicago: Year Book Medical Publishers, 1973.
Watanabe Y, Dreifus L. Cardiac arrhythmias: Electrophysiologic basis for clinical interpretation. New York: Grune & Stratton, 1977.
Gillette PG, Garson AJ. Electrophysiologic and pharmacologic characteristics of automatic ectopic atrial tachycardia. Circulation 1977; 56:571.

SINUS TACHYCARDIA

AMI E. ISKANDRIAN, M.D.

The normal resting sinus rate varies between 60 and 100 beats per minute, although much lower rates are not unusual in well-trained athletes and higher rates are common in infancy and childhood. Traditionally, sinus tachycardia has been defined as a sinus rate in excess of 100 beats per minute.

Changes in the sinus rate are mediated by changes in sympathetic and parasympathetic tone and local and systemic levels of catecholamines. Under basal conditions, vagal tone prevails. Thus, vagal withdrawal and sympathetic stimulation can result in an increase in sinus rate, which electrophysiologically is mediated by an increased rate of diastolic depolarization.

Sinus tachycardia can be viewed as a result of altered activity of the autonomic nervous system rather than as a primary disorder of the sinus node. A rare exception may be seen in patients who have chronic sinus tachycardia, which may be a manifestation of sinus node reentry. The P waves in these cases resemble the normally conducted sinus P waves.

Sinus tachycardia characteristically is gradual in onset and gradual in termination. Vagal maneuvers and carotid massage may decrease the rate, but the rate invariably increases when these maneuvers are terminated. The causes of sinus tachycardia are summarized in Table 1.

EXERCISE IN NORMAL SUBJECTS

Many studies have shown an age-related decline in peak exercise heart rate, which may account for the age-related decline in cardiac output. The peak exercise heart rate can roughly be calculated as 220

Table 1   Causes of Sinus Tachycardia

Physiologic
  Physical or mental stress

Pathologic
  Acute myocardial infarction, bacterial endocarditis, congestive heart failure, cardiac tamponade, pulmonary embolism, aortic dissection, dehydration, hypovolemia, shock
  Postoperative conditions: cardiac and noncardiac—fever, excess catecholamines, fluid imbalance, anxiety
  Endocrine disorders: hyperthyroidism, pheochromocytoma
  Infectious diseases and fevers
  Anemias
  Drugs: atropine, catecholamines, thyroid hormones, alcohol, nicotine, caffeine, theophylline, dopamine

bpm minus age. Thus, the peak exercise heart rate is 200 bpm for a person aged 20 years and is only 150 bpm for a person aged 70 years. It has been postulated that a decrease in responsiveness to circulating catecholamines may explain the decline in peak exercise heart rate.

In patients with cardiac diseases, other factors may also modify the heart rate response during exercise. Obviously cardiac medications, especially beta blockers and calcium channel blockers, may modify the heart rate response. In general, in patients with left ventricular dysfunction, the increase in heart rate may be the only mechanism by which the cardiac output is modulated during exercise, as the stroke volume often does not change in these patients. On the other hand, increases in both stroke volume and the heart rate contribute to the augmentation of cardiac output in normal subjects, especially during exercise in the upright position. After training, there is a decrease in heart rate, both at rest and at each level of submaximal exercise, although at peak exercise, the heart rate is generally unchanged. The cardiac output remains unchanged at submaximal exercise after training because of left ventricular dilatation and an increase of stroke volume. Obviously, in patients with coronary artery disease, exercise-induced tachycardia causes an increase in myocardial oxygen demand, myocardial ischemia, and deterioration in the regional and global functions of the left ventricle.

In some patients with coronary artery disease, chronotropic incompetence has been observed; i.e., these patients fail to increase their heart rate during exercise. In fact, the peak heart rate during exercise has been found to have prognostic significance in such patients. Patients who fail to achieve an adequate heart rate response to exercise have a worse prognosis than those who achieve a higher heart rate.

A variety of other physiologic and psychologic causes may increase the heart rate, but seldom to the extent seen during exercise (see Table 1).

PATHOLOGIC SINUS TACHYCARDIA

Pathologic sinus tachycardia is seen in a variety of circulatory, cardiac, and noncardiac disorders (see Table 1). During acute myocardial infarction, tachycardia may be caused by pain, anxiety, and a reflex mechanism to maintain the cardiac output because of the decline in stroke volume secondary to left ventricular dysfunction. As with exercise, sinus tachycardia in these patients may worsen ischemia and increase the infarct size because of the increase in myocardial oxygen demand.

In one pathologic condition, sinus tachycardia may actually be useful. This is seen in patients with acute aortic regurgitation. Sinus tachycardia in these patients may decrease the amount of aortic regurgitation per beat and thus decrease left ventricular size, filling pressure, and left atrial pressure by decreasing the diastolic filling period.

In pulmonary embolism, tachycardia may occur even in the absence of underlying cardiopulmonary disease and may account for the slight increase in cardiac output seen in patients with mild to moderately severe pulmonary embolism. In severe and extensive cases of pulmonary embolism, cardiogenic shock may occur. In postoperative patients, volume shifts, fever, infection, incisional pain, and medications may explain the tachycardia so often seen.

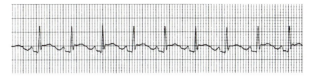

Figure 1 Sinus tachycardia. Note that a normal P wave precedes each QRS complex. The rate in this example is approximately 130 beats per minute. S-T segment elevation due to pericarditis is present and was the cause of sinus tachycardia.

DIFFERENTIAL DIAGNOSIS

Sinus tachycardia should be differentiated from supraventricular tachycardia, atrial fibrillation, and occasionally from ventricular tachycardia in patients with underlying bundle branch block. As indicated earlier, sinus tachycardia has a gradual onset and offset. The P waves have a normal configuration, duration, and axis (Fig. 1). The only difficulty is in patients with supraventricular tachycardia caused by sinus nodal reentry or when first-degree atrioventricular block obscures the P wave in the preceding T wave.

TREATMENT

The primary treatment of sinus tachycardia is directed to the treatment of the underlying cause. In patients with acute myocardial infarction and sinus tachycardia, beta-blocker therapy may be useful to decrease the myocardial oxygen demand. Such treatment has, in fact, been shown to improve survival if started early after acute infarction.

SUGGESTED READING

Iskandrian AS. Nuclear cardiac imaging: Principles and applications. Philadelphia: FA Davis, 1987.

ATRIAL FIBRILLATION

LEONARD N. HOROWITZ, M.D.

Atrial fibrillation is a relatively common arrhythmia and is the most common supraventricular tachyarrhythmia. It may occur in either a paroxysmal or a persistent (also referred to as chronic or established) form. Atrial fibrillation may coexist with other arrhythmias and conduction disturbances. Although other atrial arrhythmias are not possible during atrial fibrillation because the atria are continuously depolarized, junctional and ventricular arrhythmias may occur, and certain electrocardiographic characteristics of atrial fibrillation may cause confusion with significant ventricular arrhythmias, particularly unsustained ventricular tachycardia.

CLINICAL SETTING

Atrial fibrillation may occur in patients with or without organic heart disease. Atrial fibrillation occurs most commonly in mitral and tricuspid valvular disease, ischemic heart disease, hyperthyroidism, and hypertensive heart disease. Atrial fibrillation may also complicate the course of congenital heart disease, with or without surgical palliation or correction, hypertrophic, infiltrative, or dilated cardiomyopathy, pulmonary thromboembolic or vascular disease, and pericarditis. The occurrence of cardiac failure significantly increases the risk of developing atrial fibrillation. In any patient with atrial fibrillation of recent onset, even in the presence of organic heart disease, occult or manifest thyrotoxicosis should be excluded.

Although atrial fibrillation is usually associated with organic heart disease, it may be encountered in patients with apparently normal hearts in whom the arrhythmia is associated with a noncardiac condition. Atrial fibrillation may be observed following thoracic (cardiac and noncardiac) surgical procedures as well as after abdominal surgery. Atrial fibrillation may also occur in pneumonia, sepsis, with pulmonary or mediastinal malignancies, after severe burns, during biliary or renal colic, and following systemic arterial embolization or visceral infarction. In such cases, it is important to exclude the presence of underlying cardiac disease that may be a predisposing factor.

Atrial fibrillation may, however, occasionally occur in patients without anatomic disease of the heart or other predisposing clinical conditions. In some persons, these episodes may be related to precipitating causes such as excessive ingestion of alcohol, the use of tobacco products or recreational drugs, acute gastroenteritis, extreme fatigue, emotional stress, violent exertion, or vasovagal reactions. In some persons without organic heart disease, no precipitating cause can be identified. When atrial fibrillation occurs in the absence of underlying organic heart disease and without an identifiable cause, it is referred to as lone fibrillation, or more commonly as idiopathic atrial fibrillation.

TYPES OF ATRIAL FIBRILLATION

Atrial fibrillation may occur in paroxysmal (also referred to as recurrent) or persistent (established, chronic, or sustained) forms. Episodes of paroxysmal atrial fibrillation may be brief, lasting minutes to hours, or more prolonged, lasting several weeks. Paroxysmal atrial fibrillation may occur with any of the aforementioned disease states. It is especially typical of hyperthyroidism and the atrial fibrillation observed after thoracic surgical procedures, pneumonia, and other mediastinal and thoracic processes. Idiopathic atrial fibrillation is typically paroxysmal, although persistent atrial fibrillation may occasionally occur in patients without organic heart disease or other causes.

Mortality is not increased in patients with idiopathic paroxysmal atrial fibrillation; however, paroxysmal atrial fibrillation in patients with associated valvular or coronary artery disease does increase mortality. Chronic atrial fibrillation is associated with an increase in overall mortality in patients with hypertensive heart disease, mitral valvular disease, and recent (within 1 year) myocardial infarction. Chronic atrial fibrillation is associated with a higher mortality than paroxysmal atrial fibrillation in such patients.

Patients with atrial fibrillation, particularly the persistent form, have an increased risk of systemic embolic phenomena. Embolic stroke is the most potentially devastating complication of persistent atrial fibrillation. The risk of embolism is increased in atrial fibrillation of any origin but is especially high when the arrhythmia is caused by mitral valvular or ischemic heart disease.

SYMPTOMS AND SIGNS

Symptoms referable to atrial fibrillation vary considerably and are determined by many factors, most important the type and severity of underlying heart disease and the ventricular rate. The acute onset of atrial fibrillation may be asymptomatic but more often is associated with palpitations. There may also be precordial oppression or pain, weakness, anxiety, or lightheadedness. Symptoms of cardiac failure, shock, or syncope may occur in patients with severe underlying heart disease. Particularly in patients with severe aortic or mitral valvular disease, preexcitation syndromes, or hypertrophic cardiomyopathy, syncope may herald the onset of atrial fibrillation.

The symptoms associated with persistent atrial fibrillation are usually less severe than those associated with the acute onset of the arrhythmia. Although this is frequently related to the effects of treatment, it is at least partially due to the fact that patients become adjusted to the rhythm disturbance. Persistent atrial fibrillation causes reduction in functional capacity and symptoms of cardiac failure more often than palpitations or syncope. Occasionally, atrial fibrillation is found in patients who are completely asymptomatic.

The distinctive sign of atrial fibrillation is irregular irregularity of the heart rate. The apical rate is usually considerably higher than the pulse rate; this difference is termed the pulse deficit. During atrial fibrillation, the A waves in the jugular venous pulse are absent and the intensity of the first heart sound varies. The presence of other physical signs is determined by associated cardiac and noncardiac diseases.

ELECTROCARDIOGRAPHIC CHARACTERISTICS

Atrial fibrillation is characterized by the absence of recognizable P waves and a supraventricular rhythm with an irregularly irregular ventricular response. Usually fibrillatory waves of atrial activity of varying amplitudes can be seen (Fig. 1). These are most readily identified in the right precordial leads and leads II, III, and aVF; however, sometimes they are only visible in the right precordial leads. Flutter-fibrillation is a term applied when nearly regular P waves of varying contour and amplitude appear intermittently interspersed with typical atrial fibrillation. The ventricular response is typically rapid (greater than 100 beats per minute) but may be within the normal range during treatment or in elderly patients even without treatment.

In atrial fibrillation, QRS complexes are typically normal in configuration. It is important, however, to appreciate that aberrant ventricular conduction may produce wide and abnormal QRS complexes that may be mistaken for ventricular ectopic activity. Particularly when several aberrant complexes occur consecutively, it is important to differentiate aberration from ventricular complexes. Aberrantly conducted complexes are suggested when (1) the QRS complexes have a typical right bundle branch block morphology (rsR' in V_1), (2) the wide QRS complex occurs after a short R-R interval that follows a relatively longer R-R interval (long-short cycle sequence or Ashman's phenomenon), and (3) the initial vectors of the normal complex and the wide complex are identical. Ventricular ectopy is suggested by atypical bundle branch block patterns, fixed coupling, concordance in the precordial leads, and markedly rightward or leftward frontal plane axes.

DIAGNOSIS

The diagnosis of atrial fibrillation requires electrocardiographic documentation. In patients with persistent atrial fibrillation, this is not difficult and a standard 12-lead electrocardiogram can be obtained readily. In patients with paroxysmal atrial fibrillation, particularly when the episodes are brief, electrocardiographic documentation may be more difficult to obtain. In such cases, Holter monitoring or transtelephonic electrocardiographic monitoring may be particularly helpful.

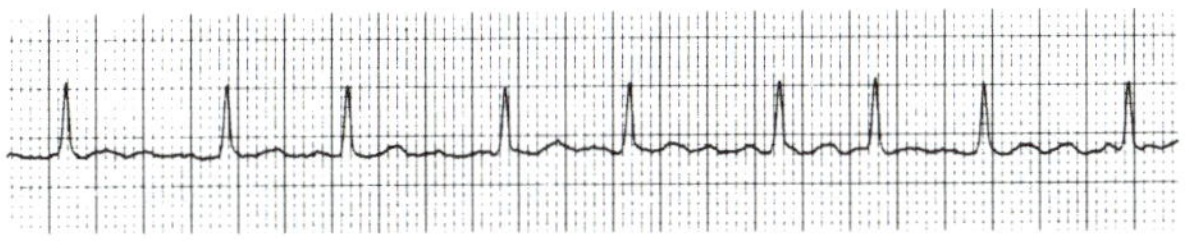

TREATMENT

Rational therapy of atrial fibrillation requires differentiation of the paroxysmal and persistent forms. If either form of atrial fibrillation is associated with a rapid ventricular rate, one goal of therapy is the slowing of the ventricular response. In paroxysmal atrial fibrillation, therapy has usually been directed at conversion of the episode to sinus rhythm and prevention of subsequent episodes. In persistent atrial fibrillation, consideration must be given to restoration of sinus rhythm, but more often therapy is directed at controlling the ventricular response.

When treating a patient with atrial fibrillation for the first time, it is important to identify underlying disease states and precipitating conditions. Once these are identified, they should be treated appropriately.

The initial therapy of patients with atrial fibrillation is determined by the patient's clinical status. A rapid assessment of cardiovascular status (blood pressure, heart rate, and respiratory rate), major organ perfusion (mental status, skin color, and temperature), presence of myocardial ischemia (symptomatic angina and/or electrocardiographic evidence of ischemia), and an evaluation of evidence of pulmonary congestion should be made. If the ventricular rate is life-threatening, as may occur in the presence of an accessory atrioventricular (AV) connection in the Wolff-Parkinson-White syndrome, or the patient is in a precarious hemodynamic state with acute cardiovascular decompensation, electrical cardioversion is the treatment of choice. In other less emergent but nonetheless serious situations, such as unstable angina associated acute atrial fibrillation, an initial attempt with rapidly acting pharmacologic therapy is appropriate prior to consideration of cardioversion. In the absence of acute decompensation, pharmacologic therapy is usually preferred.

Pharmacologic Treatment of the Acute Attack of Paroxysmal Atrial Fibrillation

When the patient is seen during an attack of atrial fibrillation, its paroxysmal nature may be recognized by a previous history of similar episodes, unless, of course, this is the first attack. In most patients, previous episodes have occurred over a period of months or years. These episodes typically

Figure 1 Atrial fibrillation with a rapid ventricular response. Note the absence of discrete P waves and the irregularly irregular ventricular response. The fibrillatory waves can be seen between QRS complexes.

terminate spontaneously and their usual duration is known. If previous experience indicates that the attack is likely to terminate within a few hours and the symptoms are tolerable, no specific therapy other than rest and sedation may be indicated. If the ventricular rate is very rapid, the symptoms are intolerable, or evidence of hemodynamic decompensation is present, therapy with intravenous drugs is indicated.

The initial goal in therapy of the acute attack of atrial fibrillation is control of the ventricular response. This can be achieved with drugs that slow AV nodal conduction, such as digitalis glycosides, beta-adrenergic blocking agents, and calcium antagonists, particularly verapamil (Table 1). Digitalis glycosides and related compounds are administered initially in a large bolus, which is then followed by a series of incremental doses. Beta-adrenergic blocking drugs are administered in increments. Esmolol, a newly introduced beta-adrenergic blocking agent that has a short half-life, is administered as a series of incremental loading boluses with a maintenance infusion. Verapamil is generally administered as an initial, small test bolus followed by a larger bolus. The goal of therapy is to reduce the ventricular rate to between 80 and 100 beats per minute. In patients with the Wolff-Parkinson-White syndrome, these agents, and particularly digitalis, are contraindicated because they may paradoxically increase the ventricular rate (see the chapter *Atrial Fibrillation in Preexcitation Syndromes*).

During the intravenous administration of any of these agents, the patient should be monitored continuously. An electrocardiographic monitor should be available. Blood pressure and heart rate should be measured frequently, and when administering agents that are given in incremental boluses, the heart rate and blood pressure should be measured prior to each bolus.

In certain circumstances, the combined use of digoxin with either a beta-adrenergic blocking agent or a calcium antagonist may be useful in slowing the ventricular rate. Caution must be exercised in adding two or more AV nodal depressing drugs because

of the possibility of AV block. Moreover, if the atrial fibrillation terminates, bradyarrhythmias caused by sinus node depression may occur in this setting.

In certain patients, the symptoms may not justify intravenous therapy. In such patients, digoxin, a beta-adrenergic blocking agent, or verapamil may be administered orally. Particularly in the patient with mild and tolerable symptoms, outpatient pharmacologic management is appropriate. Outpatient pharmacologic management should be considered only in patients without heart disease or in those with mild to moderate underlying heart disease and without significant associated conditions. If outpatient therapy is used, incremental doses of oral medications are not appropriate, as the patient is not being continuously monitored. Therapy with a standard loading dose of digoxin (1.0 mg over 24 hours) or standard doses of beta-adrenergic blockers or verapamil may be employed (Table 2).

Since most paroxysms of atrial fibrillation subside spontaneously, the initial therapy used to slow the ventricular rate is frequently credited with having restored normal sinus rhythm. Most episodes of paroxysmal atrial fibrillation terminate spontaneously within 24 hours, often in less than 12 hours. In some patients, however, episodes persist beyond 24 to 48 hours, and pharmacologic therapy must be employed to restore sinus rhythm. A quinidine preparation is most commonly used. The use of large and incremental doses of quinidine to produce conversion to normal sinus rhythm is no longer indicated. That approach is associated with a high incidence of gastrointestinal toxicity and proarrhythmia, most notably torsades de pointes. When quinidine is ineffective, poorly tolerated, or contraindicated, procainamide or disopyramide may be used. The usual clinical doses of these agents may be used (Table 3). Quinidine and quinidine-like drugs should be withheld until adequate control of ventricular response has been achieved with digoxin, a beta blocker, or verapamil, because quinidine and related agents often increase the ventricular response by facilitating AV nodal conduction.

Table 1 Intravenous Agents Used to Control Ventricular Response in Acute Atrial Fibrillation

Drug	Dose	Cautions
Digoxin	0.25–0.50 mg initially followed by 0.25 mg at 4- to 6-hr intervals to a total dose of 1.0 mg	
Propranolol	0.1–0.2 mg/kg at 0.5–1.0 mg/min	Monitor pulse and blood pressure continuously during administration
Esmolol	500 µg/kg/min for 1 minute, then 50–300 µg/kg/minute for 4 minutes (begin with 50 µg/kg/minute and increase gradually after additional 500 µg/kg/minute loads for 1 minute)	May produce more hypotension than other beta blockers
Verapamil	0.075–0.15 mg/kg over 2 minutes (3 minutes in elderly patients)	Caution should be exercised if the patient has received the beta blocker before the verapamil

Table 2 Oral Agents Used to Control Ventricular Response in Atrial Fibrillation

Drug	Initial Dose	Maintenance Dose	Comment
Digoxin	0.75–1.5 mg (total dose) given at 0.25–0.50 mg every 4–8 hr	0.125–0.5 mg daily	In the elderly patients and those with renal failure, institution of the maintenance dose without loading may be appropriate
Propranolol	10–20 mg every 6 hr	10–80 mg every 6 hr	Titrate dose to ventricular rate by gradual upward titration
Nadolol	40 mg once daily	40–320 mg once daily	Titrate dose to ventricular rate by gradual upward titration
Metoprolol	25–50 mg every 12 hr	50–200 mg every 12 hr	Titrate dose to ventricular rate by gradual upward titration
Atenolol	25–50 mg once daily or every 12 hr	50–100 mg every 12–24 hr	Titrate dose to ventricular rate by gradual upward titration
Acebutolol	200 mg every 12 hr	200–600 mg every 12 hr	Titrate dose to ventricular rate by gradual upward titration
Verapamil	40–80 mg every 6 hr	40–120 mg every 6 hr	Titrate dose to ventricular rate by gradual upward titration

The utility of class IC agents, such as flecainide and encainide, in conversion of atrial fibrillation to sinus rhythm is undergoing study at present. Although these agents have not been approved for this purpose, present evidence suggests that they will be useful when employed in appropriately selected patients. The doses that have proved successful are the same as those that have been used for the treatment of ventricular arrhythmias.

If an episode of paroxysmal atrial fibrillation is not converted to sinus rhythm by pharmacologic therapy, elective cardioversion is indicated. This is necessary infrequently.

Anticoagulation is not generally required prior

Table 3 Oral Agents Used to Terminate or Prevent Paroxysmal Atrial Fibrillation

Drug	Initial Dose	Dose Range	Dosing Interval	Comments
Quinidine				
sulfate	200 mg	200–400 mg	Every 4–6 hr	Loading dose with 600–1,000 mg (200 mg every 2 hr) rarely used at present
gluconate	324 mg	324–972 mg	Every 8–12 hr	
Procainamide				
regular	250–500 mg	250–1,000 mg	Every 3–4 hr	Can start therapy with loading dose of regular preparation
sustained release	500–750 mg	375–1,500 mg	Every 6–8 hr	
Disopyramide				
regular	100 mg	100–200 mg	Every 6 hr	Dose should be reduced in renal failure patients. Use cautiously in patients with low ejection fractions and avoid in patients with heart failure
sustained release	100–150 mg	150–300 mg	Every 12 hr	
Flecainide*	50–100 mg	50–200 mg	Every 12 hr	
Encainide*	25 mg	25–50 mg	Every 8 hr	
Propafenone*	150 mg	150–300 mg	Every 8 hr	
Amiodarone*	200 mg	200–400 mg	Every 24 hr	Treatment may be started with a loading regimen (see chapter on *Amiodarone*); not for conversion of an acute episode because of its long half-life

*Not approved for atrial fibrillation by the Food and Drug Administration.

to pharmacologic or electrical conversion of a patient with an acute episode of atrial fibrillation. If the episode has been present less than 1 week, the risk of systemic embolization is minimal, unless a complicating condition such as mitral stenosis or a prosthetic valve or a history of recent or recurrent systemic emboli is present.

Prevention of Paroxysmal Atrial Fibrillation

The typical clinical course of patients with paroxysmal atrial fibrillation is a gradually increasing frequency of episodes and a gradual increase in the duration of paroxysms. The arrhythmia may remain paroxysmal or may progress to persistent atrial fibrillation. This process may occur over a period of weeks to months but more typically occurs over many years. On the other hand, the process may remain paroxysmal for decades.

Because initially paroxysms may be separated by periods of months or years, patients who are mildly symptomatic during paroxysms may not require prophylactic therapy after restoration of sinus rhythm. Reassurance and prescription of a mild sedative to be taken during paroxysms may be sufficient. It is important to obtain electrocardiographic documentation during the episodes. Although this can be achieved by a visit to a physician's office or to an emergency medical facility, transtelephonic electrocardiographic monitors now facilitate obtaining such documentation. If episodes are infrequent but the ventricular rate is rapid during them, digoxin may be the best therapeutic alternative. Although it will not prevent recurrences of atrial fibrillation, it may reduce the ventricular rate during paroxysms and ameliorate the symptoms.

If the attacks are frequent or despite control of ventricular rate during the paroxysms the symptoms are distressing, prophylactic therapy aimed at preventing paroxysms of atrial fibrillation is indicated. A quinidine preparation is the most commonly used. A sustained-release preparation is preferable. The dose should start at 600 to 1,200 mg of quinidine base per 24 hours in appropriately divided doses. If the initial dosage is ineffective, it should be progressively increased as tolerated. An electrocardiogram should be obtained to assess the QRS complex and Q-T interval durations within 1 week of each dose increase. Increases in the QRS complex of less than 25 percent and in the Q-T interval to less than 0.55 are desirable. Procainamide or disopyramide may be employed instead of quinidine if preferred or if quinidine is not tolerated (see Table 3).

Encainide, flecainide, and related class IC antiarrhythmic agents have shown promise in the treatment of paroxysmal atrial fibrillation. Their efficacy is equal to that of quinidine in some studies, and in patients with minimal or no heart disease, they may be better tolerated. An additional advantage of these agents is that they depress conduction in the AV node and thus will slow the ventricular response during the paroxysm of atrial fibrillation. These agents are preferred in the pharmacologic management of patients with paroxysmal atrial fibrillation complicating the Wolff-Parkinson-White syndrome because they slow conduction through accessory pathways (see Table 3).

Amiodarone has been used in the treatment of patients with paroxysmal atrial fibrillation. Because of its toxicity, it should be reserved for severely symptomatic patients in whom all other pharmacologic therapy has been ineffective or not tolerated. When used for prophylactic therapy of atrial fibrillation, a low loading dose of 400 to 600 mg daily for 1 to 2 weeks should be employed. Some prefer to use no loading dose in this setting. The maintenance dose should be 200 mg daily or lower in most patients. An occasional patient may require as much as 400 mg daily to control atrial fibrillation (see Table 3).

Treatment of Persistent Atrial Fibrillation

In patients with persistent atrial fibrillation, therapy is directed initially at slowing the ventricular response. Digoxin is the drug of choice for ventricular rate control in persistent atrial fibrillation. It is preferred to beta-blocking agents and calcium antagonists because it is less expensive and generally more convenient for the patient. The purpose of digoxin therapy is to control the ventricular rate and not restore sinus rhythm. The dose of digoxin is adjusted to maintain an apical heart rate of 60 to 80 beats per minute at rest, and with moderate exertion, such as walking two flights of stairs, the heart rate should not exceed approximately 120 beats per minute. The usual dose of digoxin required to achieve this rate control is 0.25 to 0.5 mg a day. In older patients and in patients with renal insufficiency, lower doses are typically required, but occasionally higher doses are needed.

Digoxin therapy of persistent atrial fibrillation is primarily monitored with the electrocardiogram. When the ventricular response is within the desired range and evidence of digitalis toxicity is not present on the electrocardiogram, the dose can be considered appropriate. Digoxin levels may be less useful in this setting because the concentrations required for rate control are frequently within the range generally considered toxic. Occasional measurements of plasma digoxin concentration are appropriate to exclude marked elevations. Particular attention should be paid to a history of symptoms consistent with digitalis intoxication.

If digoxin does not effectively control the ventricular rate, beta-blocking drugs or calcium antagonists may be added or used instead. A variety of beta-adrenergic blocking agents are available for oral therapy. The selected agent should be started at a low initial dose and titrated upward every other day until the heart rate goal is achieved or side effects intervene. Beta-adrenergic blockers usually control the ventricular response during exercise better than digoxin. In patients who have a rapid ventricular response, particularly during exercise, beta blockers should be used instead of digoxin.

Verapamil and diltiazem are effective in controlling the ventricular response during atrial fibrillation. They can be combined with digoxin, but they should be used with caution with beta-blocking agents.

Rarely, encainide, flecainide, and similar agents are required for control of ventricular response in patients with persistent atrial fibrillation. They should be considered for this purpose only if digoxin, beta blockers, and calcium antagonists used alone and in combination have been ineffective.

Patients who remain symptomatic from rapid ventricular rates despite aggressive pharmacologic attempts to control the ventricular response during atrial fibrillation with digoxin, beta-adrenergic blockers, calcium antagonists, and, if indicated, class IC antiarrhythmic agents can be considered for His bundle ablation. With this technique, the AV node and bundle of His are damaged or destroyed. If complete heart block is produced, permanent ventricular pacing is required. With some techniques, AV nodal or His bundle modification can be produced, and a permanent pacemaker may not be necessary. Occasionally, open chest transection of the AV conduction system is required because of the failure of the closed-chest transcatheter ablation of the His bundle. If transcatheter ablation is being considered, the patient should be referred to a center with expertise in electrophysiologic studies and nonpharmacologic management of complex arrhythmias.

Chronic Anticoagulant Therapy

Another objective in the treatment of persistent atrial fibrillation is prevention of systemic atrial embolization. The incidence of systemic embolization in patients with persistent atrial fibrillation is increased, particularly in patients with rheumatic mitral valvular disease. Unless it is absolutely contraindicated, such patients should be treated with chronic warfarin sodium (Coumadin) anticoagulation. The indications for anticoagulation in other patients with persistent atrial fibrillation are not as clear. Although there is an increased risk of systemic embolization in patients with persistent atrial fibrillation compared with patients in sinus rhythm, it is not clear that the potential benefits of chronic anticoagulation outweigh its risk. Unless there is another indication for chronic anticoagulation, such as left atrial or left ventricular mural thrombus, prosthetic valve, or a history of embolization, it is probably not indicated for patients with persistent atrial fibrillation.

Because the incidence of systemic embolization is increased when persistent atrial fibrillation is converted to sinus rhythm, anticoagulant therapy should be instituted prior to an attempt at either pharmacologic or electrical cardioversion. If atrial fibrillation has been present for longer than 1 week, anticoagulation with warfarin sodium should be instituted for 2 to 4 weeks prior to the attempted cardioversion. If the attempt at cardioversion is unsuccessful or if sinus rhythm cannot be maintained, long-term anticoagulation need not be continued indefinitely unless one of the indications discussed above is present.

Restoration of Sinus Rhythm in Persistent Atrial Fibrillation

An attempt at restoration of sinus rhythm may be indicated in a variety of situations. Atrial fibrillation that has been caused by an acute process (e.g., thyrotoxicosis, cardiac surgery, pericarditis) usually converts spontaneously to sinus rhythm when the underlying condition is corrected. When it does not, an attempt to convert the atrial fibrillation to sinus rhythm is appropriate. In the presence of refractory heart failure with atrial fibrillation, restoration and maintenance of sinus rhythm may dramatically improve ventricular function and ameliorate the symptoms of cardiac failure. Restoration of sinus rhythm may also be beneficial when the ventricular response is difficult to control or there is a substantial risk of systemic embolization.

Quinidine or other class I antiarrhythmic agents can be used to convert atrial fibrillation to sinus rhythm. The drug can be administered either orally or intravenously, although the latter route is used infrequently and most commonly with procainamide. The prior custom of incremental doses of quinidine sulfate every 2 hours until conversion or toxic levels are reached should be abandoned. The hypokalemia that is produced by the diarrhea that frequently results from this method potentiates the proarrhythmic risk of quinidine. A regular or sustained-release preparation of quinidine, procainamide, or disopyramide can be employed in the usual clinical doses. They can be titrated up as tolerated by patient symptoms and electrocardiographic changes. Although conversion may occur at any interval after starting therapy, it is uncommon to observe it more than 1 week after attaining the highest tolerated dose.

As noted above, class IC antiarrhythmic agents (encainide, flecainide) and amiodarone may be used in an attempt to convert atrial fibrillation to sinus rhythm. It is uncommon to observe spontaneous conversion longer than 2 weeks after attaining maintenance doses of the class IC antiarrhythmic agents.

Because of the variable and very long half-life of amiodarone, it is unclear what duration of therapy should elapse before declaring the agent ineffective in converting the arrhythmia to normal sinus rhythm. Generally, treatment is continued for 1 to 3 months before efficacy is assessed.

Electrical Cardioversion of Persistent Atrial Fibrillation

Before considering cardioversion of persistent atrial fibrillation, any treatable underlying initiating or predisposing condition should be treated. Furthermore, an assessment should be made of the likelihood that sinus rhythm will be maintained. It is now clear that as the left atrial dimension increases above normal, the likelihood of maintaining sinus rhythm after cardioversion decreases. When the left atrial dimension exceeds 45 to 50 mm, the likelihood of maintaining sinus rhythm for more than 1 year falls significantly below 50 percent. Unless extenuating circumstances are present, the cardioversion should not be attempted in such patients. Unless the atrial fibrillation was associated with a cause that has resolved or can be eliminated, the patient's inability to take chronic prophylactic antiarrhythmic therapy is also a contraindication to cardioversion.

After a trial of pharmacologic therapy for conversion of atrial fibrillation that has been unsuccessful, the patient should be maintained on a regimen that is well tolerated. Cardioversion should be performed when the patient is on this antiarrhythmic regimen. Thus, if sinus rhythm is restored by cardioversion, the patient will be on a prophylactic regimen to prevent recurrent atrial fibrillation.

Sedation, anesthesia, and amnesia can now be provided by a variety of agents. I recommend an initial setting of 100 joules moving to 200 and then 400 on successive shocks. If a 320- to 400-joule shock does not convert the atrial fibrillation, it is unlikely that it can be converted, although occasionally a 400 to 500 joule shock may be effective, when the usual electrode configuration is ineffective, an anterior-posterior configuration may facilitate conversion.

Suggested Reading

Klein HO, Kaplinsky E. Verapramil and digoxin: Their respective effects on atrial fibrillation and their interaction. Am J Cardiol 1982; 50:894–902.

Mancini GBJ, Goldberger AL. Cardioversion of atrial fibrillation: Consideration of embolization, anticoagulation, prophylactic pacemaker, and long-term success. Am Heart J 1982; 104:617–621.

Olshansky B, Waldo AL. Atrial fibrillation: Update on mechanism, diagnosis, and management. Mod Concepts Cardiovasc Dis 1987; 56:23.

Roy R, Marchand E, Gagne P, et al. Usefulness of anticoagulant therapy in the prevention of embolic complications of atrial fibrillation. Am Heart J 1986; 112:1039–1043.

ATRIAL FLUTTER

ALBERT L. WALDO, M.D.

Atrial flutter, first described by Jolly and Ritchie in 1911, is a remarkably common arrhythmia. Nevertheless, surprisingly little was understood about the nature and mechanism of this rhythm until fairly recently. Moreover, despite our having recognized this clinical entity for so long, until recently, its management has changed remarkably little. Acute therapy during atrial flutter classically had been to use a digitalis preparation to slow and control the ventricular response rate until atrial fibrillation or sinus rhythm was produced and to use either quinidine or procainamide to prevent recurrence of the rhythm. And, in most instances, chronic therapy to prevent recurrence of atrial flutter has employed one of the class IA antiarrhythmic agents along with digitalis to control the ventricular response rate in case the atrial flutter recurs.

The last two decades have witnessed significant improvements in therapy of atrial flutter, beginning with the advent of direct current cardioversion in the 1960s. The past 15 years have seen the addition of beta-blocking agents, initially propranolol, as an adjunct to (but on occasion in lieu of) digitalis therapy in an effort to control ventricular response rate to atrial flutter. The most recent addition of esmolol, an intravenous beta-blocking agent with a short half-life, has permitted prompt and continuous control of the ventricular response rate in patients with paroxysmal atrial flutter until more definitive measures can be taken. Also, the last few years have seen the use of the so-called calcium channel blockers, verapamil and diltiazem, in the same manner as the beta blockers. In addition, there has been a growing experience, primarily in Europe and South America, with the use of amiodarone in the successful treatment of recurrent atrial flutter. And most recently, experience with the use of class IC antiarrhythmic agents, primarily flecainide has begun to appear in the prevention of recurrent atrial flutter and intravenous use of flecainide in the acute treatment of atrial flutter to convert it to sinus rhythm.

Other advances in the diagnosis and management of atrial flutter have included the use of various techniques to record atrial electrograms (intracavitary, epicardial, and esophageal) and to diagnose atrial flutter; His bundle ablation to obtain complete heart block in patients with uncontrollable paroxysmal atrial flutter in whom the ventricular response rate is clinically unacceptable and cannot be controlled by drug therapy for any number of reasons; and techniques of cardiac pacing, both acute and chronic, to interrupt atrial flutter. The most recent developments in understanding atrial flutter have been the series of studies, recently summarized, which have shown that atrial flutter is almost certainly caused by reentry in the right atrium and that the reentry circuit also seems to include a critical area of slow conduction that seems vulnerable to catheter ablation to prevent future recurrence. Also, the later understanding of atrial flutter has led to early but innovative approaches to its permanent correction using intraoperative surgical techniques.

In this chapter, I will provide a personal view on the approach to diagnosis and treatment of atrial flutter.

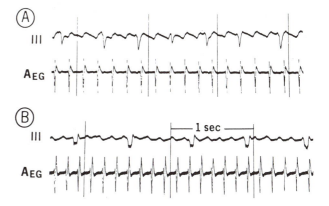

Figure 1 *A* and *B* both demonstrate the simultaneous recording of electrocardiogram lead III and a bipolar arterial electrogram (AEG) during type I atrial flutter with an atrial rate of 296 beats per minute (*A*) and type II atrial flutter and a rate of 420 beats per minute (*B*). In each example, note the constant beat-to-beat cycle length, polarity, morphology, and amplitude of recorded atrial electrogram signal characteristic of atrial flutter. See text for discussion. (Modified from Wells JL Jr, MacLean WAH, James TN, Waldo AL. Characterization of atrial flutter. Studies in man after open heart surgery using fixed atrial electrodes. Circulation 1979;60:665–673. Reprinted by permission of the American Heart Association.)

DIAGNOSIS OF ATRIAL FLUTTER

Types of Atrial Flutter

Evidence has recently been provided that there are two types of atrial flutter: type I (classic) and type II (very rapid) (Fig. 1). This classification is independent of the morphology or polarity of the atrial flutter waves in the electrocardiogram. Type I atrial flutter can always be influenced by rapid atrial pacing from sites high in the right atrium, whereas type II atrial flutter cannot. This major difference served as the initial distinction between these two types of atrial flutter. The reason for the inability to interrupt type II atrial flutter with rapid atrial pacing from high right atrial sites is unknown. It has been suggested that type II atrial flutter is caused by leading circle reentry. If that is the case, it is not surprising that rapid pacing cannot interrupt this rhythm, because this form of reentry does not have an excitable gap.

Two observations have provided additional reasons to suggest that a separation of atrial flutter into two types is valid. First, type II atrial flutter was observed to convert spontaneously to type I in a stepwise fashion in several patients. Second, on several occasions, when rapid atrial pacing from a high right atrial site was used to treat type I atrial flutter, type II was present after termination of the rapid

pacing. Thus, it would appear that type I and type II atrial flutter are not really part of a continuum of atrial flutter but rather are separate although perhaps closely related entities.

The foregoing observations permitted further differentiation between two types of atrial flutter in terms of range of atrial rates. Type I atrial flutter is characterized by a range of atrial rates from 240 to 340 beats per minute, and type II atrial flutter is characterized by a range of atrial rates from 340 to 433 beats per minute. There almost certainly is some overlap in the upper range of rates with type I atrial flutter and the lower range of rates of type II atrial flutter. Likewise, there is almost certainly some flexibility in the upper and lower ranges of atrial rates of each of these types. However, common to both types of atrial flutter is the remarkably constant beat-to-beat atrial cycle length, first noted by Lewis and coworkers and later confirmed by recording atrial electrograms over long periods. This, along with the constant beat-to-beat morphology and polarity of recorded atrial electrograms, differentiates atrial fibrillation from type I atrial flutter.

Approach to the Diagnosis of Suspected Atrial Flutter

When a patient presents with a tachycardia that is suspected to be atrial flutter, unless the tachycardia is clinically life-threatening (e.g., associated with pulmonary edema or 1:1 atrioventricular (AV) conduction, perhaps in the face of Wolff-Parkinson-White syndrome), it is recommended that the diagnosis of atrial flutter be established before initiating therapy. The demonstration of classic saw-toothed flutter waves in the electrocardiogram, particularly in leads II, III, and AVF, remains the standard for the diagnosis of type I atrial flutter and is probably the simplest way to establish the diagnosis in any event. If the diagnosis is not clear from an electrocardiogram, usually because a rapid ventricular response rate prevents clear identification of atrial events, several other diagnostic options may be used.

In patients following open heart surgery, temporary atrial epicardial wire electrodes may be used to record atrial electrograms either simultaneously or sequentially with an electrocardiogram. This should establish the diagnosis readily and definitively (Fig. 2). For other patients, any of a number of vagal maneuvers to produce transient increased AV block while recording the electrocardiogram often permits the diagnosis of atrial flutter by the appearance of atrial flutter complexes in the electrocardiogram. If a simple vagal maneuver does not work so that the diagnosis is still unclear, and the clinical situation permits it, any of the following maneuvers may be used: (1) placement of an esophageal lead to record atrial electrograms; (2) use of a pharmacologic agent (edrophonium, adenosine, esmolol, or verapamil) to increase AV conduction transiently; or (3) transvenous placement of a temporary endocardial bipolar electrode catheter. The advantages of options (1) and (3) are that not only does either one permit a definitive diagnosis but either one also permits effec-

tive treatment of atrial flutter with rapid atrial pacing techniques. The advantage to option (2) is that it does not require any invasive procedure, and by transiently slowing ventricular response rate, it gives the clinician additional time to determine the next course of therapy.

It must be emphasized that in the face of a wide QRS complex tachycardia in which it is uncertain whether the rhythm is supraventricular or ventricular, or in the face of possible 1:1 AV conduction secondary to the presence of an accessory AV connection (Wolff-Parkinson-White syndrome), drug intervention to establish the diagnosis of atrial flutter is fraught with important clinical problems and usually is contraindicated.

It is occasionally useful and possible to establish the diagnosis of atrial flutter by more indirect techniques. This includes echocardiography (flutter waves seen on the mitral valve echoes), a signal-averaged electrocardiogram, or jugular venous pulsations.

TREATMENT OF ATRIAL FLUTTER

Acute Treatment of Type I Atrial Flutter

Once the diagnosis is established, three courses of therapy are available: (1) direct current cardioversion; (2) rapid atrial pacing to interrupt atrial flutter and restore sinus rhythm; or (3) antiarrhythmic drug therapy. In our judgment, the preferable course of treatment is direct current cardioversion or rapid atrial pacing. Antiarrhythmic drug therapy may be used prior to performing either direct current cardioversion or rapid atrial pacing. When drug therapy is used, it should be to slow the ventricular response rate (with either a beta blocker or a calcium channel blocker); to enhance the likelihood that rapid atrial pacing will restore sinus rhythm (use of quinidine, procainamide, or disopyramide), or to help assure that direct current cardioversion not only will be effective but also that atrial flutter will be less likely to recur (use of a class IA or perhaps a class IC antiarrhythmic agent).

Prior to the advent of direct current cardioversion and rapid atrial pacing techniques, the usual form of treatment was aggressive administration of a digitalis preparation, usually intravenously, until conversion of the rhythm either to atrial fibrillation or to sinus rhythm. This form of treatment is acceptable but generally is not the treatment of choice. Also, it was recognized early on that administration of a class I antiarrhythmic agent, particularly procainamide or quinidine intravenously, would effectively slow the atrial rate but was not very likely to interrupt atrial flutter. Thus, unlike the use of lidocaine or procainamide for the conversion of ventricular tachycardia, there has been no drug that when

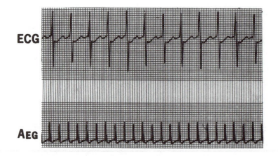

Figure 2 Monitor electrocardiogram lead recorded simultaneously with a bipolar atrial electrogram (AEG) during an episode of type I atrial flutter. The atrial rate is 280 beats per minute, and there is 2:1 AV conduction. Note that atrial complexes are not readily discernible from the electrocardiogram alone, but the bipolar atrial electrogram clearly establishes the nature of atrial activation and its relationship to ventricular activation. (From Waldo AL, MacLean WAH, Cooper TB, et al. Use of temporarily placed epicardial atrial wire electrodes for the diagnosis and treatment of cardiac arrhythmias following open heart surgery. J Thorac Cardiovasc Surg 1978;76:500–505, with permission.)

given intravenously has demonstrated a reasonable expectation of successfully converting atrial flutter to sinus rhythm. However, there have been recent reports, primarily from studies in Europe, indicating that administration of intravenous flecainide has a reasonable likelihood of restoring sinus rhythm. However, because this drug is not readily available in intravenous form, its use is impractical in any event.

Whether one chooses to initiate acute therapy of atrial flutter with direct current cardioversion or atrial pacing depends on the clinical presentation of the patient and the clinical availability of either of these techniques. Thus, for the patient with atrial flutter but who has just eaten or who has chronic lung disease, administration of an anesthetic agent(s) is usually not desirable. Such a patient is far better off undergoing rapid atrial pacing to interrupt atrial flutter. Similarly, for the patient following open heart surgery who has temporary atrial epicardial wire electrodes, rapid atrial pacing clearly is the treatment of choice.

Rapid Atrial Pacing to Interrupt Atrial Flutter

For pacing using temporary epicardial wire electrodes or catheter electrodes placed in the right atrial cavity, we currently recommend a ramp atrial pacing technique in which bipolar atrial pacing at a rate that is about 10 beats per minute faster than the spontaneous atrial rate is begun and electrocardiographic lead II is recorded continuously. Using this technique, it is preferable that pacing be performed high in the right atrium. When it is demonstrated that the atrial rate has increased to the pacing rate, the latter is gradually increased until the atrial complexes (flutter waves) in lead II, which previously had been negative, become positive. This is almost always a marker of interruption of atrial flutter, and the atrial pacing then may be abruptly terminated or the pacing rate may be quickly slowed. The latter permits control of the atrial rhythm until a desirable atrial rate such as 100 to 110 beats per minute is achieved. A representative example is illustrated in Figure 3.

A constant rate atrial pacing technique also may be used. Rapid atrial pacing is initiated at a rate faster than the spontaneous rate, and pacing at this rate is continued for 15 to 30 sec. Then pacing is either abruptly terminated or rapidly slowed to a desirable atrial rate. Because we have found that the most successful rate for interruption of type I atrial flutter is approximately 120 to 130 percent (range 111 to 135 percent) of the spontaneous atrial rate, if this second technique is used, pacing is initiated at a rate within this percentage range of the spontaneous atrial flutter rate (for example, 125 percent of the spontaneous rate) and is continued either for 15 to 30 sec or until the atrial complexes in electrocardio-

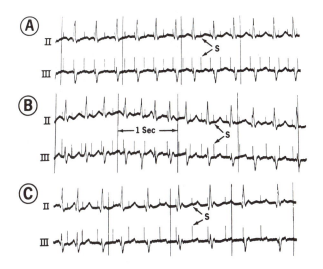

Figure 3 Electrocardiogram leads II and III recorded from a patient during rapid high right atrial pacing to treat atrial flutter (intrinsic rate 294 beats per minute. Previously, pacing had been initiated at a rate of 309 beats per minute and increased to a rate of 355 beats per minute but had failed to interrupt the atrial flutter. During this previous ramp pacing, the atrial complexes only became biphasic in leads II and III. Then, as illustrated in this figure (*A*), pacing was reinitiated at a rate of 350 beats per minute and increased to a rate of 382 beats per minute. Now, the atrial complexes became completely positive in both leads II and III, with close observation of the records in *A* revealing that this occurred at a pacing rate of about 370 beats per minute. When the pacing rate was slowed, the lower the rate of the spontaneous atrial flutter, atrial capture was maintained (*B* and *C*). In fact, atrial capture was maintained as the pacing rate was decreased to a rate of 110 beats per minute. Time lines are at 1-sec intervals. S = stimulus artifact. (From Waldo AL, MacLean WAH, Karp RB, et al. Entrainment and interruption of atrial flutter with atrial pacing. Studies in man following open heart surgery. Circulation 1977;56:737–745. Reprinted by permission of the American Heart Association.)

gram lead II change from negative to positive. If pacing at the initial rate does not interrupt atrial flutter, the atrial pacing rate is increased by increments of 5 to 10 beats per minute until successful interruption of the atrial flutter has been achieved. A similar although more conservative approach would be to initiate pacing at a rate that is 10 beats per minute faster than the spontaneous atrial rate for 15 to 30 sec. Upon termination of rapid atrial pacing, if the atrial flutter is not interrupted, the atrial pacing rate is increased by increments of 5 to 10 beats per minute until successful interruption of atrial flutter has been achieved.

With either of the two pacing techniques, when the atria are paced at rates faster than the spontaneous rate, the atrial flutter may not be interrupted even though atrial capture has been obtained. This phenomenon, called transient entrainment, should not be considered evidence that rapid atrial pacing will be unsuccessful. Rather, it provides evidence that pacing at a more rapid rate is required to interrupt the atrial flutter. Occasionally, but rarely in the presence of a class IA antiarrhythmic agent, atrial pacing rates over 400 beats per minute may be required to interrupt type I atrial flutter when using either the ramp or constant rate pacing technique. Also, when using the constant rate technique for interruption of the atrial flutter, a critical duration of pacing (average 11 sec) at the critical rate is required.

When performing either epicardial or endocardial rapid atrial pacing, it is important to remember that the stimulus strength required for atrial capture at rapid rates occasionally is rather high, and loss of capture or no atrial capture at all may occur unless a sufficient stimulus strength is used. In addition, because the stimulus strength required to maintain atrial capture increases as the pacing rate increases, particularly when using the ramp pacing technique, we generally recommend that pacing be initiated using a stimulus strength of at least 10 mA. It is unusual to require more than 20 mA, although we have on occasion required even as much as 39 mA.

Using the technique of atrial pacing via the esophagus (esophageal pacing), virtually all the above suggestions apply, with two important exceptions. First, because atrial pacing via the esophagus tends to be moderately painful (usually causing a stinging sensation), we recommend pacing for shorter periods, usually less than 15 sec at a time. In addition, we always recommend initiating pacing after first demonstrating a good atrial electrogram recording with only a minimal ventricular deflection, and then pacing at a rate sufficiently slow that if ventricular capture is inadvertently obtained, there will be no adverse effects. Thus, we do not recommend starting pacing at rates in the range generally required to interrupt atrial flutter. Also, pacing equipment must be used that permits the stimulus duration to be at least 9 to 10 msec and the stimulus strength to be up to 30 mA because the threshold for atrial capture is generally high, and it is not unusual for the stimulus strength required to be greater than 20 mA.

Precipitation of Atrial Fibrillation

In some patients, rapid atrial pacing produces atrial fibrillation. Atrial fibrillation precipitated by rapid atrial pacing is most often transient, lasting seconds to minutes before spontaneously converting to sinus rhythm. For those few patients in whom atrial fibrillation persists, it is usually a more desirable rhythm than the continuation of type I atrial flutter because atrial fibrillation is almost always associated with a slower ventricular response rate than

that occurring during atrial flutter. Also, in almost all instances, the ventricular response rate to atrial fibrillation can be easily controlled with digitalis or, occasionally, with a calcium channel blocker or a beta blocker. For those patients in whom type I atrial flutter recurs despite interruption by rapid atrial pacing, continuous rapid atrial pacing to precipitate and sustain atrial fibrillation may be indicated on a temporary basis until pharmacologic control of the recurrent atrial flutter is achieved.

It has been shown that administration of a class IA antiarrhythmic agent (procainamide, disopyramide, or quinidine) can be used effectively to augment the efficacy of rapid atrial pacing to convert atrial flutter to sinus rhythm. Thus, when clinically feasible, we recommend administration of procainamide intravenously (500 mg over about 10 minutes or 1 g over about 20 minutes). Initially, this will slow the atrial flutter rate and, consequently, usually the ventricular response rate. But more important, initiation of rapid atrial pacing following administration of the drug results in a high incidence of successful conversion of atrial flutter to sinus rhythm, avoiding a period of atrial fibrillation.

Direct Current Cardioversion to Convert Atrial Flutter

Atrial flutter is generally easy to treat by cardioversion. It often requires as little as 25 J for successful cardioversion, although at least 50 J is generally recommended because this is more often successful. Because 100 J is virtually always successful and never harmful, we recommend it as the initial shock, in order to avoid the need for delivery of a second shock in the event that the first is not successful.

Chronic Treatment of Atrial Flutter

Drug Therapy

Paroxysmal atrial flutter may be difficult to suppress clinically. Standard treatment is to administer a class IA agent, either quinidine or procainamide, in an effort to prevent recurrence. When either of these drugs is ineffective or cannot be administered for any reason (e.g., adverse effects), recent data indicate that one of the class IC agents may be effective and well tolerated. In fact, if the class IC agents continue to be shown to be more effective or at least as effective as class IA agents in the suppression of atrial flutter, class IC agents may be the drugs of choice for long-term suppression. In addition, class III antiarrhythmic agents (amiodarone or sotalol) may be effective. However, there are very few data concerning sotalol, and potential amiodarone toxicity is a well-described concern.

Permanent Antitachycardia Pacing

For patients in whom atrial flutter tends to recur, although atrial flutter per se is rarely a life-threatening problem, it is often a problem that significantly interferes with the quality of life. In such patients, consideration should be given to implantation of a permanent antitachycardia pacemaker. Although the published series of patients who have used these devices have been small, the devices have nevertheless been shown to be effective in interrupting recurrent atrial flutter in properly selected patients. These patients usually still need chronic treatment with antiarrhythmic drug therapy. Nevertheless, the ability to interrupt atrial flutter promptly whenever it recurs should provide safe and effective treatment.

A potential problem with the use of a permanent antitachycardia pacemaker is the precipitation of atrial fibrillation. If precipitation of atrial fibrillation is clinically unacceptable, this technique is probably best avoided.

Catheter Ablation Techniques

Two catheter ablation techniques have been used successfully for the treatment of chronic or recurrent atrial flutter. The first, His bundle ablation to create high-degree AV block, thereby preventing the rapid ventricular response rate to atrial flutter, is now a generally accepted technique. For patients who are intolerant of antiarrhythmic drug therapy or in whom atrial flutter with a rapid and clinically unacceptable ventricular response rate recurs despite antiarrhythmic drug therapy, producing third-degree or high-degree AV block provides a successful form of therapy without the need for any more antiarrhythmic agents. Of course, it does include the need for a chronic ventricular pacemaker, but there are a host of very acceptable pacemakers available for use, including various forms of DDD pacemakers or activity mode pacemakers, whether VVI or DDD.

The second mode of catheter ablation therapy is currently investigational. It involves identification of an apparent critical area of slow conduction in the atrial flutter reentry circuit. When this area is mapped and identified during cardiac catheterization, it can be ablated. To date in a small series of patients this technique has provided successful therapy. This technique awaits further development to understand the associated short- and long-term efficacy rates and potential adverse effects.

Surgical Therapy

Acceptable surgical therapy awaits more definitive understanding of the nature of the reentrant circuit of atrial flutter in patients and a clearer un-derstanding of what type of surgical intervention (e.g., ablation, incision, excision) might prove effective when applied appropriately. Guiraudon and co-workers reported on three operated patients in whom intraoperative mapping showed an area of slow conduction or a gap in activation during atrial flutter between the coronary sinus surface and the tricuspid annulus. Cryoablation of the region successfully prevented recurrent atrial flutter in two patients, but the third had symptomatic atrial fibrillation. Clearly, this surgical series is too small to project the future, but the similarities between these data and the ablation data of Saoudi and associates seem related and promising.

One special case should be mentioned. Atrial flutter that occurs in patients who have the Wolff-Parkinson-White syndrome can be its usual troublesome self or, when associated with 1:1 AV conduction, may be life-threatening. For reasons that are not understood, ablation of the accessory AV connection is initially always associated with elimination of the atrial flutter (this is true for atrial fibrillation as well). Therefore, in this group of patients surgical ablation (or, for that matter, catheter ablation) of the accessory AV connection should be considered as a therapeutic option (it is clearly indicated when 1:1 AV conduction of atrial flutter has been demonstrated), as it will most likely effect a cure.

Supported in part by grant RO1 HL38408 from the National Institutes of Health, National Heart, Lung and Blood Institute, a Research Initiative Award from the Northeast Ohio Affiliate of the American Heart Association, and a grant from the Wuliger Foundation.

SUGGESTED READING

Allessie MA, Bonke FIM, Schopman FJG. Circus movement and rapid atrial muscle as a mechanism of tachycardia. III. The 'leading circle' concept: A new model of circus movement in cardiac tissue without the involvement of an anatomic obstacle. Circ Res 1977; 41:9.

Allessie MA, Lammers WJEP, Bonke FIM, Hollen J. Intraatrial reentry as a mechanism for atrial flutter induced by acetylcholine and rapid pacing in the dog. Circulation 1984; 70:123–135.

Barold SS, Wyndham CRC, Kappenberger LL, et al. Implanted atrial pacemakers for paroxysmal atrial flutter: Long term efficacy. Ann Intern Med 1987; 107:144–149.

Olshansky B, Okumura K, Hess PG, et al. Use of procainamide with rapid atrial pacing for successful conversion of atrial flutter to sinus rhythm. J Am Coll Cardiol 1988; 11:359–364.

Saoudi N, Atallah G, Kirkorian G, Touboul P. Catheter ablation of the atrial myocardium in human type I atrial flutter. Circulation, in press.

Scheinman MM. Catheter techniques for ablation of supraventricular tachycardia. N Engl J Med 1989; 320:460–461.

Waldo AL. Mechanisms of atrial fibrillation, atrial flutter, and ectopic atrial tachycardia—a brief review. Circulation 1987; 75:III-37–40.

Waldo AL, MacLean WAH, Cooper TB, et al. Use of temporarily

placed epicardial atrial wire electrodes for the diagnosis and treatment of cardiac arrhythmias following open heart surgery. J Thorac Cardiovasc Surg 1978; 76:500–505.

Waldo AL, MacLean WAH, Karp RB, et al. Continuous rapid atrial pacing to control recurrent or sustained supraventricular tachycardias following open heart surgery. Circulation 1976; 54:245–250.

Waldo AL, MacLean WAH, Karp RB, et al. Entrainment and interruption of atrial flutter with atrial pacing. Studies in man following open heart surgery. Circulation 1977; 56:737–745.

Wells JL Jr, MacLean WAH, James TN, Waldo AL. Characterization of atrial flutter. Studies in man after open heart surgery using fixed atrial electrodes. Circulation 1979; 60:665–673.

MULTIFOCAL ATRIAL TACHYCARDIA

PETER M. YURCHAK, M.D.

Multifocal atrial tachycardia (MAT) is an irregular supraventricular tachyarrhythmia, occurring in the setting of acute illness and best treated by correction of underlying contributory factors. Electrocardiographic criteria for its diagnosis include an atrial rate above 100 beats per minute; well-organized, discrete P waves of varying morphology, arising from at least three different foci; irregular variation in the P-P interval; and an isoelectric baseline between P waves (Fig. 1). As a rule, atrioventricular (AV) conduction is 1:1, although occasional very early P waves may not be conducted because of physiologic refractoriness of the AV conducting system. Frequent nonconducted P waves, occurring relatively late after the preceding R wave, or periods of 2:1 AV conduction are features of MAT with AV block, usually a sign of digitalis toxicity (Fig. 2).

MAT was described in 1968 as a "clinical-electrocardiographic syndrome" in 32 subjects suffering from a variety of acute medical or postoperative surgical problems. Mortality rates from the associated conditions have ranged from 50 to 75 percent. Since that time, numerous case reports and series have appeared, generally supporting the concept that MAT is a "secondary" arrhythmia provoked by dire acute disease and subsiding with correction of the clinical problems. However, subsets of individuals exhibiting MAT have also been delineated, such as infants and children and subjects with the repetitive form, interspersed with cycles of normal sinus rhythm. One group of observers stated that MAT was a precursor of atrial fibrillation, but a significant association between the two arrhythmias has not been borne out by the observations of others.

MULTIFOCAL ATRIAL TACHYCARDIA AND ATRIAL FIBRILLATION

MAT must be distinguished from atrial fibrillation in the electrocardiogram. Both are atrial tachyarrhythmias, but beyond this the similarity

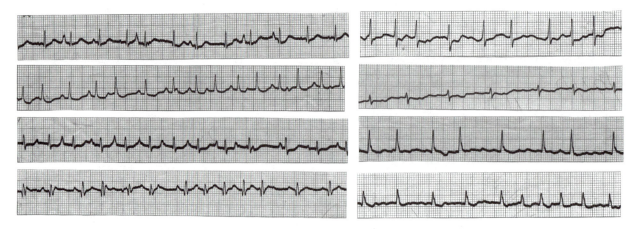

Figure 1 Representative examples of MAT from four different subjects (*left*), compared with atrial fibrillation in four other subjects (*right*), emphasizing the key features of the two arrhythmias. Note the discrete, multiform P waves in MAT, separated by an isoelectric baseline.

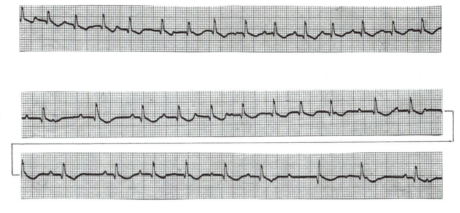

Figure 2 MAT (*top*) and MAT with AV block induced by digitalis toxicity (*lower two continuous strips*). Note the repetitive periods of 2:1 AV block and the prolonged P-R interval of conducted P waves.

ends. MAT is usually seen at rates between 140 and 160 beats per minute, although occasionally very ill patients may exhibit rates as high as 200 beats per minute. By contrast, atrial fibrillation is seen at rates of 300 beats per minute or more. A key distinction is the discrete nature of atrial deflections in MAT, with an isoelectric baseline between P waves (Fig. 3). Even at atrial rates approaching 200 beats per minute, the longer cycles show the telltale isoelectric interval. The electrocardiograms of many subjects with MAT exhibit baseline artifact owing to somatic tremor. This tends to obscure both the atrial deflections and the baseline, giving rise to confusion. A stratagem under such circumstances is to move the electrodes from the patient's extremities to the back of the shoulders and buttocks. This largely eliminates somatic tremor and permits accurate diagnosis. A small percentage of patients may shift back and forth between MAT and atrial fibrillation, also contributing to possible confusion. In atrial fibrillation many atrial depolarizations are not transmitted to the ventricles because of physiologic refractoriness of the AV conducting system. In MAT, 1:1 conduction is the rule. Figure 1 compares the two rhythms.

In doubtful cases, carotid sinus massage will expose the continuously active baseline in atrial fibrillation and the isoelectric baseline in MAT.

We have emphasized the differences between MAT and atrial fibrillation because the therapeutic implications for the two rhythms are vastly different. Atrial fibrillation may be seen in apparently normal hearts and in patients without acute medical or surgical problems — so-called lone or idiopathic atrial fibrillation. Atrial fibrillation may also be the presenting manifestation of thyrotoxicosis, rheumatic mitral stenosis, or atrial septal defect in subjects in middle life. Whatever the etiology, digitalis is considered the sovereign treatment, producing benefit by slowing the ventricular response to the rapid atrial mechanism. At times digitalis therapy may accomplish reversion to normal rhythm. On the other hand, MAT is rarely encountered outside the setting of acute medical or postoperative surgical problems, serves as an index of the very serious clinical state of the patient, and cannot be dispelled by digitalis administration alone. Indeed, injudicious administration of digitalis in a vain effort to control the arrhythmia may lead to digitalis toxicity, which can end in fatal arrhythmia.

MULTIFOCAL ATRIAL TACHYCARDIA: A SECONDARY ARRHYTHMIA

Table 1 lists the contributory factors to the genesis of MAT, drawn from published series and personal experience. Many subjects with MAT suffer from chronic and acute pulmonary disease. The bronchodilators and sympathomimetic agents used in treatment of these problems appear to be factors contributing to the genesis of MAT. Their administration should be tempered or eliminated in an effort to correct the arrhythmia. Although derangements in blood oxygen and carbon dioxide tension are common in these subjects, along with electrolyte disturbances, no single factor has been consistently

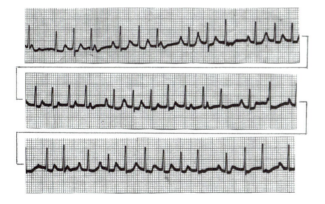

Figure 3 Very rapid MAT (180 beats per minute). Even at this rate, the isoelectric baseline is clearly seen.

Table 1 Multifocal Atrial Tachycardia Correctable
Contributory Factors

Hypoxia	Pulmonary hypertension
Hypercarbia	Right-sided heart failure
Respiratory acidosis	Right atrial distention
Hypokalemia	Left-sided heart failure
Hypomagnesemia	
Metabolic alkalosis	Infection (pulmonary or extrapulmonary)
Sympathomimetics	Postoperative abdominal processes (ileus, pancreatitis, sepsis)
Methylxanthines	

encountered in all cases. Efforts to improve these derangements serve as part of a multifaceted effort to improve the patient's condition and, with it, to dissipate the arrhythmia. The clinician's first response upon encountering MAT in a patient should be to seek the factors contributing jointly to production of this marker of an acutely ill patient. Occasionally MAT is the presenting manifestation of pulmonary embolism, and this should be considered when other conditions are not obvious.

SUBSETS OF MULTIFOCAL ATRIAL TACHYCARDIA

Rare individuals with very severe obstructive lung disease exhibit MAT as a *chronic* rhythm pattern, even when out of the hospital.

As stated, digitalis alone is not the appropriate first response to the diagnosis of MAT. A minority of patients with the rhythm may in fact have left- or right-sided heart failure, evidenced by the usual physical and radiographic findings. These individuals should be treated with digitalis and other adjunctive measures in anticipation that their rhythm will stabilize once cardiac compensation is restored. However, digitalis probably has no place in the absence of heart failure.

MAT has been reported in a handful of infants, most with significant congenital anomalies, both cardiac and noncardiac. In these cases the rhythm appears to be a manifestation of developmental immaturity of the normal pacemakers of the heart and has seldom required treatment. The prognosis of the patient is determined by the presence of associated anomalies. Whether treated or untreated, the arrhythmia tends to disappear when the infant reaches the age of 2 years.

Forty years ago, Parkinson and Papp described a *repetitive* form of paroxsymal tachycardia in which salvos of atrial or ventricular tachyarrhythmia were interspersed with one or more cycles of sinus rhythm. The arrhythmia was usually well tolerated,

except for associated palpitations, and carried a good long-term prognosis. A handful of cases of the repetitive form of MAT have been described, bearing out the above statement. The decision of whether to treat this form is determined by the nuisance value of the palpitations.

COMMENT ON ANTIARRHYTHMIC AGENTS

In general, the classic antiarrhythmic agents quinidine and procainamide have proved to be of little benefit in dealing with arrhythmias. The calcium channel blocking agent verapamil has been advocated as beneficial, by means of reduction in atrial (and secondarily ventricular) rate. However, proof is lacking that this maneuver improves patients' prognoses. Some individuals develop a fall in atrial oxygen tension coincident with the use of verapamil, and the possibility exists that patients with myocardial disease might suffer severe and prolonged hypotension in response to this agent. Verapamil does not appear to have a legitimate place in treatment of this arrhythmia.

Because many subjects with MAT have chronic lung disease, one is reluctant to employ beta-blocking agents for rhythm stabilization because of the possibility of aggravating bronchospasm. The cardiac-selective agent metoprolol has been reported to be of benefit in small series in the literature, but as with verapamil, proof of improvement in prognosis is lacking. Most of the few hemodynamic studies of metoprolol in MAT show no improvement in cardiac output coincident with cardiac slowing produced by this agent. In general, slowing the cardiac rate by means of pharmacologic agents robs the therapist of a useful marker of the patient's clinical status and tends to deflect attention from remedying the underlying contributory factors.

Cardioversion is generally agreed to be of no benefit, because the arrhythmia promptly recurs even when briefly dispelled by the technique.

One group of investigators has recorded the beneficial effect of intravenous magnesium in dispelling the arrhythmia. As with other agents, proof of improvement in prognosis is lacking. Intravenous magnesium tends to induce hypokalemia, and therefore potassium must be administered along with magnesium. This approach to therapy appears to have drawn few adherents.

MAT with AV block (see Fig. 2), as stated earlier, is generally a manifestation of digitalis toxicity. Serum glycoside levels can confirm this, but digitalis should be withheld at the first sign of the electrocardiographic pattern. If hypokalemia is present as a contributory factor to digitalis toxicity, this should be corrected with intravenous or oral repletion.

Table 2 Management of Multifocal Atrial Tachycardia

Diagnostic Measures	Definitive Measures	Invasive Monitoring
Hematocrit, white blood cell count	Stop or reduce sympathomimetics, methylxanthines	Arterial line
Urinalysis		Pulmonary artery catheter
Blood chemistry tests	Intubate, ventilate	Foley catheter
Potassium	Pulmonary physiotherapy	
Magnesium	Pressors for hypotension	
Theophylline	Volume repletion if pulmonary capillary wedge pressure is low	
Digoxin		
?Amylase	Packed blood cells for anemia	
Arterial blood gases	Antibiotics for infection	
Cultures: sputum, blood, urine	Heparin for pulmonary embolus	
Chest film	Nasogastric suction for ileus	
?Pulmonary angiogram	Digoxin, diuretics for heart failure	
	?Therapeutic bronchoscopy (atelectasis, copious secretions)	

PRINCIPLES IN MANAGEMENT

Generally speaking, the contributory factors listed in Table 1 should be eliminated or ameliorated as much as possible. Table 2 lists the diagnostic studies and corrective measures available to the therapist in improving the patient's overall condition. As a point of view, a parallel can be drawn between one's approach to MAT and one's approach to very rapid sinus tachycardia (above 140 beats per minute) in a severely ill patient. When encountering extreme sinus tachycardia, the approach should focus on identifying and correcting the underlying contributory factors, not on attempting to slow the sinus rate by pharmacologic agents.

If digitalis is to serve as part of a multifaceted program of treatment, because of the presence of heart failure, serum glycoside levels of such patients should be monitored carefully to avoid inadvertent digitalis toxicity.

SUGGESTED READING

Arsura E, Lefkin AS, Scher DL, et al. A randomized, double-blind, placebo-controlled study of verapamil and metoprolol in treatment of multifocal atrial tachycardia. Am J Med 1988; 85:519–524.

Habibzadeh MA. Multifocal atrial tachycardia: A 66 month follow-up of 50 patients. Heart Lung 1980; 9:328–335.

Shine KI, Kastor JA, Yurchak PM. Multifocal atrial tachycardia. N Engl J Med 1968; 279:344–349.

Wang K, Goldfarb BL, Gobel FL, Richman HG. Multifocal atrial tachycardia. Arch Int Med 1977; 137:161–164.

AUTOMATIC ATRIAL TACHYCARDIA AND NONPAROXYSMAL ATRIOVENTRICULAR JUNCTIONAL TACHYCARDIA

C. PRATAP REDDY, M.D.
JOHN D. ARNETT, M.D.

Ectopic automatic supraventricular tachycardia caused by abnormal or triggered automaticity constitutes a small but significant fraction of supraventricular tachycardias. Abnormal automaticity refers to the property of self-excitation in nonpacemaking fibers or to enhanced phase 4 depolarization in subsidiary pacemakers. In contrast, triggered automaticity produced by afterdepolarizations always requires a stimulus to initiate and maintain a repetitive discharge. In clinical practice, however, these mechanisms cannot be proved, and their diagnosis remains tentative.

Supraventricular tachycardias attributed to the abnormal or triggered automaticity mechanism include (1) automatic atrial tachycardia; (2) nonparoxysmal atrioventricular (AV) junctional tachycardia; (3) atrial tachycardia with AV block; and (4) multifocal atrial tachycardia. In this chapter we present the electrocardiographic and electrophysiologic features, clinical diagnosis, and approach to treatment of automatic atrial tachycardia and nonparoxysmal AV junctional tachycardia. Multifocal atrial tachycardia and atrial tachycardia with AV block are described elsewhere in this book.

AUTOMATIC ATRIAL TACHYCARDIA

Automatic atrial tachycardia may be transient, intermittent, or persistent. The more common transient and intermittent forms are found, typically, in older patients with cardiac or pulmonary disease and are self-limited, lasting for only a few seconds to minutes. In contrast, chronic persistent atrial tachycardia is often found in patients with no structural heart disease and is frequently disabling. This tachycardia has been described under various names as incessant atrial tachycardia, ectopic auricular tachycardia, persistent atrial tachycardia, and chronic atrial tachycardia. Although the first case of persistent automatic atrial tachycardia was reported more than 50 years ago, a review in 1974 by Scheinman and coworkers revealed only 22 such cases in the English literature. The true incidence of automatic atrial tachycardia is not known but is believed to constitute 2 to 5 percent of all supraventricular tachycardias. In children with supraventricular tachycardias, the incidence of automatic atrial tachycardia appears to be somewhat higher. In one study, automatic atrial tachycardia was diagnosed in 11 percent of children with supraventricular tachycardia.

Clinical Features

Unlike reentrant supraventricular tachycardia, which is characterized by abrupt onset and offset, automatic atrial tachycardia tends to be incessant or permanent, with tachycardia being present for more than half of each day. Sinus rhythm either is absent or is rarely seen. In various reported cases, tachycardia persisted from 3 months to 43 years, and the reported age of onset varied from 1 month to 36 years. In adults with automatic atrial tachycardia, structural heart disease is infrequently present. In children with this condition, the diagnosis is usually made before the age of 6 years, and a family history of supraventricular tachycardia is often present. Although most children with persistent automatic atrial tachycardia do not have underlying structural heart disease, a few have either congenital or acquired valvular heart disease. In one instance, incessant automatic atrial tachycardia was caused by an atrial tumor.

In most reported cases of persistent automatic atrial tachycardia, congestive heart failure, as evidenced by cardiac enlargement and impaired ventricular contractile function, was present at the time of initial presentation or occurred at some time during follow-up. We have followed three patients who had chronic persistent automatic atrial tachycardia of 1 to 33 years' duration and no apparent structural heart disease. In all three patients, cardiomegaly, depressed left ventricular function, and congestive heart failure appeared during the follow-up period. The presence or absence of congestive heart failure may depend on the duration and the rate of tachycardia and the presence or absence of AV block. Although congestive heart failure is common in patients with persistent atrial tachycardia, it is rare in patients with the repetitive form of atrial tachycardia. Cerebrovascular accident, probably secondary to a cerebral embolus, has been reported in a small percentage of patients with automatic atrial tachycardia.

Characteristics of the Electrocardiogram

In patients with recurrent forms of automatic atrial tachycardia, an atrial premature complex arising late in the cardiac cycle interrupts sinus rhythm and initiates tachycardia (Fig. 1). The P-wave configuration of the tachycardia-initiating complex is identical to the P waves of succeeding complexes, suggesting a common origin of the initiating premature atrial complex and the subsequent complexes of ectopic tachycardia. In contrast to the reentrant supraventricular tachycardia, the P-R interval of the tachycardia-initiating premature atrial complex is not prolonged.

After the onset, the cycle length of tachycardia first shortens progressively (warm-up phase), but once established, the P-P intervals do not vary by more than 50 msec unless an exit block from the tachycardia focus is present (Figs. 1, 2). During tachycardia, the P wave is always visible and the P wave axis is abnormal. The rate of tachycardia is usually slower than that in patients with reentrant supraventricular tachycardia, but rates as high as 270 beats per minute have been reported. The rate of tachycardia tends to vary significantly from day to day and from hour to hour, being influenced by many physiologic factors, including posture, exercise, emotion, time of the day, and state of consciousness. During sleep, the rate of tachycardia slows and AV block may occur, or when it is already present it becomes more pronounced (see Fig. 2). During exercise the rate of tachycardia increases and AV block disappears or becomes less pronounced. Atropine and isoproterenol may increase and phenylephrine and carotid sinus stimulation may decrease the rate of tachycardia. The latter maneuvers may also produce AV block without terminating the tachycardia. As a rule, sinus rhythm does not occur even when the rate of tachycardia slows.

Clinical Electrophysiology

Unlike reentrant supraventricular tachycardia, which can be initiated and/or terminated by prema-

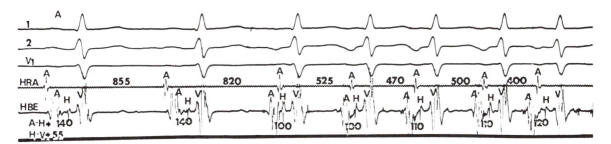

Figure 1 Initiation of automatic atrial tachycardia. The tracing shows electrocardiogram leads I, II, and V₁ and high right atrial (HRA) electrogram and His bundle (HBE) electrogram. The first two complexes are sinus, with a normal sequence of atrial activation. A premature atrial complex arising late in the cycle (third complex) initiates tachycardia. Note that (1) the sequence of atrial activation in the tachycardia-initiating premature complex is low to high and similar to that of subsequent complexes, (2) initiation of tachycardia is not dependent on A-H interval prolongation, and (3) the cycle length of tachycardia gradually shortens (warm-up) before stabilization. (From Reddy CP. Supraventricular tachycardias due to mechanisms other than re-entry. In: Surawicz B. et al, eds. Tachycardias. Hingham, MA: Martinus Nijhoff Publishing, 1984; with permission.)

ture atrial stimulation or by rapid atrial pacing, automatic atrial tachycardia can neither be initiated nor terminated by programmed atrial stimulation (Fig. 3 and Table 1). In automatic atrial tachycardia, the atrial activation sequence of the tachycardia-initiating complex is identical to that of the succeeding complexes of tachycardia, whereas in reentrant supraventricular tachycardia, the atrial activation sequence of the tachycardia-initiating complex is dif-

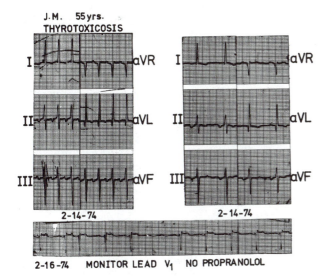

Figure 2 Automatic atrial tachycardia in a patient with thyrotoxicosis showing fluctuation of tachycardia rate because of exit block from the tachycardia focus and occurrence of AV block. Electrocardiograms recorded at different times on the same day (2-14-74) show rates of 150 bpm and 75 bpm. The slower rate most likely is due to 2:1 exit block encountered by the tachycardia focus. A monitor lead recorded 2 days later (2-16-74) during sleep shows AV block.

ferent from that of the succeeding complexes of tachycardia. During tachycardia, programmed atrial extra stimuli introduced at long coupling intervals result in a fully compensatory pause both in reentrant and automatic supraventricular tachycardias. However, at short coupling intervals, the response of automatic supraventricular tachycardia differs from that of reentrant supraventricular tachycardia in that the former becomes reset without cessation of tachycardia, whereas the latter may stop with resumption of sinus rhythm (Fig. 4). In this regard, the automatic focus behaves like an accessory sinus node. If an entrance block into the ectopic focus is present, however, a fully compensatory pause, without reset, will be observed at all coupling intervals. In contrast to reentrant supraventricular tachycardia, which can be terminated by overdrive pacing, in automatic atrial tachycardia, overdrive pacing captures the atrium but upon cessation of pacing, tachycardia immediately resumes without an intervening sinus beat (see Fig. 3). In some instances, overdrive pacing may slow the rate of atrial tachycardia or suppress the tachycardia focus transiently with the emergence of sinus rhythm for a period of a few beats.

Diagnosis

Diagnosis of ectopic automatic atrial tachycardia is important because if left untreated, it may lead to a picture of dilated cardiomyopathy. More important, in patients with this arrhythmia, a permanent cure can be effected by surgical excision or electrical ablation of the arrhythmia focus. Diagnosis is made by the analysis of resting and ambulatory electrocardiograms. Automatic atrial tachycardia is characterized by a clearly visible P wave with an abnormal axis preceding each QRS complex, a distinct P-R interval, and a progressive shortening of the cycle length (warm-up) at the onset of tachycar-

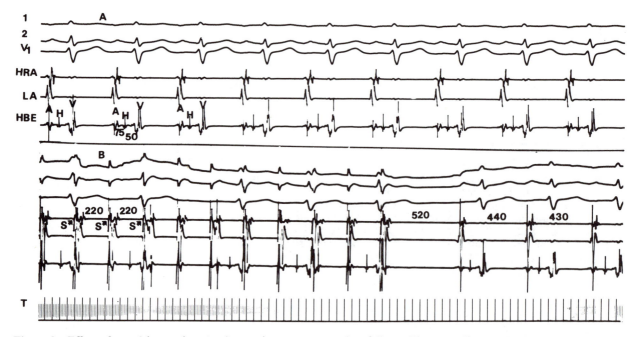

Figure 3 Effect of overdrive pacing. Analog tracings are arranged as follows: Electrocardiogram leads I, II, and V$_1$, and intracardiac electrograms from the high right atrium (HRA), left atrium (LA), and the His bundle (HBE). Panel *A* shows eccentric atrial activation during tachycardia. Overdrive atrial pacing at a cycle length of 220 msec fails to terminate tachycardia, and upon termination of pacing, ectopic atrial tachycardia promptly returns.

dia (see Fig. 1). This warm-up behavior is characteristic of automatic atrial tachycardia. When analysis of the electrocardiogram alone is not sufficient, electrophysiologic studies may be required to define the tachycardia mechanism. Automatic atrial tachycardia is neither induced nor terminated by atrial pacing or premature atrial complexes. When tachycardia starts with a premature atrial complex, the initiation is not dependent upon either a critical coupling interval or a critical P-R interval prolongation (see Fig. 1). Programmed premature atrial stimulation during automatic tachycardia will reset but does not terminate the tachycardia. Overdrive atrial pacing may increase, slow transiently, or have no effect on the rate of tachycardia. Unlike the AV

nodal or atrioventricular reentrant supraventricular tachycardia, which cannot sustain itself in the presence of AV block, automatic atrial tachycardia can perpetuate in the presence of AV block because the AV node is not an integral part of the tachycardia circuit.

Treatment

In patients with intermittent or transient automatic atrial tachycardia, treatment of underlying illness is the cornerstone of therapy. When treatment of the underlying illness does not resolve the arrhythmia, treatment with digitalis or calcium channel or beta blockers may be helpful in controlling the

Table 1 Electrophysiologic Criteria Used to Differentiate Reentrant from Automatic Supraventricular Tachycardia

Criteria	Reentry	Abnormal Automaticity	Triggered Automaticity
Initiation by premature complex	+	−	+
Initiation by rapid pacing	+	−	+
Termination by premature complex	+	−	+
Termination by overdrive pacing	+	−	+
Overdrive acceleration	?	−	+
Inverse relation between the coupling interval of tachycardia-initiating premature complex and the interval between the premature complex and the first complex of tachycardia	+	−	−
Delayed conduction of tachycardia-initiating premature complex	+	−	−

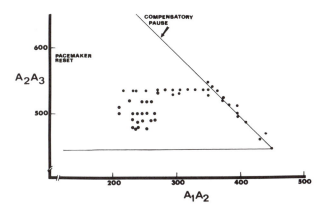

Figure 4 Response to the introduction of premature atrial extrastimuli during tachycardia. The effect of atrial premature depolarizations (APDs) (A$_2$) introduced during automatic ectopic atrial tachycardia (AET) is shown. The interval following the APD (A$_1$A$_2$) in milliseconds is plotted as a function of the coupling interval of the APD (A$_1$A$_2$) in milliseconds. The diagonal line indicates a fully compensatory pause following the APD. The area inside the diagonal line labeled pacemaker reset indicates the range of values that might be expected if A$_2$ reset the atrial cycle with a variable degree of suppression of the ectopic focus. Note that as A$_2$ is introduced progressively prematurely, all points fall within the area of pacemaker reset. (From Goldreyer BN, Gallagher JJ, Damato AN. The electrophysiologic demonstration of atrial ectopic tachycardia in man. Am Heart J 1973,85:205–212; with permission.)

ventricular rate and rarely in suppressing the tachycardia. Unlike reentrant supraventricular tachycardia, persistent automatic atrial tachycardia is refractory to medical therapy and cannot be converted to sinus rhythm by direct current countershock. Digitalis may, however, be helpful in the management of coexisting heart failure. Beta-adrenoceptor blockers, although helpful in controlling the ventricular rate of tachycardia, should be administered with caution and in low doses in patients with associated left ventricular dysfunction. Propranolol has been reported to be especially helpful in young children and infants with automatic atrial tachycardia.

In general, treatment with class IA antiarrhythmic agents, which are known to suppress automaticity and to prolong the atrial refractory period, has been disappointing. In some cases, treatment with these agents may make the tachycardia rate worse. Flecainide and encainide, class IC agents, have been reported to be effective in some patients with automatic atrial tachycardia. Moricizine, a phenothiazine derivative belonging to class IB, has also been reported to be effective in suppressing automatic atrial tachycardia, but more experience is needed before firm conclusions can be made about the efficacy of these agents. Several investigators have re-

ported a favorable response of atrial tachycardia to treatment with both intravenous and oral amiodarone in children. Because long-term treatment with amiodarone is associated with a high incidence of toxicity, we discourage its use for treatment of this arrhythmia.

When aggressive treatment with antiarrhythmic agents fails, surgical excision of arrhythmogenic focus, or cryo, or electrical ablation of ectopic focus should be considered. The experience with these ablative and surgical techniques is limited, and before these treatment modalities can be applied, electrophysiologic studies with both pre- and intraoperative mapping are required to localize the tachycardia focus. Because automatic atrial tachycardia is sensitive to temperature changes and anesthesia, the tachycardia may not be inducible, making intraoperative mapping of the tachycardia focus impossible. In children, recurrence of automatic atrial tachycardia from new foci after resection of a previously mapped automatic focus has been reported. Isolation of the left atrium and entrapment of atrial tachycardia within the left atrium have been successfully performed in some cases of automatic tachycardias with their origin in the left atrium. These techniques avoid creating AV block and permit normal sinus rhythm.

NONPAROXYSMAL ATRIOVENTRICULAR JUNCTIONAL TACHYCARDIA

AV junctional tachycardia is a relatively common arrhythmia that has been attributed to accelerated impulse formation in the AV junction with control of ventricles or of both the ventricles and the atria. However, it has been suggested recently that triggered automaticity owing to delayed afterdepolarizations may be the mechanism of this tachycardia. Although the exact site of origin and the mechanism of this tachycardia cannot be determined with certainty, the tachycardia is generally attributed to increased automaticity of the pacemaker cells in the region extending from the atrial approaches to the AV node to the end of the common bundle of His. However, the possibility cannot be ruled out that this arrhythmia originates within the atria without recognition of its atrial origin on the electrocardiogram or on intracardiac electrogram recordings. It is believed that the N region of the AV node is the least likely site of origin of nonparoxysmal AV junctional tachycardia.

Clinical Features

Nonparoxysmal AV junctional tachycardia seldom occurs in the absence of underlying heart disease. It is frequently attributable to digitalis toxicity, but other causes include inferior or posterior myocardial infarction, cardiac surgery, viral or rheumatic carditis, and hypokalemia. In the study of Pick and Dominguez, heart disease was present in 28 of 30 patients with nonparoxysmal AV junctional tachycardia, and in more than half of the patients the tachycardia was caused by digitalis toxicity. Dreifus and colleagues examined 11,000 consecutively recorded electrocardiograms and found 41 cases of nonparoxysmal AV junctional tachycardia. In 40 percent of these patients, the tachycardia was produced by digitalis intoxication, in 30 percent by cardiac surgery, and in the remaining 30 percent by acute myocardial infarction or hypokalemia. The clinical course of this arrhythmia is usually benign and self-limiting. However, in patients with significant preexisting hemodynamic impairment, cardiac output may be decreased significantly because of the loss of atrial kick.

Characteristics of the Electrocardiogram

The electrocardiogram usually shows a narrow QRS complex but may occasionally show slight aberration (Fig. 5). In either case, the QRS complex resembles that in sinus rhythm. The rate of tachycardia seldom exceeds 130 beats per minute. When the rate of tachycardia is less than 100 beats per minute, the term accelerated AV junctional rhythm is preferred to describe this arrhythmia. Because the conditions precipitating nonparoxysmal AV junctional tachycardia often impair AV nodal conduction, AV dissociation is frequently present. Retrograde conduction to the atria is present in only about 15 percent of patients, and the P wave may be positioned in front of, simultaneous with, or after the QRS complex. When the P wave is in front of the QRS complex, the P-R interval is less than 0.10 sec and when the P wave follows the QRS, the R-P interval does not exceed 0.20 sec. When AV dissociation is present, the atria may be controlled by sinus rhythm, atrial tachycardia, atrial flutter, or atrial fibrillation. In some cases, the atria and ventricles may be depolarized by two separate AV junctional pacemakers, resulting in double AV junctional tachycardia. Depending upon the severity of impairment of AV nodal conduction, the AV dissociation may be com-

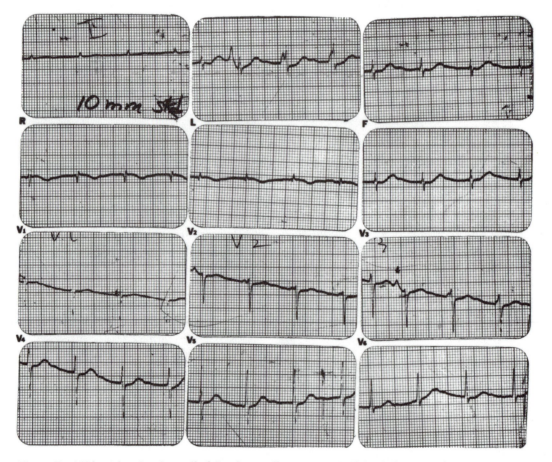

Figure 5 AV junctional tachycardia following cardiac surgery. A 12-lead electrocardiogram shows AV junctional tachycardia with incomplete AV dissociation. Sinus captures are seen in leads II and V_3. (From Reddy CP. Supraventricular tachycardias due to mechanisms other than re-entry. In: Surawicz B. et al, eds. Tachycardias. Hingham, MA: Martinus Nijhoff Publishing, 1984; with permission.)

plete with no conduction across the AV node in either an antegrade or retrograde direction or incomplete with intermittent capture of the ventricles by the atrial rhythm. Similarly, the AV junctional focus may intermittently capture the atria, depending upon the time relationship between the atrial (P wave) and ventricular (QRS complex) events.

Diagnosis

The diagnosis of nonparoxysmal AV junctional tachycardia is rarely difficult. The gradual onset and termination, slower rate of tachycardia, frequent presence of AV dissociation, and the presence of associated clinical conditions make the differentiation of nonparoxysmal AV junctional tachycardia from paroxysmal supraventricular tachycardia an easy task. When clinical evaluation and analysis of the electrocardiogram are not sufficient, electrophysiologic studies are helpful. Electrophysiologic studies with programmed atrial stimulation will reveal the nonparoxysmal AV junctional tachycardia to be an automatic rhythm (Table 1).

Treatment

Except in patients with digitalis toxicity, this arrhythmia is usually self-limiting, resolving within hours to a few days without any treatment. However, in patients with preexisting hemodynamic impairment, the arrhythmia may cause significant hemodynamic changes because of low cardiac output resulting from the loss of atrial contribution. Similar changes in cardiac hemodynamics may occur when the rate of tachycardia is fast. In these patients, institution of temporary AV sequential pacing frequently remedies the problem. We have found AV sequential pacing especially useful in patients with nonparoxysmal AV junctional tachycardia following cardiac surgery. When the rate of tachycardia is fast, administration of drugs such as propranolol or digoxin may suppress or decrease the rate of tachycardia.

Nonparoxysmal AV junctional tachycardia due to digitalis toxicity is a very serious condition requiring prompt therapeutic measures. Early recognition that the arrhythmia is caused by digitalis toxicity is of utmost importance because continued administration of digitalis can result in more serious and lethal arrhythmias. Digitalis should be discontinued at once and electrocardiographic monitoring instituted. If the rate of tachycardia is less than 100 beats per minute, the discontinuation of digoxin with electrocardiographic monitoring may be sufficient. On the other hand, if the rate of tachycardia is greater than 100 beats per minute or manifests exit block, or hemodynamic derangement is present, the tachycardia should be treated more actively. If serum potassium is in the low normal range or less than normal, potassium chloride may be given orally as 1 g every 4 hours. When oral administration is not possible because of gastrointestinal symptoms, potassium chloride can be given intravenously by mixing 40 mEq of potassium chloride in 500 ml of 5 percent dextrose in water, followed by close monitoring of the electrocardiogram and the serum potassium level. Extreme caution must be exercised during potassium administration because of the risks associated with hyperkalemia. Phenytoin, lidocaine, and propranolol are useful in the treatment of nonparoxysmal AV junctional tachycardia caused by digitalis toxicity. Phenytoin, 5 to 10 mg per kilogram of body weight, may be given intravenously at a rate of 100 mg every 5 minutes. If the arrhythmia is suppressed, an oral maintenance dose at 200 mg twice a day should be initiated. Cardiac depression, hypotension, and bradycardia are the most significant side effects of intravenously administered phenytoin. Lidocaine may be administered intravenously as a 100-mg bolus every 5 minutes until a total dose of 3 mg per kilogram is given, followed by continuous infusion at 1 to 3 mg per minute. Both phenytoin and lidocaine have no adverse effects on the sinoatrial or AV node or on the His-Purkinje system. In some patients with nonparoxysmal AV junctional tachycardia, intravenous propranolol in doses of 1 to 5 mg given at a rate of 1 mg per minute may be successful in suppressing the tachycardia. If the arrhythmia is controlled, treatment with oral propranolol, 20 to 40 mg every 6 hours, may be initiated. In serious cases in which the rate of AV junctional tachycardia is rapid, resulting in hemodynamic collapse, treatment with Fab fragments of digoxin-specific antibodies can be used.

SUGGESTED READING

Gillette PC, Garson AT. Electrophysiologic and pharmacologic characteristics of automatic ectopic atrial tachycardia. Circulation 1977; 56:571–575.

Goldreyer BN, Gallagher JJ, Damato AN. The electrophysiologic demonstration of atrial ectopic tachycardia in man. Am Heart J 1973; 85:205–215.

Pick A, Dominguez P. Nonparoxysmal A-V nodal tachycardia. Circulation 1957; 16:1022.

Rosen MR, Fisch C, Hoffman BF, et al. Can accelerated atrioventricular junctional escape rhythms be explained by delayed afterdepolarizations? Am J Cardiol 1980; 45:1272–1284.

Scheinman NM, Basu D, Hollenburg M. Electrophysiologic studies in patients with persistent atrial tachycardia. Circulation 1974; 50:266–273.

PAROXYSMAL REENTRANT SUPRAVENTRICULAR TACHYCARDIA WITHOUT PREEXCITATION: PHARMACOLOGIC THERAPY

EDWARD C. HUYCKE, M.D.
RUEY J. SUNG, M.D.

Paroxysmal supraventricular tachycardia is a rhythm disturbance commonly seen in clinical practice. Clinical consequences of such tachyarrhythmias can range from insignificant to life-threatening. Management requires termination of the acute episode of paroxysmal supraventricular tachycardia and, in selected patients, may be followed by long-term suppressive therapy to prevent future episodes.

Extensive electrophysiologic evidence suggests that paroxysmal supraventricular tachycardia is usually caused by sustained reentry involving one or more cardiac tissues. The most commonly encountered electrophysiologic mechanisms for paroxysmal supraventricular tachycardia are atrioventricular (AV) nodal reentry, and AV reciprocation. In AV nodal reentrant tachycardia, reentry is believed to take place between longitudinally dissociated AV nodal pathways. In the typical form of AV nodal reentrant tachycardia, antegrade conduction is through a slow AV nodal pathway and retrograde conduction is through a fast AV nodal pathway, whereas in the atypical form of AV nodal reentrant tachycardia, antegrade conduction is through the fast AV nodal pathway and retrograde conduction is through the slow AV nodal pathway. Likewise, there are two forms of AV reciprocation. In the orthodromic form of AV reciprocating tachycardia, antegrade impulse conduction occurs through the AV node–His Purkinje system, and retrograde conduction occurs through an anomalous AV connection (Kent fiber). In antidromic AV reciprocation, antegrade conduction is through the anomalous AV connection, whereas retrograde conduction is through the AV node–His Purkinje system or a second anomalous AV connection. However, the QRS complex morphology of antidromic AV reciprocating tachycardia reflects ventricular preexcitation and is, therefore, not considered a form of supraventricular tachycardia. Less common electrophysiologic mechanisms underlying paroxysmal supraventricular tachycardia include sinoatrial and intraatrial reentry in which the reentrant circuit is believed to involve sinus node and/or perinodal atrial tissue in the first and only atrial tissue in the second.

The electrocardiographic hallmark of paroxysmal supraventricular tachycardia is the presence of regular QRS complexes at a rate between 150 and 250 per minute. In the absence of antegrade conduction through an anomalous AV connection (ventricular preexcitation) or functional bundle branch block, the morphology of the QRS complex during tachycardia is identical to that seen during sinus rhythm. Tachycardia onset and termination are usually abrupt. Although the morphology and location of the P wave during tachycardia may be helpful in identifying the underlying electrophysiologic mechanism, definitive determination of the electrophysiologic mechanism often requires electrophysiologic study (Fig. 1).

MANAGEMENT OF ACUTE EPISODES

The initial management of an episode of paroxysmal supraventricular tachycardia is dictated by the hemodynamic state of the patient as related to the rhythm disturbance. The presence of chest pain, cerebral hypoperfusion with mental status changes, or symptomatic hypotension requires immediate QRS-synchronized, direct current cardioversion. Cardioversion energies as low as 25 joules may successfully convert paroxysmal supraventricular tachycardia to sinus rhythm. Electrical cardioversion should be avoided, however, in the presence of digitalis intoxication because of the potential development of intractable postcardioversion ventricular tachyarrhythmias.

In hemodynamically stable patients, maneuvers that transiently increase vagal tone can be useful by prolonging refractoriness and suppressing conduction through the sinoatrial node and/or the AV node. Unilateral carotid sinus massage or the Valsalva maneuver may terminate paroxysmal supraventricular tachycardia in which the sinus node or the AV node is part of the reentrant circuit (sinoatrial reentrant tachycardia, AV nodal reentrant tachycardia, and AV reciprocating tachycardia). In patients in whom the reentrant circuit is confined to the atrium, vagal maneuvers often fail to convert paroxysmal supraventricular tachycardia to sinus rhythm but instead increase the degree of AV block. In elderly patients, auscultation of the carotid arteries should be performed and carotid sinus massage deferred in those with a history of transient cerebral ischemic episodes or stroke or with demonstrable carotid arterial disease. Breath-holding coupled with facial immersion in ice water stimulates the diving reflex, increases vagal tone, and may also

The opinions or assertions contained herein are the private views of the authors and are not to be construed as official or as reflecting the views of the Department of the Army or the Department of Defense.

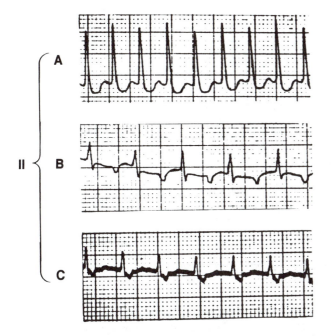

Figure 1 Three electrocardiographic (ECG) patterns of paroxysmal supraventricular tachycardia (SVT). *A*, Typical AV nodal reentry. During SVT, the retrograde P wave is inscribed within the QRS complex, hardly discernible from the surface ECG. *B*, Atypical AV nodal reentry. During SVT, the retrograde P wave is inscribed far behind the QRS complex, with an R-P interval longer than the P-R interval. *C*, Orthodromic AV reciprocation. During SVT, the retrograde P wave is inscribed immediately after the QRS complex, with an R-P interval shorter than the P-R interval. II = ECG lead II. Paper speed = 25 mm/sec.

slow or terminate paroxysmal supraventricular tachycardia. This reflex is more prominent, clinically effective, and safer in young patients than in the elderly.

Often in patients who come to medical attention with acute episodes of paroxysmal supraventricular tachycardia, vagal maneuvers are unsuccessful in restoring sinus rhythm and pharmacologic therapy must be initiated. In patients with paroxysmal supraventricular tachycardia without evidence of ventricular preexcitation, the intravenous administration of the calcium channel antagonist verapamil is usually the pharmacologic treatment of choice. In doses of 5 to 10 mg intravenously given over 2 minutes, verapamil therapy successfully converts 80 percent of patients with paroxysmal supraventricular tachycardia to sinus rhythm. In patients with AV reciprocating tachycardia, verapamil causes tachycardia termination by prolonging refractoriness and slowing conduction through the AV node; the electrophysiologic properties of the anomalous AV connection are usually unchanged. In patients with typical AV nodal reentrant tachycardia, verapamil-mediated

conversion to sinus rhythm is usually due to prolonged refractoriness in the antegrade slow AV nodal pathway, although the electrophysiologic effects of verapamil responsible for restoration of sinus rhythm may be seen in the retrograde fast AV nodal pathway. In a few patients with atypical AV nodal reentrant tachycardia, intravenous verapamil has successfully restored sinus rhythm by prolonging refractoriness in the retrograde slow AV nodal pathway. In limited numbers of patients, intravenous verapamil has also successfully terminated sinoatrial reentrant tachycardia. Verapamil should be avoided in patients with known sick sinus syndrome and those with severe left ventricular dysfunction or congestive heart failure, as its negative inotropic effects may cause further deterioration of cardiac function. In patients with a wide QRS complex tachycardia of ventricular origin (ventricular tachycardia) and/or atrial flutter-fibrillation with ventricular preexcitation, intravenous verapamil is contraindicated. Hemodynamic deterioration may occur in these patients because of verapamil-mediated peripheral vasodilation and resultant reflex sympathetic discharge, causing tachycardia acceleration.

Intravenous diltiazem,* 0.25 to 0.35 mg per kilogram, is another calcium channel antagonist that has been shown to be quite efficacious and safe when used to terminate paroxysmal supraventricular tachycardia. Similar to intravenous verapamil, it acts by prolonging refractoriness and slowing conduction through the AV node; it exerts little electrophysiologic effect on the anomalous AV connection in patients with AV reciprocating tachycardia (Fig. 2). In patients with the typical form of AV nodal reentrant tachycardia, tachycardia termination usually occurs after failed antegrade conduction in the slow AV nodal pathway. Like intravenous verapamil, intravenous diltiazem must be avoided in patients with wide QRS complex tachycardia of ventricular origin or attributable to ventricular preexcitation because tachycardia acceleration may be seen.

Intravenous edrophonium (10 mg), digoxin (0.5 mg initially followed by 0.25 mg every 6 hours to a total loading dose of 1.0 to 1.25 mg over 24 hours), and propranolol (1 mg per minute to a total dose of 0.15 to 0.20 mg per kilogram) also slow conduction and prolong refractoriness of the sinus and AV nodes and may be used to terminate paroxysmal supraventricular tachycardia. In patients with significant left ventricular dysfunction, digitalis preparations are the preferred initial pharmacologic agents. Intravenous propranolol should be used with caution in patients with left ventricular dysfunction because of its negative inotropic effects and should be

---

*Intravenous diltiazem is currently under clinical investigation in the United States.

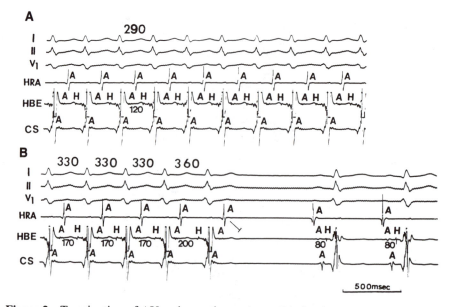

Figure 2 Termination of AV reciprocating tachycardia after intravenous diltiazem. *A,* In the control state, the AV node–His-Purkinje system is used for antegrade conduction and a left-sided lateral accessory AV connection for retrograde conduction. *B,* After intravenous diltiazem, 0.25 mg per kilogram antegrade conduction time through the AV node is prolonged from 120 to 170 msec, whereas the retrograde conduction time through the anomalous AV connection (ventriculoatrial conduction time) is unchanged compared with the control. Tachycardia termination occurs by development of block in the AV node *(arrow).* Surface electrocardiographic leads I, II, and V$_1$, were recorded simultaneously with intracardiac high right atrium (HRA), His bundle (HBE), and distal coronary sinus (CS) electrograms. A = atrial deflection; H = His bundle deflection. Numbers are in milliseconds. (Reprinted from Huycke EC, Sung RJ, Dias VC, et al. Intravenous diltiazem for termination of reentrant supraventricular tachycardia: A placebo-controlled, randomized, double-blind, multicenter study. J Am Coll Cardiol 1989; 13:538–544; with permission.)

avoided in patients with bronchial asthma or obstructive pulmonary disease because of the possibility of precipitation of acute bronchospasm in these patients.

Intravenous procainamide (50 mg per minute to a total dose of 1,000 mg) may also be used in the acute setting to terminate paroxysmal supraventricular tachycardia. Procainamide causes tachycardia termination by slowing conduction and prolonging refractoriness of the anomalous AV connection in patients with AV reciprocating tachycardia and of the retrograde fast AV nodal pathway in patients with AV nodal reentrant tachycardia (Fig. 3). Frequent blood pressure measurements must be made during bolus infusion of procainamide, as significant hypotension due to sympathetic blockade may occur.

Intravenous propafenone* is a fast inward so-

dium channel blocking agent that has been classified as a class IC antiarrhythmic agent according to the Vaughan Williams classification. Infusion of propafenone, 2 mg per kilogram over 2 minutes, has been shown to be useful in the treatment of acute paroxysmal supraventricular tachycardia, restoring sinus rhythm in 75 percent of patients treated. In patients with AV reciprocating tachycardia, propafenone causes tachycardia termination by prolonging refractoriness and slowing conduction in the anomalous AV connection (Fig. 4). In patients with the typical form of AV nodal re-entrant tachycardia, the sites of tachycardia interruption may be in the antegrade slow or retrograde fast AV nodal pathway. In a small number of patients, intravenous propafenone caused termination of intraatrial reentrant tachycardia (Fig. 5). Other class IC antiarrhythmic agents have also been shown to terminate acute episodes of paroxysmal AV nodal or AV reciprocating tachycardia.

Adenosine, a purine derivative and an intermediate of many biochemical pathways, depresses sinus

---

*Intravenous propafenone is currently under clinical investigation in the United States.

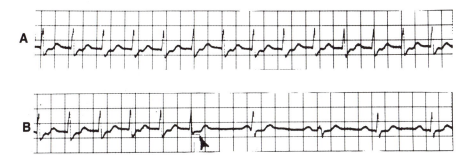

Figure 3 Termination of supraventricular tachycardia with intravenous procainamide. *A*, Carotid sinus massage and intraveous edrophonium, 10 mg, fail to terminate the tachycardia. *B*, Within 2 minutes after infusion of procainamide, 150 mg intravenously, the tachycardia is converted to sinus rhythm. The sudden disappearance of the retrograde P wave (*arrow*) before termination of tachycardia suggests the development of a retrograde conduction block in an anomalous AV connection or fast AV nodal pathway. Paper speed = 25 mm/sec.

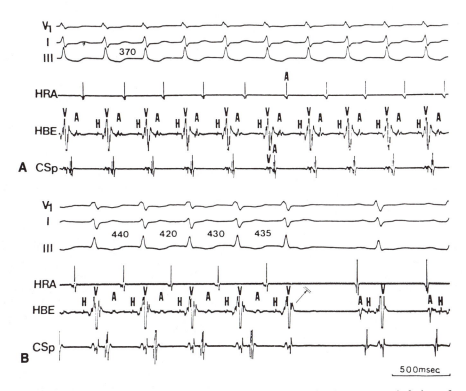

Figure 4 Termination of AV reciprocating tachycardia after intravenous infusion of propafenone. *A*, In the control state, the tachycardia uses the AV node–His-Purkinje system for antegrade conduction and a left-sided posterior paraseptal anomalous AV connection for retrograde conduction. *B*, Orthodromic AV reciprocating tachycardia in the same patient after intravenous infusion of propafenone, 2 mg per kilogram. Both the antegrade conduction time through the AV node (AH interval) and the retrograde conduction time through the anomalous AV connection (ventriculoatrial conduction time) became prolonged. Tachycardia termination occurs by development of block in the anomalous AV connection (*arrow*). Leads V_1, I, and III were recorded simultaneously with intracardiac high right atrial (HRS), His bundle (HBE), and proximal coronary sinus leads (CSp). A = atrial electrogram; H = His bundle electrogram; V = ventricular electrogram. Numbers are in milliseconds. (Reprinted from Shen EN, Keung E, Huycke, E, et al. Intravenous propafenone for termination of reentrant supraventricular tachycardia: A placebo-controlled, randomized, double-blind, crossover study. Ann Intern Med 1986; 105:655–61; with permission.)

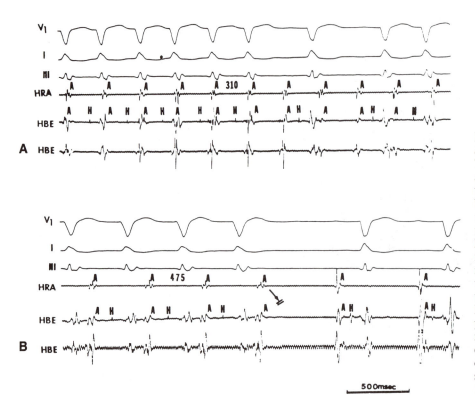

Figure 5 Termination of intra-atrial reentrant tachycardia. *A.* The atrial tachycardia has an atrial cycle length of 310 msec in the control state. Intermittent AV block is noted. *B,* After intravenous infusion of propafenone, 2 mg per kilogram, the atrial cycle length increases to 475 msec before conversion (*arrow*) to sinus rhythm. Trace layout and abbreviations are the same as for Figure 4. (From Shen EN, Keung E, Huycke E, et al. Intravenous propafenone for termination of reentrant supraventricular tachycardia: A placebo-controlled, randomized, double-blind, crossover study. Ann Intern Med 1986; 106:655–661; with permission.)

node automaticity and prolongs AV node conduction when pharmacologic doses of 6 to 12 mg are administered by rapid intravenous injection. In patients with paroxysmal supraventricular tachycardia due to AV nodal reentry or AV reciprocation, adenosine has been shown to be effective and safe. Tachycardia termination is due to block in the AV node in patients with AV reciprocating tachycardia and to block in either the antegrade slow or retrograde fast AV nodal pathway in patients with the typical form of AV nodal reentrant tachycardia. In a small number of patients with intraatrial reentrant tachycardia or sinoatrial reentrant tachycardia, adenosine administration failed to bring about tachycardia termination or to alter the atrial cycle length, but it did increase the degree of AV block. Because adenosine is metabolized within seconds of injection, the electrophysiologic effects and any side effects, which may include dyspnea or flushing or both, are transient.

Pressor agents (including phenylephrine and metaraminol) have been used to terminate paroxysmal supraventricular tachycardia in some hypotensive patients. These agents increase blood pressure, thereby stimulating carotid baroreceptors and causing a reflex increase in vagal tone. However, an exaggerated hypertensive response to pressor agents may cause clinical deterioration in patients with left ventricular dysfunction or angina pectoris in patients with coronary artery disease. Occasionally

stroke may occur with use of these agents. Electrical QRS complex synchronized cardioversion should be considered in this situation prior to use of pressor agents.

LONG-TERM MANAGEMENT

After successful control of an acute episode of paroxysmal supraventricular tachycardia, the decision to proceed with detailed evaluation of the tachycardia or to institute long-term antiarrhythmic therapy must be confronted. Infrequent, short-lived, self-limited episodes of paroxysmal supraventricular tachycardia in the absence of ventricular preexcitation that are hemodynamically well tolerated may require neither extensive evaluation nor long-term antiarrhythmic therapy. For some patients, instruction on the performance of appropriate vagal maneuvers such as the Valsalva maneuver may be all that is necessary to terminate such infrequent episodes. Further, many patients with more frequent episodes of paroxysmal supraventricular tachycardia who require or who desire long-term antiarrhythmic therapy can be managed empirically, without resorting to invasive electrophysiologic studies.

In selected patients with paroxysmal supraventricular tachycardia without ventricular preexcitation, detailed invasive electrophysiologic studies are indicated (1) to achieve rapidly an effective therapeutic regimen in those with hemodynamically serious consequences such as cardiac arrest, congestive heart failure, or angina pectoris caused by the tachycardia; (2) to characterize precisely the underlying electrophysiologic mechanism of the tachycardia in symptomatic patients whose disorder is resistant to empirical therapy in order to allow more rational drug selection; or (3) to characterize precisely paroxysmal supraventricular tachycardia that is resistant to pharmacologic therapy in order to assess the role of nonpharmacologic options, including antitachycardia pacemakers, electrode catheter ablation, or surgical intervention.

Multiple oral medications have been found to be useful in reducing the frequency of recurrence of paroxysmal supraventricular tachycardia. Verapamil (80 to 120 mg every 8 hours) is effective in preventing paroxysmal supraventricular tachycardia, but successful tachycardia termination with the intravenous form of the drug does not predict long-term efficacy with oral verapamil therapy. Oral diltiazem (60 to 90 mg every 8 or 6 hours) is also effective treatment. Oral beta-adrenergic blocking agents may also chronically suppress paroxysmal supraventricular tachycardia. A regimen of nadolol (80 to 160 mg daily) has been shown to be useful in preventing paroxysmal supraventricular tachycardia. Each of these medications must be administered cautiously to patients with left ventricular dysfunction, as clinical exacerbation of congestive heart failure may occur with therapy. Digitalis preparations also suppress recurrent episodes of paroxysmal supraventricular tachycardia, and digoxin (0.125 to 0.25 mg daily) would be the initial oral agent in patients with left ventricular dysfunction.

Premature atrial and ventricular complexes often initiate paroxysmal supraventricular tachycardia. Therefore, therapy with quinidine (gluconate, 324 to 648 mg every 8 hours), procainamide (500 to 1,000 mg every 6 hours with sustained-release preparations), disopyramide (100 to 200 mg every 8 hours), flecainide* (100 to 200 mg every 12 hours), or encainide* (25 to 50 mg every 8 hours) may be clinically efficacious by reducing or eliminating these initiating events. These antiarrhythmic medications may also work by prolonging conduction and refractoriness of the atrium, His-Purkinje system, retrograde fast AV nodal pathway, ventricular myocardium, and anomalous AV connection. Since each of these antiarrhythmic agents may induce significant proarrhythmic ventricular ectopy, a 12-lead electrocardiogram and/or 24-hour ambulatory monitoring may be indicated in selected patients shortly after initiating therapy. In addition, the negative inotropic and dromotropic effects of flecainide, encain-

ide, and disopyramide preclude the use of these agents in patients with reduced left ventricular ejection function (ejection fraction less than 40 percent) and in those with significant conduction disturbances such as complete left bundle branch block, bifascicular block, Mobitz type II block, and high-degree AV block.

In symptomatic patients whose disorder is resistant to therapy with conventional antiarrhythmic medications, amiodarone* (100 to 400 mg daily) may be effective in preventing episodes of paroxysmal supraventricular tachycardia by preventing ectopic complexes and by prolonging conduction and refractoriness in the cardiac tissues composing the reentrant circuit. Unfortunately, the side effects of amiodarone therapy, including tremor, ataxia, corneal microdeposits, thyroid dysfunction, skin discoloration and rash, hepatotoxicity, and potentially fatal pulmonary fibrosis preclude its long-term use in all but the most difficult circumstances. Nonpharmacologic approaches for the prevention of paroxysmal supraventricular tachycardia in young patients are usually preferable to long-term therapy with amiodarone. In elderly patients for whom nonpharmacologic therapy is contraindicated, amiodarone therapy to prevent recurrent, symptomatic paroxysmal supraventricular tachycardia may be desirable.

Not infrequently it may be necessary to use a combination drug therapy for better control of chronic paroxysmal supraventricular tachycardia. The concept of combination therapy is twofold: (1) to have additive or synergistic effects of two antiarrhythmic agents, and (2) to reduce side effects by lowering the dose of each agent. Various combinations can be used clinically: digoxin with a calcium channel blocking agent (e.g., diltiazem) or a beta-receptor blocking agent (e.g., propranolol), a calcium channel blocking agent with a beta-receptor blocking agent, and an AV nodal depressant agent (e.g., digoxin, diltiazem, or propranolol) with a type I antiarrhythmic agent (e.g., quinidine). The latter combination is to treat both limbs of the reentrant pathway of AV nodal reentry or AV reciprocation. In addition, type I antiarrhythmic agents suppress atrial and/or ventricular premature beats, which are commonly the initiating events for paroxysmal supraventricular tachycardia.

With combination therapy, the possibility of drug interactions should be considered. The combination of two AV nodal depressants such as digoxin with diltiazem or diltiazem with propranolol can markedly depress sinus and AV node function, thereby leading to significant sinus pause or advanced AV nodal block or both. Quinidine, verapamil, diltiazem, and amiodarone can increase serum digoxin levels, thereby inducing digoxin toxicity. Amiodarone is also known to raise serum levels of many antiarrhythmic agents (e.g., quinidine, procainamide, disopyramide, and propranolol). Conse-

---

*Flecainide, encainide, and amiodarone are approved for use in the United States only in patients with life-threatening ventricular arrhythmias.

quently, proarrhythmic effects, precipitation of AV block, and worsened congestive heart failure have been observed. To avoid these adverse side effects, dose titration and careful monitoring of serum drug levels are essential during combination drug therapy.

SUGGESTED READING

DiMarco JP, Sellers TP, Lerman BB, et al. Diagnostic and therapeutic use of adenosine in patients with supraventricular tachycardia. J Am Coll Cardiol 1985; 6:417–425.

Huycke EC, Sung RJ, Dias VC, et al. Intravenous diltiazem for termination of reentrant supraventricular tachycardia: A placebo-controlled, randomized, double-blind, multicenter study. J Am Coll Cardiol 1989; 13:538–544.

Shen EN, Keung E, Huycke E, et al. Intravenous propafenone for termination of reentrant supraventricular tachycardia: A placebo-controlled, randomized, double-blind, crossover study. Ann Intern Med 1986; 105:655–661.

Sung RJ, Chang MS, Chiang BN. Clinical electrophysiology of supraventricular tachycardia. Cardiol Clin 1983; 1:225–251.

Sung RJ, Elser B, McAllister RG. Intravenous verapamil for termination of reentrant supraventricular tachycardia. Ann Intern Med 1980; 93:682–689.

PAROXYSMAL REENTRANT SUPRAVENTRICULAR TACHYCARDIA WITHOUT PREEXCITATION: NONPHARMACOLOGIC THERAPY

GERALD V. NACCARELLI, M.D.

Supraventricular tachycardias can be subclassified into those that are primarily atrial in origin and those that are secondary to reentry utilizing the atrioventricular (AV) junction. Primary atrial tachycardias include atrial fibrillation, atrial flutter, and ectopic atrial tachycardia. Reentrant paroxysmal supraventricular tachycardias utilizing the AV junction include the typical and atypical forms of AV node reentrant tachycardia and orthodromic supraventricular tachycardia in patients with the Wolff-Parkinson-White syndrome. Other forms of supraventricular tachycardia that are uncommon and are not discussed here include sinus node reentrant tachycardia, intraatrial reentrant tachycardia, junctional ectopic tachycardia, and the permanent form of junctional reciprocating tachycardia.

The purpose of this chapter is to discuss nonpharmacologic therapies of patients with paroxysmal supraventricular tachycardia not related to the preexcitation syndromes. From a practical standpoint, the clinically common arrhythmias discussed are the primary atrial tachycardias, including ectopic atrial tachycardia, atrial fibrillation, and atrial flutter, and the most commonly occurring form of reentrant supraventricular tachycardia secondary to reentry within the AV node.

Although antiarrhythmic drugs are commonly used in patients with supraventricular tachycardia, they are not always successful in eliminating tachycardia recurrences. In addition, side effects may limit utilization of some of these drugs in selected patients. Because of this, nonpharmacologic therapies are an important part of the physician's armamentarium in treating such patients. The primary nonpharmacologic therapies used in the treatment of supraventricular tachycardia without preexcitation include cardiac pacing, catheter ablation, and surgery (Table 1). The uses and limitations of each of these therapies in patients with primary atrial and AV nodal reentrant tachycardia are addressed.

PACING TREATMENT OF SUPRAVENTRICULAR TACHYCARDIA

Pacing can be used to treat supraventricular tachycardia (1) to prevent the initiation of tachycardia, and (2) to terminate the supraventricular tachycardia once it has occurred.

Pacing has a very limited role in minimizing occurrences of primary atrial tachycardia. Overdrive pacing may play some role in preventing escape atrial complexes that can predispose to initiation of atrial tachycardias.

The primary use of antitachycardia pacing to prevent tachycardia is in patients with AV nodal reentrant tachycardia by using dual-chambered pacing devices that can be programmed to the atrial or atrioventricular synchronous mode. By synchronizing ventricular depolarizations to atrial activation, a premature complex previously able to initiate reentry is now followed by ventricular activation that can retrogradely conduct to the opposite end of the reentrant circuit and thus prevent the arrhythmia. A dual-chamber system capable of sensing either the atrial or ventricular electrograms and in turn triggering simultaneous AV stimulation (DDT pacing) has been used successfully in patients with refractory AV nodal reentrant tachycardia. All atrial and ventricular premature stimuli elicit simultaneous AV stimulation that results in impulse collision in the AV node and blocking of the initiation of the tachycardia.

The primary use of pacemakers for patients with supraventricular tachycardia has been for terminating the tachycardia once the arrhythmia has occurred. Pacing can be used successfully in terminating tachycardias that are reentrant in nature. Thus, from a practical standpoint, of the paroxysmal supraventricular tachycardias not associated with preexcitation, only atrial flutter and AV node reentrant tachycardia can be successfully treated using these techniques. Prior to implantation, the efficacy of pacing must be very carefully evaluated at the time of electrophysiologic study. The mechanism and the rate of the tachycardia and the reproducible termination with the proper antiarrhythmic pacing sequence have to be carefully studied. Avoidance of misrecognition of sinus tachycardia and the use of rate stability programs so that atrial fibrillation does not trigger the device must be considered. In patients without overt preexcitation, the risk of accelerating the tachycardia into atrial fibrillation usually does not cause significant hemodynamic compromise except for patients with a rapidly conducting AV node.

For patients with both atrial flutter and AV node reentrant tachycardia, our preferred approach is the use of antiarrhythmic drugs. However, in patients with refractory and/or rare recurrences of either of these tachycardias, properly prescribed antitachycardia pacing is appropriate. Fisher and colleagues reported a 93 percent 1-year and a 78 percent 5-year success rate of antitachycardia pacing in 15 patients with supraventricular tachycardia. In some patients, antitachycardia pacing can be used in combination with antiarrhythmic drugs. That is, in patients with very frequent episodes of tachycardia, antiarrhythmic drugs can be used to minimize the number of recurrences of tachycardia, with a pacemaker automatically treating the breakthrough recurrences.

Table 1 Nonpharmacologic Treatment of Supraventricular Tachycardia without Preexcitation

Pacing
Prevention of tachycardia recurrence
Termination of tachycardia

Catheter Ablation
AV junction modification/ablation
Ectopic focus ablation

Surgery
Excision/ablation of ectopic atrial focus
AV nodal modification/ablation
Microsurgery in AV modal reentrant tachycardia

Patient selection is critical in the proper prescription of an antitachycardia pacemaker used to automatically terminate the tachycardia. Patients with incessant tachycardia are not candidates for such treatment, since as soon as the tachycardia is terminated, the arrhythmia will be reinitiated. Patients who have frequent recurrences of tachycardia may also be a problem. Even if the device successfully terminates 95 percent of the tachycardias in a patient who is having daily recurrences, the patient may have several visits to the emergency room over 3 months. Therefore, these devices are most appropriate for patients whose tachycardia is refractory to drug treatment and who have infrequent recurrences of their arrhythmia. In certain patients who have only rare recurrences of their arrhythmia (less than 10 times per year), an antitachycardia pacemaker may be considered front-line therapy, since the patient can use this pacemaker to treat his or her arrhythmia without taking concomitant chronic antiarrhythmic therapy. Finally, in patients who have coexisting conduction abnormalities serious enough to warrant bradycardia pacing, the threshold to use an antitachycardia pacemaker in the AAIT or VVIT mode should be lower.

CATHETER ABLATION FOR SUPRAVENTRICULAR TACHYCARDIA

Catheter ablative techniques have recently been introduced as therapy for patients with drug-resistant cardiac arrhythmias (see the chapter *Ablation*). In patients with supraventricular tachycardia, catheter ablation can be used to modify or ablate the AV junction with resultant complete heart block, to ablate an ectopic atrial focus, or to alter the retrograde limb of the AV node reentrant tachycardia circuit.

In patients who are candidates for catheter ablation of the AV junction, a multiple electrode catheter is inserted by vein and placed in the region of the His bundle. A temporary pacemaker is placed in the right ventricle. Using defibrillator current, 150 to 300 joules are delivered from the catheter electrode (anode) showing the largest unipolar His deflection to an indifferent left posteroscapular patch that acts as the cathode. Radiofrequency energy can be used as an alternative to this technique, since the energy is more controllable and the patient does not require general anesthesia.

The results of AV junction ablation from the most recent report of the Percutaneous Cardiac Mapping and Ablation Registry (PCMAR) are shown in Table 2. Briefly, 65 percent of 552 patients had resultant third-degree AV block and were asymptomatic without antiarrhythmic drugs during follow-up. Modification of AV conduction without the production of complete AV block occurred in 20 percent. In 12 percent of patients, antiarrhythmic

Table 2 Percutaneous Cardiac Mapping and Ablation Registry—AV Junction Ablation

	$n = 552$
Third degree AV block	354 (65%)
Resumption of AV conduction	
Asymptomatic, no drugs	46 (8%)
Asymptomatic, drugs	64 (12%)
Unsuccessful	88 (16%)
Follow-up = 23±18 months	

drugs were required after AV modification, whereas in 8 percent drug therapy was not needed. Results of AV junction ablation using radiofrequency ablation are still preliminary. However, it appears that successful complete ablation can be attained in the majority of patients. In addition, since energy is more carefully delivered, modification of the AV junction can be attained in a higher percentage of patients. If radiofrequency energy is not effective in modifying the AV junction, we proceed with defibrillator-catheter ablation.

Catheter ablation of an atrial ectopic focus can be performed after careful mapping of the arrhythmia. Isolated case reports have suggested successful therapy. However, the success rate is not as high as with AV junction ablations, and there is concern about atrial perforation.

Recent reports predominantly using radiofrequency catheter ablation have suggested that modification of the retrograde limb of the fast pathway in patients with slow-fast AV node reentry can periodically be attained. Rare development of complete antegrade AV block has occurred as a complication of this technique.

Complications from catheter ablation have included hypotension secondary to barotrauma, cardiac perforation and tamponade, intracardiac embolization and thrombosis, pericarditis, and development of new arrhythmogenic foci. In addition, in patients who have preexisting pacemakers, damage to either the pacemaker generator or the electrode has rarely occurred.

In patients with rapid ventricular rates from their atrial tachycardias, it is our current practice to consider AV junction ablation if antiarrhythmic drugs have not been successful. Catheter ablation should be considered before cryosurgical ablation of the AV node. Obviously these patients become permanently pacemaker-dependent because of their complete heart block, and this is a limitation of this approach. Since AV synchrony cannot be maintained with pacing because of refractory atrial arrhythmias, we usually insert a ventricular demand rate-responsive permanent pacemaker following ablation of the AV junction. We feel that catheter

ablation of the AV junction is a safer and more effective alternative to catheter or surgical ablation of the primary atrial focus.

SURGICAL APPROACHES TO SUPRAVENTRICULAR TACHYCARDIA

Surgery for patients with supraventricular tachycardia has primarily involved surgical ablation of the accessory AV connections of patients with Wolff-Parkinson-White syndrome. In patients with supraventricular tachycardia not associated with the preexcitation syndromes, three main surgical operations have been performed: (1) excision and/or ablation of an atrial ectopic focus, (2) cryosurgical ablation of the AV node, and (3) microsurgery in patients with AV node reentrant tachycardia.

In patients with refractory ectopic atrial tachycardia, careful endocardial mapping in the electrophysiology lab and endocardial and epicardial mapping at the time of operation can help localize the origin of the tachycardia. Surgical excision or cryosurgical ablation of this focus can be successfully performed.

In patients with rapid atrial tachyarrhythmias that are not controlled with drugs or catheter ablation, intraoperative mapping of the His bundle can be performed followed by cryosurgery of the AV junction. In a study by Marchese and coworkers, complete AV block was produced in 86 percent of patients in the cryosurgery group and in 88 percent of patients in the catheter ablation group. Chronic antiarrhythmic therapy was required in 36 percent and 27 percent of patients in the cryosurgical and catheter ablation groups, respectively. The short-term morbidity rate was lower among patients who underwent catheter ablation—only 12 percent compared with 42 percent in patients requiring surgery. Thus, catheter ablation is associated with less short-term morbidity and avoids the need for a major surgical procedure. It is therefore the preferable approach to ablation of the AV junction when permanent abolition of AV conduction is necessary. How-

Table 3 Surgical Treatment of AV Nodal Reentrant Tachycardia: Postoperative Observations

	Ross et al (Australia)*	Cox et al (St. Louis)†
Patients	10	8
Technique	Incision	Cryosurgery
Ventriculoatrial block	5	2
Recurrent supraventricular tachycardia	0	0
Follow-up (mo)	8±4	26±21

*J Am Coll Cardiol 1985; 6:1383
†Circulation 1987; 76:1329

Table 4 Supraventricular Tachycardias: Optimal Therapeutic Techniques

| | Therapeutic Technique | | | | |
	Guided Surgical Ablation	Catheter-Guided Electro-Coagulation*	HIS Bundle† Ablation	Drugs	Anti Tachycardia Pacing Systems
Atrial fibrillation	NA	NA	+++	++++	NA
Atrial flutter	+	+++	+++	++++	+
AVNRT	++	+++	+	+++	++
Atrial tachycardia	+	++	+++	++++	NA

*Technique under development.
†Rate control. Catheter or surgical ablation.
+ = Application is site-dependent.
AVNRT = AV nodal reentrant tachycardia.
NA = Not applicable.

ever, despite the usefulness of AV junction ablation, we have had to perform surgical ablation of AV conduction in several patients who failed to have satisfactory responses to catheter ablation.

In patients with AV nodal reentrant tachycardia, operative approaches that preserve antigrade AV nodal conduction have been described by Ross and associates and Cox and coworkers (Table 3). In Ross' study, a surgical incision through the right atrial wall 2 mm above the tricuspid annulus is extended from a point lateral to the mouth of the coronary sinus to the apex of the triangle of Koch. Further appropriate surgical ablation depends on retrograde atrial activation sequence mapping during tachycardia. Cox has performed similar surgery employing a cryoprobe during normothermic cardiopulmonary bypass. In this approach, a series of cryolesions is produced in the region of the coronary sinus to the apex of Koch's triangle. The reasons for the success of these surgical procedures are unclear. Ventriculoatrial conduction was often intact although usually altered after these operations. In most patients, dual antegrade AV nodal physiology cannot be demonstrated postoperatively. Some of the success of this operation may be secondary to damaging local autonomic nervous system input to the AV node. At this time, it is our feeling that surgical approaches for AV nodal reentry should be used only in patients whose disease is refractory to other therapies since the initial results for AV node surgery are encouraging but remain investigational.

In patients with ectopic atrial tachycardia in whom antiarrhythmic drugs have failed, we prefer catheter ablation of the AV junction with good rate control in place of surgical excision or ablation of the ectopic atrial focus, since many patients have more than one focus of atrial tachycardia, and thus extensive surgical approaches with atrial excision as part of the operation may be required. We feel that this approach would be limited to patients in whom other therapies have failed.

Table 4 lists our current preferences for nonpharmacologic and pharmacologic therapy for patients with supraventricular tachycardia that is not associated with overt preexcitation.

SUGGESTED READING

Cox JL, Holman WL, Cain ME. Cryosurgical treatment of atrioventricular node reentrant tachycardia. Circulation 1987; 67:1329–1336.

Evans GT, Scheinman MM, Zipes DP, et al. The Percutaneous Cardiac Mapping and Ablation Registry, final summary of results. PACE 1988; 11:1621–1626.

Fisher JD, Johnston DR, Furman S, et al. Long-term efficacy of antitachycardia pacing for supraventricular and ventricular tachycardias. Am J Cardiol 1987; 60:1311–1316.

Fisher JD, Kim SG, Mercando AD. Electrical devices for treatment of arrhythmias. Am J Cardiol 1988; 61:45A–57A.

Marchese AC, Pressley JC, Sintetos AL, et al. Cryosurgical versus catheter ablation of the AV junction. Am J Cardiol 1987; 59:870–873.

Osborn MJ, Holmes DR. Antitachycardia pacing. Clin Prog Electrophysiol Pacing 1985; 3:239–267.

Ross DL, Johnson DC, Denniss AR, et al. Curative surgery for atrioventricular junction ("AV nodal") reentrant tachycardia. J Am Coll Cardiol 1985; 6:1383–1392.

Scheinman MM. Catheter ablation of patients with cardiac arrhythmias. PACE 1986; 9:551–564.

Seals AA, Lawrie GM, Magro S, et al. Surgical treatment of right atrial focal tachycardia in adults. J Am Coll Cardiol 1988; 11:1111–1117.

SUPRAVENTRICULAR TACHYCARDIA IN PEDIATRIC PATIENTS

ROBERT M. HAMILTON, M.D.
ARTHUR GARSON JR., M.D.

Supraventricular tachycardia (SVT) is defined as a rapid heart rate resulting from an abnormal mechanism that requires tissues proximal to the bifurcation of the bundle of His. Atrial flutter and fibrillation also fit this definition but are usually discussed separately from SVT.

The management of pediatric SVT is made unique by the developmental electrophysiologic differences present as childhood progresses. Conduction intervals through the atrioventricular (AV) node and His-Purkinje system are generally shorter in children than in adults, and tachycardia rates are faster. Retrograde conduction through the AV node is present in 80 percent of pediatric patients.

Autonomic innervation of the heart of younger patients is incomplete. Newborn and infant hearts demonstrate a higher degree of adrenergic tone. Simple vagal maneuvers are less successful in young children, particularly in those under the age of 4 years. However, the more complex dive reflex may be very effective in children.

Drug dosing for children must be modified according to age, weight, and body surface area. The profile of side effects of many antiarrhythmic medications is modified in pediatric patients.

Finally, the relative risks of surgical versus medical management are different in children. Patients with most types of SVT have excellent chances of surgical cure of their tachycardia. This approach may be preferable to the long-term risks of medical management of their tachycardia over an expected normal life span.

DIAGNOSIS

Heart rates exceeding 230 beats per minute are present in the majority (60 percent) of pediatric patients with SVT, and this is a useful figure to remember because sinus tachycardia almost never exceeds this rate. A narrow QRS complex is present in 92 percent of patients. The QRS complex is the same as in sinus rhythm in 98 percent of patients with SVT. P waves are visible in 56 percent.

The mechanism of SVT can usually be discerned from the history and the electrocardiogram (ECG) during SVT (Table 1). The most common types of paroxysmal SVT in childhood are those caused by an accessory AV connection of the Kent type (60 to 70 percent of all SVT). Approximately half of those with Kent SVT have manifest preexcitation (WPW). The next most common type is typical AV node re-entry.

The incessant tachycardias are more common in children than in adults (15 to 20 percent of all pediatric SVT). The most common is atrial ectopic SVT, followed by the permanent form of junctional reciprocating tachycardia.

Invasive electrophysiologic testing is usually reserved for preoperative evaluation. In the rare infant or toddler who requires invasive diagnosis or assessment of treatment, transesophageal pacing and recording of atrial electrograms provide a useful substitute for direct catheter recordings. Nonetheless, invasive electrophysiologic testing can be performed in infants younger than 6 months if necessary, especially using custom catheters with 1 to 2 mm interelectrode distances.

THERAPY OF ACUTE EPISODES

The approach to a new patient in tachycardia depends on the clinical presentation. All patients receive immediate preparation for possible cardioversion, including attaching monitor leads and obtaining a synchronized electrocardiographic signal. If the patient is extremely ill with absent pulses, mottled skin, or marked diaphoresis, cardioversion is performed with 0.5 to 2 watts-second per kilogram of energy. In all cases, we attempt to record a 12-lead ECG in tachycardia before conversion.

Our first choice in converting stable patients with SVT is atrial esophageal overdrive pacing with either an electrode catheter (infants) or pill electrode (older cooperative children). A portable stimulator capable of generating a wide pulse width is required, and we usually start with 9.9 msec and 10 to 20 mA of current. Sedation is required during pacing and is achieved with either midazolam, 0.035 per kilogram intravenously, or ketamine, 1 mg per kilogram intravenously. Sedation is best administered following swallowing of the pill electrode in older patients.

We consider this approach to have many advantages. Confirmation by atrial electrogram of the P-R interval in SVT provides information on the tachycardia mechanism. The reentrant nature of the tachycardia is confirmed by its response to overdrive pacing. The bradycardia following conversion that is frequently found with vagal and drug therapies can be avoided, and direct current cardioversion and its potential complications can usually be avoided.

Initiation of a dive reflex by an icebag applied to the face is also an appropriate first measure, particularly if esophageal pacing is not available or if the tachycardia mechanism has already been established by either previous diagnosis or surface ECG. This

Table 1 Electrocardiographic Characteristics of Types of Supraventricular Tachycardia

	Incessant/ Paroxysmal	Conduction	P Wave	P-R Interval	Oscillation/ Warm-up
Reentry without Bypass Tract					
Sinus node reentry	P	2°	Sinus	N to L	No
Atrial muscle reentry	P	2°	Not sinus	N to L	No
Atrioventricular node reentry	P	1:1	LSRA or absent	Zero	Osc
His Bundle reentry	P	AVD or 1:1	Sinus or LSRA	Dissoc	No
Reentry with Bypass Tract					
Wolff-Parkinson-White symdrome	P/l	1:1	Not sinus	L	Osc
Concealed Wolff-Parkinson-White syndrome	P/l	1:1	Not sinus	L	Osc
Permanent form of junctional reciprocal tachycardia	l	1:1	Late, LSRA	N to L	Osc
SVT using Mahaim-fiber	P	AVD or 1:1	Sinus or LSRA	Dissoc	No
SVT using James fiber	P	1:1	LSRA	LSRA	Osc
Automatic					
Atrial ectopic tachycardia	l	2°	High but not sinus	L	W/U
Junctional ectopic tachycardia	l	AVD	Sinus	Dissoc	W/U
Triggered					
Nonparoxysmal junctional tachycardia	l	AVD	Sinus or AF, AFl	Dissoc	No

AVD = AV dissociation, LSRA = low septal right atrium, Osc = oscillating, W/U = warm-up, No = neither oscillation nor warm-up, Dissoc = dissociation.

reflex is present from birth to adulthood. It is a strong vagal stimulating reflex and produces withdrawal of sympathetic tone. It is best produced by placing a bag of crushed ice or an ice-cold wet facecloth over the patient's face for 10 to 30 seconds. Other vagal maneuvers may also be attempted, either singly or in combination. We avoid the use of ocular pressure, since it may cause retinal detachment.

Drug dosages for termination of acute SVT are given in Table 2. We generally prefer to avoid drugs in acute SVT if possible, since complications are relatively common. For example, intravenous verapamil may cause apnea, bradycardia, and hypotension in young infants. In patients beyond the first year of age who are not in congestive heart failure,

verapamil can be used if reentrant SVT involving the AV node is suspected. Intravenous calcium chloride should be available for administration if severe bradycardia or hypotension occurs. Pretreatment with calcium chloride may be useful in attenuating the adverse hemodynamic effects in older children. We avoid the use of intravenous verapamil in any child regardless of age if we have not seen a sinus rhythm ECG. Some children have narrow QRS ventricular tachycardia, and verapamil is contraindicated in these patients. Intravenous verapamil is 90 percent effective in converting reentrant SVT and remains a useful drug therapy in acute cases in children beyond infancy with SVT.

Adenosine is frequently successful in terminating acute reentrant tachycardia involving the AV

Table 2 Pediatric Dosing of Intravenous Antiarrhythmic Agents

Drug	Loading Dose	Maintenance Dose	Therapeutic Level
Procainamide	10–15 mg/kg*†	30–80 µg/kg/min	4–10 µg/ml
Propafenone	2 mg/kg	4–7 µg/kg/min	0.5–1.5
Propranolol	0.1–0.2 mg/kg		
Verapamil	0.075–0.150 mg/kg‡		
Adenosine	0.1–0.25 mg/kg	5 µg/kg/min	
Phenylephrine	0.005–0.01 mg/kg		
Edrophonium	0.1–0.2 mg/kg		
Neostigmine	0.05 mg/kg		

*No faster than 0.5 mg/kg/min.
†Over 100 min (i.e. give 0.2 mg/kg IV every 10 min for 10 doses).
‡Over 1 min.

node. Its half-life is 10 to 15 seconds, and side effects are limited to transient dyspnea and flushing.

Propafenone has occasionally been used for the treatment of life-threatening junctional ectopic tachycardia if other methods of stabilization and therapy are insufficient. It has moderate negative inotropic effects that frequently require volume loading, and hypotension is a frequent complication in the postoperative patient in whom this arrhythmia most frequently occurs.

Intravenous procainamide prolongs the refractory period of the accessory connection and is capable of terminating and preventing reentrant SVT utilizing a Kent bundle. In addition, procainamide may occasionally be a useful agent in slowing junctional tachycardia in symptomatic patients.

Intravenous propranolol is moderately effective in the treatment of reentrant SVT, particularly if it involves the AV node in the circuit. However, its effect is limited by its negative inotropic action. It should be avoided in patients with any evidence of congestive heart failure and may result in cardiac decompensation even in patients who present without congestive heart failure.

Pharmacologic vagal stimulation may be achieved with a number of drugs. Phenylephrine induces a vagal reflex. Blood pressure may become markedly elevated, and after the tachycardia breaks, a severe bradycardia may occur. Phenylephrine increases cardiac afterload by causing vasoconstriction, and if the tachycardia does not break, cardiac output may markedly decrease. Edrophonium and neostigmine, both relatively short-acting anticholinesterases, are also capable of chemically producing vagal effects, but not without side effects, which may last from a few minutes to a few hours. Although these agents are used in some institutions, we have not used them, preferring physical methods, including synchronized cardioversion.

LONG-TERM DRUG THERAPY

In the majority of children with SVT, the arrhythmia recurs. Recurrence is not predictable in the individual patient. Death, although rare, does occur in SVT patients, including those with apparently normal hearts and uncomplicated SVT mechanisms. The sudden nature of symptoms of syncope and presyncope results in a marked alteration in daily activities in many patients. For these reasons, we treat all patients with paroxysmal SVT for 1 year after their first episode. We then discontinue the drug and reinstitute therapy only if SVT recurs. Some centers have advocated esophageal study after drug therapy has been discontinued in an attempt to assess the residual substrate for SVT. We have only rarely done this, since it may not predict the likelihood of recurrent SVT. Some teenagers are reluctant

to take antiarrhythmic drugs; if their episodes are infrequent and self-terminating, we are less insistent on treatment.

The duration of therapy depends on the likelihood that the underlying mechanism will resolve. Accessory pathways present in infancy may resolve with age. This may be related to autonomic changes or to further cardiac development and more complete insulation of the AV ring. However, our experience indicates that an accessory pathway present at 5 years of age is likely to persist. In a review of 140 patients with the Wolff-Parkinson-White syndrome, we found a 78 percent long-term recurrence rate of SVT in patients who had SVT after 5 years of age.

A small proportion of automatic tachycardias resolve with time. We continue drugs in these patients for 1 year after sinus rhythm is achieved and then discontinue the drug to see if SVT reappears. If tachycardia-related cardiomyopathy has occurred and cardiac function has not returned to normal, we may continue drugs longer than 1 year.

Historically, digitalis was the first medical treatment of SVT and was very effective in most patients. With the recognition of digitalis-related deaths in adults and some children with the Wolff-Parkinson-White syndrome, therapy was modified to include electrophysiologic study of accessory pathway conduction and its response to cardiac glycosides prior to the institution of digoxin. Those patients with acceleration of accessory pathway conduction with digoxin were treated with alternate agents. This approach was adapted to pediatrics, and esophageal pacing could be used to investigate infants. However, large patient numbers (not yet available) would be required to prove the success of this approach. Our current policy is to avoid treatment with digoxin in infants and children of any age who have the Wolff-Parkinson-White syndrome. The risk of sudden death in such children taking digoxin is 2 to 4 percent. This must be compared with the risk of taking other drugs as well as with the risk of nontreatment. At present, the use of digoxin in infants continues to be controversial; in those over 8 to 10 years of age, atrial fibrillation is more likely to occur and digoxin is used even less frequently.

Propranolol is our first line of long-term therapy in most infants and children with SVT. This drug has an extremely low incidence of complications and side effects in children and is moderately effective. However, it should not be used in children with reactive airway disease. In addition, hypoglycemia has been reported in children taking beta blockers, especially during periods of reduced oral intake.

Long-term therapy with verapamil is moderately effective in reentrant SVT with or without a bypass tract. If the above medications are not effective, quinidine therapy may be instituted, but infants and children frequently do not tolerate the gastrointestinal effects of nausea, vomiting, diarrhea, and abdominal pain. Side effects of quinidine require discontinuation of therapy in 10 to 30 percent of patients. Quinidine syncope is a dangerous side effect that is more common in children with structural heart disease, and it is considered to be secondary to torsades de pointes. Unfortunately, the QT interval is not predictive of which children will develop torsades de pointes.

Digoxin may be used in patients with AV node reentry or with true concealed Wolff-Parkinson-White syndrome (who have never demonstrated antegrade AV conduction over an accessory pathway). Patients with any evidence of antegrade accessory pathway conduction, even only during evoked potential study, are excluded.

The place of class IC agents such as flecainide has not yet been established. These drugs have been extremely effective in children with SVT. However, there have been reports of proarrhythmia.

Knowledge of the pharmacokinetics of pediatric antiarrhythmic agents is limited. Infants have decreased rates of gastric absorption and emptying, and young children have an increased volume of distribution, both leading to relatively decreased plasma concentration of drug for a given dose. However, most drug metabolic and elimination pathways have decreased function in the first 6 months of life, followed by "hyperfunction" during childhood as compared with in adulthood. In general, the summation of these factors leads to prolonged drug half-lives in the first 6 months of life, followed by shortened drug half-lives up to adolescence.

The most accurate practical method for determination of drug dosages in children is adjustment for body surface area. For some drugs, the dose per square meter of body surface area has been developed. For others, the only available measure is by body weight (Table 3).

Quinidine

Quinidine continues to be an effective drug for treatment of SVT, but it has been replaced to a large extent by medications with less apparent toxicity. Pacemaker placement is recommended in those who have or are at risk for sick sinus syndrome. This is particularly true in patients who have had a Mustard or a Senning atrial switch procedure for D-transposition of the great vessels. This is less clear after a Fontan procedure. In the presence of normal AV conduction with sick sinus syndrome, we place an AAI pacemaker. Atrial pacing is sufficient because the yearly incidence of AV conduction disease in pediatric patients with sick sinus syndrome is relatively low (2 percent per year) and does not justify the placement of a dual-chamber device.

Procainamide

Procainamide is very effective in the acute treatment of many forms of SVT. Conduction block in accessory connections can frequently be achieved, and automatic forms of tachycardia can frequently be slowed. Long-term use is usually avoided because of the risk of drug-induced systemic lupus erythematosus in a growing child.

Moricizine

Moricizine is effective in reentry but has been particularly effective in suppressing atrial ectopic tachycardia.

Flecainide

A recent preliminary report has questioned the safety of flecainide on the basis of its use in adults with myocardial infarction. The relevance of this

Table 3 Pediatric Dosing of Oral Antiarrhythmic Agents

Drug	Daily Dosage	Interval	Therapeutic Level
Quinidine	15–60 mg/kg	6(8)	2–6 μg/ml
Procainamide	50–100 mg/kg	3–4(6–8)	4–8 μg/ml
Disopyramide	6–14 mg/kg	6(12)	2–5 μg/ml
Flecainide	100–250 mg/m^2	12(8)	0.2–1.0 μg/ml
Encainide	60–120 mg/m^2	8(12)	
Propafenone	150–600 mg/m^2	8	0.5–1.5 μg/ml†
Moricizine	5–15 mg/kg	6	
Propranolol	2.5–5 mg/kg	6	
Atenolol	1–2 mg/kg	24(12)	
Nadolol	1–2 mg/kg		
Metoprolol			
Verapamil	4–7 mg/kg	8	
Amiodarone	5 mg/kg	24	1–2.5 μg/ml
Sotalol	80–320 mg*	12	

*Adult dosage available only.
†Preliminary data.

study to the use of flecainide in treatment of pediatric SVT is questionable.

In children with SVT, the slowing of accessory pathway conduction without complete block may result in more frequent or incessant tachycardia. Proarrhythmia of this type may be related to a low flecainide concentration during initiation of therapy, and if this is confirmed by a serum trough flecainide concentration, increasing the flecainide dose should be attempted. Trough drug levels should be assessed five half-lives following a dosage change. A 20 to 30 percent prolongation of the QRS complex duration with flecainide generally correlates with an excessively high concentration. If incessant SVT occurs, additional temporary arrhythmia control may be accomplished with intravenous procainamide until the flecainide concentration increases. The presence of a new ventricular arrhythmia at any drug concentration or the presence of SVT despite a therapeutic flecainide concentration indicates failure of drug treatment.

Pacemaker lead threshold increases are known to occur during flecainide therapy and warrant an increased frequency of pacemaker checks during the initiation of therapy.

Flecainide was able to control or partially control 18 of 25 (72 percent) patients with paroxysmal SVT, 7 of 7 patients with permanent junctional reciprocating tachycardia, and 7 of 8 patients with atrial ectopic tachycardia. Proarrhythmia of the incessant SVT type occurred in 5 of 25 (20 percent) of patients with SVT caused by a Kent bundle. We have had two major overdoses occur in children, one as a suicide gesture and one as a formulation error by an independent pharmacy. In both cases, serum drug levels of 2 μg/per milliliter were attained, and in both they resolved within 12 hours. Transient slow ventricular tachycardia occurred in one patient.

Propafenone

Propafenone is currently undergoing investigation in the treatment of pediatric SVT. Propafenone may produce a moderate elevation of plasma digoxin levels. Propafenone is occasionally used with some success in junctional ectopic tachycardias in children. Although control of reentrant SVT can often be achieved with propafenone, it has not yet undergone sufficient investigation in children. Because it frequently slows atrial flutter rate significantly and only mildly slows conduction through the AV node, patients may be at risk of developing 1:1 AV conduction with atrial ectopic SVT or atrial flutter. In our experience with children, drug levels above 1.5 μg/per milliliter predict proarrhythmia and should be assessed during institution of therapy. The effect of propafenone on pacemaker thresholds has not been evaluated.

Encainide

In children, encainide has a relatively high incidence of proarrhythmia, particularly in patients with severe arrhythmias and poor ventricular function. It also has an extremely short duration of action and excessive QRS interval prolongation, especially in the youngest patients with rapid sinus rates, possibly owing to its frequency-dependent effects. In our practice its use has been supplanted by other agents.

Amiodarone

We have evaluated the use of amiodarone in children for both ventricular and supraventricular arrhythmias. The drug was effective in 21 of 28 patients treated for SVT. Side effects were common, particularly photosensitive skin reaction, but all side effects resolved with discontinuation or reduction of the drug dose. Growth was unimpaired.

Sotalol

Sotalol, which combines class III effects with beta-blocking activity, is currently under investigation as an antiarrhythmic agent in children.

Verapamil

This calcium channel blocking agent has negative inotropic effects. There is some evidence that the immature myocardium is more prone to these effects. Therefore, intravenous verapamil should not be used in infants less than 1 year of age or in patients in congestive heart failure. Verapamil should not be administered in patients receiving beta blockers. Oral verapamil may be used with caution in young patients.

Digoxin

Recommendations for oral digoxin dosing are given in Table 4. Digoxin interacts with verapamil, quinidine, flecainide, amiodarone, and propafenone, and dosage adjustments may need to be made when these agents are used concomitantly.

Table 4 Recommended Oral Digoxin Dosage

Age	Digitalizing Dosage (μg/kg/24 hr)	Maintenance Dosage (μg/kg/24 hr)
Premature	20	5
Full term <2 mo	30	8–10
Infants <2 yr	40–50	10–12
Children >2 yr	30–40	8–10
Adults	1.25 mg–1.5 mg total dosage	0.25 mg/day total dosage

SURGICAL TREATMENT

Kent Bundles (Accessory AV Connections)

Patient Selection. Currently, we recommend surgical treatment in patients with Kent bundles (Wolff-Parkinson-White or concealed Wolff-Parkinson-White syndrome) in the following circumstances:

1. Syncope or cardiac arrest with the Wolff-Parkinson-White syndrome (with documentation of extremely rapid SVT or atrial fibrillation with rapid ventricular response based on electrophysiologic study).
2. Failure to control clinical episodes of SVT with conventional drugs.
3. SVT and the Wolff-Parkinson-White syndrome with short antegrade refractory period of the accessory connection and potential noncompliance with medication.
4. Patients requesting surgical cure of SVT.
5. In asymptomatic patients with a short antegrade effective refractory period of the Kent bundle, the slight increase in risk of syncope and/or sudden death is discussed and surgery is recommended only if the patient plays a hazardous sport or has a hazardous occupation.

Surgery is usually not performed in infants under 18 months of age because of the need for prior electrophysiologic catheterization, including coronary sinus mapping. The small size of the basilic vein that is entered percutaneously, the stiffness of electrode catheters, and the relatively small size of the coronary sinus make the procedure more difficult in patients under this age. Nonetheless, we have successfully performed surgery in infants as young as 3 months old with absolutely drug-refractory SVT.

At Texas Children's Hospital, atrial disconnecting operations are performed for left or right lateral free wall pathways and cryoablation is performed for septal or paraseptal pathways. This surgery is performed on cardiopulmonary bypass but requires a relatively short cardiopulmonary bypass time.

Our success rate in the surgical ablation of Kent bundles is now 95 percent, with no deaths in the last 110 patients. There have been no late recurrences and no late occurrence of atrial flutter or ventricular tachycardia. The use of a transverse inframammary incision has made this a much more cosmetically acceptable operation in female patients.

Permanent Form of Junctional Reentrant Tachycardia

Surgery for permanent junctional reentrant tachycardia involves ablation of a slowly conducting accessory connection, with its atrial connection inserting inside the mouth of the coronary sinus or in the posterior atrial septum. We have been successful at ablating this pathway in eight surgical patients by performing atrial endocardial mapping and cryoablation of the atrial location. The risk of cryoablation is the production of permanent AV block, which occurred in our smallest and youngest patient (18 months old).

Atrial Ectopic SVT

Atrial ectopic tachycardia is treated surgically when medical therapy fails to prevent symptoms or when episodes of tachycardia remain frequent and are associated with decreased ventricular function. We have also performed "elective" operations in patients who have had atrial ectopic tachycardia longer than 1 year (to be sure it does not spontaneously resolve) and who no longer wish to take medication. Preoperative mapping is particularly important in this lesion, as the rhythm disturbance is not inducible by electrical stimulation and may not be present at the time of operative mapping.

Surgical treatment of atrial ectopic tachycardia generally involves cardiopulmonary bypass with excision of the area of earliest atrial activation and cryoablation of the edges of the incision. We have successfully ablated 18 of 20 right atrial foci and 9 of 9 left atrial foci. There have been no deaths, and the tachycardia-related cardiomyopathy, when present, has resolved in all patients.

Direct current catheter ablation has been performed for atrial ectopic tachycardia. Although temporary success has been reported, these arrhythmias have recurred, and we have abandoned this technique in children.

Junctional Ectopic SVT

Surgical treatment of drug-refractory junctional ectopic tachycardia has been limited to His bundle ablation, necessitating back-up pacemaker placement. In older children, these procedures may be performed transvenously. In our experience, even aggressive surgical His bundle ablation through the right atrium has been unsuccessful at controlling some patients with this tachycardia, suggesting that the SVT is located in a left-sided His bundle, or in one of the bundle branches, or even in the summit of the ventricular septum.

AV Node Reentry

Recently we have successfully treated life-threatening, drug-resistant AV node reentry in 3 of 3 patients with cryotherapy to achieve modification of AV nodal conduction without AV block. Perinodal freezing was performed at multiple sites through a right atriotomy to the point where second-degree AV block and short periods (less than 10 seconds) of third-degree AV block were produced during the freezing. Follow-up electrophysiologic study 1 month later demonstrated no inducible SVT and loss of dual antegrade AV node conduction pattern as well as complete retrograde block.

THERAPEUTIC ALTERNATIVES

Although the current major choices for children with SVT are drug therapy or surgical cure, other therapeutic avenues continue to be explored. Antitachycardia pacemakers can potentially be used either primarily or to supplement drug therapy in the treatment of SVT, but they do not provide a cure and require repeated assessment, reprogramming, revision, and replacement.

Catheter ablation techniques are being adapted to pediatric SVT therapy. Our experience in both animal studies and clinical trials of direct current catheter ablation of atrial ectopic tachycardia suggests that this technique may be unsafe in pediatric patients because of the energies required. More controlled energy sources such as radiofrequency cath-eter ablation and laser catheter ablation should be further investigated.

We have on one occasion performed cardiac transplantation for a drug-resistant primary ventricular tachycardia with secondary cardiomyopathy in a 3-year-old child. Transplantation remains the most extreme option for life-threatening tachycardia when all other treatment options have failed.

SUGGESTED READING

Deal BJ, Keane JF, Gillette PC, Garson A Jr. Wolff-Parkinson-White syndrome and supraventricular tachycardia during infancy: Management and follow-up. J Am Coll Cardiol 1985; 5:130–135.

Gillette PC, Garson A. Pediatric cardiac dysrhythmias. Orlando: Grune & Stratton, 1981.

Moak JP. In: Garson A Jr, Bricker JT, McNamara DG, eds. Antiarrhythmic drugs in science and practice of pediatric cardiology. Philadelphia: Lea & Febiger, 1989.

Moak JP, Garson A. Newer antiarrhythmic drugs in children. Am Heart J 1987; 113:179–185.

Perry JC, McQuinn RL, Smith RT, et al. Flecainide acetate for resistant arrhythmias in the young: Efficacy and pharmacokinetics. J Am Coll Cardiol 1989; 14(1):185–191.

Schneeweiss A. Drug therapy in infants and children with cardiovascular diseases. Philadelphia: Lea & Febiger, 1986.

Webb CL, Dick M II, Rocchini AP, et al. Quinidine syncope in children. J Am Coll Cardiol 1987; 9:1031–1037.

IV PREEXCITATION SYNDROMES

PREEXCITATION SYNDROMES: DIAGNOSTIC AND MANAGEMENT STRATEGIES

MICHAEL E. CAIN, M.D.
BRUCE D. LINDSAY, M.D.

Ventricular preexcitation, based on analysis of the electrocardiogram, occurs in one to three per 1,000 individuals. Results of basic and clinical research have delineated the anatomic and pathophysiologic derangements that underlie ventricular preexcitation and have contributed immensely to formulating the clinical approach to patients with the Wolff-Parkinson-White (WPW) syndrome. The therapeutic options for the long-term management of patients with recurrent arrhythmias are summarized in Table 1. Significantly, the availability of several pharmacologic and nonpharmacologic approaches enables therapy to be tailored to the individual patient. This chapter reviews the seminal issues that are the basis of our management strategies for patients with WPW syndrome.

EMBRYOLOGY AND ANATOMY

Early during cardiac embryogenesis, atrial and ventricular myocardium are contiguous. The subsequent invagination of the atrial and ventricular septa and formation of the anulus fibrosus normally sever all atrioventricular (AV) connections except for the AV node/His bundle. Persistent AV connections that bypass all or portions of the AV node/His bundle complex are the anatomic substrates that underlie ventricular preexcitation. Defects in the continuity of the anulus fibrosus may account for the subendocardial location of many right-sided accessory pathways, particularly those associated with abnormalities in the development of the AV ring, and

may explain the high incidence of preexcitation syndromes in patients with Ebstein's anomaly. Left free wall pathways usually represent residual, subepicardial, AV bridges of myocardium that failed to regress during fetal development.

Morphologically, accessory pathways are strands of normal myocardium that bridge the AV groove at any point around the anulus fibrosus on either side of the heart except that portion of the mitral valve anulus between the right and left fibrous trigones. Because of the anatomic limitations imposed by the valve anulus and the epicardium overlying the AV groove, the atrial and ventricular insertions of accessory pathways must be between the valve anulus and the atrial and ventricular epicardial reflections, respectively. Accessory pathways are not located outside the epicardium or within the valve anulus but are confined to locations near the valve anulus, either within the fat pad of the AV groove or just beneath the epicardium overlying the AV groove.

Moreover, accessory pathways at posterior septal and anterior septal sites have complex anatomic relationships to the coronary circulation and normal AV conduction system. Posterior septal pathways occur within the pyramidal space bound anteriorly by the insertion of the atrial extension of the membranous septum into the right fibrous trigone and posteriorly by the epicardium overlying the crux of the heart. The lateral boundaries are formed by divergent walls of the left and right atria. Within this space is the AV nodal artery, the tendon of Tadaro, epicardial fat, and the proximal portion of the coronary sinus. The AV node and its proximal penetrating bundle lie within the triangle of Koch, immediately adjacent to the pyramidal space. Anterior septal pathways, which typically are located just anterior to the AV node, pass through the fat pad between the right and left fibrous trigones and the insertion of the right coronary artery into the AV groove. This path lies anterior to the membranous portion of the interatrial septum and is bounded by the pericardial reflection of the ascending aorta and medial wall of the right atrium. Understanding the anatomy of the AV groove is essential for the continued development of nonpharmacologic procedures as well as the explicit definition of the type of

Table 1 Therapeutic Options for Long-Term Management of Arrhythmia Patients

Pharmacologic Therapy
  Empirically versus electrophysiologically-guided selection
  Prophylactic versus intermittent administration

Nonpharmacologic Therapy
  Surgery
  Catheter ablation
  Antitachycardia devices

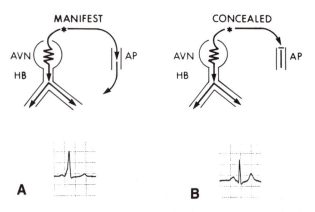

Figure 1 Atrioventricular conduction patterns and QRS morphologies during sinus rhythm for manifest (*A*) and concealed (*B*) accessory pathways. AVN = atrioventricular node, HB = His bundle, AP = accessory pathway.

damage to key structures that may result from surgical or catheter ablative techniques.

Several congenital abnormalities are associated with preexcitation syndrome. Foremost is Ebstein's anomaly, in which the incidence of WPW syndrome has been reported to be as high as 25 percent. Accessory pathways are most often located at right free wall or posterior septal sites. Moreover, multiple accessory pathways have been detected in up to 50 percent of these patients. In addition, Mahaim fibers have been described alone or in combination with an accessory pathway in patients with Ebstein's anomaly. Ventricular preexcitation has also been described in patients with coarctation of the aorta, hypertrophic cardiomyopathy, ventricular septal defects, and D-transposition of the great arteries.

PATHOPHYSIOLOGY

Accessory pathways may conduct antegrade, retrograde, or in both directions (Fig. 1). During sinus rhythm in patients with manifest preexcitation, the ventricles are activated through both the normal conduction system and the accessory pathway. Because accessory pathways do not usually exhibit the conduction delay characteristic of the AV node, ventricular activation adjacent to the accessory pathway occurs before propagation through the normal AV conduction system is complete. In contrast to the sharp onset and relatively narrow QRS characteristic of simultaneous activation of the right and left ventricles through the normal AV conduction system, eccentric activation of the ventricles through the accessory pathway slurs the QRS upstroke and prolongs its duration. This eccentric and premature activation of the ventricle is responsible for the altered QRS morphology and short P-R interval that are the electrocardiographic hallmarks of WPW syndrome.

The QRS pattern and the P-R interval depend on the relative contribution of conduction through the accessory pathway to ventricular activation and may show considerable temporal variation. Perturbations that delay conduction through the AV node, such as premature atrial depolarizations or an increase of vagal tone, result in preferential conduction through the accessory pathway and enhance-

ment in the degree of preexcitation evident on the electrocardiogram.

In contrast, antegrade ventricular activation during sinus rhythm is normal in patients having accessory pathways that conduct only retrogradely (concealed), and the electrocardiogram does not demonstrate preexcitation.

Patients with WPW syndrome are prone to orthodromic supraventricular tachycardia (SVT), antidromic SVT, and atrial fibrillation (Fig. 2). Orthodromic SVT (Fig. 3) is most common and accounts for 90 to 95 percent of the arrhythmias encountered clinically and induced in the electrophysiology laboratory. During orthodromic SVT,

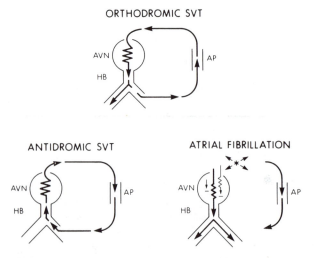

Figure 2 Schematic representation of the patterns of conduction through an accessory pathway (AP) and the normal conduction system (AVN-HB) during orthodromic SVT, antidromic SVT, and atrial fibrillation.

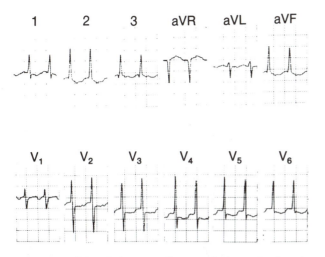

Figure 3 12-Lead electrocardiogram during orthodromic SVT. The QRS complex is normal in the absence of aberration in the His-Purkinje system or other underlying cardiac abnormalities. During SVT, atrial activation begins 70 to 110 msec after the onset of the QRS complex and requires 50 to 60 msec for completion. Consequently, the P wave occurs after the QRS complex and typically distorts the S-T segment in the first half of the R-R interval.

antegrade conduction to the ventricles is through the AV node/His-Purkinje system, and retrograde conduction to the atria is through the accessory pathway. The morphology of the QRS complex is normal unless aberration due to bundle branch block occurs. Orthodromic SVT utilizes a macro-reentrant circuit involving the atria, ventricles, the normal AV conduction system, and the accessory pathway, and it is terminated by AV or ventriculoatrial (VA) conduction block.

Antidromic SVT (Fig. 4) occurs spontaneously in 5 percent of patients and is inducible in 10 percent of patients with WPW syndrome. The antegrade limb is the accessory pathway, and the retrograde limb is either the normal conduction system or a second accessory pathway. Because the ventricles are activated exclusively through the accessory pathway, the QRS complex is maximally preexcited and may mimic that seen during ventricular tachycardia. Antidromic SVT also utilizes a macro-reentrant circuit that is terminated by AV or VA conduction block.

Atrial fibrillation is detectable in approximately 30 percent of patients with WPW syndrome and develops de novo or as a consequence of orthodromic or antidromic SVT. During atrial fibrillation, the ventricles are activated through the AV node/His-Purkinje system, the accessory pathway, or both, depending on the intrinsic electrophysiologic prop-

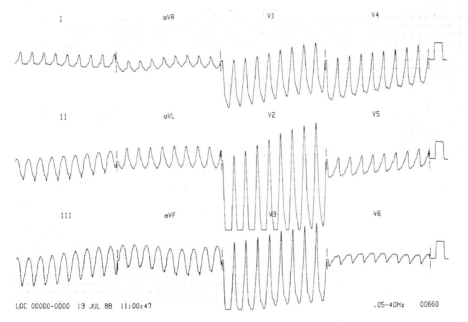

Figure 4 12-Lead electrocardiogram during antidromic SVT. Maximal preexcitation is evident. Retrograde P waves may be detectable during the first half of the R-R interval but may be difficult to appreciate because of the marked repolarization abnormality associated with preexcited complexes. When evident, P waves have a 1:1 relationship with the QRS, since AV or VA block would terminate the tachycardia.

erties of each (Fig. 5). Accordingly, the QRS morphology during atrial fibrillation varies with the relative contribution of conduction through the normal and anomalous AV pathways to ventricular activation. In patients with accessory pathways having short refractory periods, ventricular activation occurs predominantly through the accessory pathway, the QRS reflects maximal preexcitation, and ventricular rates exceeding 250 beats per minute may be observed. The resultant short diastolic filling times reduce cardiac output and may result in profound hypotension, impaired coronary perfusion, and ventricular fibrillation.

Patients with concealed pathways are prone to orthodromic SVT (see the chapters *Paroxysmal Atrioventricular Reentrant Tachycardia: Pharmacologic Therapy* and *Paroxysmal Atrioventricular Reentrant Tachycardia: Nonpharmacologic Therapy*). Because the accessory pathway conducts only retrogradely, antidromic SVT cannot occur. During atrial fibrillation, antegrade conduction is exclusively through the AV node/His-Purkinje system. The ventricular rate and QRS morphology are similar to those from patients without accessory pathways.

DIAGNOSIS

The diagnosis of WPW syndrome can usually be established by analysis of the 12-lead electrocardiogram obtained during sinus rhythm. The electrocar-

diographic features of WPW syndrome include (1) a short P-R interval (<120 msec); (2) an initial slurring of the QRS complex (delta wave); (3) an abnormally wide QRS complex (≥120 msec); and (4) secondary S-T and T-wave abnormalities. Distinguishing electrocardiographic features during orthodromic SVT, antidromic SVT, and atrial fibrillation are detailed in Figures 3 through 5. If the diagnosis of WPW syndrome is in doubt, perturbations such as exercise that facilitate conduction through the accessory pathway may enable the characteristic electrocardiographic features to be more readily detectable. Obtaining the definitive diagnosis may necessitate an invasive electrophysiologic study (Fig. 6).

The electrocardiographic patterns of preexcitation during sinus rhythm can be used to regionalize the location of accessory pathways to left lateral, left posterior, posterior septal, right free wall, and anterior septal sites (Figs. 7 through 11). It has been suggested that analysis of ventricular wall motion using radionuclide ventriculography and echocardiography is useful in estimating the location of accessory pathways, but in our experience, neither modality offers a distinct advantage over analysis of the 12-lead electrocardiogram. Definitive identification of the location of an accessory pathway requires invasive electrophysiologic study (see Fig. 6).

Ideally, spontaneous arrhythmias should be documented before contemplating therapy or a change in the antiarrhythmic regimen. Patients with frequent arrhythmias that are associated with severe

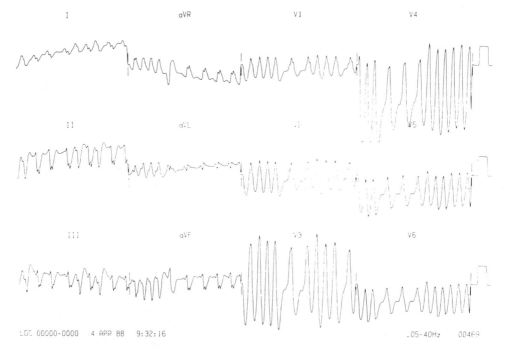

Figure 5 12-Lead electrocardiogram during atrial fibrillation. The ventricular rate is rapid and the QRS morphologies are varied because of fusion through the accessory pathway and normal AV conduction system as well as exclusive conduction through the accessory pathway.

symptoms may require observation in a telemetry unit. In most patients, arrhythmias occur infrequently and are not severe enough to warrant hospitalization. Because they occur capriciously, they are unlikely to be detectable by 24-hour ambulatory monitoring. In our experience, arrhythmias are provoked by exercise testing in less than 10 percent of patients with WPW syndrome. Patient-activated transtelephonic monitoring devices represent a practical method of documenting spontaneous arrhythmias. Clinical arrhythmias can be induced reproducibly during electrophysiologic testing in the majority of patients with WPW syndrome.

Clinical symptoms and the shortest R-R interval between two preexcited complexes during atrial fibrillation that occurs spontaneously or is induced during electrophysiologic study are the most definitive measures of risk for life-threatening arrhythmias. Stable hemodynamics and shortest R-R intervals (>250 msec) imply a low risk for sudden death. Intermittent preexcitation or abrupt loss of preexcitation with normalization of the QRS complex during exercise or during the intravenous administration of procainamide is a characteristic of patients at low risk for sudden death.

MANAGEMENT OBJECTIVES

The goals of therapy in patients with WPW syndrome are to eliminate or lessen symptoms associated with arrhythmias using approaches that are safe, efficacious, and cost effective. Therapeutic options for long-term management are outlined in Table 1 and include both pharmacologic and nonpharmacologic approaches. Decisions regarding the clinical approach to patients with WPW syndrome

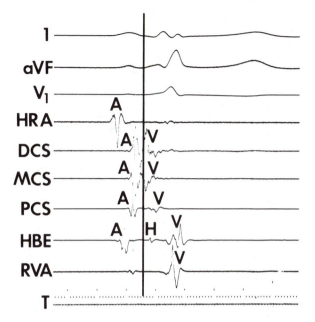

Figure 6 Intracardiac recordings during sinus rhythm from a patient with WPW syndrome. The figure is organized from top to bottom with electrocardiographic leads I, aVF, and V₁ and recordings from the high right atrium (HRA), distal (DCS), middle (MCS), and proximal (PCS) coronary sinus, His bundle region (HBE), right ventricular apex (RVA), and time (T) lines. The vertical line demarcates the onset of the delta wave in the electrocardiogram. The diagnosis of ventricular preexcitation is based on detection of delta waves and an abnormally short or negative HV interval. Ventricular activation is eccentric, with local ventricular (V) electrograms at the DCS and MCS recording sites coincident with the onset of the delta wave. This pattern is diagnostic of a left free wall accessory pathway.

Figure 7 Representative electrocardiograms recorded during sinus rhythm from three patients with left lateral accessory pathways. Characteristic features include negative delta waves in aVL and, frequently, lead I, a normal QRS axis in the frontal plane, and early precordial R wave transition. (Reproduced with permission from Lindsay BD, Crossen KJ, Cain ME. Concordance of distinguishing electrocardiographic features during sinus rhythm with the location of accessory pathways in the Wolff-Parkinson-White syndrome. Am J Cardiol 1987; 59:1093–1102.)

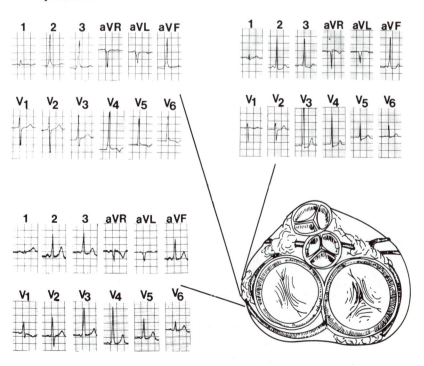

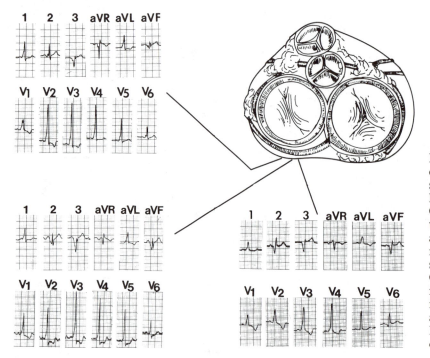

Figure 8 Representative electrocardiograms recorded during normal sinus rhythm from three patients with left posterior accessory pathways. Characteristic features include negative delta waves in the inferior leads and a prominent R wave in V_1 (R:S ration >1). (Reproduced with permission from Lindsay BD, Crossen KJ, Cain ME. Concordance of distinguishing electrocardiographic features during sinus rhythm with the location of accessory pathways in the Wolff-Parkinson-White syndrome. Am J Cardiol 1987; 59:1093–1102.)

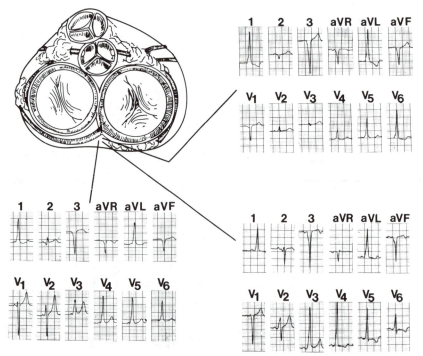

Figure 9 Representative electrocardiograms recorded during sinus rhythm from three patients with posterior septal accessory pathways. Characteristic features include negative delta waves in the inferior leads, left superior QRS axis, and an R:S ration of less than 1 in V_1. (Reproduced with permission from Lindsay BD, Crossen KJ, Cain ME. Concordance of distinguishing electrocardiographic features during sinus rhythm with the location of accessory pathways in the Wolff-Parkinson-White syndrome. Am J Cardiol 1987; 59: 1093–1102.)

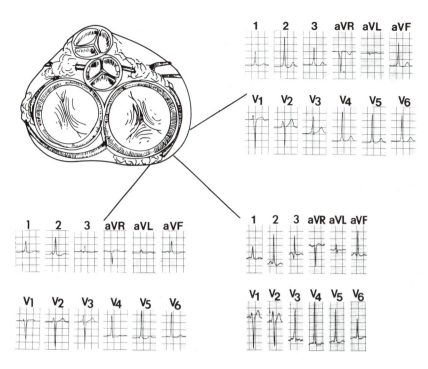

Figure 10 Representative electrocardiograms recorded during normal sinus rhythm from three patients with right free wall accessory pathways. Characteristic features include a negative delta wave in lead aVR, normal QRS axis, and precordial R wave transition in V₃ to V₅. (Reproduced with permission from Lindsay BD, Crossen KJ, Cain ME. Concordance of distinguishing electrocardiographic features during sinus rhythm with the location of accessory pathways in the Wolff-Parkinson-White syndrome. Am J Cardiol 1987; 59:1093–1102.)

Figure 11 Representative electrocardiograms recorded during sinus rhythm from three patients with anterior septal accessory pathways. Characteristic features include negative delta waves in V₁ and V₂, normal QRS axis, and precordial R wave transition in V₃ to V₅. (Reproduced with permission from Lindsay BD, Crossen KJ, Cain ME. Concordance of distinguishing electrocardiographic features during sinus rhythm with the location of accessory pathways in the Wolff-Parkinson-White syndrome. Am J Cardiol 1987; 59:1093–1102.)

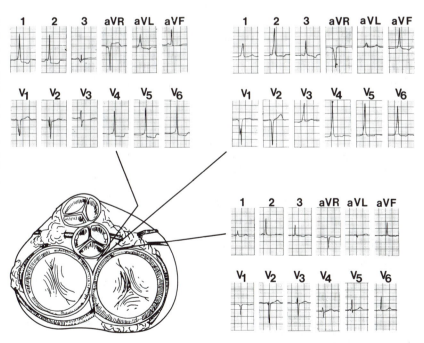

require (1) understanding of the potential morbidity and mortality of WPW syndrome; (2) consideration of patient age, general health, and the severity and frequency of symptoms; (3) awareness of the efficacy and adverse effects of pharmacologic and nonpharmacologic therapies; and (4) appreciation of the value of electrophysiologic studies.

Natural History

Many patients with WPW syndrome first experience symptoms caused by arrhythmias early in life. Congestive heart failure may complicate recurrent or prolonged episodes of tachycardia, whereas incessant tachycardias may lead to left ventricular dysfunction. Although the incidence of sudden death in infants with WPW syndrome has been estimated to be less than 1 percent, it is likely that the true incidence of life-threatening arrhythmias has been underestimated because of the difficulty in documenting specific arrhythmias in this young age group. Only a paucity of studies have examined the natural history of patients with arrhythmias. Results that are available suggest that at least 50 percent of children with arrhythmias will continue to experience them as adolescents and adults.

Most arrhythmias in patients with WPW syndrome are troublesome but not life-threatening. A small percentage of patients are at risk of sudden death, most commonly caused by ventricular fibrillation. Although the incidence is low, ventricular fibrillation may be the first manifestation of WPW syndrome. Patients who have experienced ventricular fibrillation have a greater prevalence of both atrial fibrillation and reciprocating tachycardia than those without a history of ventricular fibrillation. Ventricular fibrillation most commonly develops as a consequence of atrial fibrillation with a rapid ventricular rate. The incidence of atrial fibrillation in patients with WPW syndrome increases during adolescence.

The natural history of patients having electrocardiographic evidence of WPW syndrome but no symptomatic arrhythmias has not been completely defined. Results that are available indicate that asymptomatic adults with WPW syndrome are at low risk for morbidity or mortality.

Patient Characteristics

Clinical factors that require careful analysis include (1) patient age and sex; (2) likelihood of pregnancy; (3) type of employment; (4) emotional status; (5) presence or absence of symptoms; (6) severity and frequency of symptoms; (7) effectiveness of prior treatment regimens; (8) the type of clinical arrhythmia; (9) presence or absence of concomitant heart disease; and (10) patient preference for palliative or curative therapy. These issues have a great impact on estimations of the benefit-risk ratio and cost effectiveness of each management approach in an individual patient.

Antiarrhythmic Drugs

The major sites of action of antiarrhythmic drugs used in the treatment of patients with WPW syndrome are shown in Figure 12. Drugs affect the normal conduction system, the accessory pathway, or both limbs of the macro-reentrant circuit. Three key issues pertinent to pharmacologic therapy are efficacy, toxicity, and cost.

The relative long-term efficacy of several drugs for the prevention of orthodromic SVT are summarized in Figure 13. Digoxin is generally not effective and has been implicated in the acceleration of the ventricular rate during atrial fibrillation. Although beta-adrenergic antagonists entail less risk in patients with atrial fibrillation, they have limited efficacy as single agents in the long-term treatment of orthodromic SVT. Verapamil is effective, but concerns persist about its safety in patients with manifest preexcitation prone to atrial fibrillation. Procainamide, quinidine, and disopyramide have comparable efficacy and prevent SVT in up to 45 percent of patients. Flecainide, encainide, propafenone, and sotalol may be effective in up to 60 percent of patients, whereas amiodarone may be effective in up to 85 percent of patients.

A major goal of drug therapy in patients with WPW syndrome and a rapid ventricular rate during atrial fibrillation is prolongation of the antegrade refractory period of the accessory pathway. The percent increase in values of the antegrade refractory period expected during treatment varies among antiarrhythmic drugs (Fig. 14). A 30 percent increase in the effective refractory period of an accessory pathway that was initially 180 msec from a patient who suffered a cardiac arrest during atrial fibrillation

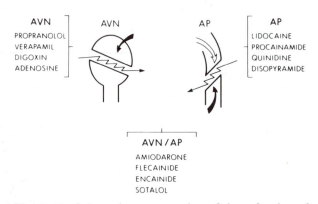

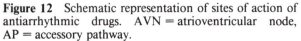

Figure 12 Schematic representation of sites of action of antiarrhythmic drugs. AVN = atrioventricular node, AP = accessory pathway.

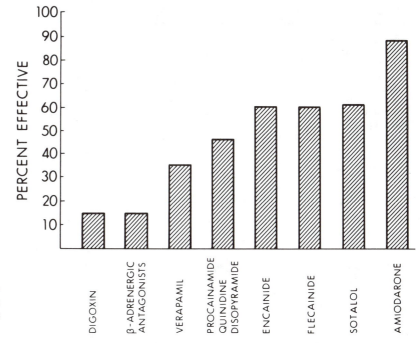

Figure 13 Comparison of the relative efficacies of antiarrhythmic drugs for the prevention of orthodromic SVT.

may not be sufficient to prevent a recurrent arrest. Moreover, the expected increases in the effective refractory period of accessory pathways in response to drugs appear to be a function of the baseline measurements. The shorter the effective refractory period, the less likely that treatment with antiarrhythmic drugs will result in a clinically important increment.

The incidences of adverse effects and the percentages of drug trials in which antiarrhythmic drugs are discontinued because of side effects are presented in Table 2. Although there are no substantial differences among drugs with regard to these issues, there are important differences in the types of side effects and extent of long-term toxic effects (Table 3). With procainamide, quinidine, and especially amiodarone, well-recognized end-organ damage is associated with long-term administration. The long-term safety of flecainide, encainide, propafenone, and sotalol in patients with WPW syndrome has not yet been established.

The monthly costs to the patient for each drug are summarized in Table 4. Costs are those charged by the Barnes Hospital Pharmacy (St. Louis, Mis-

Figure 14 Comparison of the relative percent increases in the antegrade effective refractory periods of the accessory pathway during treatment with antiarrhythmic drugs.

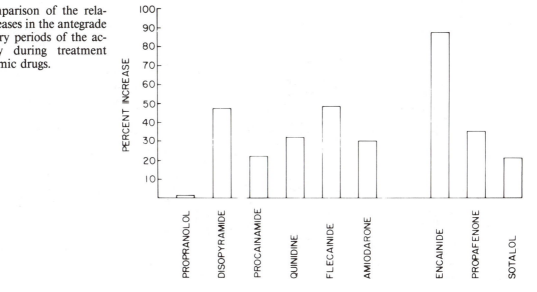

Table 2 Adverse Effects of Antiarrhythmic Drugs

Drug	Adverse Effects (%)	Discontinuation (%)
Flecainide	55	18
Encainide	57	8
Procainamide	55	22
Quinidine	64	24
Disopyramide	48	30
Amiodarone	47	30

Table 4 Monthly Costs of Antiarrhythmic Drugs

Drug	Cost/Month
Procan SR (procainamide)	$ 84.20
Cardioquin (quinidine)	$ 70.10
Norpace (disopyramide)	$128.00
Tambacor (flecainide)	$ 61.60
Enkaid (encainide)	$ 68.70
Cordarone (amiodarone)	$104.00

souri) for brand-name preparations. An individual who is 18 years old, for example, could pay up to $61,440 for disopyramide over 40 years.

Nonpharmacologic Approaches

Refinements in surgical techniques, improved understanding of the electrophysiologic-anatomic determinants of WPW syndrome, and the demonstration of the feasibility of transvenous catheter ablation have contributed to the evaluation and development of nonpharmacologic techniques for the treatment of patients with WPW syndrome. In contrast to the objectives of medical therapy, nonpharmacologic approaches are designed to ablate permanently or to alter the electrophysiologic-anatomic derangements responsible for arrhythmias, thus obviating lifelong treatment with antiarrhythmic drugs.

Surgery. At present, surgery is the best approach to effect a cure for patients with the WPW syndrome. Surgical procedures divide accessory pathways at either their atrial or ventricular inser-

Table 3 Noncardiovascular Adverse Effects of Antiarrhythmic Agents

	Most Common Effects	Long-Term Effects
Procainamide	GI Dermatologic	Lupus erythematosus Granulocytopenia
Quinidine	GI	Hemolytic anemia Thrombocytopenia Agranulocytosis
Disopyramide	Anticholinergic GI	Cholestatic jaundice
Flecainide	CNS	
Encainide	CNS	
Amiodarone	Dermatologic CNS Ocular	Pulmonary fibrosis Thyroid dysfunction Skin discoloration Hepatic dysfunction Neuropathy Myopathy

GI = gastrointestinal; CNS = central nervous system.

tions rather than at their midsection because of the difficulty of establishing a reproducible plane of dissection in the middle of the AV groove. The endocardial approach, employed at Washington University, severs the ventricular end of accessory pathways by establishing a plane of dissection between the AV groove fat pad and the ventricle. The epicardial approach is designed to sever the atrial end of accessory pathways by establishing a plane of dissection between the AV groove fat pad and the atrium.

The surgical correction of the WPW syndrome now approaches 100 percent, with an operative mortality for elective, uncomplicated cases that ranges from 0 to 0.5 percent. There has been only one recurrence following surgery in which the endocardial technique was utilized in our own series, which now includes 287 consecutive accessory pathways, and the recurrence rate following the epicardial technique is acceptably low. Moreover, the inadvertent creation of heart block is no longer a problem with either technique.

Catheter Ablation. Closed chest catheter ablation, in principle, is appealing in that it offers a way to interrupt conduction through the accessory pathway without cardiac surgery. The feasibility of this approach was demonstrated initially in experimental animals using synchronous discharges of 20 to 240 joules delivered through a catheter positioned in the coronary sinus or abutting the right atrial septum. Pathophysiologic specimens demonstrated extensive scarring of atrial tissue adjacent to the site of discharge. The coronary sinus exhibited varying degrees of stenosis and was occluded in up to 50 percent of animals. Moreover, perforation of the coronary sinus was observed after high energy shocks. Nearly 20 percent of animals were found to have evidence of intimal hyperplasia of the circumflex coronary artery.

The experience with catheter ablation of accessory pathways in humans is limited. Attempts to ablate left free wall pathways using catheters positioned in the coronary sinus have, for the most part, been unsuccessful and associated with an unacceptable risk of coronary sinus rupture and pericardial tamponade. Overall, this approach has not been successful in patients with accessory pathways at left free wall or right free wall sites. Success has been reported in up to 71 percent of patients with posterior septal pathways. The complex anatomy of the AV groove and the potential for permanent injury to the coronary sinus and arteries remain serious limitations of this approach.

Recently, catheter ablation using radiofrequency energy has been evaluated in experimental animals and humans. Preliminary results have shown that the area of necrosis is more focused and the incidence of occlusion of the coronary sinus reduced when compared with that produced by electrical shock energy. These results demonstrate the potential feasibility of this approach for ablation of accessory pathways in patients.

Electrophysiologic Studies

The goals of an electrophysiologic study are to (1) document the presence of an accessory pathway; (2) confirm that the accessory pathway participates in the clinical arrhythmia; (3) identify the location and number of accessory pathways; (4) determine the functional properties of the accessory pathway and normal AV conduction system; and (5) provide an objective end point for assessing the effectiveness of pharmacologic and nonpharmacologic therapies. The electrophysiologic properties of the normal AV conduction systems and accessory pathways in patients with WPW syndrome measured before and during treatment with antiarrhythmic drugs may explain drug efficacy. Determination of the antegrade and retrograde refractory periods of these tissues, together with the anticipated effects of antiarrhythmic drugs, provides insight into the likelihood that specific drugs will be effective, not effective, or proarrhythmic (Fig. 15).

MANAGEMENT STRATEGIES

There are a variety of treatment options for patients with WPW syndrome and symptomatic arrhythmias (see Table 1). Previously we have reviewed separately the key issues that are the foundations for clinical decision making. This section integrates these issues and summarizes our approach to the management of patients with WPW syndrome.

Empirically Versus Electrophysiologically Guided Drug Therapy

The clinical circumstances may favor empirically guided drug therapy (Table 5). We consider this trial and error approach only for patients with frequent and well-tolerated arrhythmias. Patients with frequent arrhythmias do not require prolonged drug

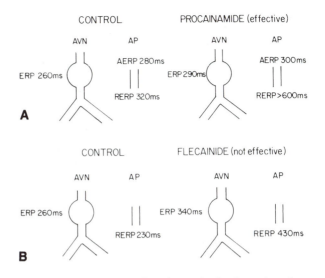

Figure 15 Selection of antiarrhythmic drugs based on results of electrophysiologic measurements. *A*, Schematic of atrioventricular node (AVN) and accessory pathway (AP) from a patient with manifest preexcitation and orthodromic SVT. During the control study the effective refractory period (ERP) of the AVN was 260 msec, the antegrade (A) ERP of the AP was 280 msec, and the retrograde (R) ERP of the AP was 320 msec. Antegrade, the ERPs of the AVN and AP differ by only 20 msec. The RERP of the AP is relatively long. SVT was induced by a programmed atrial extrastimulus at 270 msec that blocked antegrade in the AP, conducted through the AVN with sufficient delay (>320 msec) to enable retrograde activation of the AP. The goal of antiarrhythmic drug therapy is to alter the electrophysiologic properties of one or both limbs of the reentrant circuit so that completion of the reentrant loop is prevented. In this example, a selective increase in the RERP would be antiarrhythmic. Procainamide primarily alters the electrophysiologic properties of the AP, especially the RERP. During treatment with procainamide, the RERP of the AP increased dramatically (>600 msec), whereas the AERP of the AP and ERP of the AVN changed to a lesser extent and reentry was precluded. *B*, Schematic of AVN and AP from a patient with a concealed AP and orthodromic SVT. The ERP of the AVN and RERP of the AP are short and differ by only 30 msec. Flecainide, which affects both the AVN and AP, would not be an ideal drug in this patient. As predicted, flecainide increased the ERP and RERP in parallel and facilitated the initiation of SVT.

Table 5 Empirically Guided Treatment of Arrhythmias

Indications
    Frequent arrhythmias
    Hemodynamically stable arrhythmias

Concealed Accessory Pathway
    Digoxin, verapamil
    Flecainide, encainide
    Disopyramide, quinidine, or procainamide

Mainfest Accessory Pathway
    Flecainide, encainide
    Disopyramide, quinidine, or procainamide

trials to determine failure of drug treatment. Moreover, recurrences would not be expected to be associated with morbidity or mortality. Recurrences of clinical arrhythmias serve as objective end points for assessing drug efficacy. In contrast, we do not rely on this approach for patients with infrequent arrhythmias in whom potentially toxic drugs could be administered for protracted intervals before determining they were not effective or for patients having arrhythmias accompanied by severe or life-threatening symptoms in whom a clinical recurrence is likely to result in significant morbidity or mortality.

Our preferences for antiarrhythmic drugs for patients with concealed and with manifest accessory pathways are outlined in Table 5. Patients with concealed accessory pathways are treated first with digoxin or verapamil, not because they are the most effective drugs but because they are the least harmful. Class IC drugs, if ever approved for WPW syndrome, exert electrophysiologic properties and have a side effect profile that makes them particularly well suited for the treatment of orthodromic SVT, antidromic SVT, or atrial fibrillation. However, the long-term efficacy and safety of these drugs in patients with WPW syndrome are not yet known. Of the class IA drugs, we prefer disopyramide for young patients. It is well tolerated, and sustained-release preparations permit convenient dosing. Quinidine and procainamide are not ideal for young patients because of frequent side effects and a high propensity for causing organ damage with their long-term use. Patients with manifest preexcitation should not receive digoxin or verapamil unless an electrophysiologic study has first documented that they are at low risk for developing a life-threatening ventricular rate during atrial fibrillation. Based on side effect profile and relative efficacy, class IC drugs offer several advantages over class IA agents, particularly in young individuals.

There are several indications for performing electrophysiologic studies in patients with WPW syndrome (Table 6). Patients should be studied (1) if the diagnosis is in question, particularly those with concealed accessory pathways; (2) if symptoms are severe and recurrent episodes would be expected to result in significant morbidity or mortality; (3) if

clinical arrhythmias occur infrequently; (4) if empirically derived approaches have failed. Electrophysiologic studies are essential to the care of patients who have already demonstrated a life-threatening ventricular rate during atrial fibrillation. Comprehensive studies are required in those patients considered for nonpharmacologic therapy.

Prophylactic Versus Intermittent Pharmacologic Therapy

Most patients with symptomatic arrhythmias require a treatment regimen that affords continuous protection against recurrences. However, some patients with infrequent episodes of orthodromic SVT may prefer intermittent oral therapy with a combination of diltiazem and propranolol only at the time of their attacks. Episodes must be well tolerated and last at least 30 minutes to enable systemic drug absorption. Patients with infrequent, brief, self-terminating episodes of SVT without debilitating symptoms may not require treatment.

Pharmacologic Versus Nonpharmacologic Therapy

Selection of patients with the WPW syndrome for nonpharmacologic therapy is predicated on several factors, including the clinical arrhythmia, the patient's age and general health, the presence of other cardiac abnormalities that require surgical intervention, the patient's emotional status, consideration of issues such as pregnancy and type of employment, and the assumption that pharmacologic therapy is unlikely to afford lifelong protection against recurrence of arrhythmias or freedom from side effects.

Our indications for nonpharmacologic therapy in patients with WPW syndrome are summarized in Table 7. The benefits of surgery are established. Surgery is the nonpharmacologic approach of first choice for curing WPW syndrome. Because of the success of surgery at Washington University, we have liberalized the indications and offer surgery to some young patients as a first-line alternative to medical therapy. For example, a young patient who remains anxious about the insecurity that medical treatment may fail and result in the occurrence of symptomatic arrhythmias during vacations or business meetings may prefer a surgical cure. Or a young woman in whom arrhythmias are well controlled by

---

Table 6 Indications for Electrophysiologic Studies

To establish a diagnosis
With arrhythmias associated with severe symptoms
With infrequent arrhythmias
When empirical therapy is unsuccessful
With atrial fibrillation with rapid ventricular rate
To assess ventricular rate during atrial fibrillation
To guide nonpharmacologic therapy:
    Surgery
    Catheter ablation
    Antitachycardia devices

Table 7 Indications for Surgical Treatment of WPW Syndrome

Life-threatening ventricular rate during atrial fibrillation or flutter
AV reentrant tachycardia refractory to medical therapy
Intolerance to medical therapy
Alternative first-line therapy in young patients

drugs that are potentially toxic to a fetus may elect to have surgery before becoming pregnant.

The information to date on the efficacy and safety of catheter ablation is too preliminary to permit definitive conclusions regarding the eventual role of this approach. Based on our interpretation of available data, catheter ablation, using current techniques, should not be performed in patients with left-sided accessory pathways. Catheter ablation in patients who have accessory pathways at right free wall locations is investigational. It appears that shocks of sufficient intensity to ablate accessory pathways can be delivered to the right atrium without producing perforation of the right atrial wall or septum. However, a factor further limiting the feasibility of ablation of right-sided pathways is the difficulty in determining their precise location. Although catheter ablation has had limited success in patients with posterior septal pathways, we still regard this approach as investigational and limit it to patients who require a nonpharmacologic approach but refuse or are not candidates for surgery.

Approach to Patients Without Symptoms

Present strategies for defining risk for sudden death are based on retrospective analyses of patients with WPW syndrome who have survived an episode of ventricular fibrillation. The merits and limitations of exercise testing and invasive electrophysiologic studies for the identification of asymptomatic patients with preexcitation syndrome at risk of ventricular fibrillation already have been described. At present, there is no objective evidence that results of these tests have a beneficial influence on the management of asymptomatic patients. Accordingly, we do not perform routine electrophysiologic studies in all asymptomatic patients with WPW syndrome. It is our practice, however, to evaluate asymptomatic patients with preexcitation syndrome whose occupation (e.g., pilot, professional athlete) places them or others at considerable risk of injury if an arrhythmia supervenes. In such patients, an exercise test is performed first. Abrupt loss of preexcitation during exercise implies a low risk of ventricular fibrillation. Patients with persistent preexcitation throughout exercise are advised to undergo an invasive electrophysiologic study. For asymptomatic patients, the decision to advise pharmacologic or nonpharmacologic therapy based on results of exercise testing or electrophysiologic studies should be balanced by recognition that the treatment may be attended by greater risk than the underlying disorder.

Supported in part by NIH Grant HL17646, SCOR in Ischemic Heart Disease.

SUGGESTED READING

Berkman NL, Lamb LE. The Wolff-Parkinson-White electrocardiogram: A follow-up study of five to twenty-eight years. N Engl J Med 1968; 278:492–494.

Cain ME, Cox JL. Surgical treatment of supraventricular arrhythmias. In: Platia E, ed. Management of cardiac arrhythmias: The nonpharmacologic approach. Philadelphia: JB Lippincott, 1987:304.

Fisher JD, Brodman R, Kim SG, et al. Attempted nonsurgical electrical ablation of accessory pathways via the coronary sinus in the Wolff-Parkinson-White syndrome. J Am Coll Cardiol 1984; 4:685–694.

Klein GJ, Yee R, Sharma AD. Longitudinal electrophysiologic assessment of asymptomatic patients with the Wolff-Parkinson-White electrocardiographic patterns. N Engl J Med 1989; 320:1229–1233.

Lindsay BD, Branyas NA, Cain ME. The pre-excitation syndrome. In: El-Sherif N, Samet P, eds. Cardiac pacing and electrophysiology. 3rd ed. Philadelphia: WB Saunders, 1990.

Lindsay BD, Crossen KJ, Cain ME. Concordance of distinguishing electrocardiographic features during sinus rhythm with the location of accessory pathways in the Wolff-Parkinson-White syndrome. Am J Cardiol 1987; 59:1093–1102.

Lundberg A. Paroxysmal atrial tachycardia in infancy: Long-term follow-up study of 49 subjects. Pediatrics 1982; 70:638–642.

Sharma AD, Yee R, Guiradon G, Klein GJ. Sensitivity and specificity of invasive and noninvasive testing for risk of sudden death in Wolff-Parkinson-White syndrome. J Am Coll Cardiol 1987; 10:373–381.

Wellens HJJ, Bar FW, Dassen WRM, et al. Effect of drugs in the Wolff-Parkinson-White syndrome. Importance of initial length of effective refractory period of the accessory pathway. Am J Cardiol 1980; 46:665–669.

PAROXYSMAL ATRIOVENTRICULAR REENTRANT TACHYCARDIA: PHARMACOLOGIC THERAPY

MASOOD AKHTAR, M.D.

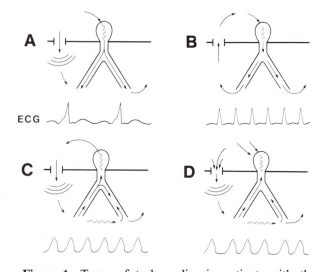

Figure 1 Types of tachycardias in patients with the Wolff-Parkinson-White syndrome. *A* provides a schematic explanation for the short P-R interval and delta wave (ventricular preexcitation) during sinus rhythm. The resulting complex is fusion, where the initial part of the QRS complex is caused by rapid conduction via the accessory pathway (the delta wave). *B* depicts the circuit of orthodromic tachycardia, which shows no evidence of preexcitation, since the ventricles are activated exclusively via the normal pathway. In *C*, the proposed circuit of antidromic tachycardia is depicted. This would produce regular wide QRS tachycardia. During atrial fibrillation (*D*), the wide QRS complex has irregular R-R intervals. See Figure 3 for labeling of anatomic structures shown. The solid horizontal lines represent the AV junction.

Patients with the Wolff-Parkinson-White syndrome are prone to a variety of supraventricular tachycardias. The most common arrhythmia in these cases is the so-called orthodromic tachycardia (Fig. 1*B*), during which the antegrade conduction is over the normal pathway; i.e., the atrioventricular (AV) node and His-Purkinje system and the retrograde conduction are along the accessory pathway. This type of circus movement tachycardia produces a narrow QRS complex with no evidence of ventricular preexcitation during the arrhythmia (Fig. 2). In the event that there is a functional block in either the left or the right bundle branches, aberrant conduction could result in QRS widening. A rare form of circus movement tachycardia has been described in which the direction of impulse propagation is reversed, i.e., the ventricles are activated via the accessory pathway and the atria by way of the AV node and His-Purkinje system (see Fig. 1*C*). This so-called antidromic tachycardia has to be distinguished from wide QRS tachycardia caused by other mechanisms, particularly ventricular tachycardia. The other clinically important arrhythmias in patients with the Wolff-Parkinson-White syndrome are atrial in origin, such as atrial flutter and atrial fibrillation, especially when the ventricular response is controlled by conduction along the accessory pathway (see Fig. 1*D*).

A discussion of the pharmacologic therapy of AV reentrant tachycardia follows. The two types of circus movement tachycardias shown in Figure 1*A* and *B* would ordinarily be classified as AV reentrant tachycardia. However, the orthodromic variety is far more common and better understood. When the ventricular activation occurs via the accessory pathway in a regular tachycardia, the term preexcited tachycardia is preferred, since the antidromic reentry tachycardia is only one of the mechanisms (see Fig. 2*C*). Other types include atrial tachycardia with 1:1 AV response via the accessory pathway (Fig. 3*A*), AV nodal reentry tachycardias with incidental accessory pathway activation (Fig. 3*B*), and circus movement tachycardia, in which one accessory pathway is used in the antegrade and the other in the retrograde direction. Therefore I use the term preexcited tachycardia, and a specific reference is given to antidromic reentry tachycardia when appropriate.

PHARMACOLOGIC TREATMENT OF ORTHODROMIC TACHYCARDIA

Management of Acute Episodes

Since effective propagation along the AV node–His-Purkinje system in the antegrade direction is an essential part of the circuit, one approach is to use intravenous medications known to depress AV

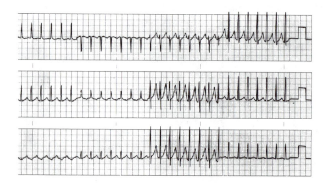

Figure 2 A 12-lead ECG of patient with orthodromic tachycardia. Note the narrow QRS complex and the absence of any evidence of ventricular preexcitation.

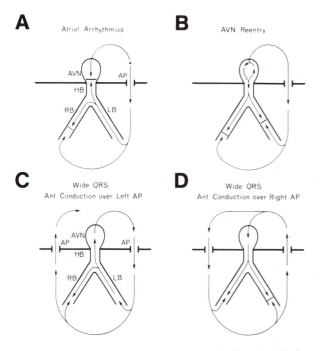

Figure 3 The circuits of reentry are depicted, and the reason for the wide QRS complex is obvious. See the text for explanation. AVN = atrioventricular node, AP = accessory pathway, HB = His bundle, LB = left bundle, RB = right bundle.

nodal conduction (Fig. 4). These include digitalis, beta blockers, and calcium channel blockers. Among the last group, verapamil has been used more extensively. The usual dose of verapamil by the intravenous route is 0.1 mg per kilogram initially, and the dose can be repeated in 15 minutes if necessary. Caution should be used in older patients, in whom it is advisable to administer the drug over several minutes.

Propranolol can be administered in similar doses of 0.1 mg per kilogram. Both beta blockers and

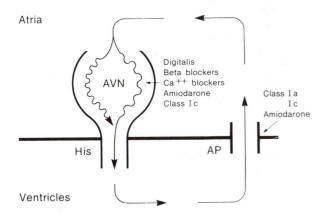

Figure 4 Schematic depiction of the location of action of various antiarrhythmic drugs in a typical circuit of orthodromic reentry to tachycardia. AVN = atrioventricular node, AP = accessory pathway.

calcium channel blockers can cause myocardial depression, significant slowing of the sinus rate, and advanced degree of AV block.

Digitalis is seldom used as a first line of therapy in these acute settings because of its delayed onset of action and less potent depression of AV nodal conduction compared with either verapamil or propranolol.

Adenosine could become the drug of choice when released (see the chapter *Adenosine*). This agent is a potent depressant of AV nodal conduction and has the advantage of a short half-life, lasting for only a few seconds. Although amiodarone given intravenously can also produce AV nodal block, terminating the reentry process, its use in this situation is not necessary in most instances.

Among the class I agents, procainamide is used frequently by intravenous route. Procainamide rarely depresses antegrade AV nodal conduction, but it does slow conduction and prolong the refractory period in the accessory pathway. Therefore, conduction block occurs in the retrograde limb of the reentry circuit (see Fig. 4). The usual dose is 50 to 100 mg per minute for a total of 10 to 15 mg per kilogram with careful monitoring of blood pressure.

In the event that excessive depression of the sinus rate or AV nodal conduction occurs with intravenous drugs following termination of AV reentry, intravenous catecholamines such as isoproterenol can readily reverse these effects. However, it should be noted that following termination of supraventricular tachycardia, sinus slowing and transient AV nodal block can occur even in the absence of drugs. Such asymptomatic episodes are usually caused by baroreceptor stimulation secondary to large stroke volume immediately after termination of tachycardia and require no intervention. It is pertinent to point out that combined use of intravenous beta blockers and calcium channel blockers is not recommended. Severe depression of sinus node and AV node can result, and ventricular standstill may follow.

Long-Term Therapy

Pharmacologic control of AV reentry tachycardia on a long-term basis involves two considerations: (1) Since these arrhythmias are triggered by spontaneous atrial and ventricular premature complexes, suppression of such triggering events could potentially prevent recurrences. Although complete suppression of premature complexes is generally not possible, class I agents are more effective in this regard. Class IC agents such as flecainide and encainide are considered the most potent suppressants of premature complexes. The alternatives would include class IA drugs such as quinidine, procainamide, and disopyramide. (2) Drugs that produce depression of AV nodal conduction in the antegrade direction and accessory pathway conduction in the retrograde direction are considered more suitable for control of AV reentry tachycardia. The usual drugs and their location of action are depicted in Figure 4. Even though amiodarone is listed, this agent should be reserved for difficult cases because of its side effect profile. On the basis of the recent data and our own experience with class IC agents, we view these drugs as the most effective in the management of patients with orthodromic tachycardia. Class IC agents (flecainide and encainide) seem to produce marked depression of conduction along the accessory pathway, and in orthodromic tachycardia the block occurs along the retrograde direction i.e., accessory pathway. Depression of conduction along the accessory pathway seems important for control of AV reentry, since we have had less success with agents that depress only AV nodal conduction (see Fig. 4).

Long-term treatment is initiated with class IC agents as the first line of therapy. We prefer flecainide because of its less frequent dosing schedule (twice a day, versus encainide, which has to be administered three times a day). Furthermore, flecainide has no active metabolites, which in the case of encainide could produce somewhat variable results. Nonetheless, both drugs are equally potent and can be substituted for each other if any intolerance to one or the other is observed. The side effects are minor and are usually neurologic, such as dizziness and blurred vision. Serious ventricular proarrhythmic effects seen in patients with ventricular arrhythmias are uncommon in patients with the Wolff-Parkinson-White syndrome in the absence of ventricular scarring and when ventricular function is normal. The usual dose of flecainide is 100 to 150 mg every 12 hours and for encainide 25 to 50 mg three times a day at 8-hour intervals.

In the case of class IA drugs, we prefer long-acting quinidine preparations. This consideration is important, since AV reentry tachycardia is an arrhythmia of the younger population, and compliance with drug therapy is a problem. Sustained-release preparation of disopyramide could also be employed. We do not use procainamide routinely because of its frequent long-term side effects, such as lupus erythematosus and arthritis.

When amiodarone is chosen for difficult cases, a relatively low daily dose may be sufficient, i.e., 200 mg or less every day. Because of its long half-life and the increased sun sensitivity it produces, amiodarone can be temporarily discontinued during the summer months. However, this approach can only be used in patients in whom the tachycardia does not produce severe symptoms, such as syncope.

One of the main reasons we prefer either class I or amiodarone in the Wolff-Parkinson-White syndrome is that patients with orthodromic tachycardia may also suffer from other arrhythmias. The most important of these are atrial flutter and atrial fibrilla-

tion. In the event that atrial arrhythmias occur and the AV response starts over the accessory pathway, class I agents and amiodarone also produce slowing of ventricular response via the accessory pathway. Furthermore, class I agents are more likely to suppress triggering mechanisms such as atrial and ventricular premature beats. Agents known to influence only AV nodal conduction (Fig. 4) either will not affect accessory pathway conduction (beta blockers) or will potentially accelerate AV response via the accessory pathway (digitalis). Calcium channel blockers in the chronic setting may be associated with less tolerance of the tachycardia (owing to hypotension from vasodilation), even if the accessory pathway properties are not markedly altered.

Reversal of Therapeutic Drug Effect

An important consideration in the pharmacologic therapy of arrhythmias is the reversal of drug effects with catecholamines. Clinical recurrences in patients who have apparent pharmacologic control may be related to the reversal of therapeutic benefit owing to the rise in endogenous catecholamine levels. In the electrophysiology laboratory, infusion of isoproterenol reverses drug-induced depression of conduction. Isoproterenol in doses sufficient to increase sinus rate to 15 percent or more of the baseline reverses encainide-induced depression of both AV nodal and accessory pathway conduction, which results in induction of tachycardia suppressed by the therapeutic agent. This effect is not unique to encainide, and we have seen it with virtually all drugs, including amiodarone. Reversal of AV nodal depression can be almost complete and that of the accessory pathway somewhat less so when compared with the baseline values. These findings provide one explanation for recurrences of drug-controlled tachycardia in the clinical settings caused by activity-related release of endogenous catecholamine. The main clinical value of these findings is twofold: (1) drugs that affect only AV nodal conduction (see Fig. 4) may not be able to maintain therapeutic effect in ambulatory settings and hence are less effective, and (2) the addition of beta blockers may prevent recurrences by preventing the reversal of therapeutic class I drug effects.

Therefore, when clinical recurrences are noted, beta blockers can be added to the class I regimen. We have been able to control recurrences of clinical tachycardia in several patients with this combination when both agents alone failed, including those with AV reentry tachycardia.

PHARMACOLOGIC TREATMENT OF PREEXCITED TACHYCARDIA

As pointed out above, the electrocardiographic patterns of preexcited tachycardia can be produced by several different mechanisms (see Figs. 1 and 3).

When the so-called true antidromic reentry tachycardia (see Fig. 1C) occurs, the same therapeutic approach can be taken as outlined for orthodromic reentry tachycardia. Even though the direction of impulse propagation is reversed, there is no reason to believe that qualitatively similar effects on the circuit will not be exerted by the same agent on the same site. It should be pointed out that in our experience, true antidromic reentrant tachycardia is rather rare. Other mechanisms such as atrial tachycardia (see Fig. 3A), AV nodal reentry tachycardia (see Fig. 3B), and incorporation of two accessory pathways (see Fig. 3C and D) should also be considered.

In both AV nodal reentry and atrial tachycardias, the AV response via the accessory pathway can be controlled with class IA and IC agents or amiodarone. Similarly, a preexcited tachycardia using two accessory pathways can be controlled with the same drugs. Again our preference is class IC agents. If these agents are not well tolerated, class IA drugs can be tried, and amiodarone can be used as a last resort. Digitalis and calcium channel and beta blockers alone have no place in the management of these cases.

In the acute setting the recommended therapy is intravenous procainamide in the same dosage as used for orthodromic tachycardia.

In patients with wide QRS tachycardia, ideally the mechanism should be studied and the arrhythmias treated accordingly. Unfortunately, in the case of a preexcited regular tachycardia, the true underlying mechanism is difficult to diagnose from surface electrocardiograms and hence the therapy is somewhat empirical.

In the acute setting, intravenous procainamide, and in chronic situations, flecainide or encainide is considered the best form of pharmacologic therapy in preexcited tachycardia. In patients with orthodromic tachycardia, the same therapeutic agents are adequate, but in addition verapamil or diltiazem (and adenosine in the future) can be employed for termination of acute conditions. These statements apply to only the pharmacologic agents available at the present time. Recommendations may change as more effective drugs become available.

SUGGESTED READING

Akhtar M, Niazi I, Naccarelli GV, et al. Role of adrenergic stimulation by isoproterenol in reversal of effects of encainide in supraventricular tachycardia. Am J Cardiol 1988; 62:45L.

Chamberlain DA, Clark ANG. Atrial fibrillation complicating Wolff-Parkinson-White syndrome treated with amiodarone. Br Med J 1977; 2:1519.

Gulamhusein S, Ko P, Carruthers SG, et al. Acceleration of the ventricular response during atrial fibrillation in the Wolff-Parkinson-White syndrome after verapamil. Circulation 1982; 65:348.

Kerr CR, Prystowsky EN, Smith WM, et al. Electrophysiologic effects of disopyramide phosphate in patients with Wolff-Parkinson-White syndrome. Circulation 1982; 65:869.

Niazi I, Naccarelli G, Dougherty A, et al. Treatment of atrioventricular node reentrant tachycardia with encainide: Reversal of drug effect with isoproterenol. J Am Coll Cardiol 1989;13:904.

Prystowsky E, Miles WM, Heger JJ, Zipes DP. Preexcitation syndromes: Mechanisms and management. Med Clin North Am 1984; 68:831.

Rinkenberger RL, Prystowsky EN, Heger JJ, et al. Effects of intravenous and chronic oral verapamil administration in patients with supraventricular tachyarrhythmias. Circulation 1980; 62:996.

Rosenbaum MB, Chiale PA, Ryba D, et al. Control of tachyarrhythmias associated with Wolff-Parkinson-White syndrome by amiodarone hydrochloride. Am J Cardiol 1974; 34:215.

Sellers TD, Bashore TM, Gallagher JJ. Digitalis in the preexcitation syndrome: Analysis during atrial fibrillation. Circulation 1977; 56:260.

Sellers TD, Campbell RWF, Bashore TM, et al. Effects of procainamide and quinidine sulfate in the Wolff-Parkinson-White syndrome. Circulation 1977; 55:15.

Wellens HJJ, Bar FW, Dassen WRM, et al. Effect of drugs in the Wolff-Parkinson-White syndrome: Importance of initial length of effective refractory period of the accessory pathway. Am J Cardiol 1980; 46:665.

Wellens HJJ, Durrer D. Effect of procainamide, quinidine, and ajmaline in the Wolff-Parkinson-White syndrome. Circulation 1974; 50:114.

Wellens HJJ, Lie KI, Bar FW, et al. Effect of amiodarone in Wolff-Parkinson-White syndrome. Am J Cardiol 1976; 38:189.

PAROXYSMAL ATRIOVENTRICULAR REENTRANT SUPRAVENTRICULAR TACHYCARDIA: NONPHARMACOLOGIC THERAPY

JONATHAN J. LANGBERG, M.D.
JERRY C. GRIFFIN, M.D.
MELVIN M. SCHEINMAN, M.D.

Paroxysmal atrioventricular reentry tachycardia is the most common arrhythmia affecting patients with the Wolff-Parkinson-White syndrome. With antegrade block in the accessory pathway (usually the result of an atrial premature complex), ventricular activation proceeds exclusively over the atrioventricular (AV) node–His axis. Ventricular excitation, in turn, produces retrograde activation of the accessory pathway and atria, resulting in a continuous circus movement tachycardia.

This arrhythmia is unique by virtue of the large size of the reentrant pathway and the fact that each portion of the circuit is anatomically and electrophysiologically distinct. These features make many patients with orthodromic AV reentry tachycardia potential candidates for catheter or surgical ablation as well as for antitachycardia pacing.

CATHETER ABLATION FOR THE TREATMENT OF ATRIOVENTRICULAR REENTRY TACHYCARDIA

Patient Selection

In general, patients with the Wolff-Parkinson-White syndrome whose disease has proved refractory to or who are intolerant of antiarrhythmic drugs should be considered for catheter ablation (see the chapter *Catheter Ablation*). We have also opted to use catheter ablation of an accessory pathway as initial therapy in some patients because of concern about poor compliance. This is especially true in patients at risk for malignant arrhythmias, such as those with a history of syncope, cardiac arrest, or hypotension during supraventricular tachycardia or those with very rapid accessory pathway conduction during induced atrial fibrillation (see the chapter *Atrial Fibrillation in the Wolff-Parkinson-White Syndrome*).

A complete electrophysiologic evaluation, including mapping of retrograde atrial activation during induced AV reciprocating tachycardia to determine accessory pathway location, must precede consideration of catheter ablation. We also perform phase image analysis of a radionuclide ventriculogram or cine computed tomographic scan during atrial pacing. By detecting the earliest site of ventricular contraction during systole, the ventricular insertion site of the accessory pathway can be inferred. These radiographic examinations serve as independent confirmation of the electrical activation mapping and help to exclude a second accessory pathway that may be difficult to detect on electrophysiologic study.

Posteroseptal Accessory Pathway Ablation

Approximately 25 percent of patients with the Wolff-Parkinson-White syndrome have an accessory pathway located in the posteroseptal region. These bypass tracts may be amenable to catheter ablation by virtue of their close proximity to the ostium of the coronary sinus.

If the initial electrophysiologic study and subsequent radiologic examinations confirm the presence of a single posteroseptal accessory pathway, an ablation should be considered. Electrode catheters are inserted in the femoral vein and positioned in the right ventricular apex for back-up ventricular pacing and across the tricuspid annulus to record the His potential. A No. 6 French quadripolar lumen electrode catheter is inserted via the internal jugular or subclavian vein and advanced into the coronary sinus. Contrast venography is performed, and the location of the ostium of the coronary sinus is carefully marked on the fluoroscopic screen. The catheter is positioned so that pole 3 is at the ostium and pole 4 (the most proximal) is outside the coronary sinus. Reciprocating tachycardia is induced in order to reconfirm that poles 3 and 4 record the earliest retrograde atrial activation. A short-acting barbiturate is used to produce general anesthesia. Poles 3 and 4 are made electrically common and are connected to the cathodal output of a standard defibrillator. A large-diameter skin electrode affixed to the posterior chest wall serves as the anode. Two or three shocks of 200 to 300 joules are applied to poles 3 and 4 of the coronary sinus catheter.

Using this technique, about two-thirds of patients have complete elimination of accessory pathway conduction and supraventricular tachycardia. An additional 10 percent of patients have attenuation of accessory pathway function such that tachycardia no longer occurs or is controllable with therapy that was previously ineffective.

Serious complications of posteroseptal accessory pathway ablation are uncommon, but persistent AV block and pericardial tamponade have been reported. The incidence of pericardial bleeding is probably less than 3 percent if meticulous attention is paid to positioning the ablating electrodes just outside the coronary sinus. Transient hypotension and ventricular arrhythmias also can occur, presumably as the result of barotraumatic injury to the ventricle.

Ablation of the Atrioventricular Junction in Patients With the Wolff-Parkinson-White Syndrome

Although it represents an indirect approach to the problem, ablation of the AV junction eliminates the antegrade limb of the AV reentry circuit and prevents any possibility of accessory pathway tachycardia. Selected patients with manifest preexcitation may be candidates for this therapy. Only those whose tachycardia is refractory to drug therapy should be considered. Patients with accessory pathways capable of rapid conduction are not suitable, since interruption of the AV node–His access does not prevent dangerously rapid rates during atrial arrhythmias. Patients with poor antegrade accessory pathway function (e.g., intermittent preexcitation in sinus rhythm) and refractory tachycardia can be successfully treated with ablation of the AV junction. After ablation, conduction proceeds exclusively over the accessory pathway, and the electrocardiogram is fully preexcited. Because the long-term stability of accessory pathway conduction is uncertain, we implant a permanent pacemaker at the time of the procedure. Surgical interruption of the accessory pathway should be considered as an alternative, since this preserves the normal conduction system.

Future Trends in Accessory Pathway Ablation

The majority of accessory AV connections are located in the left free wall of the heart. These pathways traverse the AV sulcus in close proximity to the coronary sinus. Since direct current shock ablation within the coronary sinus is associated with an unacceptably high risk of coronary sinus perforation and tamponade, several innovative approaches are being explored. Transseptal puncture is being used to position an electrode catheter within the left atrium. Although localizing the accessory pathway with this technique is technically demanding, the success rate with an experienced operator approaches 90 percent.

Radiofrequency current is being explored as an alternative to direct current shock as an ablative energy source. Between 10 and 30 watts of high frequency (500 to 1000 kHz) current is applied for 10 to 60 seconds. Unlike defibrillator discharges, radiofrequency causes localized injury exclusively through resistive heating. There is no explosive gas formation or shock wave, minimizing the risk of cardiac perforation. Radiofrequency ablation has been shown to be safe when applied within the coronary sinus in experimental animals. Preliminary reports of ablation of both left and right free-wall accessory pathways with radiofrequency are encouraging and suggest that this technique may be safely used in thin-walled areas of the heart.

PACING FOR LONG-TERM MANAGEMENT OF ATRIOVENTRICULAR REENTRANT TACHYCARDIA

To achieve success in pacing for the management of tachyarrhythmias, one must amortize the initial cost and morbidity of pacemaker implantation over many years and delay a second operative intervention as long as possible. This is especially the case in the management of supraventricular tachycardias in which the risks are low. Although many reports of pacemakers for tachycardia are available, the most important are those providing long-term follow-up data stratified by tachycardia mechanism (see the chapter *Antitachycardia Pacemakers*).

Patient Selection

Patients considered candidates for permanent antitachycardia pacing should undergo complete electrophysiologic evaluation. The electrophysiologic study is used to define the arrhythmia mechanism, to quantify the conduction and refractoriness of each limb of the tachycardia circuit both at baseline and during catecholamine infusion, and to assess the safety and efficacy of pacing termination.

Unlike patients with AV nodal reentry, important limitations and contraindications to pacemaker therapy exist for those in whom an accessory pathway is present, since there is a low but significant incidence of sudden death in patients having pacemakers for control of orthodromic AV reentrant supraventricular tachycardia. Occasional atrial fibrillation is an almost predictable consequence of pacing for tachycardia termination. If the accessory AV connection is capable of rapid antegrade conduction, the induction of atrial fibrillation may result in rapid, life-threatening ventricular rates. Pacing is therefore contraindicated in such patients. Although there is no consensus for a particular cutoff with regard to antegrade accessory pathway refractoriness, we consider an effective refractory period of 330 to 350 msec or greater *during catecholamine infusion* to be acceptable for chronic pacing therapy.

It is also significant that a disproportionate number of patients dying suddenly with an antitachycardia pacemaker for AV reentrant supraventricular tachycardia had the lead placed in the ventricle. Although the cause of death was not always known in these patients, we do not recommend ventricular pacing for termination of chronic AV reentrant tachycardia.

Antitachycardia Pacemaker Evaluation and Follow-Up

Careful and repeated testing of tachycardia termination should be performed in all patients considered for permanent implants. We do approximately 50 to 100 induction/terminations of supraventricular tachycardia before implantation and assess the effectiveness of various pacing modalities and burst cycle lengths. An explanted nonsterile device is very useful for this purpose. After implantation, the permanent device is used for further testing.

One must also not neglect careful postimplant measurements of pacing threshold and sensing level both in sinus rhythm *and during* supraventricular tachycardia. The most effective stimulus pattern is useless if capture is lost or if undersensing occurs. We use output levels 20 to 30 percent greater than the usual 100 percent voltage safety margin for pacing. Bradycardia pacing is programmed off unless it is specifically needed.

Implanted pacemakers can potentially benefit patients with paroxysmal supraventricular tachycardia but seem less effective for long-term management of patients with AV reentrant accessory pathway tachycardias than of those with other mechanisms. Attrition in the use of implanted pacemakers has been due to sensing problems, tachycardia frequency, and atrial fibrillation. The success of pacing therapy may also reflect the level and sophistication of lead and device technology. Capabilities such as rate adaptation of the terminating burst, multiple tachycardia detection algorithms, the ability to program bradycardia pacing off (OAOT mode), and better atrial lead systems may, in the future, contribute to improved results in AV reentrant arrhythmias.

SURGERY FOR PATIENTS WITH THE WOLFF-PARKINSON-WHITE SYNDROME

Surgery is clearly recommended for patients with the Wolff-Parkinson-White syndrome and life-threatening cardiac arrhythmias that are refractory to drug therapy. More recently, surgical interventions have been applied to patients with the Wolff-Parkinson-White syndrome in order to obviate the need for lifelong drug therapy.

Endocardial Studies

All surgical candidates must have detailed electrophysiologic studies prior to ablation. These studies include endocardial mapping in order to locate the site(s) of the accessory pathway(s). It is critical to obtain as much information as possible relating to pathway location and function *prior* to surgery. In addition, we leave a multipolar electrode catheter in the coronary sinus in order to facilitate mapping of the left free wall in the operating room. As with candidates for catheter ablation, we attempt to confirm the results of endocardial catheter mapping with noninvasive nuclear scintigraphic or cine computed tomographic techniques.

Epicardial Mapping

At surgery, the heart is exposed using a sternum-splitting approach. A pair of electrodes is sutured on to the right atrium and right ventricle. We first pace the right atrium to determine the cycle length associated with maximum preexcitation but without deleterious hemodynamic effects. During atrial pacing, a roving probe is used to explore the ventricle at the level of the annulus in order to detect the earliest area of ventricular preexcitation. After completion of the ventricular map, the ventricle is paced and retrograde atrial mapping is achieved by exploring the atrial myocardium adjacent to the annulus. Mapping may be performed during induced supraventricular tachycardia provided the patient remains hemodynamically stable during the arrhythmia. Mapping may be continued under cardiopulmonary bypass but must be abbreviated in order to minimize the duration of extracorporeal support.

Surgical Technique

Currently, two surgical techniques are used for ablation of accessory pathways. The traditional approach involves dividing the pathway(s) using an endocardial incision and extending the dissection to the epicardial reflection on the ventricle. Another approach, used by Guiraudon and colleagues, uses an epicardial approach with dissection into the fat pad over the annulus. In both surgical procedures, the ends of the incision are "closed" in order to provide for pathways immediately subjacent to the annulus. Both surgical procedures are associated with a success rate of 90 to 100 percent and a mortality rate of less than 1 percent. Surgery has become the treatment of choice for patients with the Wolff-Parkinson-White syndrome and malignant arrhythmias. Patients with the Wolff-Parkinson-White syndrome with the shortest preexcited R-R interval during atrial fibrillation of less than 250 msec appear to be at increased risk for sudden death. In addition, surgery is currently more widely offered to patients with tachycardia who do not wish to be dependent on lifelong drug therapy. Surgical therapy affords an improved quality of life for such patients compared with those treated with long-term medical therapy. These considerations are particularly important for adolescents with ambivalent feelings about long-term oral therapy or for women who are planning pregnancies.

SUGGESTED READING

Cox JL, Gallagher JJ, Cain ME. Experience with 118 consecutive patients undergoing operation for the Wolff-Parkinson-White syndrome. J Thoracic Cardiovasc Surg 1985; 90:490–501.

Guiraudon GM, Klein GJ, Sharma AD, et al. Closed-heart technique for Wolff-Parkinson-White syndrome: Further experience and potential limitations. Ann Thorac Surg 1986; 42:651–657.

Morady F, Scheinman M, Kou W, et al. Long-term results of catheter ablation of a posteroseptal accessory atrioventricular connection in 48 patients. Circulation 1989; 79:1160–1170.

Newman D, Evans GT, Scheinman MM. Catheter ablation of cardiac arrhythmias. Curr Probl Cardiol 1989; 14:119–155.

Scheinman MM. Catheter ablation for patients with cardiac arrhythmias. PACE 1986; 9:551–564.

Schnittger I, Lee JT, Hargis J, et al. Long-term results of antitachycardia pacing with the Cybertach-60 (Intermedics, Inc.) in patients with supraventricular tachycardia. PACE, 1989; 12:936–941.

PREEXCITATION SYNDROMES: NONPHARMACOLOGIC MANAGEMENT

SANJEEV SAKSENA, M.D.
HUANLIN AN, M.D.

Serious and symptomatic supraventricular tachyarrhythmias are frequently observed in patients with preexcitation syndromes. Therapy has been designed to alleviate symptoms as well as to improve patient survival. The scientific basis for identifying effective therapy has been advanced with increasing knowledge of the electrophysiologic mechanisms underlying supraventricular tachyarrhythmias in this condition. Experimental and clinical investigations have established that the fundamental abnormality in preexcitation syndromes is a congenital cardiac anomaly in which one or more abnormal pathways of electrical impulse propagation exist. In the most common type of preexcitation syndrome, the Wolff-Parkinson-White syndrome, the abnormal pathway connects the atrium and ventricle, functioning as an atrioventricular bypass tract. In other variants, structures connected can include the atrium, the normal specialized conduction system or the ventricle, or abnormally rapid transmission in the normal specialized conduction system may be present. In most instances, bypass tract conduction is unusually rapid although slowly conducting pathways are now well described. Arrhythmogenesis occurs either by reentrant mechanisms involving the bypass tract(s) or by abnormally rapid atrioventricular conduction of a supraventricular tachyarrhythmia such as atrial flutter, atrial fibrillation, or atrial tachycardia (reentrant or ectopic). In either instance, abnormally rapid heart rates may be achieved with increasingly ineffective ventricular function and impaired cardiac output. Symptoms associated with the tachyarrhythmia can range from a total absence of symptoms to a perception of rapid heart action (palpitations), compromise of forward cardiac output with evidence of a low cardiac output state (presyncope and syncope), and in the most significant state, induction of ventricular fibrillation and cardiac arrest.

An individual patient with ventricular preexcitation can, however, be asymptomatic and remain asymptomatic. Thus, the natural history of the preexcitation syndromes is of importance in designing treatment. Asymptomatic patients usually have a low incidence of major cardiac events. During longitudinal follow-up, a significant proportion of these asymptomatic patients (perhaps up to 30 percent) may lose the capacity for preexcitation and antegrade conduction over the accessory pathway. This is most often observed in older patients who have prolonged antegrade bypass tract refractory periods. Disappearance of antegrade preexcitation is frequently also observed in children during the first year of life. However, a significant proportion may develop spontaneous supraventricular tachyarrhythmias. One study indicated that 7 percent of patients developed supraventricular tachyarrhythmias within a 3-year period. In symptomatic patients, a relapsing and recurring course is the usual pattern. Periods of remission, however, are not uncommon. Similarly, paroxysmal exacerbation even to the point of incessant tachycardias can be observed. The true incidence of recurrent cardiac arrest in patients with atrial fibrillation and rapid antegrade atrioventricular conduction or a history of prior cardiac arrest remains unknown. Finally, ventricular fibrillation can be the presenting manifestation of the Wolff-Parkinson-White syndrome. With these limitations in our knowledge of the natural history of this disorder, selecting the appropriate point in time for therapeutic intervention is often debated. It is our general practice to recommend antiarrhythmic therapy in patients in whom there is a reasonable expectation that survival may be prolonged or significant symptoms may be relieved. In each instance, a careful analysis of the benefits of the therapy versus its risks must be undertaken. The duration of therapy as well as its impact on the psychological, social, and economic aspects of the patient's life needs to be carefully considered. These latter issues assume importance because the vast majority of patients are young, active, and often gainfully employed.

Therapeutic options for these arrhythmias include pharmacologic and nonpharmacologic (interventional) therapy. Interventional therapy may consist of ablation of the arrhythmogenic substrate (intraoperative or catheter) or implantation of an antitachycardia device. Interventional therapy is generally employed in several different clinical situations. In our practice, this approach is restricted to symptomatic patients with supraventricular tachyarrhythmias associated with the preexcitation syndromes and generally not applied to asymptomatic patients. Infrequent exceptions may be made in instances in which asymptomatic patients wish to pursue employment or pursuits in which elimination of the arrhythmogenic substrate is a prerequisite. The indications we currently employ for interventional therapy are as follows:

1. Supraventricular tachyarrhythmias with severe symptoms or life-threatening electrical or hemodynamic consequences. This includes patients with hypotensive supraventricular tachyarrhythmias with or without syncope, induction of ischemia or ventricular failure with the tachyarrhythmia, documented ventricular fibrillation or cardiac arrest, or evidence of a tachycardia-induced cardiomyopathy with progressive cardiac failure.
2. Patients with limited symptoms associated with these supraventricular tachyarrhythmias that are not of a life-threatening nature but are refractory to trials of antiarrhythmic drugs. In general, a trial of two or more antiarrhythmic drugs is undertaken prior to consideration of such therapy.
3. Patients with supraventricular tachyarrhythmias in whom nonpharmacologic therapy is preferred to pharmacologic therapy by the patient. These preferences are usually based on the need for continuous and prolonged antiarrhythmic drug therapy that may not be acceptable to the patient, particularly in a young individual. Alternatively, the patient's inability to comply with such a regimen, the long-term economic cost, or limitations in employment may elicit such an indication.
4. Patients who are intolerant to antiarrhythmic drugs even though the selected agent(s) may be effective in arrhythmia control.

A more formalized approach for patient selection using individual scores for a variety of clinical, social, psychological, and demographic factors has been employed at some centers. The highest priority for interventional therapy is given to patients who fall into the above categories. The scoring system permits quantification and may be helpful in patient selection. Other centers differentiate patients for interventional therapy into those who require direct intervention and those who are candidates for such intervention. The former group of patients have life-threatening arrhythmias or highly symptomatic drug-refractory arrhythmias. Patients who are moderately or minimally symptomatic are considered candidates for interventional therapy as one of their choices during selection of definitive treatment. We prefer an individualized approach to each patient. A careful explanation of the benefits and risks of interventional therapy permits the opportunity of eliciting patient and family response, if necessary, before the final decision to undertake an intervention is completed. Often, it is necessary to discuss immediate short-term therapy with a view to more definitive long-term therapy, particularly in patients who are not highly symptomatic. Pharmacologic therapy is often a bridge during this short-term period until the decision to undertake definitive interventional therapy has been completed. Conversely, clinical observation and follow-up of a patient may provide significant direction as to the need for interventional therapy. Prolonged remission after a temporary exacerbation may result in deferring this form of therapy and, conversely, a relapsing recurrent course may precipitate the decision toward this treatment.

INTERVENTIONAL TECHNIQUES

Ablation

Ablation of the arrhythmogenic substrate in the preexcitation syndromes has been most widely applied to supraventricular tachyarrhythmias associated with the Wolff-Parkinson-White syndrome. It has been less frequently applied to uncommon varieties of the preexcitation syndrome such as Lown-Ganong-Levine syndrome (enhanced atrioventricular nodal conduction), Mahaim fibers, or the permanent form of junctional reciprocating tachycardia utilizing retrogradely conducting septal accessory tracts. This is related to the greater prevalence of WPW syndrome and a better definition of the anatomic substrate for arrhythmogenesis. The mechanisms of the supraventricular tachyarrhythmias in the Wolff-Parkinson-White syndrome have now been extensively defined. These have been discussed in earlier chapters in this text.

Interruption of the tachycardia circuit in atrioventricular reentrant tachycardia can be accomplished at four different levels, namely, the atrium, atrioventricular node and His-Purkinje system, ventricle, or accessory bypass tract. In general, the specialized conduction system and the accessory pathway have been considered the vulnerable links for ablative purposes. These structures are amenable to focal and limited ablation and are critical to arrhythmogenesis. Although the earliest attempt at controlling supraventricular tachycardia utilized interruption of the specialized conduction system, in recent years interruption or modification of conduction in the accessory bypass tract has become the procedure of choice. This is aimed at preserving normal physiologic transmission of the sinus node impulse with the advantages of modulated atrioventricular conduction owing to the presence of the atrioventricular node. In addition, the long-term stability of accessory pathway conduction is unknown. Although ablation had been performed almost exclusively intraoperatively using a variety of different techniques, it has now been performed using cardiac catheterization techniques.

A prerequisite for either type of ablation is accurate identification of the target tissue. This is achieved by cardiac mapping. Cardiac mapping can be performed by the catheter technique alone or in conjunction with intraoperative electrical mapping techniques. Identification of the normal specialized atrioventricular conduction system and the accessory pathway is usually sought. Intraoperative ablation is accomplished by mechanical resection or cryothermal or laser energy. Catheter ablation is accomplished by the delivery of a direct current shock or radiofrequency current.

Catheter Ablation

Catheter ablation procedures for accessory bypass tracts are currently performed under an investigational device exemption protocol at our institution. The protocol is approved by the Institutional Review Board and the Food and Drug Administration. The device used for ablation is a standard quadripolar pacing and recording electrode catheter. Use of this device for ablation is currently considered an experimental application in the United States. Thus, informed consent for a catheter ablation procedure is obtained after explanation of the nature of the procedure as well as the risks and benefits associated with it. The efficacy of catheter ablation for bypass tracts is often dependent on the exact location of the bypass tract. Since this is not precisely known prior to the mapping procedure, it becomes necessary to have good localization of the bypass tract in order to obtain truly informed consent. Nevertheless, we routinely inform patients that the final decision to perform catheter ablation is taken during the procedure and is based on the final determination of the location of the bypass tract in relation to surrounding structures and its accessibility to catheter ablation.

A significant amount of information has to be obtained prior to undertaking the ablation proce-

dure. Prior electrophysiologic studies should elucidate a reproducible mode of initiation as well as interruption of the tachyarrhythmia. Hemodynamic monitoring during the cardiac arrhythmia is essential. A full cardiac catheterization with angiographic studies to define ventricular function, coronary artery anatomy, and the structure and function of the coronary sinus needs to be undertaken. Most often, this is performed as a separate procedure prior to the catheter ablation. On occasion, we have combined angiographic and electrophysiologic studies. We have found this particularly valuable in the case of posteroseptal accessory tracts where ablation of the tract is influenced by its proximity to the coronary artery and coronary sinus. In these instances, an electrode catheter is located at the site of the bypass tract. With the electrode catheter in situ, usually in the vicinity of the coronary sinus, left coronary angiography with prolonged arterial and venous phase imaging is performed. During the coronary sinus phase, the vein is defined and the anatomic location of the electrode closest to the bypass tract in relation to the coronary sinus can be clearly visualized.

A catheter ablation procedure at our center is generally performed when ablation of a posteroseptal accessory tract or a right-sided accessory tract is being considered. Infrequently, we have attempted ablation of a left-sided accessory tract using a transseptal catheterization of the left atrium through a patent foramen ovale. Multipolar electrode catheters are inserted in the right atrium, atrioventricular junction, right ventricular apex, and coronary sinus. In the instance of left-sided accessory tracts, transseptal placement of an electrode catheter through a patent foramen ovale has been attempted. Alternatively, retrograde catheterization of the left ventricle with the Judkins technique, and retrogradely of the left atrium, has been reported. Atrioventricular reentrant tachycardia is initiated by standard programmed electrical stimulation techniques. Catheter endocardial mapping is performed to localize the site of earliest retrograde atrial activation along the atrioventricular groove. Retrograde ventriculoatrial conduction intervals of 100 msec or less should be obtained at this site. The exact interval depends on tachycardia cycle length, concomitant antiarrhythmic drug therapy, and the presence or absence of bundle branch block. We have generally avoided accepting retrograde atrial activation in ventricular pacing as equivalent and will make every effort to initiate atrioventricular reentry, including the use of multiple stimulation sites or sympathomimetic agents (Fig. 1). In some instances, potentials from the accessory tract can be identified (Fig. 2).

After localization of the atrial insertion of the accessory tract in the atrioventricular groove, the precise anatomic location of this tract should be determined. Posteroseptal accessory tracts that are located at or outside the os of the coronary sinus are amenable to the direct current shock catheter abla-

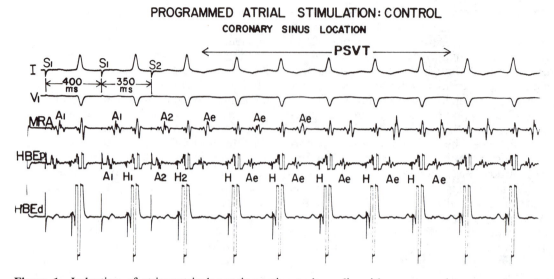

PROGRAMMED ATRIAL STIMULATION: CONTROL
CORONARY SINUS LOCATION

Figure 1 Induction of atrioventricular reciprocating tachycardia with coronary sinus programmed electrical stimulation. In this patient, conventional high right atrial stimulation was ineffective in stimulating tachycardia. Tachycardia cycle length is 350 msec. Abbreviations: MRA = mid right atrium; HBep = proximal His bundle electrogram; HBed = distal His bundle electrogram; AA = atrial electrogram; AE = atrial echo; S = pacing stimulus; H = His bundle electrogram. (From Saksena S, et al. Role of electrophysiologic studies with acute drug testing in refractory supraventricular tachycardia. In: Steinbach K, Glogar D, Laskowitz A, et al, eds. Cardiac pacing. Darmstadt, West Germany: Steinkopff Verlag, 1989, with permission.)

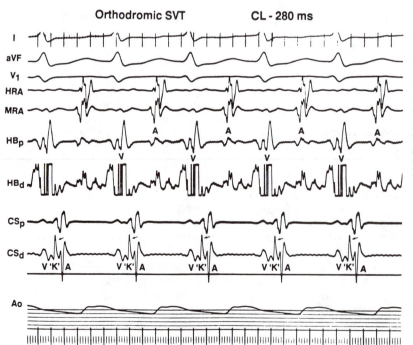

Figure 2 Catheter endocardial mapping during induced orthodromic supraventricular tachycardia. Note that the retrograde atrial activation pattern indicates a left lateral atrioventricular bypass tract. A high frequency Kent potential is recorded at this site. Abbreviations: HRA = high right atrium; MRA = mid right atrium; HB = His bundle; p = proximal; d = distal; CS = coronary sinus; Ao = aorta; K = Kent potential; A = atrial electrogram; V = ventricular electrogram.

tion technique. Atrial endocardial ablation for right- or left-sided tracts can be attempted along the atrioventricular groove. At present, we do not attempt direct current shock ablation through electrodes placed within the coronary sinus. High-frequency current delivery in the coronary sinus has been reported to be effective in modifying accessory tract conduction in selected patients. For the direct current shock technique, we commonly employ an initial shock energy of 160 to 250 J. The catheter electrode is used as the cathode, and an interscapular backplate is used as the anode. Prior to ablation, temporary ventricular pacing through a previously positioned catheter electrode is established. Arterial blood pressure is monitored during the entire procedure. Intravenous thiopental is used for short-term general anesthesia. Ablation is usually performed during sinus rhythm, although it could be performed during induced tachycardia. In our experience, rapid heart motion during tachycardia complicates precise catheter positioning and maintenance during ablation. After general anesthesia is induced, the first shock is delivered. In most instances of posteroseptal accessory tract ablation, complete atrioventricular block of a transient nature can be expected. For free wall pathway ablation, disappearance of the delta wave with resumption of normal atrioventricular conduction may appear. If this is not observed, further mapping for more precise bypass tract localization is indicated. Following the first ablative shock, a second equivalent or incremental shock is delivered through an adjoining set of electrodes after repositioning of the catheter at the ablative site. Delivery of both shocks is accomplished within a few minutes, and general anesthesia is then terminated. Serial measurements of cardiac enzymes and electrocardiograms are performed in all patients, and continuous hemodynamic monitoring is maintained.

Immediately after the ablative procedure, reinduction of tachycardia may be attempted and reevaluation of atrioventricular and ventriculoatrial conduction patterns may be undertaken. However, in all instances, this should be recognized as being an acute effect, and the chronic effect of the ablative procedure will be apparent only after several days. When radiofrequency current is used, multiple pulses of low to moderate power output ranging from 2 to 20 W are employed. Hemodynamic compromise is uncommon with radiofrequency current delivery. General anesthesia is also not necessary during this procedure. In our experience, most currently available catheter electrodes are unsuitable for radiofrequency energy delivery. The results of radiofrequency catheter ablation of accessory tracts in several centers are summarized in Table 1.

At the end of the catheter ablative procedure, the patient is transferred to the intensive care unit where he or she is monitored for 24 to 48 hours to ensure hemodynamic and electrical stability. Particular attention is paid to the development of hypotension with the possibility of pericardial tamponade, ventricular arrhythmias related to ventricular injury, or atrioventricular block. Recovery of preexcitation within the first 24 hours usually predicts failure of the ablative attempt, and a second attempt is considered. The option of surgical ablation should be considered as well at the time of failure of the catheter ablative procedure. A cardiac surgeon is usually involved in the decision to perform catheter ablation as opposed to surgical ablation and in the discussion of the risks of the catheter ablation procedure. This individual is usually available in case emergency surgical exploration is necessary for treatment of complications. Figure 3 shows an example of a patient undergoing catheter ablation of the posteroseptal accessory tract. Preoperative elec-

Table 1 Clinical Studies in Radiofrequency Ablation

Cardiac Tissue	Author	Number of Patients	Immediate Results		Long-Term Results	
			Complete Success (%)	Partial Success (%)	Complete Success (%)	Partial Success (%)
Atrioventricular junction	Goy	3	1 (33)	0 (0)	1 (33)	0 (0)
	Lavergne et al	2	1 (50)	0 (0)	1 (50)	1 (50)
	Huang et al	1	1 (100)	0 (0)	1 (100)	0 (0)
	Davis et al	3	2 (67)	0 (0)	1 (33)	0 (0)
	Scanu et al	3	3 (100)	0 (0)	3 (100)	0 (0)
	Borggrefe et al	10	6 (60)	2 (20)	5 (50)	1 (10)
	Bowman et al	3	3 (100)	0 (0)	3 (100)	0 (0)
	Saksena et al	4	3 (75)	0 (0)	1 (25)	2 (50)
	Total	31	22 (71)	2 (6)	18 (58)	4 (13)
Bypass tract	Goy	3	1 (33)	0 (0)	1 (33)	1 (33)
	Huang et al	1	0 (0)	0 (0)	0 (0)	0 (0)
	Borggrefe et al	7	2 (29)	0 (0)	1 (14)	0 (0)
	Saksena et al	1	0 (0)	0 (0)	0 (0)	0 (0)
	Total	14	5 (36)	0 (0)	3 (21)	2 (14)

trophysiologic study confirms the presence of such a tract and baseline atrioventricular conduction intervals show a P-A interval of 20 msec, an A-H interval of 65 msec, and an H-V interval of 60 msec. Atrioventricular reentrant tachycardia was induced and the shortest retrograde ventriculoatrial conduction interval was measured at the os of the coronary sinus at 85 msec (Fig. 3A). Two 150 J direct current shocks were delivered at this site (Fig. 3B). After the first shock, the patient developed transient atrial flutter followed by sinus bradycardia. After the second shock, the patient developed junctional tachycardia for 15 sec, followed by sinus rhythm with frequent premature ventricular complexes. Postoperatively,

bypass tract conduction was abolished and no inducible supraventricular tachycardia was elicited (Fig. 3C).

Intraoperative Ablation

Intraoperative ablation can be employed for interruption of the accessory bypass tract or the normal specialized conduction system. In the majority of instances, the former is practiced. Currently, the latter approach is reserved for special circumstances in which the arrhythmia is not amenable to accessory bypass tract ablation alone or if bypass tract ablation has failed. Permanent pacemaker implanta-

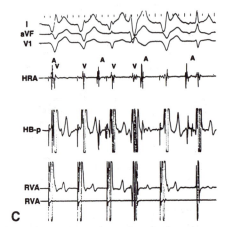

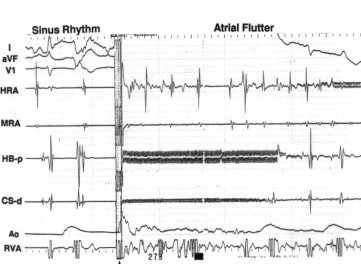

Figure 3 A, Mapping of orthodromic supraventricular tachycardia using catheter endocardial techniques. The earliest retrograde atrial activation during atrioventricular reentrant tachycardia is noted in the proximal coronary sinus electrogram almost coincidentally with the His bundle electrogram. The measured ventriculoatrial time (VA) is 85 msec. Coronary angiography with a venous phase localized this electrode to be at the os of the coronary sinus. B, Catheter ablation of the posteroseptal accessory tract identified in A. Synchronous 150 J direct current shock was delivered at the os of the coronary sinus through the proximal pair of electrodes in the coronary sinus catheter. This results in induction of atrial tachyarrhythmias with antegrade atrioventricular nodal conduction. C, Postoperative electrophysiologic study after catheter ablation of the posteroseptal tract shows absence of retrograde ventriculoatrial conduction consistent with successful ablation of the bypass tract. I, aVF, V1 = ECG leads, HRA = high right atrium, MRA = mid right atrium, HB-p = His bundle—proximal, HB-d = His bundle—distal, CS-p = coronary sinus—proximal, CS-d = coronary sinus—distal, RVA = right ventricular apex, Ao = aortic pressure, CL = cycle length, MS = milliseconds.

tion is necessary if the latter procedure is performed. Concomitant performance of both procedures is rarely undertaken, although it is often discussed. Prior to undertaking an intraoperative procedure, preoperative screening includes a full cardiac catheterization and endocardial mapping, usually during the induced tachycardia. Preoperative electrophysiologic studies are performed using standard techniques employed for patients with preexcitation syndromes. Individual arrhythmias are induced and their mechanisms analyzed. Reproducible initiation of the arrhythmia with programmed electrical stimulation should be demonstrated. At this time, the induction mode and the site used for programmed stimulation should be carefully noted. Preoperative catheter endocardial mapping is usually performed during induced atrioventricular reentrant tachycardia. Retrograde atrial activation is mapped during this rhythm, and the shortest ventriculoatrial conduction interval is determined. The site of this observation in our laboratory is recorded on videotape or on cineangiographic film in two perpendicular planes.

Intraoperative epicardial mapping is performed using a multipolar strip electrode that permits simultaneous recording along the entire atrioventricular groove (Fig. 4). More recently, a band electrode has been employed to obtain recording from the anterior and posterior aspects of the atrioventricular groove and analyzed using computerized mapping techniques. Mapping is performed during induced orthodromic supraventricular tachycardia. It can occasionally be observed that this tachycardia may not be inducible or unsustained at the time of surgical mapping. Computerized mapping techniques are useful in unsustained arrhythmias, and preoperative catheter endocardial mapping is essential to the ablative procedure if intraoperative mapping cannot be performed. In some instances, retrograde atrial activation patterns are determined during ventricular pacing. Although these may be similar to activation mapping during orthodromic tachycardia, atrioventricular conduction intervals are rarely as short as during induced tachycardia. Localization of the bypass tract achieved is often similar to that obtained with induced atrioventricular reentrant tachycardia, but specific pitfalls exist. Simultaneous retrograde activation of the bypass tract and the specialized atrioventricular conduction system during ventricular pacing provides two pathways for retrograde atrial activation. Thus, early activation in the interventricular groove and the posterior right atrium can be expected during ventricular pacing.

After analysis of ventriculoatrial conduction intervals and localization of the bypass tract, several different surgical approaches can be undertaken for tract ablation. In the classic endocardial ablation technique, different approaches are utilized for right-sided and left-sided accessory tracts. In the former, a right atriotomy is performed along the lateral margin of the right atrium. Right atrial endocardial mapping is performed to localize the bundle of His, usually using a hand-held probe. The atrium is incised along the atrioventricular groove at the site of the bypass tract, which can be reconfirmed by endocardial mapping prior to resection. Atrial ablation can be performed with standard mechanical incision techniques coupled with atrioventricular groove dissection by cryoablation or the use of pulsed argon laser discharges. In each instance, after completion of the atriotomy and atrial ablation, dissection in the atrioventricular groove is usually performed until the epicardial surface is reached. This is generally done to eliminate the possibility of strands of accessory bypass tract that may exist in a subepicardial location. In the case of posteroseptal accessory tracts, the posterior septum of the right atrium is excised, carefully avoiding the His bundle location. Dissection is performed in the posterior interatrial triangle to complete the procedure. In left-sided accessory tracts, a standard left posterior atriotomy is performed for exposure of the mitral valvular apparatus and supravalvular endocardium. Endocardial atriotomy can be performed by mechanical or laser techniques (Fig. 5), and endocardial ablation can be performed by cryothermal techniques. Atrioventricular groove dissection can be performed up to the epicardium. The atriotomy is repaired. For left-sided tract ablation, hypothermic cardioplegic arrest is essential. In right-sided ablation techniques, partial cardiopulmonary bypass may be adequate.

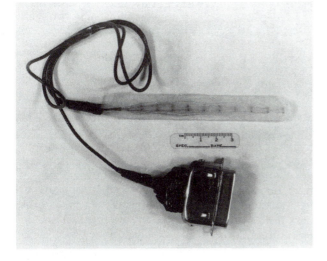

Figure 4 Prototype intraoperative epicardial plaque electrode used for mapping along the atrioventricular groove. This prototype enables multiple recordings along the atrioventricular groove to be obtained from the atrial or ventricular aspect during sinus rhythm, ventricular pacing, and induced orthodromic atrioventricular reentrant tachycardia.

NSR with preexcitation   RVP induction   Orthodromic SVT

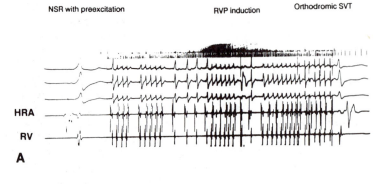

HRA

RV

A

Orthodromic SVT (V00 pacemaker)

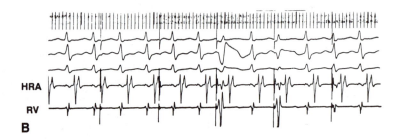

HRA

RV

B

5 second Argon Laser Pulse

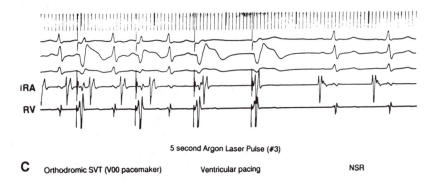

IRA

RV

5 second Argon Laser Pulse (#3)

C   Orthodromic SVT (V00 pacemaker)   Ventricular pacing   NSR

Figure 5 Ablation of a right anterior septal accessory pathway in a normothermic patient during induced orthodromic supraventricular tachycardia associated with the Wolff-Parkinson-White syndrome. During sinus rhythm (top panel), ventricular preexcitation is clearly evident. The tachycardia is induced by bursts of rapid ventricular pacing in the uppermost panel. Pulsed argon laser ablation is commenced during the induced tachycardia. A non-sensing ventricular paced beat from a previously implanted pacemaker is intermittently seen (middle panel) with maintenance of retrograde accessory pathway conduction. After the third laser pulse, the tachycardia terminates due to retrograde accessory pathway block (bottom panel) and a subsequent sinus beat shows elimination of preexcitation. This patient with incessant supraventricular tachycardia has had no postoperative spontaneous recurrences of tachycardia nor any inducible tachycardia on laboratory testing. The postoperative electrocardiograms continue to show normal antegrade atrioventricular conduction.

Alternative approaches utilize closed heart techniques for ablation. In this approach, epicardial ablation of the atrium and the atrioventricular groove is performed. This can be done using cryoablation techniques. Dissection of the atrioventricular groove from the epicardial surface is undertaken, and then cryoablation is performed along the groove. This can be performed in nearly all locations in the atrioventricular groove, except for certain specific types of septal accessory tract locations. This technique avoids the need for prolonged cardiopulmonary bypass and in many cases eliminates the need for cardiopulmonary bypass. Hypothermic cardioplegic arrest is not necessary, and the effect of the ablative technique can be directly assessed in the normothermic heart. Epicardial laser discharges are being evaluated for the same purpose. Upon completion of the ablative procedure, programmed atrioventricular stimulation is usually repeated to reevaluate bypass tract conduction and the inducibility of supraventricular tachycardia. Often, additional bypass tracts are demonstrated at this time, requiring repeated mapping and ablation. This procedure is essential for assessment of failure of surgical ablation and the demonstration of additional bypass tracts. It should be routinely performed unless precluded by the patient's clinical condition.

Implantation of Antitachycardia Device

Device therapy is considered for patients with reentrant supraventricular tachycardias. In the preexcitation syndromes, this has been predominantly employed for atrioventricular reentrant tachycardia. In specific instances, atrioventricular nodal reentrant tachycardia associated with the preexcitation syndromes and atrial flutter has been treated in this fashion. However, this is usually in the setting of no manifest or provokable ventricular preexcitation. Antitachycardia devices employed in this fashion sense tachycardia primarily based on rate with secondary criteria, such as rate stability, being employed in specific instances. The sensing rate is programmed at the time of device implant. Electrical termination modes used in patients with atrioventricular reentrant tachycardia include programmed extrastimuli as well as burst pacing, decremental or incremental pacing performed either from the atrium or the ventricle, or simultaneous dual-chamber pacing performed in the atrium and ventricle. In some instances, coronary sinus pacing, i.e., left atrial pacing, is performed. Although a variety of devices have been used over the years, the most recent and sophisticated antitachycardia devices include the Cordis Orthocor Model 284A, Intermedics Intertach, Medtronic Model 7008 Interactive Tachycardia System, and the Telectronics Pasar. With the exception of the Medtronic Model 7008 unit, these are single-chamber devices. The lead is positioned in the chamber to be stimulated. Bipolar and unipolar

pacing and sensing configurations are available in most units. In the instance of the Medtronic Symbios 7008, atrial and ventricular leads are inserted. Termination is usually accomplished by overdrive atrial pacing (Fig. 6) or less commonly, ventricular extrastimulation (Fig. 7).

Prospective evaluation of a candidate for an implantable antitachycardia device involves careful assessment of the clinical history to determine the frequency of tachycardia episodes. Because tachycardia episodes may or may not be perceived by the patient, these can be potential limitations of the patient history. Nevertheless, information as to the frequency of tachycardia episodes should be determined on this basis, as well as the use of more objective means such as ambulatory electrocardiographic monitoring and the record of the patient's past hospitalizations. The hemodynamic consequences of the arrhythmia can be elicited. The occurrence of presyncope or syncope after the onset of the arrhythmia should be determined. Immediate onset of hemodynamic compromise eliminates the possibility of using manually triggered devices and emphasizes the need for rapid arrhythmia reversion. Clinical examination should be directed at the status of the patient's cardiac disease. The presence of an-

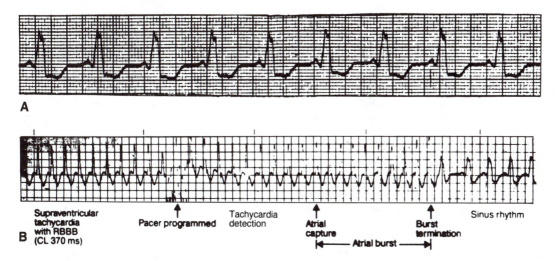

Figure 6 Management of supraventricular tachycardia in a patient with the Wolff-Parkinson-White syndrome using a dual-chamber antitachycardia pacemaker. *A*, In this patient with incessant supraventricular tachycardia, a Medtronic Model 7008 Symbios pacemaker was inserted, and bipolar stimulation was used to achieve permanent paced preexcitation. Atrioventricular sequential pacing was established in the DVI mode with an atrioventricular interval of 100 msec. This resulted in a marked decrease in the frequency of supraventricular tachycardia episodes. *B*, Recurrent paroxysmal supraventricular tachycardia was occasionally observed, and the same antitachycardia device as shown in *A* is now programmed to the automatic mode using atrial burst pacing for tachycardia termination. Supraventricular tachycardia with a right bundle branch block configuration with a cycle length of 370 msec occurred spontaneously. The pacemaker is programmed to the predetermined antitachycardia device termination mode. Automatic tachycardia detection ensues within the next 2 seconds and is followed by the delivery of an atrial burst that resets the tachycardia and results in antegrade atrioventricular nodal block with penetration of the accessory pathway antegradely and failure of maintenance of the tachycardia wavefront. The patient subsequently reverts to sinus rhythm with antegrade preexcitation. (From Saksena S, Goldschlager N. Electrical therapy of cardiac arrhythmias, Philadelphia: W.B. Saunders, 1990, with permission.)

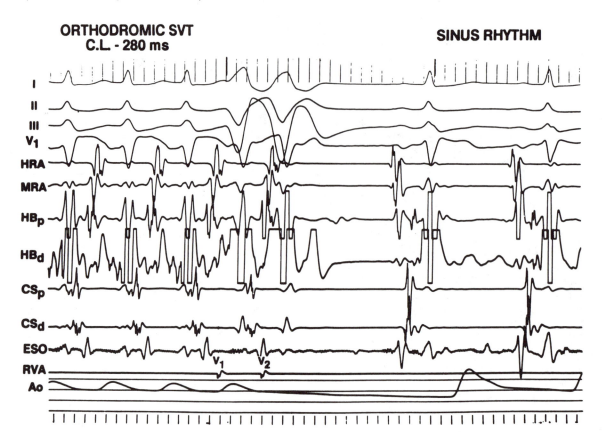

Figure 7 Termination of orthodromic SVT by paired ventricular extrastimuli. The tachycardia is terminated by two ventricular extrastimuli at close coupling intervals (V_1, V_2). V_1 results in retrograde atrial activation, which is advanced, and V_2 results in retrograde ventriculoatrial (VA) block. This results in interruption of the tachycardia. In this instance, resetting precedes termination. Abbreviations: HRA = high right atrium; MRA = mid right atrium; LRA = low right atrium; HB_p = proximal His bundle electrogram; HB_d = distal His bundle electrogram; RVA = right ventricular apex; Ao = aorta; C.L. = cycle length; SVT = supraventricular tachycardia; CS_p = proximal coronary sinus electrogram; CS_d = distal coronary sinus electrogram; ESO = esophageal electrogram; V_1, V_2 = ventricular extrastimuli. (From Saksena S, An H. Electrophysiologic mechanisms underlying management of supraventricular tachycardia by electrical stimulation. In: Saksena S, Goldschlager N eds. Electrical therapy of cardiac arrhythmias, Philadelphia: W.B. Saunders, 1990, with permission.)

gina pectoris, congestive heart failure, or valvular incompetence needs to be considered. The patient's own intrinsic sinus rate is important, particularly when pacing in the ventricle is contemplated. In patients with concomitant sinus node dysfunction or bradycardia, demand ventricular pacing could result in pacemaker syndrome, worsening of congestive heart failure, or increased valvular incompetence. In addition, the use of rapid pacing modes in a patient with significant angina pectoris may precipitate an ischemic syndrome. These latter consequences must be considered relative contraindications to the use of device therapy.

Additional clinical information is obtained from noninvasive studies. Exercise testing to assess the sinus node response is valuable in defining the programmed sensing rate. Spontaneous recordings of

tachycardia on a definitive drug regimen are often valuable for the same purpose. Holter monitoring provides information regarding the number of episodes of unsustained and sustained tachyarrhythmias observed during the recording period as well as the variations in native sinus rate. This information is also used in programming the device. Although cardiac catheterization and coronary angiography are not essential parts of the preimplant evaluation, a complete and thorough assessment of the patient's native cardiac disease is essential. Because most patients with supraventricular tachyarrhythmias in the preexcitation syndromes are young, this information may be obtained most often by noninvasive methods. In older patients, the need for invasive evaluation is more frequent. Electrophysiologic evaluation, however, is an essential part of patient assessment. Baseline electrophysiologic studies should be performed in the absence of antiarrhythmic drug therapy using standard techniques. Multipolar electrode catheters and programmed electrical stimulation are employed. The mechanism of the supraventricular tachyarrhythmia as well as the essential components of the tachycardia circuit are defined. The antegrade and retrograde conduction patterns of the accessory bypass tract and the normal specialized conduction system are determined. Induction modes used for this purpose are carefully noted. Furthermore, termination techniques for the supraventricular tachycardia are studied. Exact stimulation intervals used in tachycardia induction and termination as well as some refractory periods are recorded. This may involve the use of single, double, triple or multiple extrastimuli, rapid burst pacing techniques that may be adaptive or nonadaptive, autodecremental rate-adaptive pacing, and simultaneous dual-chamber pacing in the atrium and ventricle.

After a decision is made to undertake antitachycardia device therapy, preimplant electrophysiologic evaluation of the discharge antiarrhythmic drug regimen is mandatory. In some instances, concomitant drug therapy is not necessary. Drug therapy is most often employed to reduce the frequency of supraventricular tachycardia, to reduce its rate to make it more amenable to pacing termination, or to limit the hemodynamic consequences of the tachycardia by slowing its rate. At the preimplant electrophysiologic study, repeated arrhythmia induction and reproducible arrhythmia termination need to be demonstrated. In most patients, a minimum of 50 episodes of induced arrhythmia should be reproducibly terminated by the selected mode. Although this may be difficult to achieve at a single study, it may be feasible by using a combination of laboratory testing and spontaneous arrhythmia termination in the monitored unit. After demonstration of reproducible arrhythmia termination, the antitachycardia device is implanted. Standard implantation pacemaker techniques are used. At the same time, temporary electrode catheter(s) are inserted for arrhythmia induction. After device implant and programming, repeated arrhythmia induction is undertaken, and a minimum of ten tachycardia terminations are demonstrated in our practice. After completion of the implant procedure, the patient is transferred back to a monitored unit. Cardiac monitoring is continued for a minimum of 72 hours to evaluate termination of spontaneous supraventricular tachycardia. This information can also be derived from the event counters in many antitachycardia devices. In many devices the capability for noninvasive arrhythmia induction using a triggered mode is available. Using this feature, serial arrhythmia induction and termination can be assessed. Typically, we perform our postimplant procedure for arrhythmia induction and termination by the implanted device. Patients with implanted antitachycardia devices are followed in an arrhythmia clinic. Periodic clinical follow-up at approximately 3-month intervals is performed to assess the clinical status of the cardiac arrhythmia and heart disease. In addition, device interrogation and evaluation can be undertaken at this time. In many instances, serial assessment of device function is performed using noninvasive arrhythmia induction and termination by the implanted device. In patients with supraventricular tachyarrhythmias with the preexcitation syndrome, this can most often be accomplished in the clinic itself. The clinic should have capabilities for electrical cardioversion as well as for immediate treatment of hemodynamic compromise and malignant ventricular arrhythmias on an emergency basis.

CLINICAL OUTCOME OF INTERVENTIONAL THERAPIES

The results of interventional therapies can now be assessed to some extent. Significant long-term experience exists with intraoperative ablation procedures using the endocardial approach. Perioperative mortality rates vary, depending on the presence or absence of concomitant cardiac disease. In the absence of any primary cardiac disease, perioperative mortality is 1 percent or less. However, in our experience and that of other centers, significant perioperative mortality can be expected in patients with advanced structural heart disease and the preexcitation syndrome. The extent of perioperative mortality is determined by the extent of cardiac disease, and complications are most often attributed to the latter condition. There is no currently available information that suggests that mapping and bypass tract resection ipso facto contribute to the negative outcome. Similar observations are in order with respect to perioperative morbidity. The epicardial closed heart technique has been widely advocated to reduce perioperative surgical risk with a high degree of efficacy. Guiraudon and colleagues have reported no perioperative mortality in over 200 cases operated on for preexcitation syndrome with this approach. With both approaches, long-term elimination of the ventricular preexcitation is apparent. Although ectopic atrial and ventricular arrhythmias may persist and be perceived by the same patients, elimination of symptomatic atrioventricular reentrant tachycardia and rapid bypass tract conduction may be expected in more than 90 percent of patients. Postoperative assessment of patient lifestyle and symptoms confirms a high degree of superiority of this approach. The outcome of catheter ablation procedures is currently being evaluated. Morady and coworkers reported the initial results of direct current shock ablation of posteroseptal accessory bypass tracts in eight patients. Successful interruption of bypass tract conduction was achieved in 75 percent of patients, with elimination of spontaneous tachycardia. More limited experience is available with other accessory tract locations primarily because of limited accessibility with conventional catheterization techniques and concern regarding damage to surrounding vascular structures. Nevertheless, early experience with radiofrequency catheter ablation has been encouraging with right-sided and certain left-sided bypass tracts. Radiofrequency ablation has been safe, but its efficacy remains to be examined in large studies. Direct current shock ablation of left-sided accessory tracts cannot be safely performed for the coronary sinus, and left atrial catheterization is usually necessary. Warin and colleagues have recently reported high success rates using transseptal or retrograde catheterization techniques and high energy direct current shocks. However, a small procedure-related mortality and morbidity rate has been reported and needs to be evaluated. At least one sudden death has also been reported during follow-up. At the present time, these approaches must be considered experimental, with long-term outcome awaiting critical evaluation.

Several antitachycardia pacemakers have been employed for management of atrioventricular reentrant tachycardia. Only atrial pacing modes are currently recommended, and the absence of antegrade preexcitation is required. Inducible atrial flutter/fibrillation is a contraindication to this therapy. Implantation is associated with no greater risk than for a conventional pacemaker implantation. Device efficacy has been rated from good to excellent in different series, but objective quantitative information is generally unavailable. Rare reports of sudden death have appeared, particularly in patients utilizing ventricular stimulation modes or having persistent antegrade bypass tract conduction. The use of such devices has remained infrequent in current medical practice, and implant rates have been relatively low.

It is reasonable to expect significant and continuing advances in interventional techniques. Increasing efficacy and safety of ablation techniques will result in wider and earlier application. Catheter ablation should prove increasingly acceptable for patients and physicians and may eventually compete with surgical ablative techniques. However, the surgical approach remains the current gold standard for effective and safe therapy. The epicardial approach may achieve greater popularity in the future. Device therapy remains a limited and second-line option for selected patients. Patterns of use currently suggest a small role for this therapy in clinical practice. With the availability of actual cardioversion/defibrillation devices this may change, but this remains to be established.

SUGGESTED READING

Borggrefe M, Budde T, Podczeck A, et al. High frequency alternating current ablation of an accessory pathway in humans. J Am Coll Cardiol 1987; 10:576.

Den Dulk K, et al. A versatile pacemaker system for termination of tachycardia with a programmable patient activator. Circulation 1982; 66 (Suppl II):217.

Fisher JD. Clinical results with implanted antitachycardia pacemakers. In: Saksena S, Goldschlager N, eds. Electrical therapy for cardiac arrhythmias. Philadelphia: WB Saunders, 1989:525.

Fisher JD, Brodman R, Kim SG, et al. Attempted nonsurgical electrical ablation of accessory pathways via the coronary sinus in the Wolff-Parkinson-White syndrome. J Am Coll Cardiol 1984; 4:685.

Gallagher JJ, et al. Wolff-Parkinson-White syndrome: The problem, evaluation and surgical correction. Circulation 1975; 51:767.

Gallagher JJ, et al. Epicardial mapping in the Wolff-Parkinson-White syndrome. Circulation 1978; 57:854.

Gallagher JJ, et al. The pre-excitation syndromes. Prog Cardiovasc Dis 1978; 20:285.

Gallagher JJ, Sealy WC, Cox JL, et al. Results of surgery for preexcitation caused by accessory atrioventricular pathways in 267 consecutive cases. In: Josephson ME, Wellens HJJ, eds. Tachycardias: Mechanisms, diagnosis, treatment. Philadelphia: Lea & Febiger, 1984:259.

Harrison L, et al. Cryosurgical ablation of the A-V node-His bundle: A new method of producing A-V block. Circulation 1977; 55–463.

Klein H, Saksena S. Diagnostic evaluation of the prospective antitachycardia device patient. In: Saksena S, Goldschlager N, eds. Electrical therapy for cardiac arrhythmias. Philadelphia: WB Saunders, 1989:p 439.

Krikler D, Curry P, Buffet J. Dual-demand pacing for reciprocating atrioventricular tachycardias. Br Med J 1976; 1:1114.

Levy S. Role of pacing in treatment of supraventricular tachycardia (supraventricular tachycardia, Wolff-Parkinson-White, flutter). In: Josephson ME, Wellens HJJ, eds. Tachycardias: Mechanisms, diagnosis, treatment. Philadelphia: Lea & Febiger, 1984:223.

Levy S, et al. Refractory supraventricular tachycardias: Successful therapy with double-demand sequential pacing. Am J Cardiol 1980; 45:457.

Morady F. A perspective on the role of catheter ablation in the management of tachyarrhythmias. PACE 1988; 11:98.

Morady F, Scheinman MM, Winston SA. Efficacy and safety of transcatheter ablation of posteroseptal accessory pathways. Circulation 1985; 72:170.

Saksena S, Hussain SM, Gielchinsky I, et al. Intraoperative mapping-guided argon laser ablation of malignant supraventricular tachycardia in Wolff-Parkinson-White syndrome. Am J Cardiol 1987; 60:196.

Sealy WC, Hattler BG, Blumenschein SD, et al. Surgical treatment of Wolff-Parkinson-White syndrome. Ann Thorac Surg 1969; 8:1.

Sowton E, Balcon R, Preston T, et al. Long-term control of intractable supraventricular tachycardia by ventricular pacing. Br Heart J 1969; 31:700.

Spurrell RAJ, Nathan AW, Bexton RS, et al. Implantable automatic scanning pacemaker for termination of supraventricular tachycardia. Am J Cardiol 1982; 49:753.

Sung RJ, Styperek JL, Castellanos A. Complete abolition of reentrant supraventricular tachycardia zone using a new modality of cardiac pacing with simultaneous atrioventricular stimulation. Am J Cardiol 1980; 45:72.

Tullo NG, An H, Saksena S. Ablation using radiofrequency current and low-energy direct-current shocks. In: Saksena S, Goldschlager N, eds. Electrical therapy for cardiac arrhythmias. Philadelphia: WB Saunders, 1989:684.

Wellens HJJ, Brugada P. Value of programmed stimulation of the heart in patients with the Wolff-Parkinson-White syndrome. In: Josephson ME, Wellens HJJ, eds. Tachycardias: Mechanisms, diagnosis, treatment. Philadelphia: Lea & Febiger, 1984:199.

Wellens HJJ, Durrer D. Relation between refractory period of the accessory pathway and ventricular frequency during atrial fi-

brillation in patients with the Wolff-Parkinson-White syndrome. Am J Cardiol 1974; 33:178.

Wellens HJJ, et al. Effect of drugs in the Wolff-Parkinson White syndrome. Importance of initial length of effective refractory period of the accessory pathway. Am J Cardiol 1980; 46:665.

ATRIAL FIBRILLATION IN THE WOLFF-PARKINSON-WHITE SYNDROME

K. ATTA BOAHENE, M.D.
GEORGE J. KLEIN, M.D.
RAYMOND YEE, M.D.
ARJUN D. SHARMA, M.D.
OSAMU FUJIMURA, M.D.

Atrial fibrillation (AF) without associated structural heart disease occurs frequently (12 to 34 percent) in the Wolff-Parkinson-White (WPW) syndrome. This arrhythmia has the potential to become life-threatening if a rapid ventricular response results from accessory pathway conduction (Fig. 1). It has been found that the risk of sudden death in the WPW syndrome is related to the shortest preexcited R-R interval during AF. A shortest preexcited R-R interval of less than 250 msec (240 beats per minute) was observed in all of a series of 25 patients presenting with ventricular fibrillation in the absence of heart disease. Patients with concealed accessory pathways (no antegrade preexcitation) have a lower prevalence of clinical AF (3 percent) and a lower incidence of sustained AF induced at electrophysiologic study (15 percent versus 47 percent) and they are not at increased risk of sudden death from AF.

Sudden death has been occasionally reported complicating AF or flutter in patients with short P-R intervals but is generally not of concern in the absence of antegrade preexcitation. Sudden death has not been described in patients with Mahaim pathways.

ELECTROCARDIOGRAPHIC RECOGNITION

The QRS complex of the WPW pattern represents "fusion" of ventricular activation via the normal atrioventricular conduction system and the accessory pathway. The degree of fusion is a function of the relative distances of the atrioventricular node and accessory pathway from the site of impulse for-

mation and their respective conduction velocities. In atrial fibrillation, relative conduction over the normal atrioventricular conduction system or over the accessory pathway depends primarily on their respective refractory periods. In AF, one sees either all preexcited QRS complexes (Fig. 2), all normal QRS complexes (Fig. 3), or a combination of preexcited complexes alternating with normal complexes (Fig. 4).

PATHOGENESIS

The pathogenesis of AF in the WPW syndrome is not completely understood. Abnormalities such as Ebstein's anomaly of the tricuspid valve and mitral leaflet prolapse may be associated with preexcitation but do not account for the increased frequency of AF in the absence of structural heart disease. Extensive atrial disease, which usually provides the electrophysiologic substrates for AF, is not more common in the WPW syndrome. Similarly, sinus node dysfunction with consequent tachy-brady syndrome is also infrequently responsible for AF in the WPW syndrome.

The accessory pathway is important in the pathogenesis of atrial fibrillation, although a specific role in the initiation or maintenance of AF is not clearly understood. In the absence of structural heart disease, patients with AF who have successful surgical ablation of the accessory pathway generally do not have recurrence of AF during follow-up. Whether this is attributable to elimination of the accessory pathway per se or the elimination of concomitant reciprocating tachycardia is not clear. Recent observations using direct accessory pathway recording suggest that, in some cases at least, accessory pathways may be branched and could theoretically support microreentry. However, other observations in the electrophysiology laboratory suggest that AF generally begins with a rapid atrial tachycardia that degenerates into AF (Fig. 5). This atrial tachycardia usually starts at the right atrium regardless of accessory pathway location.

The presence of clinical AF in the WPW syndrome usually correlates with the presence of concomitant reciprocating tachycardia. Transition of reciprocating tachycardia to AF has been demon-

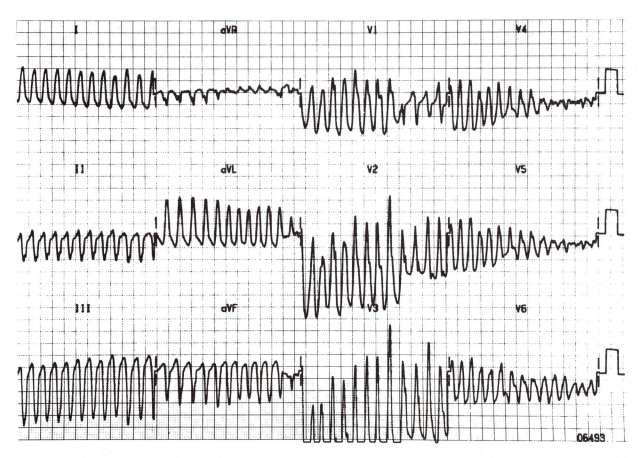

Figure 1   12-Lead electrocardiogram showing AF with rapid conduction over an accessory pathway induced by atrial pacing during electrophysiologic study. AF degenerated into ventricular fibrillation by lead V$_4$.

strated in the laboratory, with AF usually beginning with atrial ectopic activity (Fig. 5). In general, patients with clinical AF also have longer intraatrial conduction times (PA interval), shorter atrial functional refractory periods, and a higher incidence of atrial vulnerability than patients without AF. This suggests that reciprocating tachycardia may be important as a trigger, but only in the patient with intrinsic atrial abnormalities.

CLINICAL PRESENTATION

AF with the WPW syndrome may vary from an incidental finding on an ambulatory monitor to overt cardiac arrest. The most frequent presentation, however, is as a paroxysmal arrhythmia in a patient who also has had reciprocating tachycardia. Chronic persistent AF is rare in the WPW syndrome. The major determinant of the mode of presentation is the rapidity of the ventricular response during AF,

modified by factors such as age and concomitant heart disease.

The typical patient with AF secondary to the WPW syndrome may have had minimally symptomatic episodes of tachycardia that terminated spontaneously or may have been treated empirically for more symptomatic paroxysmal reciprocating tachycardia. Thus, there is frequently a history of preceding tachycardia. When AF supervenes, patients usually present with irregular tachycardia that is recognized by them as being different from their preceding tachycardia. In general, their symptoms include rapid heart beating, diaphoresis, dizziness, near-syncope, or syncope when rapid ventricular conduction is present. Patients with exclusive atrioventricular nodal conduction or slower ventricular rates during AF (see Figs. 3 and 4) may not feel incapacitated. Rarely, a patient may present with ventricular fibrillation and have preexcitation documented only after successful resuscitation (see Fig. 1). The occurrence of AF may be related to exercise or alcohol ingestion but is frequently unexplained.

MANAGEMENT OF ACUTE AF (Table 1)

The electrophysiologic properties of the atrium, ventricle, atrioventricular conduction system and, mainly, the accessory pathway, determine the ventricular response during AF (Fig. 6). A 12-lead electrocardiogram should be obtained if possible, since this may provide valuable information (risk of sudden death, number and location of accessory pathways) that will assist in future management. The major goals of acute therapy are initially to slow the ventricular response and then to terminate the arrhythmia.

Synchronized cardioversion is indicated in the patient who is markedly hypotensive or otherwise unstable.

Initial drug therapy depends on the proportion of normal and preexcited QRS complexes during AF.

The patient with predominantly or entirely normal QRS complexes during AF (Figs. 3 and 7*A*) should be treated as any other patient with AF in the absence of preexcitation (see the chapter *Atrial Fibrillation*). Here, the normal atrioventricular conduction system (Fig. 6) is responsible for the ventricular response, which can be slowed in the usual way with drugs that prolong atrioventricular nodal refractoriness, such as digoxin, verapamil, and beta blockers. A membrane-active drug, such as procainamide, disopyramide, or quinidine, can then be given to restore sinus rhythm once the ventricular rate has been controlled.

The patient with predominantly preexcited QRS complexes during tachycardia (see Figs. 2 and 7*B*) is treated entirely differently, since the accessory pathway is essentially responsible for atrioventricular conduction. In this situation, the initial therapy is directed at slowing the ventricular response by prolonging accessory pathway refractoriness using membrane-active drugs such as procainamide (see Fig. 6). The same membrane-active drugs may also revert the AF to normal sinus rhythm. In these patients it is important to avoid atrioventricular nodal blocking drugs, especially digitalis and verapamil,

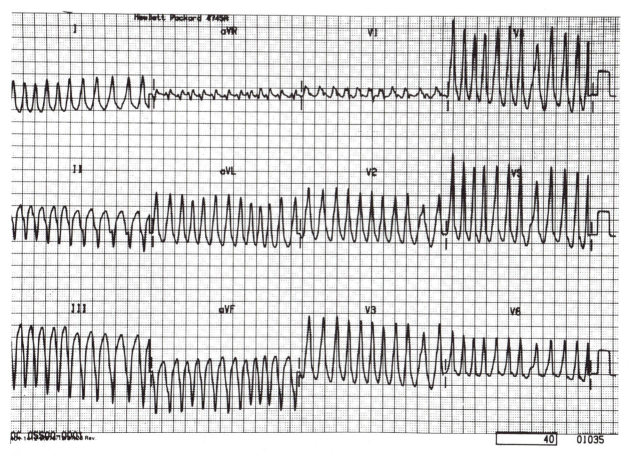

Figure 2 AF in a patient with exclusive conduction over the posteroseptal accessory pathway with a shortest R-R interval between two consecutive preexcited beats of 200 msec.

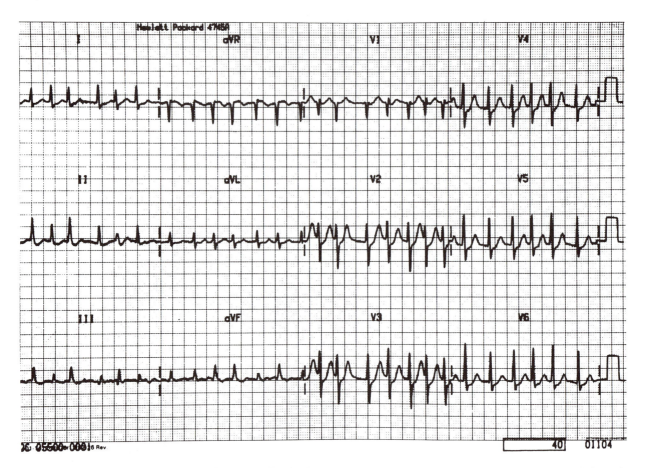

Figure 3 This patient has evidence of preexcitation in sinus rhythm, but the accessory pathway does not participate in conduction during AF. All QRS complexes are normal, implying a shorter effective refractory period of the atrioventricular conduction system relative to the accessory pathway.

since they will not prolong accessory pathway refractoriness and will not slow the ventricular response. In fact, they may increase the ventricular response by direct effect on the accessory pathway or secondarily by slowing competitive atrioventricular nodal conduction. In addition, a negatively inotropic drug such as verapamil given to such a patient may in fact increase the ventricular response and lead to cardiac arrest.

Membrane-active drugs of class IA (procainamide, disopyramide) or IC group (propafenone, flecainide) have been shown to slow the ventricular response in patients with predominantly preexcited QRS complexes and may also result in conversion to sinus rhythm (see Table 1). The class IB agent lidocaine has not been shown to be useful in this context and may in fact accelerate the ventricular response in AF. Intravenous procainamide is useful given in doses of 10 to 12 mg per kilogram intravenously. The drug is infused at a rate of 100 mg every 2 to 3 minutes, with careful attention paid to the blood pressure reading and the ventricular response. This results in the slowing of the ventricular response in the great majority of patients and reversion to sinus rhythm in over 50 percent. Intravenous disopyramide in a dose of 1 to 2 mg per kilogram given over 10 minutes provides similar results, although this agent is not available in the intravenous form in the United States. Similarly, the class IC agent propafenone used intravenously in a dose of 1 to 2 mg per kilogram infused over 15 minutes slows the ventricular response and restores sinus rhythm in the majority of patients.

MANAGEMENT OF CHRONIC ATRIAL FIBRILLATION (Table 2)

Further investigation and therapy after the acute episode depend greatly on the frequency and severity of the patient's symptoms. If the ventricular rate is

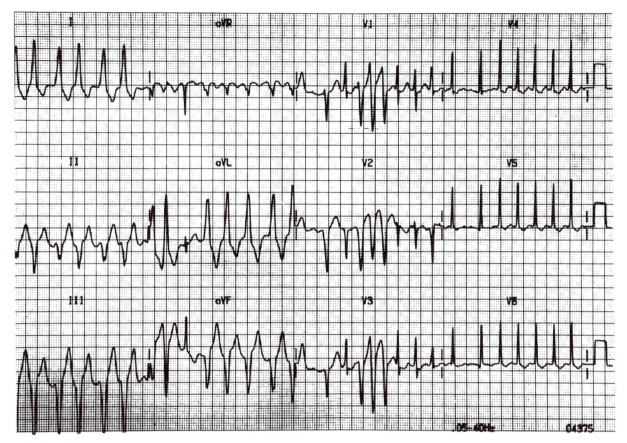

Figure 4 AF in a patient in which the accessory pathway and atrioventricular nodal refractory periods allow for conduction over both pathways. The preexcited morphology suggests a right lateral accessory pathway.

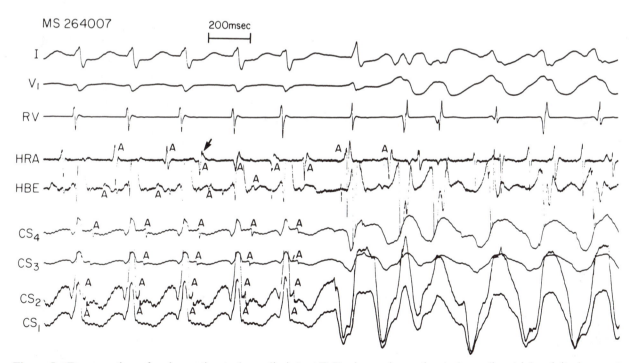

Figure 5 Degeneration of reciprocating tachycardia into AF. During reciprocating tachycardia, atrial activity began at the distal coronary sinus, the site of the accessory pathway (CS$_1$), and occurred last at the right atrial site (HRA). The atrial activity denoted by the arrow is out of sequence, occurring earlier than expected for the reciprocating tachycardia and followed by multiple rapid atrial activity at this site, leading to AF with wide QRS complexes. This premature atrial activity that initiated AF is at a site different from that of the accessory pathway. CS$_1$–CS$_4$ = coronary sinus electrodes from the most distal (CS$_1$) to the most proximal (CS$_4$) electrodes; HBE = His bundle electrogram; HRA = high right atrial electrogram; RV = right ventricular apex electrogram; I, V$_1$ = surface electrocardiographic leads.

Table 1   Drugs for Treatment of Acute AF With Predominantly Preexcited Complexes in WPW Syndrome

Drug	Dose	Beneficial Effects	Major Adverse Effects
Disopyramide (class IA)	1–2 mg/kg in 10 minutes	Slows ventricular response in AF Terminates AF in majority of cases Prolongs ERP of AP, atrium, ventricle, and His-Purkinje system	Hypotension Urinary retention, blurred vision, dry mouth because of potent anticholinergic action
Procainamide (class IA)	10–12 mg/kg at 100 mg every 2–3 minutes	Slows ventricular response in AF Terminates AF in majority Prolongs ERP of AP, atrium, ventricle, and His-Purkinje system	Hypotension
Propafenone (class IC)	1–2 mg/kg over 10 minutes	Slows ventricular response in AF Prolongs ERP in AP, atrium, and ventricle Terminates AF in about half of cases	Hypotension Nausea, vomiting rash
Flecainide (class IC)	1–2 mg/kg over 15 minutes	Slows ventricular response in AF Prolongs conduction in AP, atrium, ventricle, and His-Purkinje system	Hypotension

AF = atrial fibrillation, AP = accessory pathway, ERP = effective refractory period.

Table 2   Drugs for Treatment of Chronic AF in WPW Syndrome

Drug	Dose	Major Adverse Reactions
Quinidine (class IA)	200–400 mg every 6 hr	Nausea, vomiting, diarrhea, abdominal pain, anorexia, tinnitus, confusion, visual disturbances, allergic reactions such as rash, fever, thrombocytopenia, and hemolytic anemia, proarrhythmia (torsades de pointes)
Procainamide (class IA)	2–6 g daily in divided doses at 4-hr intervals	Myalgias, skin rashes, giddiness, psychosis, hallucinations, fever, agranulocytosis, lupus syndrome
Disopyramide (class IA)	100–200 mg (up to 1.2 g/day) every 6 hr	Depression of left ventricular function, proarrhythmia (torsades de pointes), constipation, dry mouth, urinary retention, blurred vision
Flecainide (class IC)	200–400 mg/day in divided doses at 12-hr intervals	Depression of left ventricular function, proarrhythmia, visual blurring, tinnitus, sleep disturbances, dizziness, nervousness
Encainide (class IC)	Begin at 25 mg every 8 hr (maximal dose of 200–300 mg/day)	Blurred vision, headache, nausea, lightheadedness, fatigue
Propafenone (class IC)	450–900 mg daily in divided doses every 8–12 hr	Metallic taste, anorexia, nausea, vomiting, dizziness, blurred vision, cholestatic hepatitis
Sotalol (beta blocker class III activity)	Begin with 80 mg b.i.d.; can increase up to maximal dose of 320 mg b.i.d.	Hypotension, bradycardia, bronchospasm, headache, dizziness, fatigue, mental depression, vertigo, nightmares
Amiodarone (class III)	200–400 mg/day; after-loading dose of 12–16 g	Pulmonary fibrosis, hepatitis, hypo- and hyperthyroidism, neuropathy, corneal deposits, bluish skin discoloration

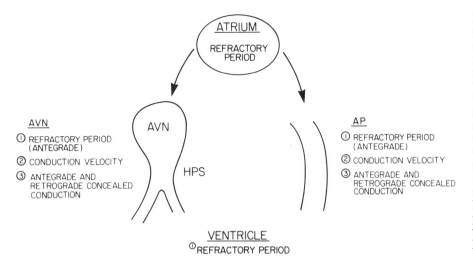

Figure 6 Factors determining the ventricular response during AF. If the refractory period of the accessory pathway is short and that of the atrioventricular node is long, the ventricular response will be rapid because of exclusive accessory pathway conduction. On the other hand, if the atrioventricular node refractory period is much shorter than that of the accessory pathway, only normal QRS complexes will be seen in AF. AP = accessory pathway, AVN = atrioventricular node, HPS = His-Purkinje system.

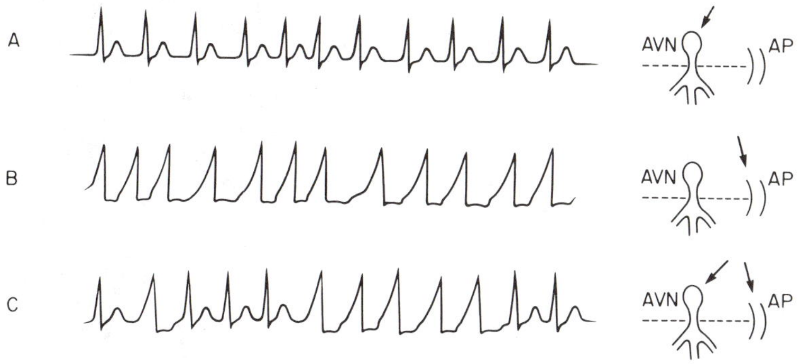

Figure 7 Possible combination of complexes that can be seen during AF in a patient with an accessory pathway, depending on the interplay of factors enumerated in Figure 6. In *A*, the relative refractory periods of the accessory pathway (AP) and atrioventricular node (AVN) favor exclusive conduction over the normal atrioventricular conduction system. In *B*, the accessory pathway is favored, with only preexcited complexes seen. In *C*, both accessory pathway and atrioventricular node are able to conduct because of accessory pathway and atrioventricular conduction that permits conduction in both pathways.

relatively slow (shortest preexcited R-R interval greater than 250 to 300 msec) and well tolerated, one may consider no therapy or empirical therapy on a trial and error basis. If empirical therapy is chosen, a membrane-active drug that would be expected to slow the ventricular response, such as the class IA and class IC agents should be chosen. Treatment guided by electrophysiologic testing is strongly recommended if the ventricular rate is rapid (shortest preexcited R-R intervals less than 250 msec) and especially if the patient is severely symptomatic or hypotensive. Electrophysiologic testing allows an objective assessment of the efficacy of a chosen therapy to prevent reciprocating tachycardia, which is a usual concomitant of AF, and also assesses the ability of the drug to slow the ventricular response in the event that AF recurs. The ability of the drug to prevent the induction of sustained AF can also be tested. Combination drug therapy can be tested, although one part of the combination should generally be a membrane-active drug.

Operative therapy in experienced hands should have a success rate greater than 95 percent and mortality approaching 0 percent. Operative therapy directed at ablation of the accessory pathway should be seriously considered in any patient who has sustained a cardiac arrest as a result of AF with a rapid ventricular response and should be seriously entertained in any patient with a potentially life-threatening arrhythmia (preexcited shortest R-R interval less than 250 msec) or for whom compliance with drug therapy may be a problem. Transcatheter ablation techniques for accessory pathways are currently being investigated and may replace operative therapy in many patients in the future (see the chapter *Catheter Ablation*).

SUGGESTED READING

Bauernfeind RA, Wyndham CR, Swiryn SP, et al. Paroxysmal atrial fibrillation in the Wolff-Parkinson-White syndrome. Am J Cardiol 1981; 47:562–569.

Gallagher JJ, Pritchett ELC, Sealy WC, et al. The preexcitation syndromes. Prog Cardiovasc Dis 1978; 20:285–327.

Klein GJ, Bashore TM, Sellers TB, et al. Ventricular fibrillation in the Wolff-Parkinson-White syndrome. N Engl J Med 1979; 301:1080–1085.

Prystowsky EN. Diagnosis and management of the preexcitation syndromes. Curr Probl Cardiol 1988; 13:231–310.

V VENTRICULAR ARRHYTHMIAS

VENTRICULAR ARRHYTHMIAS: CLASSIFICATION AND GENERAL PRINCIPLES OF THERAPY

J. THOMAS BIGGER JR., M.D.

Ventricular arrhythmias are a common clinical problem causing troublesome or severe symptoms. These arrhythmias are also of great importance because they are involved in most sudden cardiac deaths, killing a person almost every minute in the United States. Interestingly, many of the ventricular arrhythmias that predict sudden cardiac death are asymptomatic, occurring in patients with previous myocardial infarction or with cardiomyopathy and congestive heart failure. This chapter serves to introduce some of the problems related to ventricular arrhythmias, their mechanisms, diagnosis, clinical significance, and management.

CLASSIFICATION OF VENTRICULAR ARRHYTHMIAS BY MECHANISM

If we could classify each clinical arrhythmia by mechanism, we would be in a better position to develop relevant animal models and drugs targeted to specific mechanisms. This would permit better clinical control of ventricular arrhythmias. Unfortunately, we are a long way from understanding the mechanism of each of the ventricular arrhythmias encountered clinically, but we do have some important insights and better tools for investigating arrhythmias than ever before. As a result, knowledge is accruing faster than ever before.

By definition, ventricular arrhythmias are abnormalities of rhythm arising in the ventricles. Table 1 classifies ventricular arrhythmias by mechanism predominantly based on findings in animal models.

Ventricular arrhythmias may arise as a result of abnormalities of impulse generation, abnormalities of impulse conduction, or a combination of the two.

Abnormalities of Automaticity

Electrolyte abnormalities or enhanced sympathetic nervous system activity can lead to increased frequency of automatic firing due to enhanced normal automaticity, i.e., automaticity arising from diastolic depolarization of Purkinje fibers that have normal high values for maximal diastolic transmembrane voltage. Enhanced normal automaticity is suppressed by overdrive pacing and lidocaine administration. Purkinje fibers injured by ischemia or mechanical damage can depolarize and demonstrate abnormal automaticity, i.e. automaticity at such a low value of maximal diastolic transmembrane voltage that normal automatic mechanisms are inoperable. Experimentally, abnormal automaticity does not suppress and may even accelerate with overdrive pacing and does not respond uniformly to lidocaine. It remains to be proved whether episodes of accelerated idioventricular rhythm are caused by normal or abnormal automaticity.

Table 1 Mechanisms Responsible for Cardiac Arrhythmias

I. Abnormalities of Impulse Generation
  A. Alterations of normal automaticity
  B. Abnormal automaticity
  C. Triggered activity
    1. Early afterdepolarizations
    2. Late afterdepolarizations
II. Abnormalities of Impulse Conduction
  A. Slowing of conduction and block
  B. Unidirectional block and reentry
    1. Ordered reentry
    2. Random reentry
    3. Summation and inhibition
  C. Conduction block, electrotonus, and reflection
III. Combined Abnormalities of Impulse Generation and Conduction
  A. Conduction slowed by phase 4 depolarization
  B. Parasystole

Triggered Activity

Repetitive firing in heart muscle can be triggered by early or delayed afterdepolarizations. Triggered activity is *not* a form of automaticity but can cause a sustained tachyarrhythmia. Early afterdepolarizations are secondary depolarizations that occur before repolarization is complete, often from the action potential plateau. Delayed afterdepolarizations are secondary depolarizations that occur after repolarization is complete. In ventricular tissues, either early or delayed afterdepolarizations can reach threshold and cause a single premature complex or trigger a series of impulses. Unlike normal automatic behavior, triggered activity is critically dependent on the previous action potential and can occur in ordinary ventricular muscle as well as Purkinje fibers.

Early Afterdepolarizations. Experimentally, early afterdepolarizations can be induced in cardiac Purkinje fibers by mechanical injury, low K^+, high Ca^{2+}, catecholamines, and drugs (e.g., quinidine, sotalol, or N-acetyl procainamide). Torsades de pointes ventricular tachycardia in humans is thought to be the counterpart of triggered activity caused by early afterdepolarizations. Torsades de pointes in humans is strongly associated with the factors that can produce early afterdepolarizations in animal models such as the congenital long Q-T syndrome and the acquired long Q-T syndrome caused by hypokalemia and/or hypomagnesemia or drugs that prolong the Q-T interval.

Delayed Afterpolarizations. Experimentally, delayed afterdepolarizations can be easily induced by digitalis toxicity in the His-Purkinje system and with more difficulty in specialized atrial or ordinary ventricular cells. In Purkinje fibers, Ca^{2+} overload can induce delayed afterdepolarizations. In the atria, coronary sinus, and mitral valve, delayed afterdepolarizations and triggered activity can be caused by catecholamines. Also, delayed afterdepolarizations and triggered activity are seen early in experimental myocardial infarction. Some digitalis-induced junctional or ventricular arrhythmias in humans have characteristics that resemble triggered activity produced by digitalis in isolated tissue preparations. These rhythm disturbances are the best clinical candidates for triggered activity initiated by delayed afterdepolarizations in humans.

Reentrant Ventricular Arrhythmias

Experimentally, a long line of research indicates that slow conduction, one-way block, and reentry can cause single ventricular ectopic complexes or continuous rhythms. By now many nuances of the reentrant process have been described, e.g., circus movement around an obstacle, leading circle reentry without an anatomic obstacle, and complex forms in which the circuit constantly changes. Circus movement around an obstacle often has an excitable gap, i.e., there is always tissue in the continuous circuit that is excitable. Many important ventricular arrhythmias in humans have characteristics that indicate they are reentrant in nature, e.g., ventricular tachycardia and fibrillation. In humans, the reentrant nature of ventricular tachycardia has been supported by starting and stopping the rhythm reproducibly using programmed electrical stimulation of the ventricle and by entrainment of the ventricular tachycardia with ventricular pacing at a rate faster than the intrinsic tachycardia.

An example of combined abnormality of impulse generation and conduction is ventricular parasystole. An automatic focus in the ventricle that fires more slowly than the dominant rhythm (usually sinus rhythm) is permitted to express itself in the electrocardiogram because of entrance block. The propagating wavefront from sinus rhythm does not penetrate the ectopic focus to depolarize and reset it. When the pacemaker in the ectopic ventricular focus reaches threshold, it propagates out to activate the ventricles, unless they are refractory. The unidirectional block is critical to the expression of the automatic rhythm.

ELECTROCARDIOGRAPHIC DIAGNOSIS OF VENTRICULAR ARRHYTHMIAS

Some of the patterns of ventricular arrhythmias recognized electrocardiographically in humans are listed in Table 2. The ventricular nature of the rhythm is diagnosed by the wide, bizarre QRS complex and atrioventricular dissociation. However, there are exceptions to the rule. Ventricular rhythms arising in the bundle of His or bundle branches may have a normal QRS duration. Also, if ventriculoatrial conduction is present, atrioventricular dissociation may not be present. Ventricular arrhythmias are classified electrocardiographically by the number of consecutive ventricular complexes and by the rate of continuous rhythms. Three or more consecutive ventricular complexes at a rate of 100 per minute or more are called ventricular tachycardia (VT). VT

Table 2 Electrocardiographic Types of Ventricular Arrhythmias

Isolated ventricular premature complexes
Unsustained ventricular tachycardia
Accelerated idioventricular rhythm
Ventricular parasystole
Uniform sustained ventricular tachycardia
Multiform sustained ventricular tachycardia
Torsades de pointes ventricular tachycardia
Ventricular flutter
Ventricular fibrillation

lasting up to 15 to 30 sec (definitions vary) is called unsustained, whereas VT of longer duration is called sustained. Important distinctions also are made according to the morphology of the complexes in continuous ventricular rhythms. When each QRS complex in a run of VT is identical, uniform VT is diagnosed. If there is marked variability of the QRS morphology during VT, multiform VT is diagnosed. Torsades de pointes has a characteristic twisting of the points and is associated almost invariably with a prolonged Q-T interval. Many ventricular rhythm patterns are recognized to have characteristic clinical associations that are useful for assigning prognosis and for directing management. Uniform VT with a left bundle branch block pattern and superior axis has been recognized as originating in the right ventricular outflow tract and as being unusually drug-responsive. Accelerated idioventricular rhythm suggests acute myocardial infarction, digitalis toxicity, or hypokalemia. The acquired form of torsades de pointes suggests hypokalemia, hypomagnesemia, or drug toxicity. This rhythm responds to treatment with ventricular pacing, catecholamine infusion, and treatment with K^+ and/or Mg^{2+} but not to treatment with drugs having class I antiarrhythmic action.

Often the ventricular rhythm can be diagnosed from an electrocardiogram. Clinical associations and the morphology of the QRS complexes in 12-lead electrocardiogram recordings are quite helpful for distinguishing VT from a supraventricular rhythm with aberrant conduction or preexisting bundle branch block or intraventricular block conduction defect. Atrial activity may be hard to define during a tachycardia with a prolonged QRS complex. Special body surface leads, esophageal leads, or intracavitary leads placed in the right atrium may be needed to detect atrial activity. The nature of the tachycardia may not be clear even when all atrial and ventricular complexes are identified, e.g., wide complex QRS tachycardia with a rate of 180 per minute, 1 : 1 atrioventricular relationship, and P wave midway in the R-R interval could be paroxysmal supraventricular tachycardia or VT. A bundle of His electrogram can easily distinguish between these two possibilities.

Intermittent arrhythmias can be detected by long-term acquisition of continuous or intermittent samples of electrocardiograms. Holter recorders, real-time intermittent sampling by recorders with on-board computers; or memory loop patient-activated recorders can all be helpful for documenting arrhythmias as the cause of symptoms.

When symptoms are severe, e.g., syncope, the signal-averaged electrocardiogram and electrophysiologic studies are effective and safe methods to determine whether sustained ventricular arrhythmias are responsible. Signal-averaged electrocardiography is a diagnostic test to detect the cardiac "substrate" that supports sustained ventricular arrhythmias. The presence of delayed, low amplitude activation in the terminal portion of the amplified QRS signal, the late potential, seems to be a moderately sensitive and very specific indicator for inducible VT during electrophysiologic study in patients with syncope but no documented ventricular arrhythmias. Preliminary data suggest that the signal-averaged electrocardiogram is more predictive than Holter monitoring–detected arrhythmic events. The combination of an abnormal signal-averaged electrocardiogram, abnormal left ventricular ejection fraction, and the presence of "high-grade" ventricular arrhythmias in Holter recordings identified a small subset at very high risk for sustained VT or sudden cardiac death. The method is not accurate when bundle branch block or intraventricular conduction defect is present. The signal-averaged electrocardiogram is not useful for guiding drug therapy. If a sustained ventricular arrhythmia was responsible for syncope, an electrophysiologic study has an excellent chance of inducing a sustained ventricular arrhythmia. The test is safe and involves minimal discomfort. Sustained uniform VT induced by programmed ventricular stimulation has almost 100 percent specificity in syncope patients; the sensitivity varies with the etiologic form of heart disease and severity of left ventricular dysfunction.

CLINICAL SIGNIFICANCE OF VENTRICULAR ARRHYTHMIAS

The clinical significance of ventricular arrhythmias lies in their potential to produce troublesome symptoms and sudden cardiac death. Prognostically insignificant ventricular arrhythmia can produce symptoms so severe that they are a source of great distress to patients. At the other extreme are totally asymptomatic ventricular arrhythmias that increase the risk of sudden cardiac death many fold. The presence and severity of symptoms attributable to ventricular arrhythmias can be detected and quantified by a careful history. The assessment of prognosis requires a comprehensive evaluation and synthesis of information about the arrhythmia per se and about the etiology and severity of associated heart diseases.

The Prognostic Classification of Ventricular Arrhythmias

We and others have previously described a prognostic classification of ventricular arrhythmias based principally in the arrhythmia's potential for causing sudden cardiac death. This classification system (Table 3) is used to clarify the risk-benefit ratio for antiarrhythmic drug therapy, to predict antiarrhythmic drug efficacy and cardiac adverse effect rates, and to select the methods used to evaluate therapy. The principal features used to classify prognosis of

Table 3 Prognostic Classification of Ventricular Arrhythmias

	Benign	Potentially Malignant	Malignant
Risk for sudden death	Very low	Low to moderate	High
Clinical presentation	Palpitations; detected by routine examination	Palpitations; detected by routine examination or screening	Palpitations; syncope; cardiac arrest
Heart disease	Usually absent	Present	Present
Cardiac scarring and/or hypertrophy	Absent	Present	Present
LVEF	Normal	Moderately decreased	Markedly decreased
VPC frequency	Low to moderate	Moderate to high	Moderate to high
Paired VPCs and/or unsustained VT	Absent	Common	Common
Sustained VT	Absent	Absent	Present
Hemodynamic effects of arrhythmia	Absent	Absent to mild	Moderate to severe

LVEF = left ventricular ejection fraction; VPC(s) = ventricular premature complex(es); VT = ventricular tachycardia.
*The characteristics listed in this table are typical but do not represent the full range of observations. For example, benign ventricular arrhythmias can be frequent and occasionally repetitive.

ventricular arrhythmias are (1) the characteristics of the arrhythmia, and (2) the severity of underlying structural heart disease. Prognosis has been related to these features by previous follow-up studies.

Benign Ventricular Arrhythmias. Ventricular arrhythmias are termed "benign" when they are unsustained, produced no hemodynamically important effects, and are not associated with structural heart disease. Such arrhythmias are not associated with an increase in the risk of sudden cardiac death. The benign class accounts for about 30 percent of patients with ventricular arrhythmias. Before starting therapy for symptomatic benign ventricular arrhythmias, the physician usually should demonstrate an association between the arrhythmia and symptoms by electrocardiographic recordings. Exercise testing may provoke unsustained or sustained VT when a continuous 24-hour electrocardiographic recording is unremarkable. Electrophysiologic testing is not indicated for patients with benign arrhythmias.

Potentially Malignant Ventricular Arrhythmias. Approximately 65 percent of ventricular arrhythmias can be classified as potentially malignant (also called prognostically significant). These arrhythmias are unsustained and are associated with significant underlying structural heart disease and often with substantial left ventricular function deficits. These arrhythmias, per se, rarely have important hemodynamic effects. This class is quite heterogeneous and the risk of sudden cardiac death ranges from modest to high. There is no doubt that asymptomatic, unsustained ventricular arrhythmias after

myocardial infarction are independent predictors of death. Four large studies done after myocardial infarction used 24-hour continuous electrocardiographic (Holter) recordings to assess ventricular arrhythmia frequency and radionuclide or angiographic methods to measure left ventricular ejection fraction (Table 4). In these studies, there was no statistical interaction between ventricular arrhythmias and left ventricular ejection fraction with respect to their mortality effects, i.e., the mortality effect of each risk predictor was independent. Also, left ventricular ejection fraction predicted early deaths (less than 6 months) better, whereas ventricular arrhythmias predicted late deaths (more than 6 months) better. There is much less information available about the prognostic significance of asymptomatic, unsustained arrhythmias in patients with heart failure. However, all of the studies available suggest that ventricular arrhythmias increase the risk of dying in patients with heart disease about two- to threefold. Since ventricular arrhythmias in patients with structural heart disease predict death independent of left ventricular ejection fraction or clinical heart failure, the presence of clinical heart failure or left ventricular ejection fraction of less than 0.30 multiplies the risk of death. A positive signal-averaged electrocardiogram also seems to multiply the mortality risks of patients with ventricular arrhythmias after myocardial infarction. The large increase in risk of sudden cardiac death of patients with asymptomatic ventricular arrhythmias after myocardial infarction or in heart failure independent

Table 4 Relationship Between Ventricular Arrhythmias, Left Ventricular Dysfunction, and Mortality After Myocardial Infarction

Study	Total Number of Patients	Left Ventricular Ejection Fraction <40%						Left Ventricular Ejection Fraction >40%					
		VPC <10/hour		VPC >10/hour		Relative Risk		VPC <10/hour		VPC >10/hour		Relative Risk
		N	Mortality Rate	N	Mortality Rate			N	Mortality Rate	N	Mortality Rate	
MPIP*	766	184	17.3%	72	32.2%	1.87		432	6.3%	78	11.7%	1.84
MILIS†	533	141	19.1%	40	40.0%	2.09		314	5.1%	38	18.4%	3.61
MDPIT*	955	203	15.2%	75	30.2%	1.99		589	7.0%	88	12.6%	1.81
UCSD SCOR‡	749	84	17.9%	101	26.7%	1.50		357	5.0%	207	14.5%	2.87

*The values for MPIP and MDPIT are Kaplan-Meier estimates of mortality rates at 24 months of follow-up.
†The values for MILIS are crude mortality rates with an average follow-up of 18 months.
‡The UCSD SCOR arrhythmia data are partitioned by Lown grade <2 and ≥2, and thus many patients with low frequency and no repetitive ventricular arrhythmias are in the ≥2 group. The mortality values are crude rates at the end of 12 months of follow-up.
  MPIP = Multicenter Post-Infarction Program, MILIS = Multicenter Investigation of the Limitation of Infarct Size, MDPIT = Multicenter Diltiazen Post-Infarction Trial, UCSD SCOR = University of California, San Diego Specialized Center of Research.

of other risk factors provides a rationale for treatment of asymptomatic ventricular arrhythmias. Electrophysiologic testing has been advocated by some to decide whether patients with low left ventricular ejection fractions and unsustained VT should be treated. If uniform sustained VT is induced, therapy is given under electrophysiologic guidance; if VT is not induced, no therapy is given. The data to support this approach have been contradictory, and this approach is still not established practice. Large-scale controlled clinical studies are needed to evaluate this approach.

Malignant Ventricular Arrhythmias. Only about 5 percent of ventricular arrhythmias are malignant or immediately life-threatening. These include sustained uniform VT, torsades de pointes VT, or ventricular fibrillation. The ventricular arrhythmias in this category nearly always produce hemodynamically important signs or symptoms such as acute heart failure, myocardial ischemia, hypotension, or syncope. Patients with sustained ventricular arrhythmias usually have severe forms of heart disease and have the highest risk of sudden cardiac death. Left ventricular ejection fraction partitions patients with malignant ventricular arrhythmias into high and very high risk groups; a value of 30 percent seems best for this purpose. Therapy is always indicated in these patients to control symptoms and to reduce the risk of sudden cardiac death. These patients should be thoroughly evaluated with coronary angiography, perfusion scans, measurement of left ventricular ejection fraction, Holter recordings, exercise testing, and electrophysiologic studies.

TREATMENT OF VENTRICULAR ARRHYTHMIAS

Decisions about treatment should be based on the severity of symptoms, the risk posed by the arrhythmia, and the risk-benefit of treatment options.

Benign Ventricular Arrhythmias

Antiarrhythmic drug therapy for benign ventricular arrhythmias is indicated only to eliminate symptoms that are severe enough to significantly impair the quality of life. When antiarrhythmic drug therapy is indicated, a beta blocker is the agent of choice because of lack of organ toxicity and low risk of noncardiac or cardiac adverse effects. If beta blockers fail, drugs with class IC antiarrhythmic action are a better choice than drugs with class IA and IB action because they have greater efficacy, lower risk of noncardiac or cardiac adverse effects, and lower risk of organ toxicity. Although the Cardiac Arrhythmia Suppression Trial (CAST) has raised questions about the safety of drugs with class IC

antiarrhythmic action, the adverse effect seems to be related to structural heart disease. Flecainide was reviewed by the Cardiovascular and Renal Drugs Advisory board of the Food and Drug Administration since the CAST results were published and recommended for use in patients without structural heart disease who have symptomatic supraventricular arrhythmias.

Potentially Malignant Ventricular Arrhythmias

The approach to symptomatic patients with potentially malignant ventricular arrhythmias is similar to the approach to those with benign ventricular arrhythmias except in patients with clinical heart failure. In heart failure, a drug that will suppress the arrhythmia without aggravating the heart failure is needed. There are no outstanding drugs for this purpose on the United States market but moricizine and dl-sotalol will be available soon and may fill this need. Treatment of asymptomatic, prognostically significant ventricular arrhythmias is a conundrum. Surveys done in 1985 and 1989 show that about half of the cardiologists were treating these arrhythmias with drugs having class I antiarrhythmic action. In 1989, the CAST presented us with information suggesting that this practice is wrong. Treatment of prognostically important ventricular arrhythmias after myocardial infarction with the drugs shown to be the most effective at suppressing arrhythmias and best tolerated increased the mortality rate over 10 months of follow-up by about 2.5 fold. This finding was concordant with smaller randomized controlled studies that previously showed that drugs with class IA or IB action increased mortality. These studies emphasize our lack of understanding of how the asymptomatic but prognostically significant ventricular arrhythmias after myocardial infarction relate to sustained ventricular arrhythmias that are responsible for sudden cardiac death. They also point out the need to demonstrate directly that a drug that suppresses ventricular arrhythmias will reduce mortality in randomized controlled trials. Controlled clinical trials have shown that beta blocker treatment reduces mortality after myocardial infarction, especially in patients who have ventricular arrhythmias. Beta blockers have modest potency for suppressing ventricular arrhythmias, minimal risks for organ toxicity, noncardiac adverse effects, or cardiac adverse effects such as proarrhythmia. Most important, they reduce the risk of sudden cardiac death after myocardial infarction. Therefore, patients with recent myocardial infarction and aysmptomatic ventricular arrhythmias should be treated for several years with a beta blocker that lacks intrinsic sympathomimetic activity. Additional clinical trials are badly needed to determine whether other drugs that suppress ventricular arrhythmias have a beneficial effect on mortality in patients with unsustained ventricular arrhythmias after myocardial infarction.

Another group of patients have asymptomatic but prognostically significant ventricular arrhythmias—those with congestive heart failure. Converting enzyme inhibitors reduce the mortality rate in patients with class IV heart failure. Furthermore, treatment with converting enzyme inhibitors significantly reduces the frequency of ventricular arrhythmias in patients with heart failure. Therefore, I recommend that ventricular arrhythmias in heart failure be treated with converting enzyme inhibitors. Clinical trials are required to establish whether or not treatment with antiarrhythmic drugs can reduce mortality and whether they are well tolerated in patients with heart failure. Their safety and suppression of ventricular arrhythmias should be documented using 24-hour continuous electrocardiographic recordings and exercise testing.

Malignant Ventricular Arrhythmias

In patients with malignant ventricular arrhythmias, drugs with class IA action appear to be the most appropriate for initial therapy followed by combination of drugs with IA and IB action and finally drugs with class IC antiarrhythmic action. Because encainide and flecainide have higher rates of proarrhythmia and flecainide has more negative inotropic effect than drugs with class IA and IB actions, they should be used just before the most toxic antiarrhythmic drug, amiodarone. dl-Sotalol has class II and class III antiarrhythmic actions and is more likely to covert inducible, sustained VT to noninducible VT than any other drug. Therefore, it may become a drug of choice for malignant ventricular arrhythmias. Drug efficacy and safety for malignant ventricular arrhythmias usually are assessed using electrophysiologic studies. Symptomatic, sustained ventricular arrhythmias should be rendered noninducible or, at least, slowed and made asymptomatic. The ESVEM trial should provide controlled data comparing the predictive accuracy of electrophysiologic methods and noninvasive evaluation using 24-hour electrocardiographic recordings and exercise testing. We know that electrophysiologic studies can predict whether patients will do well, but we still do not know whether they are capable of assessing drug efficacy, e.g., they may select for severity of illness more than for drug efficacy. In about half the cases, no drug is found that is predicted to be satisfactory for long-term treatment. These patients have nonpharmacologic options for treatment. Patients with anterior scars and ventricular aneurysms are the prime candidates for resection of the endocardial tissue that is critical for the sustained arrhythmia. There is about an 80 percent chance for a cure, with a surgical mortality rate of about 8 percent. Many patients have problems that raise the surgical mortality risk and lower the chance for cure by surgery. For these patients, the automatic implantable cardioverter defibrillator* is the best choice for treatment. The mortality rate for patients with malignant ventricular arrhythmias treated with automatic implantable cardioverter defibrillators is remarkably low, but the technology is complex and interferes significantly with lifestyle in many patients. Now that there are so many patients with automatic implantable cardioverter defibrillators surviving and doing well, these patients could help us to determine the ability of drugs to reduce the sudden cardiac death rate. Patients with implanted documenting defibrillators could be randomized to groups given drugs predicted to be effective by electrophysiologic studies or to a group given a corresponding placebo. Differences between the two groups for documented episodes of sustained ventricular arrhythmias and sudden cardiac death would give us the answer to an important unanswered question. The answer would permit us to improve drug therapy as the primary treatment and to use antiarrhythmic drugs correctly as adjuncts to surgery or implanted defibrillators. Experimental methods for nonsurgical ablation include radiofrequency or direct current shocks delivered via electrode catheters or ablative chemicals delivered into the appropriate coronary artery via selective catheterization.

We have learned much about the mechanisms, prevalence, significance, and management of ventricular arrhythmias over the past 25 years. However, it is evident that we still have much to learn about these challenging arrhythmias and their management in the years to come. Every year significant progress is made and additional tools become available for attacking the problem of ventricular arrhythmias and sudden cardiac death. It seems clear that, through better understanding, the morbidity and mortality burden of ventricular arrhythmias will be substantially reduced in the near future.

SUGGESTED READING

Akhtar M, Shenasa M, Jazayeri M, et al. Wide QRS complex tachycardia. Reappraisal of a common clinical problem. Ann Intern Med 1988; 109:905–912.

Allessie MA, Bonke FIM, Schopman FJG. Circus movement in rabbit atrial muscle as a mechanism of tachycardia. II. The role of nonuniform recovery of excitability in the occurrence of unidirectional block as studied with multiple microelectrodes. Circ Res 1976; 39:168–177.

Bigger JT. Identification of patients at high risk for sudden cardiac death. Am J Cardiol 1984; 54:3D–8D.

Bigger JT Jr. Why patients with congestive heart failure die:

---

*The automatic implantable cardioverter defibrillator is manufactured by Cardiac Pacemakers, Inc. This term has been used in a generic sense throughout the text.

Arrhythmias and sudden cardiac death. Circulation 1987; 75(Suppl 4):28–35.

Bigger JT Jr, Fleiss JL, Kleiger R, et al. The relationship among ventricular arrhythmias, left ventricular dysfunction and mortality in the 2 years after myocardial infarction. Circulation 1984; 69:250–258.

Coromilas J, Bigger JT Jr, Kleiger RE, et al. Relations among left ventricular dysfunction, ventricular arrhythmias, and mortality after myocardial infarction. Circulation 1989; 80(Suppl II):48.

Cranefield PF. The conduction of the cardiac impulse. The slow response and cardiac arrhythmias. Mt Kisco, NY: Futura, 1975.

Cranefield PF. Action potentials, afterpotentials, and arrhythmias. Circ Res 1972; 41:415–423.

Dangman KH, Hoffman BF. Studies on overdrive suppression of canine cardiac Purkinje fibers: Maximal diastolic potential as a determinant of the response. J Am Coll Cardiol 1983; 2:1183–1190.

Dargie HJ, Cleland JG, Leckie BJ, et al. Relation of arrhythmias and electrolyte abnormalities to survival in patients with severe chronic heart failure. Circulation 1987; 75:IV-98–107.

Denniss AR, Richards DA, Cody DV, et al. Prognostic symptoms of ventricular tachycardia and fibrillation induced at programmed stimulation and delayed potential detected on the signal–averaged electrocardiograms of survivors of acute myocardial infarction. Circulation 1986; 74:731–745.

Gomes JA, Winters SL, Stewart D, et al. A new noninvasive index to predict sustained ventricular tachycardia and sudden death in the five years after myocardial infarction based on signal-averaged electrocardiogram, radionuclide ejection fraction and Holter monitoring. J Am Coll Cardiol 1987; 10:349–357.

Gorgels APM, Vos MS, Brugada P, Wellens HJJ. The clinical relevance of abnormal automaticity and triggered activity. In: Brugada P, Wellens HJJ, eds. Cardiac arrhythmias: Where to go from here? Mount Kisco, NY: Futura Publishing Co 1987:pp 147–169.

Johnson NJ, Rosen MR. The distinction between triggered activity and other cardiac arrhythmias. In: Brugada P, Wellens HJJ, eds. Cardiac arrhythmias: Where to go from here? Mount Kisco, NY: Futura, 1987:129.

Josephson ME, Seides SF. Clinical cardiac electrophysiology: Techniques and interpretation. Philadelphia: Lea & Febiger, 1979.

Kuchar DL, Thorburn CW, Sammel NL. Late potentials detected after myocardial infarction: Natural history and prognostic significance. Circulation 1986; 74:1280–1289.

Mitchell LB, Duff HJ, Manyari DE, Wyse DG. A randomized clinical trial of the noninvasive and invasive approaches to drug therapy of ventricular tachycardia. N Eng J Med 1987; 317:1681–1687.

Morganroth J. Premature ventricular complexes; diagnosis and indications for therapy. JAMA 1984; 252:673–676.

Morganroth J, Bigger JT Jr, Anderson J. Treatment of ventricular arrhythmias by United States cardiologists: A survey before the Cardiac Arrhythmia Suppression Trial (CAST) results were available. Am J Cardiol 1990; 65:40–48.

Mukherji J, Rude RE, Poole KE, et al. Risk factors for sudden death after acute myocardial infarction: Two-year follow-up. Am J Cardiol 1984; 54:31–36.

Nicod P, Gilpin E, Dittrich H, et al. Prognostic significance of complex ventricular arrhythmia for cardiac death during the first year after myocardial infarction. J Electrophysiol 1987; 1:93–102.

Tchou P, Young P, Mahmud R, et al. Useful clinical criteria for the diagnosis of ventricular tachycardia. Am J Med 1988; 84:53–56.

The Cardiac Arrhythmia Suppression Trial (CAST) Investigators. Increased mortality due to encainide or flecainide in a randomized trial of arrhythmia suppression after myocardial infarction. N Engl J Med 1989; 321:406–412.

The CONSENSUS Trial Study Group. Effects of enalapril on mortality in severe congestive heart failure. Results of the Cooperative North Scandinavian Enalapril Survival Study (CONSENSUS). N Engl J Med 1987; 316:1429–1435.

The ESVEM Investigators. The ESVEM Trial. Electrophysiologic study versus electrocardiographic monitoring for selection of antiarrhythmic therapy of ventricular tachyarrhythmias. Circulation 1989; 79:1354–1360.

Vlay S. How the university cardiologist treats ventricular premature beats: A nationwide survey of 65 university medical centers. Am Heart J 1985; 110:904–909.

Waldo AL, Olshansky B, Okumura K, Henthorn RW. Current perspective on entrainment of tachyarrhythmias. In: Brugada P, Wellens HJJ, eds. Cardiac arrhythmias: Where to go from here? Mount Kisco, NY: Futura, 1987:171.

Wellens HJJ, Bar FW, Lie KI. The value of the electrocardiogram in the differential diagnosis of a tachycardia with a widened QRS complex. Am J Med 1978: 64:27–33.

Wellens HJJ, Brugada P, Stevenson WG. Programmed electrical stimulation of the heart in patients with life threatening ventricular arrhythmias: What is the significance of induced arrhythmias and what is the correct stimulation protocol? Circulation 1985; 72:1–7.

Winkle RA, Thomas A. The automatic implantable cardioverter defibrillator: The US experience. In: Brugada P, Wellens, HJJ, eds. Cardiac arrhythmias: Where to go from here? Mount Kisco, NY: Futura, 1987:663.

Wit AL, Cranefield PF. Triggered and automatic activity in the canine coronary sinus. Circ Res 1977; 41:435–445.

Worley SJ, Swain JL, Colavita PG, et al. Development of an endocardialepicardial gradient of activation rate during electrically induced, sustained ventricular fibrillation in dogs. Am J Cardiol 1985; 55:813–820.

Yusuf S, Peto J, Collins R, Sleight P. Beta blockade during and after myocardial infarction: An overview of the randomized trials. Prog Cardiovasc Dis 1985; 27:335–371.

Zeldis SM, Levine BJ, Michelson EL, Morganroth J. Cardiovascular complaints: Correlation with cardiac arrhythmias on 24-hour monitoring. Chest 1980; 78:456–462.

VENTRICULAR PREMATURE COMPLEXES AND UNSUSTAINED VENTRICULAR TACHYCARDIA: NONINVASIVE APPROACH

JOEL MORGANROTH, M.D.

DEFINITIONS AND CLASSIFICATION

Ventricular premature complexes (VPCs) can occur as a normal phenomenon or be a marker of electrical heart disease. A study in normal individuals by Kostis and colleagues can be used to define the frequency threshold of VPCs in order to identify their presence in healthy individuals. That threshold of VPC frequency is less than 100 total VPCs per day or less than 5 per hour. A frequency exceeding these limits or the presence of VPCs in repetitive form (such as unsustained ventricular tachycardia) would define an individual with electrical heart disease. Unsustained ventricular tachycardia (USVT) is defined as the presence of three or more VPCs in a row at a rate of at least 100 to 120 per minute.

The presence of frequent VPCs and/or USVT in a patient without structural heart disease does not increase the risk of sudden cardiac death. The ventricular arrhythmia in these patients is classified as "benign." Such patients are identified by chance electrocardiographic recording or because they have symptoms that suggest the presence of a ventricular arrhythmia. Unfortunately, there is a poor correlation between the complaints of palpitations, lightheadedness, or dizziness and the presence of ventricular arrhythmias. More often than not, ventricular arrhythmias produce no symptoms, and frequently these complaints correlate with sinus tachycardia, atrial premature complexes, or no specific dysrhythmia. Some patients clearly sense the presence of VPCs and/or long runs of USVT, and at times lifestyle-limiting symptoms can occur that may even justify antiarrhythmic drug therapy for relief.

Patients with structural heart disease and particularly those with a depression of left ventricular function (especially with an ejection fraction below 0.40) appear to have an increased risk of sudden cardiac death when VPCs and/or USVT are present. In a post–myocardial infarction patient, the mere presence of six VPCs per hour increases the risk of sudden death, and even a single ventricular triplet can markedly increase the 1-year mortality rate. Patients with VPCs and/or USVT occurring in the presence of left ventricular dysfunction can be considered to have potentially lethal or prognostically significant ventricular arrhythmias. Patients with potentially lethal ventricular arrhythmias may present with symptoms as described above for the benign class but usually are asymptomatic.

Individuals who have milder forms of structural heart disease without a depression of ventricular function fall into a "gray zone" between the benign and potentially lethal ventricular arrhythmia classes. Examples include patients with mitral valve prolapse or coronary artery disease without active ischemia. It is important to note that overt ischemia is not usually the mechanism responsible for initiating VPCs and/or USVT. In addition, some patients may develop ventricular arrhythmias, particularly USVT, as a result of increased catecholamine levels. These individuals do not tend to have structural cardiac disease although underlying ischemia is always questioned. The overall prognostic classification for ventricular arrhythmias is detailed in Table 1.

Table 1 Classification of Ventricular Arrhythmias

	Benign	Potentially Lethal		Lethal
		LVEF ≥ .30	LVEF < .30	
Risk of sudden cardiac death	Lowest	Moderate	High	Highest
Structural heart disease	0	Moderate	Moderately severe	Severe
Hemodynamic symptoms	0	0	0	Present
Method of evaluation	Holter	Holter	Holter (or EP)	EP
Where to initiate therapy	Out of hospital	Out of hospital	Out of/in hospital	In hospital

LVEF = left ventricular ejection fraction, EP = Electrophysiologic testing, IC = a drug belonging to class IC antiarrhythmic agents, IA = a drug belonging to class IA antiarrhythmic agents.

DIAGNOSIS

The diagnosis of VPCs and USVT requires a quantitative evaluation, especially if therapy is contemplated. The noninvasive approach using long-term electrocardiographic ambulatory recording (Holter monitoring) provides the principal method of defining the presence or absence of ventricular arrhythmias, of correlating the arrhythmias with symptoms (if present), and of quantifying their frequency. The Holter monitoring used for these purposes should be of the continuous 24-hour format, since accurate quantitation of arrhythmia frequency is necessary. Real-time electrocardiographic systems have generally been found to produce less accurate results in quantifying VPC frequency and identifying USVT.

Exercise testing is complementary to Holter monitoring, since it often detects USVT attributable to a "catecholamine mechanism" or occasionally identifies the unusual patient with ventricular arrhythmias that are directly correlated with ischemia. VPC frequency should be reported as the mean number of VPCs per hour, which is defined by dividing the total number of VPCs by the length of the recording in hours. USVT is commonly reported as the number of events per day (irrespective of the number of beats in each run) as well as the number of beats in the form of USVT per day. Comparative quantitation is essential for defining therapeutic efficacy, inefficacy, or proarrhythmia.

INDICATIONS FOR TREATMENT

There are only two indications for the treatment of ventricular arrhythmias. The first is to relieve arrhythmia-induced symptoms as a means of improving the quality of life. It is important to remember that in patients with benign or potentially lethal ventricular arrhythmias, the symptoms never cause hemodynamic consequences (syncope or worse), and therefore symptoms in this setting only affect the overall quality of life, whereas control of hemodynamically important symptoms in lethal ventricular arrhythmias is essential to preserve life. The second indication for treatment of ventricular arrhythmias is the hope of preventing the increased risk of sudden cardiac death in patients with potentially lethal or lethal ventricular arrhythmias.

Unfortunately, studies to date have not clearly defined whether the suppression of ventricular arrhythmias achieves this benefit. Currently the National Institutes of Health's Cardiac Arrhythmia Suppression Trial (CAST) is evaluating this potential in post–myocardial infarction patients, and it is hoped that by the mid-1990s we will have a final answer to this important question. Until that time, the only firm indication for therapy of ventricular arrhythmias is for the elimination of associated symptoms.

An interim report from CAST in April 1989 identified that patients randomized to groups taking encainide or flecainide had an enhanced mortality rate from arrhythmic death compared with those on placebo. These results indicate that the suppression of asymptomatic VPCs in the post–myocardial infarction patient does not automatically decrease the risk of sudden cardiac death. Since the CAST trial is continuing to evaluate moricizine (Ethmozine), and since encainide and flecainide (class IC antiarrhythmic agents) profoundly delay cardiac conduction, it may well be that suppression of sudden cardiac death, if demonstrated, is drug-specific. The findings from CAST indicate that physicians should have a very high threshold for treating patients with asymptomatic ventricular arrhythmias and should carefully consider the risks versus the benefits of class I antiarrhythmic therapy.

APPROACH TO THERAPY

Symptomatic Benign or Potentially Lethal Ventricular Arrhythmias

Until we know whether sudden cardiac death can be prevented by the suppression of potentially lethal ventricular arrhythmias, the only benefit of treating VPCs or USVT is to improve the patient's quality of life. This benefit is thus only of minimal to moderate importance. Therefore the risk of antiarrhythmic drug therapy must be clearly defined and carefully considered. A comparison of the potency and risks of the currently approved oral antiarrhythmic agents in the United States is provided in Table 2. This comparison reveals that there is a high prevalence of noncardiac adverse effects and a relatively high potential for important organ toxicity with the use of quinidine, procainamide, and tocainide. There is a high noncardiac side effect rate for disopyramide and mexiletine. Oral amiodarone should not be used in patients with benign or potentially lethal ventricular arrhythmias in light of its high rate of organ toxicity. Thus our approach to therapy of patients with VPCs and USVT is to use beta blockers as the principal first-line drugs when such arrhythmias warrant the use of drug therapy. In patients with benign ventricular arrhythmias in whom there is no potential benefit other than reducing nonhemodynamically important symptoms, we tend to rely particularly on beta-blocking agents as the antiarrhythmic drug of choice. Only when beta blockers fail and symptoms continue to affect the quality of the patient's life do we consider other antiarrhythmic agents. Beta-blocking drugs appear to be effective irrespective of their beta-1 receptor selectivity or the presence or absence of intrinsic

Table 2

AA Drug Class	Efficacy		% Risk of NCAE	Risk of Organ Toxicity	Risk of Serious Proarrhythmia		Risk of CHF	
							B/PL	L
	B/PL	L			B/PL	L	EF ≥ .30 NYHA I & II	EF < .30 III & IV
IA								
Quinidine	3+	2+	25	Moderate	Highest	Moderate	0	0
Procainamide	2+	2+	25	High	Moderate	Moderate	0–1+	1+
Disopyramide	2+	1+	35	None-Low	Moderate	Moderate	2+	4+
IB								
Tocainide	2+	1+	40	High	Low	Low	0	0
Mexiletine	2+	1+	40	Low	Low	Low	0	0
IC								
Encainide	4+	2+	10	None-low	Low	Highest	0	1+
Flecainide	4+	2+	10	None-low	Low	Highest	1+	3+
II								
Beta blocker	2+	1+	10	None-low	Low	Low	1+	3+
III								
Amiodarone	N/A	3+	N/A	Highest	N/A	Low	0–1+	1+

AA = Antiarrhythmic agent, B = Benign ventricular arrhythmia class, PL = Potentially lethal ventricular arrhythmia class, L = Lethal ventricular arrhythmia class, CHF = Congestive heart failure, EF = Ejection fraction, NYHA = New York Heart Association, NCAE = Noncardiac adverse effects, N/A = Not applicable.

sympathomimetic activity. We tend to choose a once-a-day beta blocker for enhanced compliance and generally select either nadolol or atenolol as the drug of choice. We have found that low doses (10 to 40 mg per day) of nadolol may be effective in some patients, whereas atenolol generally requires a dose of 50 or 100 mg per day to achieve efficacy. The beta blockers specifically approved by the FDA for ventricular arrhythmia management are propranolol and acebutalol. Outpatient initiation of beta blockers is safe and effective in patients with benign ventricular arrhythmias, since the incidences of all adverse reactions are very low.

In patients with potentially lethal ventricular arrhythmias, the same approach to therapy is generally applicable. Many of these patients are already taking beta blockers because of the presence of underlying problems such as ischemic heart disease or hypertension, and thus when ventricular arrhythmias require therapy in such patients for symptom relief, at present we select a class I antiarrhythmic agent. The best agent to select cannot yet be defined pending availability of data from CAST or moricizine or the release of new class III agents such as sotalol. These agents can be administered safely to outpatients as long as the following conditions are not present: (1) marked depression of left ventricular function (usually ejection fractions less than 0.30), (2) New York Heart Association class III or IV symptomatic congestive heart failure, (3) sick sinus syndrome, or (4) an elderly and debilitated patient. Patients with lethal or malignant ventricular arrhythmias such as USVT with hemodynamic symptoms (e.g., syncope)

or sustained ventricular tachycardia require antiarrhythmic drug therapy to suppress such life-threatening symptoms. In this group of patients beta blockers tend to be ineffective, and class IC antiarrhythmic agents have significant cardiac adverse effects, such as serious or fatal proarrhythmias. Thus, in this population we choose as first-line therapy drugs belonging to the IA class (e.g., quinidine or procainamide), followed by class IA and IB drug combinations. Class IC agents and amiodarone should be considered second-line agents.

Definition of Response for Benign or Potentially Lethal Ventricular Arrhythmias Using the Noninvasive Approach

Once patients are appropriately started on antiarrhythmic drugs for the treatment of VPCs and USVT, it is important to determine whether or not the antiarrhythmic agent is effective. The presence of symptomatic relief is not sufficient, in my opinion, to justify continuation of an antiarrhythmic drug, unless it can be demonstrated that the reduction in symptoms is attributable to suppression of the VPCs and/or USVT as previously quantitated before therapy. Thus it is important to repeat a 24-hour quantitative Holter monitor while the patient is on therapy to be certain that adequate arrhythmia suppression is the cause of the symptom relief (and not a placebo effect) and to be certain that asymptomatic proarrhythmia has not occurred. Adequate suppression requires a rather high degree of arrhythmia reduction in light of the marked spontaneous variability in

VPC and USVT frequency. We require at least a 75 to 80 percent reduction in the frequency of VPCs and a 90 to 100 percent reduction in the presence of USVT to define drug efficacy.

Asymptomatic proarrhythmia is usually defined as an increase in USVT by at least tenfold on therapy compared with baseline and/or an increase in VPC frequency of threefold if the average VPC frequency at baseline was over 100 per hour and tenfold if the average baseline VPC frequency was less than 100 per hour. It is important to interrupt therapy by discontinuing medication every 6 to 12 months to be certain the patient still requires arrhythmia suppression. Approximately 25 percent of the time we find that such discontinuation of antiarrhythmic drugs reveals that the ventricular arrhythmia is no longer present, and thus the antiarrhythmic drug therapy need no longer be continued. We believe this procedure can safely be performed in an outpatient setting by abruptly discontinuing the antiarrhythmic drug and asking the patient to return in 1 to 2 weeks for a repeat Holter recording if necessary.

SUGGESTED READING

Kostis JB, McCrone K, Moreya AE, et al. Premature ventricular complexes in the absence of identifiable heart disease. Circulation 1981; 63:1351–1356.

Morganroth J. Premature ventricular complexes: Diagnosis and indications for therapy. JAMA 1984; 252:673–676.

Morganroth J. Ambulatory ECG monitoring in the evaluation of new antiarrhythmic drugs. Circulation 1986; 73:II92–97.

Morganroth J, Anderson JL, Gentzkow GD. Classification by type of ventricular arrhythmia predicts frequency of adverse cardiac events from flecainide. J Am Coll Cardiol 1986; 8:607–615.

Morganroth J, Horowitz LN. Antiarrhythmic drug therapy 1988: For whom, how and where? Am J Cardiol 1988; 62:461–465.

VENTRICULAR PREMATURE COMPLEXES AND UNSUSTAINED VENTRICULAR TACHYCARDIA: INVASIVE APPROACH

STEPHEN L. WINTERS, M.D.
J. ANTHONY GOMES, M.D.

OVERVIEW OF COMPLEX VENTRICULAR ECTOPY

Classically, the term complex ventricular ectopy has been used to describe the presence of frequent ventricular premature complexes (VPCs; greater than 10 to 30 VPCs per hour), repetitive VPCs, and/or unsustained ventricular tachycardia (three or more repetitive VPCs) on ambulatory electrocardiographic monitoring. Although initially introduced in an effort to stratify patients at risk for sustaining lethal forms of ventricular tachyarrhythmias, such a grading scheme in itself does not necessarily portend a higher risk. Thus, an alternative way of viewing VPCs has been proposed. This grading system considers ventricular arrhythmias as benign, potentially lethal, and lethal. Whereas the risk of sudden cardiac death is thought to be minimal in the group with benign arrhythmias, the greatest risk occurs in patients with arrhythmias that are believed to be potentially lethal or lethal. Both benign and potentially lethal arrhythmias that are usually recorded on a routine electrocardiogram may result in no symptoms or in complaints of awareness of extra beats. In contrast, lethal ventricular arrhythmias are often recorded in patients who have survived a prior episode of cardiac collapse or sustained ventricular tachycardia. Clearly, evaluation and treatment should be concentrated in patients with potentially lethal and lethal arrhythmias.

Often the presence of complex ventricular ectopy is an extremely anxiety-provoking finding, not only for patients but frequently also for the treating physicians. Several reasons exist for not utilizing antiarrhythmic therapy in all patients with complex ventricular ectopy. The antiarrhythmic drugs frequently employed are expensive and often cause a variety of systemic side effects, some of which may be fatal. They may be a nuisance in the daily schedule of individual patients. However, the most significant reason for not utilizing antiarrhythmic agents in all patients with complex ventricular ectopy is the concern about arrhythmia aggravation or proarrhythmia. The potential for antiarrhythmic drugs to cause arrhythmia aggravation or proarrhythmogenesis has been documented from electrophysiologic studies as well as electrocardiographic monitoring and/or exercise treadmill testing follow-up. Over the past decade, arrhythmia aggravation has been documented in up to 12 percent of antiarrhythmic drug trials in patients with ventricular ectopy. Furthermore, in patients undergoing multiple drug trials for suppression of ventricular ectopy, up to 35 percent have experienced at least one proarrhythmic effect. Perhaps the most compelling argument against empirical antiarrhythmic drug therapy are the data derived from the Cardiac Arrhythmia Suppression Trial. In this study of more than 1,400 patients randomized for drug treatment of ventricular arrhythmias after myocardial infarction, 9 percent receiving one of the two most suppressive antiarrhythmic agents (flecainide or encainide) experienced the development of sustained ventricular tachycardia or sudden cardiac death, as compared with 33 percent of patients treated with placebo.

ASYMPTOMATIC COMPLEX VENTRICULAR ECTOPY IN PATIENTS WITH NORMAL VENTRICULAR FUNCTION

In various subgroups of individuals as well as in the general population, the occurrence of VPCs has been noted in up to 75 percent or more of individuals. As continuous ambulatory electrocardiographic monitoring techniques are employed more frequently, the chances of diagnosing ventricular ectopy increase. As many as 25 percent of patients with no significant symptoms and no significant organic heart disease may have episodes of unsustained ventricular tachycardia documented on ambulatory electrocardiographic monitoring. However, several long-term follow-up studies have revealed no significant increase in the incidence of sustained ventricular tachycardia or sudden cardiac death in individuals with asymptomatic complex ventricular ectopy in the absence of abnormal ventricular function.

It is important to point out that both the right and left ventricle need to be assessed as normal, since diseased states of either ventricle may increase subsequent morbidity and mortality. Studies have documented no increased risk for sustained ventricular tachyarrhythmias or sudden death in such individuals over a period of 10 years. Thus, in individuals with complex ventricular arrhythmias, efforts should be made to exclude any systemic processes or organic heart disease of which the ectopy may be a marker. However, more invasive assessments of

complex ventricular ectopy in patients with no overt heart disease are rarely indicated.

EVALUATION OF COMPLEX VENTRICULAR ECTOPY IN PATIENTS FOLLOWING MYOCARDIAL INFARCTION

The knowledge that complex ventricular ectopy after myocardial infarction is associated with subsequent increased mortality and the development of sustained ventricular tachycardia stems from data that have been well known for the past decade. The frequently published and cited data stemming from a study of more than 1,700 post–myocardial infarction patients reported by Ruberman and colleagues revealed that over 3 years of follow-up, the cumulative probability of sudden cardiac death was as high as 15 percent in patients with complex VPCs. It was less than 5 percent in patients with simple VPCs or no VPCs.

Two large-scale studies reported in the mid-1980s evaluated the independent and interactive roles of complex ventricular ectopy and left ventricular systolic dysfunction in patients' status following myocardial infarction. Table 1 summarizes the pertinent findings from these two studies. As can be ascertained, the likelihood of subsequent sudden cardiac death or the development of sustained ventricular tachyarrhythmias is very low in patients with no VPCs and left ventricular ejection fractions that are normal or near normal. The incidence of sudden death rises exponentially if systolic left ventricular function is impaired and complex VPCs are present. At one extreme, the incidence of sudden cardiac death was found to be 18 percent within 6 months if these two prognostic indicators were present together.

COMPLEX VENTRICULAR ECTOPY IN THE PRESENCE OF OTHER CARDIAC CONDITIONS

Various other cardiac conditions may exist in which complex ventricular ectopy may herald the potential for malignant ventricular tachyarrhythmias. Idiopathic hypertrophic subaortic stenosis rep-

Table 1 Ventricular Ectopy After Myocardial Infarction

	No. of Patients	Follow-up	Mortality	Sudden Deaths	No VPCs/ Pr LVEF	Complex VPCs/ Abnl LVEF
MPIRG*	766	24 mo	89 (12%)	54 (7%)	3%	38% Mortality
MILIS†	583	6 mo	66 (11%)	29 (5%)	2%	18% Sudden deaths

*The Multicenter Post-Infarction Research Group.
†The Multicenter Investigation of the Limitation of Infarct Size.
Abnl LVEF = Relatively low left ventricular ejection fractions.
Pr LVEF = Relatively preserved left ventricular ejection fractions.

resents an extremely serious condition if complex ventricular ectopy, in particular unsustained ventricular tachycardia, is present on electrocardiographic recording or ambulatory electrocardiographic monitoring. Whereas unsustained ventricular tachycardia has been recorded in 19 to 28 percent of patients with idiopathic hypertrophic subaortic stenosis, the incidence of sudden death may be as high as 8 percent per year in such patients. In individuals without unsustained ventricular tachycardia who have idiopathic hypertrophic subaortic stenosis, the incidence of sudden cardiac death is not significantly higher than that for the general population. Thus, numerous studies have been evaluated to determine whether there is a role for antiarrhythmic drug therapy in individuals with idiopathic hypertrophic subaortic stenosis and complex ventricular ectopy. Unfortunately, most trials of conventional antiarrhythmic agents have not shown any improvement in survival in those in the high-risk category. However, promising data, although still preliminary, have been reported on improved survival in amiodarone-treated patients thought to be at high risk for sudden cardiac death because of the presence of unsustained ventricular tachycardia with idiopathic hypertrophic subaortic stenosis. The prognostic value of programmed ventricular stimulation in patients with idiopathic hypertrophic subaortic stenosis and unsustained ventricular tachycardia is under evaluation at present.

Another setting in which complex ventricular ectopy may have significant relevance is in individuals with idiopathic dilated cardiomyopathy. With a 1- to 2-year mortality rate of as high as 50 percent in these patients, the two leading causes of death are embolic phenomena and sudden cardiac death. Although it is not proved, it is assumed that most cardiac sudden deaths in such individuals are due to ventricular tachyarrhythmias. However, other arrhythmias, including high-degree or complete heart block, may also play a role. In addition, because of the negative inotropic effects of many antiarrhythmic drugs, use of most antiarrhythmic agents on an empirical basis may hasten the decline in overall well-being in such patients.

No conclusive data are available regarding the value of empirical antiarrhythmic drug therapy in prolonging life in patients with complex ventricular arrhythmias and dilated cardiomyopathy. However, a debate is emerging with respect to empirical amiodarone treatment in patients with complex ventricular ectopy and dilated cardiomyopathy. Although no clear evidence supports a role for the use of amiodarone in such patients, there are theoretical reasons to avoid its empirical use. These include the systemic toxicities associated with amiodarone as well as its potential for the precipitation of heart block in patients who often have profound disease of the entire conduction system.

Other conditions exist in which complex ventricular ectopy may be a harbinger of future problems. The detection of complex ventricular ectopy may lead to diagnoses of right ventricular dysplasia, mitral valve prolapse, or systemic sarcoidosis. A subgroup of patients with right ventricular dysplasia may develop significant ventricular tachycardia giving rise to the condition known as arrhythmogenic right ventricular dysplasia. Although these patients often respond to antiarrhythmic drug therapy, the recurrence rate of ventricular tachycardia is high. Nonetheless, overall survival has been good with antiarrhythmic drug therapy.

Usually, the presence of complex ventricular ectopy in association with mitral valve prolapse should not be of concern. The only documented high-risk group of patients with mitral valve prolapse and complex ventricular ectopy is composed predominantly of women with the long Q-T interval syndrome, a family history of sudden death, and diffuse T-wave changes. Finally, the presence of infiltrative myocardial processes such as sarcoidosis may be associated with complex ventricular arrhythmias that may deteriorate to more sustained forms of tachycardia. However, exact means of identifying patients in this latter subgroup who are at risk for the development of sudden cardiac death are unknown at present.

ROLE OF VENTRICULAR STIMULATION IN THE ASSESSMENT OF PATIENTS WITH COMPLEX VENTRICULAR ECTOPY

At the time of this writing, at least eight studies have examined the role of invasive electrophysiologic testing in the evaluation and treatment of patients with complex ventricular ectopy. These studies, summarized in Table 2, have included reasonable but relatively small numbers of patients with respect to the population at risk. With the exception of one study, the rest of the studies included patients with a variety of organic heart conditions as well as those with no significant heart disease. Overall, the percentage of patients with no inducible ventricular tachyarrhythmias ranged from 39 to 80 percent. In contrast, the percentage of patients with inducible ventricular tachyarrhythmias of significance ranged from 20 to 55 percent. In most of these studies, a breakdown of the number of patients studied with a history of a prior myocardial infarction could be performed. In such patients, the incidence of inducible ventricular tachyarrhythmias of significance ranged from 33 to 57 percent, with a mean of approximately 44 percent. Although not assessed in each study, data suggest that induction of ventricular tachycardia may be more common in the setting of diminished left ventricular systolic function.

Table 2 Programmed Ventricular Stimulation in Patients With Complex Ventricular Ectopy

Study	No. of Patients	Number Noninducible	Number Inducible	Number Myocardial Infarction Inducible
Gomes (1984)	73	53 (73%)	20 (27%)	17/40 (43%)
Veltri (1985)	33	19 (58%)	14 (42%)	—
Zheutlin (1986)	88	55 (63%)	33 (37%)	24/53 (45%)
Sulpizi (1987)	61	24 (39%)	37 (61%)	—
Buxton (1987)	62	34 (55%)	28 (45%)	28/59 (46%)
Winters (1988)	53	40 (75%)	13 (25%)	11/27 (41%)
Kharsa (1988)	40	32 (80%)	8 (20%)	7/21 (33%)
Klein (1989)	40	18 (45%)	22 (55%)	19/33 (57%)

The follow-up in patients with no inducible ventricular tachyarrhythmias ranged from 14 to 30 months, as illustrated in Table 3. With the exception of two studies in which the incidence of a significant ventricular tachyarrhythmic event was 29 percent and 12 percent in patients with no significant inducible ventricular tachyarrhythmias, the incidence of the development of significant tachyarrhythmic events or sudden death ranged from 0 to 8 percent. In contrast, with follow-up of similar periods of time, the incidences of development of significant, sustained ventricular tachyarrhythmias or sudden death in the group of patients with inducible ventricular tachyarrhythmias ranged from 4 to 40 percent.

Compliance with recommendations of withholding antiarrhythmic therapy (in patients with no inducible ventricular tachyarrhythmia of significance) and the use of electrophysiologically-guided antiarrhythmic therapy (in patients with induced ventricular tachycardia) was not always carried out in these studies. Furthermore, in many instances, appropriate electrophysiologically-guided antiarrhythmic therapy could not be documented. In the study of Klein and coworkers, only patients who had had a prior myocardial infarction were evaluated, and the incidence of subsequent sustained ventricular tachycardia or sudden cardiac death in patients

who received therapy not guided by electrophysiologic assessment was approximately 64 percent. Again, this does not necessarily imply that recommendations were not adhered to but also applies to circumstances in which no effective suppressive antiarrhythmic drug regimen could be identified.

In evaluating the numerous studies on the role of invasive electrophysiologic testing and programmed ventricular stimulation in patients with complex ventricular arrhythmias, several inconsistencies need to be considered. To begin with, the patient populations in these studies varied dramatically. The history of prior syncopal episodes also varied significantly from one study to the other. In fact, it has been shown that syncope in the setting of unsustained ventricular tachycardia or complex ventricular arrhythmias may be an independent risk factor for the subsequent induction of a sustained ventricular tachycardia at the time of programmed ventricular stimulation. In addition, the stimulation protocols utilized varied from one study to the other. Whether the appropriate stimulation protocol should be nonaggressive with the use of only two premature stimuli or should utilize an aggressive protocol with three premature stimuli and/or the use of agents such as isoproterenol is unknown.

One further limitation in evaluating these various studies centers on the end point of the stimulation protocol. One group considered the inducibility of only three repetitive ventricular responses as a significant end point for induction of a ventricular tachyarrhythmia and had poor predictive accuracy. Some of the studies included reproducible, unsustained ventricular tachycardia of a monomorphic nature, lasting for five or more beats, as an end point for classifying induction of a significant ventricular tachyarrhythmia. Several other studies included only patients with induced sustained ventricular tachycardia of a monomorphic nature. Thus, recommendations as to the true end point from an electrophysiologic study in patients with complex ventricular ectopy cannot be stated with certainty.

The cause for the high incidence of the development of sustained ventricular tachyarrhythmias or

Table 3 Programmed Ventricular Stimulation in Patients With Complex Ventricular Ectopy

Study	Noninducible		Inducible	
	Follow-up (mo)	Arrhythmic Events	Follow-up (mo)	Arrhythmic Events
Gomes (1984)	30	1 (2%)	30	5 (32%)
Veltri (1985)	23	4 (29%)	23	3 (21%)
Zheutlin (1986)	22	0	17	4 (12%)
Sulpizi (1987)	26	3 (8%)	26	1 (4%)
Buxton (1987)	28	4 (12%)	28	7 (25%)
Winters (1988)	15	2 (5%)	17	2 (15%)
Kharsa (1988)	17	0	16	0
Klein (1989)	14	0	14	9 (40%)

sudden death in patients who had induced ventricular tachycardia is unknown. One possibility is that these patients had poor results because appropriate electrophysiologically-guided antiarrhythmic agents were not utilized in many cases or simply could not be found. Alternatively, one must consider that some of the agents utilized may have had proarrhythmic effects, despite the beneficial results suggested with programmed ventricular stimulation. It is possible that these patients would have been more likely to develop ventricular tachyarrhythmias or experience sudden death if antiarrhythmic therapy had not been utilized. However, the use of non-electrophysiologically-guided antiarrhythmic therapy appears to be associated with a higher arrhythmic mortality.

Thus, although there is increasing evidence to support the use of electrophysiologic testing with programmed ventricular stimulation in the evaluation of patients with complex ventricular arrhythmias, it remains unclear whether antiarrhythmic therapy significantly alters the arrhythmic mortality in the high-risk inducible group. At least one large multicenter study, with randomized forms of therapy in inducible patients, is planned for the future.

ROLE OF SIGNAL-AVERAGED ELECTROCARDIOGRAPHY IN SELECTING PATIENTS WITH COMPLEX VENTRICULAR ECTOPY FOR PROGRAMMED VENTRICULAR STIMULATION

As discussed previously, it is clear that for the most part, patients with normal ventricular function do not need electrophysiologic testing. Furthermore, such testing may not be as sensitive and specific in individuals with conditions such as dilated cardiomyopathies. However, such testing does play a role in patients who have had prior myocardial infarctions. Some use also may be found in patients with specific organic cardiac conditions such as sarcoidosis in association with ventricular arrhythmias.

One cannot propose that all individuals with complex ventricular ectopy undergo programmed ventricular stimulation. To begin with, the test is expensive, time-consuming, and often unpleasant for the patient. Furthermore, the resources available do not permit such testing on the enormous number of patients who present with complex ventricular ectopy. Thus, screening methods for selecting patients for invasive electrophysiologic testing are needed.

Signal-averaged electrocardiography has been evaluated as such a screening method. The assumption that recording of late potentials from surface electrocardiograms might help in stratifying patients into those at high risk or low risk for the development of sustained ventricular tachyarrhythmias in the setting of complex ventricular ectopy is based on extrapolation from data known in patients with sustained ventricular tachycardia. In essence, most patients who are unresponsive to antiarrhythmic drug therapy and who require endocardial resection and/or ventricular aneurysmectomy to treat sustained ventricular tachyarrhythmias have late potentials that can be recorded epicardially and endocardially. These late potentials are believed to reflect areas of slow conduction that comprise the underlying substrate capable of sustaining ventricular tachycardia.

Several studies have evaluated the role of signal-averaged electrocardiography in the prediction of inducibility or lack of inducibility of ventricular tachycardia at electrophysiologic testing. Although limited data is available from patients with nonischemic cardiomyopathies, the largest series have focused on patients with prior myocardial infarctions. Among patients referred for evaluation to major arrhythmia centers where signal-averaged electrocardiography and electrophysiologic testing were available, the incidence of abnormal signal-averaged electrocardiograms in patients with complex ventricular ectopy was as high as 42 percent. Of those patients with abnormal signal-averaged electrocardiograms, ventricular tachycardia was induced in up to 61 percent. The greatest sensitivity, specificity, and predictive accuracy of signal-averaged electrocardiography were 73 to 91 percent, 82 to 89 percent, and 78 to 84 percent, respectively. Thus, it appears that signal-averaged electrocardiography can be used as an adjunctive tool to stratify all patients with complex ventricular ectopy into groups of patients who are likely to have induction of ventricular tachycardia or lack of induction of ventricular tachycardia at programmed ventricular stimulation.

Particular attention has been focused on the occurrence of complex ventricular ectopy in post-myocardial infarction patients. In one study of patients evaluated for complex ventricular ectopy with programmed ventricular stimulation after transmural myocardial infarctions, almost two-thirds had abnormal signal-averaged electrocardiograms. Presentation with an abnormal signal-averaged electrocardiogram did not appear to be different, regardless of the ejection fraction or the presence of akinetic and/or dyskinetic left ventricular segments suggestive of a ventricular aneurysm. In one study, ventricular tachycardia was induced in 50 percent of those patients with an abnormal signal-averaged electrocardiogram. In contrast, none of the post-infarction patients with normal signal-averaged electrocardiograms had significant ventricular tachycardia induced at programmed ventricular stimulation.

When particular attention is focused on post-infarction patients who have abnormal signal-averaged electrocardiograms in the presence of complex ventricular ectopy, the history of a prior syncopal episode represents an independent risk factor for the induction of a ventricular tachyarrhythmia at programmed ventricular stimulation. Low-risk patients may be identified utilizing signal-averaged electrocardiography as a means to stratify patients for programmed ventricular stimulation if they have complex ventricular arrhythmias and organic heart disease. These individuals have been documented to do well without antiarrhythmic therapy. Thus, withholding antiarrhythmic therapy and/or further invasive electrophysiologic testing in individuals with normal signal-averaged electrocardiograms can be considered. Although an abnormal signal-averaged electrocardiogram may be associated with only a 50 percent risk of inducible ventricular tachycardia, if electrophysiologic guidance of antiarrhythmic therapy is adhered to, programmed ventricular stimulation may be justified in these patients.

SUGGESTED READING

Bigger J, Fleiss JL, Hager R, et al. Multicenter Post-infarction Research Group. The relationship among ventricular arrhythmia, left ventricular dysfunction, and mortality in the two years after myocardial infarction. Circulation 1984; 69:250–258.

Buxton AE, Marchlinski FE, Flores BT, et al. Nonsustained ventricular tachycardia in patients with coronary artery disease: Role of electrophysiologic study. Circulation 1987; 75:1178–1185.

Buxton AE, Simson MB, Falcone RA, et al. Results of signal-averaged electrocardiography and electrophysiologic study in patients with nonsustained ventricular tachycardia after healing of acute myocardial infarction. Am J Cardiol 1987; 69:80–85.

Fananapazir L, Tracy CM, Leon MB, et al. Electrophysiologic abnormalities in patients with hypertrophic cardiomyopathy: A consecutive analysis in 155 patients. Circulation 1989; 80:1259–1268.

Gomes JA, Hariman RI, Kang PS, et al. Programmed electrical stimulation in patients with high-degree ventricular ectopy: Electrophysiologic findings and prognosis for survival. Circulation 1984; 70:43–51.

Kennedy HL, Whitlock JA, Sprague MK, et al. Long-term follow-up of asymptomatic healthy subjects with frequent and complex ventricular ectopy. N Engl J Med 1985; 4:193–202.

Kharsa MH, Gold RL, Moore M, et al. Long-term outcome following programmed electrical stimulation in patients with high-grade ventricular ectopy. PACE 1988; 11:603–609.

Klein RC, Machell C. Use of electrophysiologic testing in patients with nonsustained ventricular tachycardia: Prognostic and therapeutic implications. J Am Coll Cardiol 1989; 14:155–161.

Lown B, Wolf M. Approaches to sudden death from coronary heart disease. Circulation 1971; 44:130–142.

Maron BJ, Savage DD, Epstein SE. Prognostic significance of 24-hour ambulatory electrocardiographic monitoring in patients with hypertrophic cardiomyopathy: A prospective study. Am J Cardiol 1981; 48:252–257.

McKenna WJ, Oakley C, Kikler DM, et al. Improved survival with amiodarone in patients with hypertrophic cardiomyopathy and ventricular tachycardia. Br Heart J 1985; 53:412–416.

Mukharjij, Rude RE, Poole K, et al. Risk factors for sudden death after myocardial infarctions: Two-year follow-up. Am J Cardiol 1984; 54:31–36.

Preliminary report: Effect of encainide and flecainide on mortality in a randomized trial arrhythmia suppression after myocardial infarction. N Engl J Med 1989; 321:406–412.

Ruberman W, Wenblatt E, Goldberg JD, et al. Ventricular premature beats and mortality after myocardial infarction. N Engl J Med 1979; 297:750–757.

Sulpizi AM, Friehling TD, Kowey PR. Value of electrophysiologic testing in patients with nonsustained ventricular tachycardia. Am J Cardiol 1987; 59:841–845.

Turitto G, Fontaine JM, Ursell SN, et al. Value of the signal-averaged electrocardiogram as a predictor of the results of programmed stimulation in nonsustained ventricular tachycardia. Am J Cardiol 1988; 61:1272–1278.

Velebilt V, Podrid PJ, Lown B, et al. Aggravation of ventricular arrhythmia by antiarrhythmic drugs. Circulation 1982; 65:886–894.

Veltri EP, Platia EV, Griffith LSC, Reid PR. Programmed electrical stimulation and long-term follow-up in asymptomatic, nonsustained ventricular tachycardia. Am J Cardiol 1985; 56:309–314.

Winters SL, Greenberg S, Deshmukh P, et al. Ventricular tachycardia associated with sarcoidosis: The anatomic substrate, natural history, and role of the A.I.C.D. Chest 1989; 96:1506.

Winters SL, Stewart D, Targonski A, et al. Late potentials identify patients post myocardial infarction with left ventricular dysfunction and complex ventricular ectopy who have inducible ventricular tachycardia. Abstract. Circulation 1988; 78:II–578.

Winters SL, Stewart D, Targonski A, et al. Role of signal averaging of the surface QRS complex in selecting patients with nonsustained ventricular tachycardia and high-grade ventricular arrhythmias for programmed ventricular stimulation. J Am Coll Cardiol 1988; 12:1481–1487.

Zheutlin TA, Roth M, Cleua W, et al. Programmed electrical stimulation to determine the need for antiarrhythmic therapy in patients with complex ventricular ectopy activity. Am Heart J 1986; 111:860–867.

SUSTAINED VENTRICULAR TACHYCARDIA

ROBERT C. BERNSTEIN, M.D.
FRANCIS E. MARCHLINSKI, M.D.

Sustained ventricular tachycardia most often (approximately 70 percent) occurs in patients with chronic coronary artery disease with a history of myocardial infarction. However, it is important to recognize that ventricular tachycardias can occur in patients with normal hearts as well as in patients with mitral valve prolapse, right ventricular dysplasia, hypertrophic or idiopathic cardiomyopathy, or congenital heart disease. Ventricular tachycardias can also be mimicked by antegrade conduction over a bypass tract during supraventricular tachycardias (Fig. 1).

We will focus on the overall approach to the management of patients with sustained ventricular tachycardia as well as provide specific recommendations for caring for patients with uniform sustained ventricular tachycardia following remote myocardial infarctions. The identification and specific management of patients with ventricular tachycardias occurring in the other disease settings noted above are discussed in later chapters.

Current management of sustained ventricular tachycardia is selected from three treatment approaches: arrhythmia prevention and/or control (pharmacologic therapy), arrhythmia cure (ablative therapy), and rapid termination of arrhythmia recurrence (device implantation). Often, the best treatment for a given patient may be a combination of more than one treatment modality.

Selection of the proper approach to treatment must be individualized (Tables 1 and 2). The underlying arrhythmia substrate, the frequency of tachycardia recurrence, tolerance of the arrhythmia, the response to prior therapy, and the patient's personal philosophy regarding the treatment options and their associated acute and chronic risks and their effect on patient lifestyle all necessarily have an impact on treatment decisions. Therefore, it is important that the patient be included in formulating the management plan for his or her disease.

No one treatment strategy or algorithm is correct for all patients with ventricular tachycardia. Outlined below is our general approach to the evaluation and treatment of patients with sustained uniform ventricular tachycardia.

PHARMACOLOGIC THERAPY

In only 30 to 40 percent of patients with sustained uniform ventricular tachycardia can induction of their arrhythmias during programmed ventricular stimulation be prevented by antiarrhythmic drug therapy. Despite this low percentage, a trial of drug therapy is still the initial treatment choice for most patients. The risks of side effects from initiating therapy are low, and although serial noninvasive and/or invasive electrophysiologic studies are necessary to assess treatment efficacy, these risks and inconveniences are preferable in most situations to more aggressive forms of ablative or device therapy.

We feel that most patients with sustained uniform ventricular tachycardia should have antiarrhythmic therapy assessed by electrophysiologic testing (see the chapter entitled *Electrophysiologic Testing*). This is of paramount importance for those patients with tachycardias that result in acute hemodynamic embarrassment or patients with ventricular tachycardias occurring while they are taking antiarrhythmic agents. Initial assessment (electrophysiologic studies, Holter monitoring, exercise testing) should be performed in the baseline state (when the patient is not taking antiarrhythmic agents). This is necessary in order to determine whether electrophysiologic studies or other diagnostic modalities will be useful for assessing drug effect. In patients not found to have inducible ventricular tachycardia (5 to 10 percent) in response to programmed ventricular stimulation or sufficient baseline ectopy on Holter monitoring (approximately 50 percent), that particular modality could not be utilized to assess drug efficacy.

Table 1 Clinical Factors Considered in Selecting Appropriate Therapy for Ventricular Tachycardia

Hemodynamic tolerance of presenting clinical arrhythmia(s)
Number of distinct ventricular tachycardia morphologies seen clinically
Characterization of underlying arrhythmia substrate
Assessment of left ventricular function
Significance and severity of coronary artery disease
Frequency of clinical recurrences on antiarrhythmic therapy

Table 2 Electrophysiologic Factors Considered in Selecting Appropriate Therapy for Ventricular Tachycardia

Morphologic characteristics of the ventricular tachycardia
Inducibility of ventricular tachycardia in the absence of drug therapy
Number of distinct ventricular tachycardia morphologies induced
Hemodynamic tolerance of induced ventricular tachycardia(s)
Comparison of induced and spontaneous ventricular tachycardia morphologies

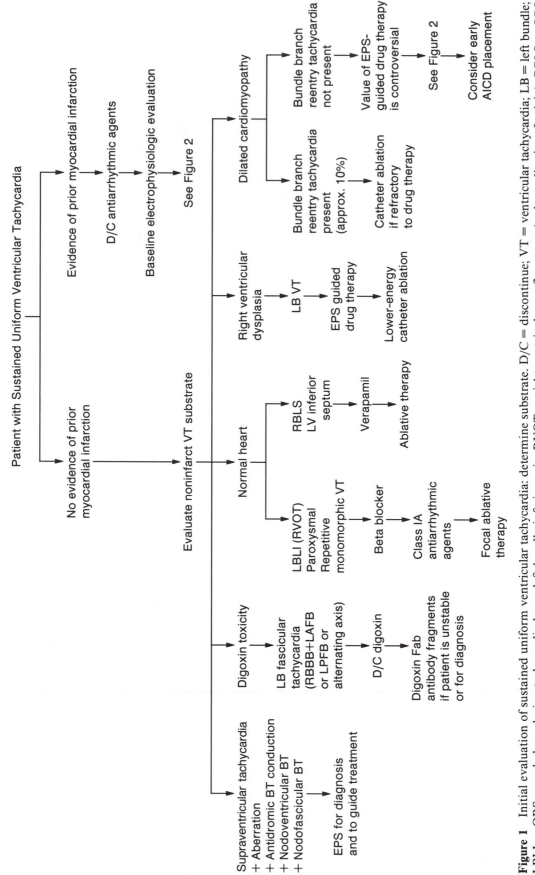

Figure 1 Initial evaluation of sustained uniform ventricular tachycardia: determine substrate. D/C = discontinue; VT = ventricular tachycardia; LB = left bundle; LBLI = QRS morphology during tachycardia has a left bundle inferior axis; RVOT = right ventricular outflow tract (tachycardia site of origin); RBLS = QRS morphology during tachycardia has a right bundle left superior axis; BT = bypass tract; RBBB = right bundle branch block; LAFB = left anterior fascicular block; LV = left ventricle (LV inferior septum is the tachycardia site of origin); LPFB = left posterior fascicular block; EPS = electrophysiology study; AICD = automatic implantable cardioverter defibrillator.

During the initial electrophysiologic study, we attempt to initiate as many distinct ventricular tachycardia morphologies as possible by completing a protocol that includes single, double, and triple premature ventricular extrastimuli delivered at a minimum of two drive cycle lengths, from at least two right ventricular sites and rapid ventricular pacing to a paced cycle length of 250 msec performed from one right ventricular site.

During the baseline evaluation (Fig. 2), if ventricular tachycardia is reproducibly initiated, we administer a procainamide load as a dose of 15 mg per kilogram, at an infusion rate of 50 mg per minute, followed by a 0.11 mg per kilogram per minute infusion to attempt to maintain stable serum pro-

cainamide concentrations. We have found that this method for infusing procainamide reliably results in serum procainamide levels of 6 to 12 mg per deciliter. If the patient has a history of ventricular tachycardia during procainamide treatment or a history of a prior adverse reaction, quinidine can be administered intravenously. We prefer procainamide for this initial study because the intravenous administration of quinidine is frequently limited by hypotension. It appears that prevention of inducibility following intravenous procainamide generally predicts efficacy of procainamide and other class IA agents administered orally.

For patients whose arrhythmias remain inducible on procainamide (approximately 80 percent), we

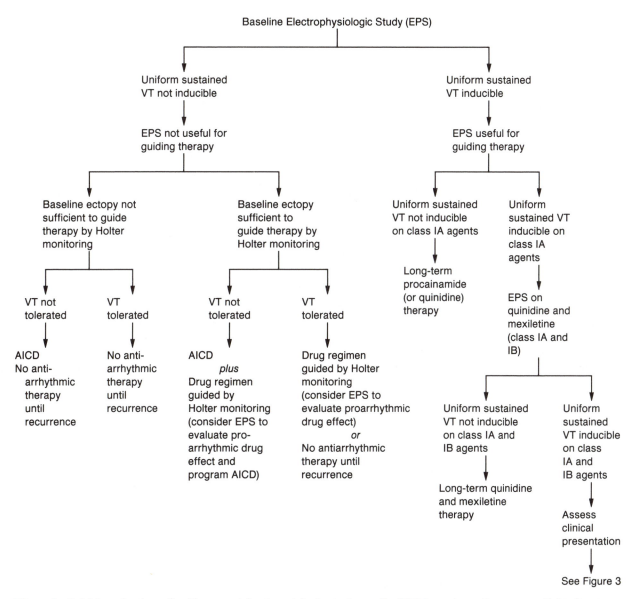

Figure 2 Initial evaluation of uniform sustained ventricular tachycardia (VT) in patient after myocardial infarction. AICD = automatic implantable cardioverter defibrillator.

do not generally try other class IA agents alone because there is less than 10 percent likelihood that another class IA agent will be successful. We therefore usually try a different class IA drug in combination with a class IB drug, usually quinidine and mexiletine. For patients whose arrhythmias continue to be inducible on procainamide and quinidine/mexiletine, decisions regarding therapy become much more difficult (Fig. 3).

The clinical parameters that influence selection among further treatment options are patient tolerance of their tachycardias at presentation, status of left ventricular function, severity of coronary artery disease, frequency of spontaneous recurrent episodes off and on antiarrhythmic medications, and persistence of an inducible poorly tolerated ventricular tachycardia. How well the patient tolerated the ventricular tachycardia at the time of presentation is, in our opinion, one of the most important parameters for guiding therapy. Patients with tachycardias that are well tolerated hemodynamically generally have a good prognosis (they are less likely to die from recurrence of their ventricular tachycardia than patients with tachycardias that are not well tolerated).

For patients with a tolerated uniform sustained ventricular tachycardia, one might consider following the patient clinically as long as no rapid arrhythmias are induced during programmed stimulation. Drug therapy could be adjusted to control frequent recurrences of the tachycardia. Ablative therapy or device therapy (antitachycardia pacing/automatic implantable cardioverter defibrillator combination) would be considered for patients with ventricular tachycardias that are refractory to pharmacologic therapy.

Patients with hemodynamically poorly tolerated ventricular tachycardias need to have all such tachycardias that are initiated during programmed ventricular stimulation rendered noninducible or sufficiently slowed (so that they become tolerated) by pharmacologic or ablative therapy. An automatic cardioverter defibrillator device should be implanted in patients with nontolerated uniform ventricular tachycardia(s) when hemodynamically poorly tolerated ventricular arrhythmias still persist on all drug regimens, unless they are ideal candidates for surgical ablative therapy.

We utilize amiodarone and amiodarone in combination with class IA and/or class IB antiarrhythmic agents for patients with clinical recurrences on the other antiarrhythmic regimens discussed above. Trials of the class IC agents, are reserved for patients with ventricular tachycardia and preserved left ventricular function. Amiodarone alone might be tried in a patient with a depressed ejection fraction and a tolerated ventricular tachycardia that is refractory to other regimens. Although amiodarone rarely prevents arrhythmia induction by programmed ventricular stimulation, it can be effective in preventing clinical ventricular tachycardia recurrence in some patients. Patients with tolerated ventricular tachycardias who have recurrence of their tachyarrhythmia on amiodarone are likely to have a well-tolerated ventricular tachycardia. This is in contrast to patients with ventricular tachycardia that is poorly tolerated hemodynamically. Such patients are at higher risk of recurrence of a nontolerated tachycardia even if found to have only hemodynamically tolerated ventricular tachycardias induced at the time of electrophysiologic study while on amiodarone. We therefore recommend that they consider automatic implantable cardioverter defibrillator placement or ablative therapy, unless no hemodynamically unstable ventricular tachycardia(s) can be induced following a complete stimulation protocol while the patient is on amiodarone therapy (Fig. 4).

ABLATIVE THERAPY

Surgical ablation and catheter ablation of a ventricular tachycardia "site of origin" are the only methods of "curing" a patient with ventricular tachycardia. Surgical ablation involves resecting a subendocardial layer of tissue identified by preoperative and intraoperative endocardial mapping to be the site(s) of origin of the sustained ventricular tachycardia. Cryoablation is used as an adjunct to subendocardial resection when sites of origin cannot be adequately accessed by the latter technique. We recommend map-guided subendocardial resection because 5 to 15 percent of ventricular tachycardias are localized to areas up to 5 cm away from the infarct border zone and would therefore be missed by nondirected subendocardial resection of abnormal regions of visible endocardial scar.

Because intraoperative endocardial mapping is performed while the patient is on normothermic cardiopulmonary bypass, hemodynamic tolerance of the tachycardia is not relevant during this procedure. Therefore patients with nontolerated tachycardias can undergo surgical ablation but not catheter ablation. It is still important to perform preoperative mapping in the electrophysiology laboratory in these patients to identify the site(s) of origin of all the morphologically distinct tachycardias that are hemodynamically tolerated. This is essential because not all ventricular tachycardias can be reproduced in the operating room when the patient is under general anesthesia, on cardiopulmonary bypass, with his or her chest and ventricle opened.

Surgical ablation is successful in eradicating the tachycardia in 70 percent of patients and in changing the tachycardia substrate in an additional 20 percent of patients who survive surgery so that drug therapy that was not helpful preoperatively can be effective postoperatively. However, since the procedure involves a left ventriculotomy, usually through

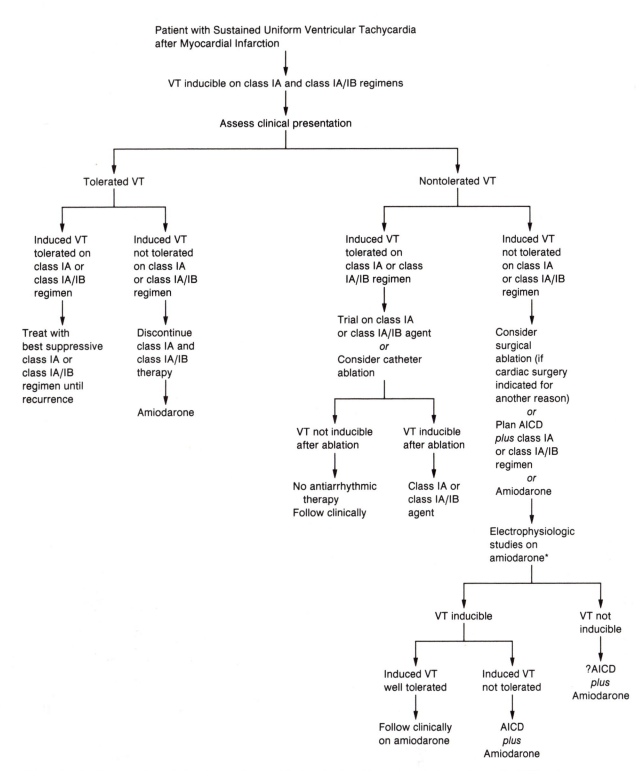

Figure 3 Evaluation of postinfarction patients with sustained uniform ventricular tachycardia (VT) refractory to class IA and class IA/IB therapy. AICD = automatic implantable cardioverter defibrillator.

*Clinical data are controversial regarding the role of electrophysiologic studies in predicting long-term outcome for patients on amiodarone.

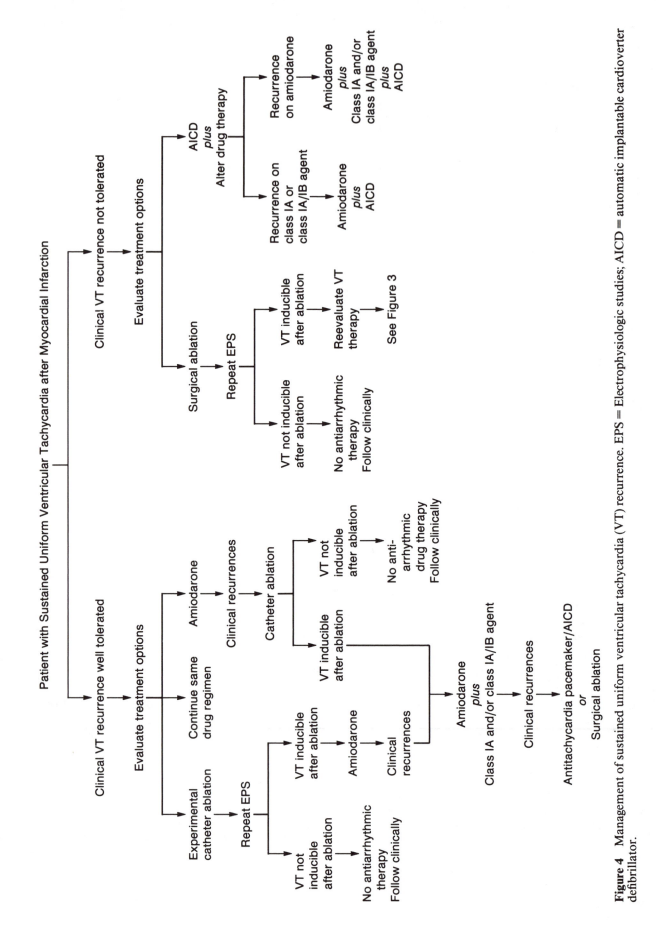

Figure 4 Management of sustained uniform ventricular tachycardia (VT) recurrence. EPS = Electrophysiologic studies; AICD = automatic implantable cardioverter defibrillator.

152

a left ventricular aneurysm, in general only patients with prior myocardial infarctions are good candidates. In addition, the perioperative mortality is high, 10 to 15 percent, making this form of ablative therapy appropriate only for patients who have had recurrent life-threatening uniform ventricular tachycardias or incessant ventricular tachycardias (tolerated or nontolerated) that have been refractory to multiple drug regimens and are not amenable to catheter ablation. Patients with ventricular tachycardia who are undergoing cardiac surgery for another reason should also be considered for surgical ablation if they have had life-threatening arrhythmias that have not been suppressed by antiarrhythmic agents.

Catheter ablation, which is still experimental, is performed in the electrophysiology laboratory following detailed ventricular endocardial catheter mapping during ventricular tachycardia to identify the appropriate site for ablation (the site of earliest local diastolic electrical activity during the ventricular tachycardia). A short-acting general anesthetic is administered before direct current catheter ablation is performed. A direct current discharge of 200 to 300 joules or radiofrequency energy is passed through a catheter positioned at the identified site of origin of the tachycardia. A direct current shock of this magnitude only destroys an area of approximately 1 cm^2 (with a variable depth). Thus, eradicating ventricular tachycardia by this technique is dependent upon precisely identifying a site that results in interruption of a necessary part of the reentrant circuit when it is ablated (see the chapter entitled *Catheter Ablation*).

It is anticipated that this mode of treatment will become the treatment of choice as the initial therapy for many patients with sustained uniform ventricular tachycardia. However, we would anticipate that only 20 to 40 percent of patients with ventricular tachycardias would be candidates for catheter ablation. Patients who are candidates for catheter ablation must have tachycardias that can be reproducibly initiated with programmed ventricular stimulation and well tolerated hemodynamically in order to allow sufficient time for detailed endocardial activation mapping of each ventricular tachycardia morphology. Often patients who initially present with a poorly tolerated tachycardia can have the rate of their ventricular tachycardia slowed sufficiently by antiarrhythmic drug therapy so that the ventricular tachycardia becomes hemodynamically tolerated. Left ventricular mapping studies and ablation can then be performed in these patients. Candidates for catheter ablation also must have no contraindication to placement of a catheter in the left or right ventricle, such as a left ventricular thrombus identified by echocardiography or ventriculography or a history of embolic stroke and left ventricular aneurysm.

Catheter ablation has been shown to be success-

ful in preventing ventricular tachycardia induced by programmed stimulation 40 to 60 percent of the time. Following the first ablation, attempts to reinitiate the ventricular tachycardia by programmed stimulation are performed. If the tachycardia is still inducible or a second morphologically distinct ventricular tachycardia is induced, repeat mapping is done prior to the second ablation attempt. Generally, no more than two or three direct current shocks are delivered during one session.

We have found direct current catheter ablation to be a relatively low-risk procedure. In addition to the risks typically associated with left- and right-sided heart catheterization during electrophysiologic studies, this procedure can be complicated by ventricular rupture at the ablation site or electromechanical dissociation and death. Although we have not seen these as clinical complications, we do maintain formal operating room back-up support for these procedures. Patients need to be made aware of these potentially life-threatening complications. Despite these risks, we feel that catheter ablation may be the treatment of choice for appropriately selected patients.

The efficacy of both surgical and catheter ablation is assessed by observing the patient on telemetry while off all antiarrhythmic medications for 3 to 10 days after the procedure. The patient then undergoes repeat programmed ventricular stimulation. If the tachycardia recurs spontaneously or remains inducible in patients who underwent surgical ablation, drug therapy can be instituted and repeat electrophysiologic studies performed to assess efficacy. The disease of two-thirds of such patients can now be controlled by antiarrhythmic medications that proved ineffective prior to the ablation. Patients who have undergone catheter ablation and who develop spontaneous episodes of ventricular tachycardia or have inducible tachycardia at their follow-up study are offered repeat ablation.

Occasionally a "failed" ablation is associated with an inducible morphologically distinct tachycardia not previously seen, despite the successful ablation of the original tachycardia morphology. Theoretically, this can result from two mechanisms. First, by eradicating the original more easily induced tachycardia, the previously unrecognized tachycardia has been unmasked. Second, the tissue substrate has been altered by the ablation attempt, resulting in the presence of a new morphologic ventricular tachycardia despite successful elimination of the original.

Although published data are lacking for the population that has undergone catheter ablation, in our experience it appears that patients with dilated cardiomyopathies and/or many ventricular tachycardia sites of origin may be less likely to have all such sites successfully treated by catheter ablation alone than patients with ventricular tachycardia and coronary artery disease, a history of myocardial infarction, and one ventricular tachycardia morphology. Similar findings have been described for such patients undergoing surgical ablation.

Patients with ventricular tachycardia occurring in association with other disease substrates may also be candidates for catheter ablation. We have successfully ablated an incessant uniform ventricular tachycardia in a patient with a normal heart. The tachycardia had a right bundle superior axis morphology and originated from the inferior aspect of the left ventricular septum midway from apex to base. Successful ablation has also been reported in patients with right ventricular dysplasia and ventricular tachycardia.

DEVICE IMPLANTATION

Devices available for the management of patients with sustained ventricular tachycardia include antitachycardia pacemakers, automatic implantable cardioverter defibrillators, and devices combining both antitachycardia pacing and back-up cardioverter defibrillator capability. Patients with recurrent ventricular tachycardias that are hemodynamically tolerated are candidates for antitachycardia pacemakers, and patients with nontolerated tachycardias, without frequent recurrences, are candidates for automatic implantable cardioverter defibrillators.

Patients with recurrent, well-tolerated ventricular tachycardia that is refractory to pharmacologic therapy or those who are not good candidates for ablative therapy are candidates for antitachycardia pacing devices. In order for the antitachycardia pacing to be effective, ventricular tachycardias must be reproducibly terminated with pacing techniques. Patients are studied in the electrophysiology laboratory to evaluate which pacing modalities are most effective in reproducibly terminating their tachycardia(s). The antitachycardia pacing device can then be programmed to introduce the most effective stimulation for terminating the tachycardia. The most sophisticated device can deliver multiple extrastimuli or burst pace, adapt to changes in the tachycardia rate, and scan, pacing with decremental intervals until the tachycardia terminates. We also implant automatic implantable cardioverter defibrillators in any patient who will have an antitachycardia pacemaker device functioning in the automatic mode (does not require physician activation of the device) to protect them from the small but finite risk of accelerated, poorly tolerated ventricular tachycardias that may result from attempts to terminate their tolerated ventricular tachycardias (see the chapter entitled *Antitachycardia Pacing*). In the near future, devices will have both antitachycardia and automatic cardioverter defibrillation capabilities.

Implanting an antitachycardia pacemaker is similar to implanting a bradycardia pacemaker. The procedure is usually performed using local anesthesia. The leads are positioned under fluoroscopic guidance. In addition to assessing routine pacemaker functions, i.e., pacing threshold and R-wave amplitude, programmed stimulation is performed. The patient's ventricular tachycardia(s) are initiated several times in order to ensure that the device both recognizes the ventricular tachycardia(s) and is able to terminate the tachycardia by proceeding through its set of preprogrammed stimulation protocols. We generally reevaluate the device function in the electrophysiology laboratory prior to patient discharge.

Patients with poorly tolerated ventricular tachycardias that are not suppressed by medical therapy but do not recur frequently are candidates for automatic implantable cardioverter defibrillator placement. All patients undergo exercise testing and/or cardiac catheterization prior to device implantation, so that if it is necessary, coronary artery bypass surgery can be performed at the same time. Preimplantation electrophysiologic testing is useful in determining the rate cut-off for automatic tachycardia recognition by the cardioverter defibrillator device on the antiarrhythmic regimen thought to suppress the patient's clinical tachycardia best.

The automatic implantable cardioverter defibrillator is implanted in the operating room under general anesthesia via a left thoracotomy, median sternotomy, or subcostal approach. Two patch leads used for energy delivery are placed directly over the epicardium or outside the pericardium, anteriorly and posteriorly. A bipolar rate sensing system that usually consists of two unipolar screw-in leads is placed on the lateral aspect of the left ventricular epicardium. Signal amplitudes, pacing thresholds, and defibrillation and ventricular tachycardia cardioversion thresholds are determined. The leads are repositioned if necessary to ensure a defibrillation threshold that is 15 joules or less (if at all possible). The generator is then connected to the leads and implanted subcutaneously in the left upper quadrant of the abdomen. The effectiveness of the generator in recognizing and terminating ventricular tachycardia and fibrillation is then demonstrated. Device function is assessed prior to discharge in the electrophysiology laboratory. Patients are seen bimonthly for routine assessment of battery life, then monthly as generator replacement time approaches (see chapter entitled *Automatic Implantable Cardioverter Defibrillator*).

The most serious complication associated with placement of automatic implantable cardioverter defibrillators has been infection of the leads or generator pocket, the incidence of which is between 2 and 5 percent. Device discharge in the absence of symptoms occurs in approximately 20 percent of patients and can be distressing. Both serious, rapid, ventricular arrhythmias and supraventricular tachycardias or unsustained ventricular tachycardia have been documented to be the cause. The long-term efficacy of the device in recognizing and defibrillating or cardioverting patients' tachyarrhythmias successfully is higher than 94 percent.

Programmable automatic implantable cardioverter defibrillators that allow postimplantation changes in rate cut-off, the use of probability density function criteria for ventricular tachycardia morphology sensing, alteration of the energy for cardioversion, and increases (decreases) in the delay time (the duration that the tachycardia must be present before the device considers it a sustained arrhythmia) are currently being tested in human subjects. Future automatic implantable cardioverter defibrillators will be smaller, have a longer battery life, and have lead systems placed subcutaneously and/or transvenously. By eliminating the need for a thoracotomy and frequent generator replacements, the morbidity and cost are reduced. This may eventually lead to expanded indications for device implantation.

Combination devices that incorporate both antitachycardia pacing and cardioverter defibrillator capability in one device are also being implanted experimentally in patients and will soon be widely available.

SUGGESTED READING

Gottlieb CD, Berger MD, Miller JM, et al. What is the acceptable risk for cardiac arrest patients treated with amiodarone? Circulation 1988; 78:500.

Herre JM, Sauve MJ, Malone P, et al. Long-term results of amiadarone therapy in patients with recurrent sustained ventricular tachycardia or ventricular fibrillation. J Am Coll Cardiol 1989; 13:442–449.

Marchlinski FE. Ventricular tachycardia associated with coronary artery disease. In: Zipes DP, Rowlands DJ, eds. Progress in cardiology 1/1. Philadelphia: Lea & Febiger, 1988:231.

Marchlinski FE, Flores BJ, Buxton AE, et al. The automatic implantable cardioverter-defibrillator: Efficacy, complications, and device failures. Ann Intern Med 1986; 104:481–488.

Miller JM, Kienzle MG, Harken AH, Josephson ME. Subendocardial resection for ventricular tachycardia: Predictors of surgical success. Circulation 1984; 70:624–631.

VENTRICULAR FLUTTER AND VENTRICULAR FIBRILLATION

ALBERTO INTERIAN, JR., M.D.
ROBERT J. MYERBURG, M.D.

Ventricular flutter or fibrillation is the most common arrhythmia identified in cardiac arrest patients. The number of survivors after out-of-hospital cardiac arrest has increased with expansion of community-based emergency rescue systems and with increasing numbers of lay persons trained in bystander cardiopulmonary resuscitation. However, recurrence of ventricular fibrillation in survivors of cardiac arrest can be as high as 30 percent in the first year. Given this high recurrence rate, we have designed a multilevel approach, adaptable to each patient's individual requirements. This requires evaluation of the patients by highly specialized, trained individuals who focus their efforts on diagnostic and pathophysiologic evaluation and the design of a long-term management plan.

ETIOLOGIES AND CLINICAL SETTINGS

Coronary heart disease is the major culprit, accounting for over 80 percent of the cases of ventricular fibrillation and flutter. Cardiomyopathies, valvular heart disease, and congenital heart disease are the other cardiac disorders that are commonly identified in this population. Primary ventricular fibrillation and flutter in patients without detectable cardiac disease may represent a subclinical disorder that is not observable by present diagnostic modalities, or may be a neural or a hormonally mediated event (Table 1).

GENERAL EVALUATION AND MANAGEMENT

Identifying the etiology and functional status and planning for long-term management of patients who survive ventricular fibrillation or flutter depend largely on central nervous system recovery and identification of factors known to lead to cardiac arrest. Those patients whose central nervous system function is severely impaired or are on maximal cardiovascular support for a failing circulation do not undergo an extensive work-up. Arrhythmias resulting from identifiable reversible causes such as proarrhythmic drug effect or electrolyte imbalances commonly require only correction of the underlying cause rather than extensive patient work-up. In patients whose cardiac arrest was triggered by an acute transmural myocardial infarction, work-up is no different than that for other patients with acute myocardial infarction. However, a more aggressive eval-

Table 1 Etiologies and Clinical Settings of Ventricular Flutter and Ventricular Fibrillation

Coronary artery disease
  With acute myocardial infarction
  Without acute myocardial infarction
Myopathies
  Hypertrophic
    obstructive
    nonobstructive
  Congestive
Valvular heart disease
Myocarditis
Wolff-Parkinson-White syndrome
Congenital heart disease
Functional causes
  Long Q-T syndrome
  Autonomic nervous system
  Metabolic, toxic, electrolyte imbalance
Idiopathic ventricular tachycardia or fibrillation

uation is indicated in the majority of patients with ventricular flutter or fibrillation in whom the underlying cause is coronary heart disease *not* associated with acute transmural myocardial infarction or other cardiac disease that can be managed by medical or surgical intervention.

Procedures employed for diagnoses include cardiac catheterization with angiography and possible biopsy when myocarditis is clinically suspected. Programmed electrical stimulation and noninvasive monitoring serve as the basis for evaluation of susceptibility to life-threatening arrhythmias.

The ultimate care of patients with life-threatening arrhythmias is dictated by the specific etiology and contributing pathophysiologic factors. Optimizing therapy for left ventricular function, control of myocardial ischemia, and general medical management is addressed simultaneously with determination of a specific antiarrhythmic approach.

Invasive Management Techniques

All patients who suffer from ventricular fibrillation or flutter require a definitive evaluation for coronary or reversible structural heart disease. This is best done by cardiac catheterization and left ventricular angiography. When borderline to insignificant coronary artery lesions are found, strong consideration should be given to ergonovine provocation and/or myocardial biopsy in order to rule out the possibility of coronary spasm or myocarditis as the triggering event or substrate for the underlying arrhythmia. Management in these cases would be limited to control of spasm or resolution of the inflammatory process.

Noninvasive diagnostic techniques, such as thallium stress imaging, serve as an estimation of functional significance of coronary lesions and the contribution of stress and catecholamines to arrhythmia

induction. Other noninvasive techniques, such as echocardiography, multigated angiogram, and gallium imaging can serve as adjunct diagnostic modalities in decision-making in these complex patients.

After anatomic and functional cardiac evaluation, electrophysiologic testing using the programmed electrical stimulation technique consisting of up to three extrastimuli at two drive cycles from the right ventricular apex and right ventricular outflow tract is carried out. If this fails to reproduce the clinical event, isoproterenol provocation and/or left ventricular stimulation may be added to the protocol.

Antiischemic Therapy

The indication for medical or surgical antiischemic therapy depends on the anatomy and physiology of the coronary lesions. Although limited data suggest that revascularization by surgery may improve recurrence and total mortality following cardiac arrest, no properly controlled prospective studies have been done. Our indications for surgery are limited to three groups of patients: (1) those who have uncontrolled angina pectoris, significant triple vessel disease, and/or left main coronary disease; (2) those who are candidates for antiarrhythmic surgery (e.g., those with discrete ventricular aneurysms and inducible lethal arrhythmias that are refractory to medical therapy); and (3) those who have clinical and/or electrophysiologic indications that their ventricular fibrillation event was ischemicly mediated. Angioplasty is also used as a means for revascularization in patients felt to have an ischemic trigger with single- or two-vessel disease. There is currently no controlled prospective study documenting the value of angioplasty for this purpose.

Medical antiischemic therapy with beta blockers, calcium channel blockers, nitrates, and antiplatelet agents is an interesting topic. These drugs may be a contributing factor in the better outcome of these patients today compared with data from the early 1970s, which had demonstrated a 30 percent 1-year and a 45 percent 2-year recurrence rate. Without arrest control data, it is difficult to determine whether these drugs are contributing to the improved outcome seen today in this patient population. At our institution, beta blockers are among the more commonly used agents in patients with ventricular fibrillation or flutter not only for their antiischemic effect but for their influence on sympathetic stimulation, which may play an important role in the pathogenesis of potentially lethal arrhythmias. Although current studies support a role for antiischemic agents in only a limited number of patients with ventricular tachycardia/ventricular fibrillation, data suggesting antiischemic therapy for such patients are convincing.

Therapy Directed at Left Ventricular Dysfunction

Decompensated left ventricular function is a known cause of ventricular arrhythmias. In patients with myopathic ventricles, long-term management by preload and afterload reduction and by inotropic agents is routinely used. Angiotensin-converting enzyme inhibitors are our first-line drugs given the benefit of both preload and afterload reduction. These have produced improved survival in patients with myopathic hearts in long-term follow-up. Digitalis and diuretics have been a recent subject of controversy. Data from the Multiple Risk Factor Intervention Trial suggest a higher mortality in the diuretic-treated group. This is felt to be secondary to potassium depletion, supporting other data regarding the relationship between potassium depletion and arrhythmias. Data on the use of digoxin is more clouded, with two studies reporting a higher mortality rate in postmyocardial infarction patients, whereas others concluded that the increased mortality was attributable to differences in patient population. Digitalis and diuretics should be used in patients with ventricular flutter or fibrillation who have marked depressed left ventricular systolic function or require these agents for other specific needs. Periodic monitoring of electrolyte status and digoxin level should be done, with potassium supplementation employed as needed.

Antiarrhythmic Therapy

Using programmed electrical stimulation as a mode of evaluating drug efficacy, serial drug testing is performed after establishing a reproducible sustained ventricular arrhythmia induced in the electrophysiology laboratory. Results from our institution support the use of beta-blocking agents alone, or in combination with other antiarrhythmic agents, as first-line therapy in some patients with ventricular flutter or fibrillation. Data on long-term follow-up using beta blockers as the antiarrhythmic agents in this patient population are unavailable at this time. If isoproterenol is used to evoke arrhythmia inducibility, it is titrated to a 25 percent increase in baseline heart rate. Intravenous propranolol is then administered in 1-mg increments every 2 minutes until adequate beta blockade is achieved or hemodynamic instability limits the further administration of this drug. The programmed electrical stimulation protocol is then repeated. If no significant ventricular arrhythmias are induced (less than 10 consecutive ventricular complexes), the patient is started on oral propranolol and drug dosing is titrated to beta blockade or hemodynamic intolerance, whichever comes first.

When beta blockade fails to control inducibility of ventricular flutter or ventricular fibrillation, a class IA antiarrhythmic agent such as procainamide or quinidine is started orally and titrated to therapeutic levels with careful monitoring of daily electrocardiograms and drug levels. An attempt is made to limit the increase of the QRS complex or Q-T interval prolongation to less than or equal to 25 percent. Patients with atrioventricular conduction delay and bundle branch block, in combination with a low ejection fraction, appear to be at highest risk of proarrhythmic effect and require increased attention. If the ejection fraction is only moderately depressed (greater than 35 percent), class IC agents such as flecainide, encainide, or propafenone or a class III antiarrhythmic such as sotalol is used. Continuous 24-hour monitoring should be carried out while titrating antiarrhythmics in order to observe the patient for early signs of proarrhythmia. Repeat testing is then done on one or combination therapy with these agents. If type I or type III antiarrhythmic failure is demonstrated in the electrophysiology laboratory, intravenous propranolol may be administered again. If this is successful, repeat testing is done on combination oral therapy. Because of its toxicity, amiodarone is currently reserved at our institution for patients with frequently occurring episodes of ventricular flutter or fibrillation that cannot be controlled by any other agent or for patients who have not responded to serial drug testing and who refuse or are not candidates for antiarrhythmic surgery or for an automatic implantable cardioverter defibrillator. When amiodarone is required along with the automatic implantable cardioverter defibrillator for suppression of frequent arrhythmic events, the drug is instituted after defibrillator implantation, given the reported morbidity from acute lung toxicity when implants are done while patients are taking amiodarone.

Management Based on Programmed Electrical Stimulation

This approach has gained popularity in the management of ventricular flutter or fibrillation, having demonstrated encouraging results when used within the limits of our present knowledge. Its use in patients with ventricular flutter or fibrillation is accompanied by problems of standardization related to sensitivity and specificity of pacing protocols and uncertainties about the end point. Combining data from five studies, induction of sustained ventricular tachycardia or fibrillation at baseline study ranged from 31 to 58 percent, and successful suppression of induction ranged from 18 to 78 percent. The mortality rate during follow-up of those patients whose inducibility was suppressed by antiarrhythmic therapy ranged from 0 to 22 percent (mean = 9 percent) when compared with a range of 22 to 78 percent (mean = 43 percent) in those patients who remained inducible. Present data indicate that in at least 40 percent of unselected survivors of cardiac arrest ventricular tachycardia or fibrillation can be induced at a baseline electrophysiologic study. Among those with a discrete ventricular aneurysm, inducibility is higher than 80 percent.

The implication of noninducibility at baseline electrophysiologic testing is controversial. It is the authors' opinion that in those patients in whom a demonstrable structural cause is identified, the use of programmed electrical stimulation is limited.

Although it is generally agreed that programmed electrical stimulation is an invaluable tool for assessing patients with ventricular flutter or fibrillation, like most interventional procedures it is not without complications (Table 2).

Table 2 Complications of Electrophysiologic Testing

Types of Complication	Number	% of Studies
Venous thrombosis	8	0.63
Arterial damage	1	0.08
Significant hemorrhage	1	0.08
Cardiac perforation	6	0.47
Pulmonary embolus	1	0.08
Myocardial infarction	1	0.08
Pneumothorax	0	0.00
Deaths	1	0.08

Number of studies = 1,270. Data from University of Miami, Jackson Memorial Hospital, 7/85–12/89.

Management Stages

Because of the multiple options and different disease states among patients with ventricular flutter or fibrillation, the authors use a stepwise, systematic approach to management. Stage I: Patients whose ventricular flutter or fibrillation was precipitated by an acute transmural myocardial infarction, correctable, noncoronary structural heart disease (e.g., valvular disease), acquired prolonged Q-T syndrome, or reversible causes (e.g., electrolyte abnormality, proarrhythmic drug effect), and those who suffer severe irreversible central nervous system impairment, reach their final management in stage I (Fig. 1). The remaining patients enter management stage II (Fig. 2). Electrophysiologic testing with programmed electrical stimulation is performed unless contraindicated. The subgroup of patients whose ar-

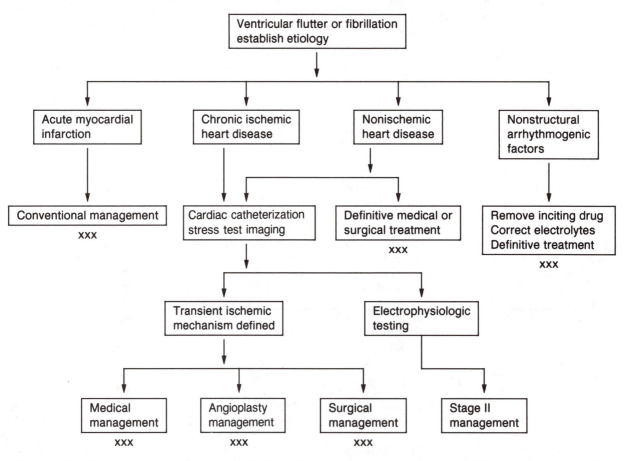

Figure 1 Stage I: Management of ventricular flutter or fibrillation. xxx = end point. (Modified from Myerburg RJ, Kessler KM: Modern Concepts of Cardiovascular Disease 1986; 55:61–66; by permission of the American Heart Association.)

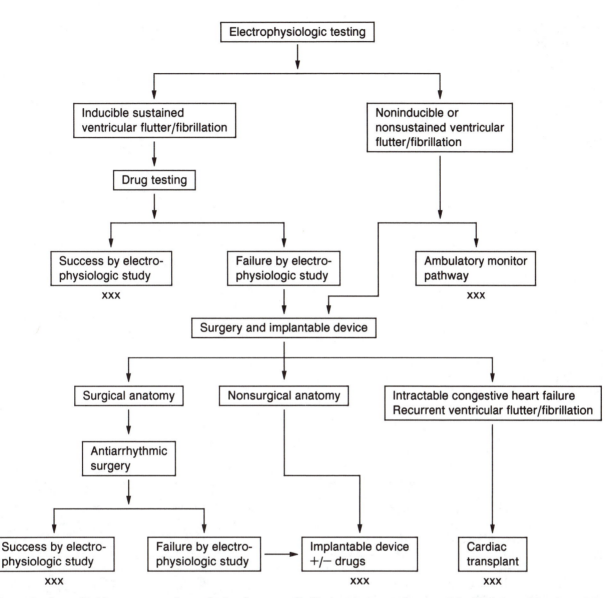

Figure 2 Stage II: Management of ventricular flutter or fibrillation. xxx = end point. (Modified from Myerburg RJ, Kessler KM: Modern Concepts of Cardiovascular Disease 1986; 55:61–66; by permission of the American Heart Association.)

rhythmias are noninducible are referred for automatic implantable cardioverter defibrillator placement, along with coronary bypass surgery if needed. In the group with reproducibly inducible sustained ventricular flutter or fibrillation, serial drug testing is done until noninducibility is attained or a hemodynamically stable ventricular tachycardia is produced that is tolerated by the patient. Once one of these goals is attained, drug serum plasma concentrations should be measured when available and monitored periodically.

Patients whose arrhythmia fails to respond to drug testing are referred for antiarrhythmic surgery if the anatomy is suitable (e.g., significant coronary disease and/or discrete aneurysm), with the place-

ment of defibrillator patches at the time. Implantable devices are recommended for patients with nonsurgical anatomy or who have had unsuccessful surgery for the arrhythmia. Prior to discharge, programmed electrical stimulation is performed on all patients who undergo arrhythmia surgery or receive an automatic implantable cardioverter defibrillator to test the efficacy of the surgical procedure or device in eradicating or terminating the ventricular arrhythmia.

Many patients whose arrhythmias are noninducible at baseline electrophysiologic study or fail to respond to serial drug testing, and patients who are deemed high risk for surgery because of multisystem failure, who have another disease state with a short-term poor prognosis, or who refuse surgery have their therapy guided by ambulatory monitoring rather than electrophysiologic testing. Suppression of complex ventricular ectopy by antiarrhythmic therapy, with concomitant antiischemic therapy, should be employed for such patients.

In the small group of patients with intractable arrhythmias and/or failure to respond to drugs, cardiac transplantation may be the only solution.

Implantable Devices

The emergence of antitachycardia pacemakers and implantable defibrillators has added a new dimension to the management of patients with ventricular flutter or fibrillation. Use of these devices currently has a highly acceptable 1-year sudden death mortality rate of less than 4 percent although total death rates are somewhat higher. The task of finding the appropriate device or combination of devices will become more complex with the advent of fully programmable units with antitachycardia pacing.

Guidelines that we recommend are as follows: Individuals with primary induced ventricular fibrillation refractory to drug therapy are treated with simple nonprogrammable or energy programmable only units. Those with a bradycardic episode of more than 3 seconds following defibrillation have a bipolar VVI pacemaker implanted along with the defibrillator or a defibrillator with bradycardic pacing capability. Finally, those patients with an inducible ventricular tachycardia (on or off antiarrhythmic therapy) that can be reproducibly terminated in the electrophysiology laboratory by a stimulation program have an antitachycardia pacemaker implanted along with a defibrillator or one of the newer generation automatic implantable cardioverter defibrillators with antitachycardia pacing capability. This is done to minimize the number of shocks delivered to the patient, which in turn increases the life of the unit and patient comfort. These devices are very effective automatic interventions but usually require

concurrent antiarrhythmic therapy to limit the number of events.

Psychosocial Management

Patients who have survived cardiac arrest usually have a prolonged traumatic course requiring multiple interventional procedures, which leave these patients in a depressed and psychologically impaired state. To help them overcome their psychological and physical limitations and adapt to the boundaries of their diseased state, these individuals require intense psychological therapy, initially on an individual basis while hospitalized followed by group therapy toward the end of their hospitalization and as outpatients. This support structure should be led by trained psychologists and social workers in this field and appears to be invaluable in helping the patients and their families acclimate to as near a normal lifestyle as possible. In severe cases of depression and psychosis, antidepressive and neuroleptic drugs may be needed and should be administered under the supervision of a trained psychiatrist in conjunction with the clinical cardiologist, given the arrhythmogenic potential of these drugs.

SUGGESTED READING

Josephson ME, Harken AH, Horowitz LN. Endocardial excision: A new surgical technique for the treatment of recurrent ventricular tachycardia. Circulation 1979; 60:1430.

Myerburg RJ, Castellanos A. Cardiac arrest and sudden death. In: Braunwald E, ed. Heart disease: A textbook of cardiovascular medicine. 3rd ed. Philadelphia: WB Saunders, 1988:pp 742–747.

Wellens HJJ, Brugada P, Stevenson WG. Programmed electrical stimulation of the heart in patients with life-threatening ventricular arrhythmias: What is the significance of induced arrhythmias and what is the correct stimulation protocol? Circulation 1985; 72:1–7.

Wilder DJ, Garan H, Finkelstein D, et al. Use of electrophysiologic testing in the prediction of long-term outcome. N Engl J Med 1988; 318:19–24.

PATIENTS AT HIGH RISK OF SUDDEN CARDIAC DEATH

RODOLPHE RUFFY, M.D.

Sudden cardiac death is a common manifestation of heart disease. In most cases it is caused by a cardiac electrical "accident" culminating in ventricular fibrillation. It may be unexpected, as in the case of an apparently healthy individual who develops an immediately fatal myocardial infarction, or it may be the end point of an overt, protracted cardiovascular disorder. A strict definition of sudden cardiac death is difficult to compose because of the uncertainty that often surrounds the occurrence of an unexpected fatality. One can tentatively describe it, however, as death occurring within 1 hour of onset of symptoms in an otherwise clinically stable individual who has known heart disease or in whom a cardiac cause is strongly suspected. Since it is the most common mode of death of adults in Western society, sudden cardiac death has been the focus of much research in a variety of health-related disciplines in an effort to control what can be considered the number one enemy of middle-aged men.

Most patients who die suddenly have underlying coronary artery disease. However, many other cardiac disorders may be the source of a fatal cardio-electrical accident occurring either as an isolated manifestation or as a terminal event taking place in a patient with severely altered cardiovascular status. From a therapeutic point of view, it is evident that because of its cataclysmic and often final nature, sudden cardiac death is better prevented than remedied. Unfortunately, our ability to identify prospective victims of sudden cardiac death is poor. Particularly problematic are the apparently healthy individuals whose first and only manifestation of coronary artery disease is an acute ischemic event immediately followed by ventricular fibrillation. Al-though precise statistics on this kind of occurrence are not available, it is clear that it represents a significant proportion of all cases of sudden cardiac death. Attempts to control this mode of death fall in the realm of primary prevention of coronary atherosclerosis, which is outside the scope of this chapter. The rest of our discussion concentrates on the management of patients who are known or are perceived to be at risk of sudden cardiac death. The most important disorders or situations known to be associated with a measurable risk of sudden cardiac death are shown in Table 1.

SURVIVORS OF OUT-OF-HOSPITAL CARDIAC ARREST

The deployment of trained and well-equipped paramedical and rescue squads has, at least in parts of the Western world, increased the number of survivors of out-of-hospital cardiac arrest. These survivors, particularly those who have obvious structural heart disease, are at high risk of fatal recurrences. Although much emphasis was placed initially on the diagnosis and management of spontaneous or inducible arrhythmias, it became gradually apparent that sudden cardiac death was commonly a consequence of complex interactions involving cardiac electrical function, coronary arterial function, and myocardial mechanical function. As a result, the management of patients at risk of sudden cardiac death, including survivors of out-of-hospital cardiac arrest, must be broad-based and include, in addition to specific antiarrhythmic therapy, meticulous care of myocardial ischemia and optimal control of chronic congestive heart failure.

Cardiac Arrest Occurring in the Midst of Acute Myocardial Infarction

It is important to establish as precisely as possible whether the out-of-hospital cardiac arrest was precipitated by an acute myocardial infarction or not. Several studies have found that ventricular fibrillation occurring as an immediate consequence of an acute myocardial infarction does not, in itself, indicate a poor *long-term* prognosis. These studies, however, have also shown that patients who suffer a cardiac arrest within the first 24 to 48 hours of myocardial infarction have a higher *in-hospital* mortality, mostly from pump failure, than patients who remain electrically stable.

Cardiac Arrest Caused by Acute Myocardial Ischemia

Among patients being evaluated after an out-of-hospital cardiac arrest, a small although important group has been noted to have collapsed as a result of

Table 1 Principal Situations or Conditions Associated with Measurable Increase in Risk of Sudden Cardiac Death in the Adult

Survival from out-of-hospital cardiac arrest
Development of sustained ventricular tachyarrhythmias in the recovery period of myocardial infarction
Survival from large myocardial infarction without symptomatic arrhythmias
Cardiac myopathic disorders—transplant candidacy
Prolonged Q-T interval syndrome
Status after repair of tetralogy of Fallot
Severe valvular disease
Right ventricular dysplasia
Anomalous origin of coronary artery

a severe, reversible ischemic episode. Patients in this category are usually found in ventricular fibrillation after developing classic symptoms of acute myocardial ischemia, or they have collapsed during a bout of anger, fright, or excitement or during vigorous physical exercise. These patients typically have severe coronary artery disease but preserved ventricular function and, when they undergo programmed ventricular stimulation, no arrhythmia is induced. In a few cases coronary disease may be insignificant, but coronary artery spasm can be provoked by ergonovine testing. The proper recognition of this distinct syndrome is essential, since its therapy consists of operative or percutaneous myocardial revascularization or of coronary spasmolysis and not of specific antiarrhythmic therapy. Failure to correct the primary disorder, i.e., coronary arterial dysfunction, is certain to be followed by recurrences of cardiac arrest.

Cardiac Arrest Occurring in the Absence of Acute Myocardial Infarction or Ischemia

Most patients admitted to the hospital after successful reanimation from a cardiac arrest do not show evidence of having sustained an acute myocardial infarction. Some elevation of creatine kinase-MB enzyme is the rule following out-of-hospital collapse and should not be interpreted as indicative of fresh myocardial infarction, unless the enzymatic rise is characteristic of significant myocardial necrosis or is accompanied by electrocardiographic changes typical of evolving myocardial infarction.

Among victims of out-of-hospital cardiac arrest, a small minority have no structural or functional cardiac abnormalities. In such cases, a carefully taken history may reveal the existence of circumstantial factors that may have led to the near-fatal arrhythmic event. The most common factors that we have identified in our own patient population are

Table 2 Circumstantial Factors That May Cause Sudden Arrhythmic Death

Arrhythmogenic effects of medicinal drugs
Arrhythmogenic effects of recreational drugs, most notably cocaine
Profound electrolyte abnormality secondary to factors such as gastrointestinal disorder, starvation diet, endurance race
Extraordinary physical effort in an otherwise unfit individual

listed in Table 2. Removal or avoidance of such precipitating factors is usually sufficient to eliminate the risk of cardiac arrest recurrences on a long-term basis. Rarely, individuals may sustain cardiac arrest in the absence of cardiac abnormality and of precipitating circumstances. These patients must undergo provocative testing in the form of maximal exercise and programmed ventricular stimulation to identify an inducible arrhythmia. If such an arrhythmia cannot be induced, the risk of recurrence is undefined yet probably low. These patients should be considered as candidates for the placement of an automatic, implantable cardioverter defibrillator.

The general decision-making steps we suggest in the management of survivors of out-of-hospital cardiac arrest, according to whether or not they have significant coronary artery disease, are summarized in Figures 1A and 1B.

It was shown several years ago that long-term prognosis is poor in patients who have sustained a cardiac arrest in the presence of structural heart disease, but in the absence of myocardial infarction, the death rate from arrest recurrences is as high as 20 to 30 percent per year. This recognition spurred the development and refinement of several diagnostic and therapeutic interventions aimed at protecting survivors of aborted sudden cardiac death against long-term recurrences. Some of these techniques, listed in Table 3, are quite effective, and it is no

Table 3 Contemporary Approaches to Sudden Cardiac Death

	Diagnostic Method	Therapeutic Intervention
Electrical function	Surface electrocardiography Exercise stress testing Electrophysiologic testing	Antiarrhythmic drugs Beta blockade Implantable devices Surgical ablation Closed chest ablation Remote site defibrillation
Coronary arterial function	Thallium exercise stress testing Thallium dipyridamole testing Coronary angiography	Coronary vasodilation Beta blockade Thrombolysis Percutaneous angioplasty Surgical revascularization
Mechanical function	Echocardiography Radionuclide/dye angiography Endomyocardial biopsy	Preload and afterload reduction Inotropic support Revascularization Immunosuppressive therapy?

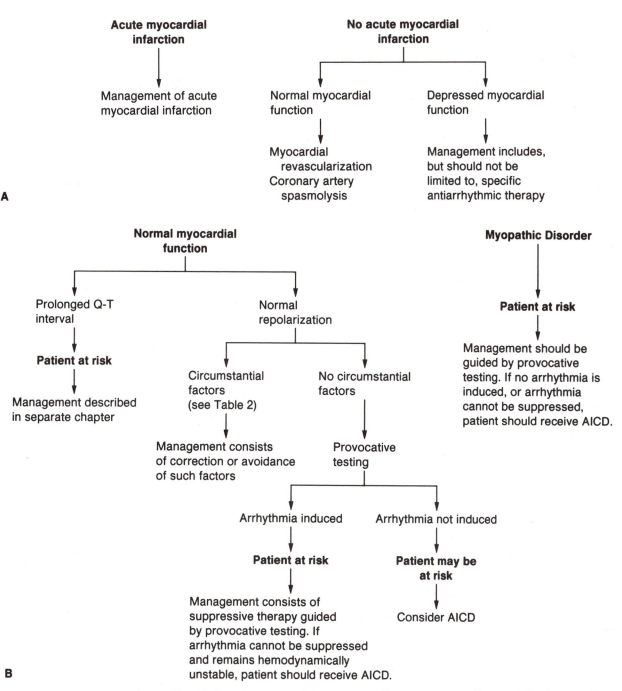

Figure 1 Management of out-of-hospital cardiac arrest. *A,* In presence of coronary artery disease. *B,* In absence of coronary artery disease.

longer appropriate to manage empirically patients who have survived an out-of-hospital cardiac arrest.

Recommended Strategy

As they are recovering from the immediate sequelae of their collapse, survivors of out-of-hospital cardiac arrest should be placed in a cardiac-monitored unit for observation. Unless they suffer from repetitive episodes of sustained ventricular tachyarrhythmias, antiarrhythmic therapy should be initially withheld. Because of the multiplicity of disorders that may underlie the occurrence of life-threatening ventricular electrical instability, it is essential to establish the nature of the patient's heart disease as precisely as possible. Diagnostic tests that are essential or useful in the characterization of patients who have survived an out-of-hospital cardiac arrest are listed in Table 4. Most if not all of the necessary information can be acquired from a detailed history (including interview of relatives and witnesses of the episode), a thorough physical examination, a 12-lead electrocardiogram, an exercise stress test, continuous cardiac monitoring, contrast angiography, and electrophysiologic testing.

Our recommended strategy for the management

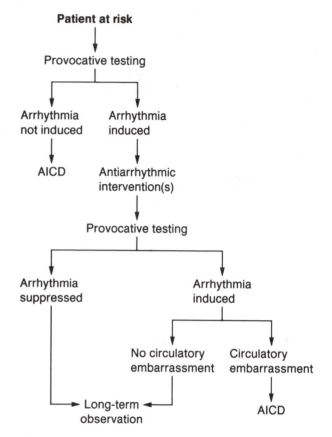

Figure 2 Recommended general strategy for the management of patients at risk for sudden arrhythmic death.

Table 4 Use of Diagnostic Tests in the Evaluation of Patients at Risk of Sudden Cardiac Death

Test	Information Contributed
Essential	
12-Lead electrocardiogram	Old or evolving myocardial infarction
	Repolarization abnormality
	Cardiac chamber enlargement
	Conduction abnormality
	Ventricular preexcitation
Exercise stress testing	Exercise-induced ischemia
	Exercise-induced arrhythmia
	Exercise-related Q-T interval prolongation
24-Hour ambulatory ECG	Qualitative/quantitative analysis of ambient arrhythmia
Cardiac ultrasonography	Segmental/diffuse ventricular dysfunction—left ventricular aneurysm
	Concentric segmental left ventricular hypertrophy
	Valvular dysfunction
	Right ventricular dysplasia
Contrast angiography	Presence/distribution of coronary artery disease—anomalous anatomy
	Segmental/global ventricular dysfunction
	Left ventricular aneurysm
	Right ventricular dysplasia
Electrophysiologic testing	Inducibility of sustained ventricular tachyarrhythmia
	Atrioventricular transmission abnormalities
	Inducibility of sustained supraventricular tachyarrhythmias
	Sinoatrial dysfunction
Complementary	
Radionuclide angiography	Ventricular dysfunction
	Left ventricular aneurysm
	Atrioventricular valve insufficiency
ECG signal averaging	Depolarization abnormality
Endomyocardial biopsy	Acute myocarditis
	Other reversible myopathic disorders

of survivors of near-fatal ventricular tachyarrhythmias perceived to be at risk of long-term recurrences is described in Figure 2. Provocative testing of tachyarrhythmias generally consists of physical exercise or programmed ventricular stimulation. The choice of the most appropriate test depends, of course, on the type of patient studied. In general, programmed ventricular stimulation is a more reliable and reproducible provocative test. However, in patients without coronary artery disease whose clinical event occurred during intense physical exercise or emotional stress, exercise stress testing may be a useful diagnostic end point. Studies are currently under way to compare invasive programmed ventricular stimulation with 24-hour ambulatory electrocardiographic monitoring as diagnostic end points in the management of patients with serious ventricular tachyarrhythmias. Until the results of these studies become available, our bias is in favor of electrophysiologic testing, which, in our judgment, provides a more rigorous representation of the patient's cardiac electrical status before and during or after antiarrhythmic interventions.

PATIENTS DEVELOPING SUSTAINED SYMPTOMATIC VENTRICULAR TACHYARRHYTHMIAS IN THE RECOVERY PHASE OF ACUTE MYOCARDIAL INFARCTION

Among patients recovering from acute myocardial infarction, those who develop spontaneous episodes of sustained ventricular tachyarrhythmias have a particularly poor prognosis and are at very high risk of sudden arrhythmic death. These patients, who often have large anterior infarctions with aneurysms in formation, must undergo early, aggressive diagnostic evaluation and therapeutic planning. We and others have found that survival can be substantially improved in this particular subset of patients if they can undergo surgical therapy. The best results appear more likely if the operation can be delayed until 3 to 4 weeks after myocardial infarction. Meanwhile, these patients may require intensive hemodynamic support and antiarrhythmic protection, including intraaortic balloon counterpulsation and intravenous amiodarone. Although intraoperative mapping has been advocated by some, we have found that the operative and long-term survival of these patients seems more dependent on an expeditious operation consisting of aneurysmectomy, subendocardial resection of additional infarcted tissue, limited endocardial encircling ventriculotomy, and complete revascularization. The epicardial electrodes of the automatic implantable cardioverter defibrillator are implanted at the same time, but implant of the pulse generator is not performed unless sustained ventricular tachyarrhythmias remain inducible during postoperative electrophysiologic testing.

USE OF SPECIFIC ANTIARRHYTHMIC MODALITIES

After the patient's cardiac disorder has been carefully characterized and he or she is perceived to be at risk of recurrences, protective antiarrhythmic efforts should be undertaken. Contemporary antiarrhythmic options include drug therapy, automatic device implantation, and surgical or closed chest ablation. These options, all of which are discussed in separate chapters of this book, are not mutually exclusive and must often be combined to offer the highest level of protection.

Drug Therapy

Prevention of sudden cardiac death by pharmacologic methods on a long-term basis is limited by the propensity for cardiac disease to change its characteristics and evolve with time. Hence, a drug predicted successful by provocative testing may eventually fail because of evolution of the underlying disease process. This is not to say that antiarrhythmic drugs have lost their place in the management of patients at risk of sudden cardiac death. Long-term success of antiarrhythmic drug therapy is more likely in patients whose mechanical and coronary arterial functions are not gravely compromised. Furthermore, a favorable long-term survival can be achieved not only when pharmacologic therapy suppresses inducibility of arrhythmias but also when it is capable of transforming a hemodynamically unstable arrhythmia into one that is well tolerated. The use of antiarrhythmic drugs demands careful titration of doses under continuous in-hospital monitoring and according to the pharmacologic characteristics of each agent chosen. This requires thorough familiarity on the part of the prescribing physician with the pharmacologic properties of antiarrhythmic drugs and with their expected therapeutic effects and adverse effects. In the balance, no drug can be put forth as being a superior agent, although amiodarone has received the most enthusiastic reports from the standpoint of efficacy.

The Automatic Implantable Cardioverter Defibrillator

The development of the automatic implantable cardioverter defibrillator (AICD) represents the single most important therapeutic advance in the treatment of recurrent out-of-hospital cardiac arrest. From the largest series of patients published thus far and from our own experience, the 3-year mortality from sudden cardiac death has been reduced to less than 5 percent in patients wearing AICDs. Because this form of therapy has its own liabilities—morbidity and toxicity—its discriminate utilization remains critical (see the chapter *Automatic Implantable Cardioverter Defibrillator*). We generally prescribe the AICD to three distinct categories of patients: (1) those at risk of sudden cardiac death whose arrhythmia cannot be provoked under controlled conditions; (2) those whose inducible tachyarrhythmia remains hemodynamically unstable despite vigorous surgical or pharmacologic antiarrhythmic efforts; and (3) those who are intolerant of drug therapy and whose arrhythmia cannot be eradicated by surgical methods.

Surgical Therapy

As a result of elegant experimental and clinical studies, the surgical treatment of tachyarrhythmias has made great progress in the last decade. Both "blind" surgical interventions and operations guided by intraoperative mapping techniques have been applied successfully in patients suffering from life-threatening ventricular tachyarrhythmias secondary to coronary artery disease. As discussed earlier, we consider as prime candidates for surgical management patients who develop recurrent sustained ventricular tachycardia in the recovery phase of myocardial infarction. In the chronic phase of coronary artery disease, the best results are achieved in patients who have anterior aneurysms and a single morphologic type of tachycardia.

Closed Chest Ablation of Ventricular Tachycardia

Delivery of high energy direct current shocks or of radiofrequency energy through a catheter placed percutaneously inside a cardiac chamber is capable, in selected cases, of destroying myocardial tissues responsible for the appearance or the sustenance of tachyarrhythmias. Results in patients with life-threatening ventricular arrhythmias have been mixed. At this time, closed chest ablation of ventricular arrhythmias plays only a small role in the management of patients at risk of sudden cardiac death. It should be considered only after more traditional therapeutic modalities have failed and should be viewed as palliative and unlikely to succeed on a long-term basis as a single therapy.

SURVIVORS OF ACUTE MYOCARDIAL INFARCTION WITHOUT SYMPTOMATIC ARRHYTHMIAS AT RISK OF SUDDEN CARDIAC DEATH

Among patients who have sustained a myocardial infarction, a subgroup without symptomatic arrhythmias can be identified which, on a long-term basis, is at increased risk of cardiac death, sudden and nonsudden. These patients have sustained large myocardial infarctions and have depressed left ventricular function. The risk of death becomes measurably increased when the left ventricular ejection fraction is less than 40 percent. The coexistence of depressed left ventricular function and complex ventricular arrhythmias, particularly unsustained ventricular tachycardia, is associated with a first-year postinfarction mortality as high as 25 percent. Several risk stratification schemes have been studied in an effort to increase our ability to identify patients at the highest risk of sudden cardiac death after myocardial infarction. The noninvasive index, which in early reports appears to be the most discriminate, combines a signal-averaged electrocardiogram, a radionuclide left ventricular ejection fraction, and a 24-hour ambulatory electrocardiogram. In a study of 102 patients, 8 of 16 (50 percent) patients who had a left ventricular ejection fraction less than 40 percent, 10 or more ventricular premature complexes per hour, and the presence of late QRS potential (in the signal-averaged electrocardiogram) had major ar-

rhythmic events within a few weeks after myocardial infarction. Conversely, none of the nine patients who had a preserved ejection fraction, less than 10 ventricular premature complexes per hour, and a normal signal-averaged electrocardiogram had an arrhythmic event during the first year of follow-up.

Some have proposed invasive programmed ventricular stimulation to induce sustained ventricular tachyarrhythmias as a risk-stratifying method in the recovery phase of myocardial infarction. Results thus far are controversial. Although programmed ventricular stimulation appears to have a good negative predictive value, its low specificity, high cost, and invasive nature make its widespread application unjustifiable for the time being.

The issue of post–myocardial infarction stratification is further complicated by the evolutionary nature of the disease process, which makes it difficult to judge the optimal timing of diagnostic testing. Moreover, once the patient is thought to be at risk, we are currently ill-equipped to offer preventive therapy. The first properly designed, large-scale attempt to study the effects of prophylactic antiarrhythmic drug therapy after myocardial infarction was recently shattered by the finding of an increased mortality in the groups of patients receiving the two drugs found most effective in suppressing ambient ventricular ectopic activity in comparison with placebo. Although this may be a drug-specific phenomenon, it will be a long time, if ever, before an antiarrhythmic drug can be declared safe and effective in the prevention of sudden cardiac death in otherwise asymptomatic, high-risk post–myocardial infarction patients. Although in a few particular cases the implant of an AICD may be appropriate, extension of this practice to all high-risk post–myocardial infarction patients on a prophylactic basis is unjustifiable until the device has become easily implantable without performing a thoracotomy.

Therefore at present the identification of patients at high risk of sudden cardiac death after myocardial infarction remains a frustrating diagnostic exercise with little therapeutic return. Meticulous care of myocardial dysfunction and residual ischemic manifestations, including, whenever possible, beta blockade, appear to be maneuvers as important as any specific antiarrhythmic intervention. Since most major arrhythmic events tend to occur within the first few months after infarction, confinement of the patient to a protected environment, including relatives trained in cardiopulmonary resuscitation and in the use of an automatic external defibrillator, may be an appropriate option in selected cases.

SUGGESTED READING

Bigger JT, Fleiss JL, Rolnitzky LM. Multicenter post-infarction research group: Prevalence, characteristics and significance of ventricular tachycardia detected by 24-hour continuous electrocardiographic recordings in the late hospital phase of acute myocardial infarction. Am J Cardiol 1986; 58:1151–1160.

Gomes JA, Winters SL, Stewart D, et al. A new noninvasive index to predict sustained ventricular tachycardia and sudden death in the first year after myocardial infarction: Based on signal-averaged electrocardiogram, radionuclide ejection fraction and Holter monitoring. J Am Coll Cardiol, 1987; 349–357.

Waller TJ, Kay HR, Spielman SR, et al. Reduction in sudden death and total mortality by antiarrhythmic therapy evaluated by electrophysiologic drug testing: Criteria of efficacy in patients with sustained ventricular tachyarrhythmia. J Am Coll Cardiol 1987; 83–89.

Winkle RA, Mead RH, Ruder MA, et al. Long-term outcome with the automatic implantable cardioverter-defibrillator. J Am Coll Cardiol 1989; 1353–1361.

Zee-Cheng CS, Kouchoukos NT, Connors JP, Ruffy R. Treatment of life-threatening ventricular arrhythmias with non-guided surgery supported by electrophysiologic testing and drug therapy. J Am Coll Cardiol 1989; 153–162.

TORSADES DE POINTES AND MULTIFORM VENTRICULAR TACHYCARDIA

CHARLES D. GOTTLIEB, M.D.

In a recent North American Society of Pacing and Electrophysiology policy statement, polymorphic ventricular tachycardia has been defined as a "ventricular tachycardia with an unstable (continuously varying) QRS complex morphology in any recorded ECG lead." This all-encompassing definition results in the grouping of at least several distinct clinical entities whose etiology, arrhythmogenic substrate, and response to specific interventions may vary dramatically. To distinguish among the various forms of polymorphic ventricular tachycardia is therefore important not only to understand their underlying mechanisms better but also to effect appropriate therapy.

In 1966, Dessertenne first described a distinctive form of polymorphic ventricular tachycardia occurring in a patient with complete heart block which he termed "torsades de pointes." Although the features necessary and sufficient to diagnose torsades de pointes remain controversial, the following characteristics are generally present: (1) The surface electrocardiogram demonstrates basic variation in the electrical polarity of the QRS complex such that the QRS complexes appear to be twisting around an isoelectric baseline (Fig. 1). Frequently it is necessary to obtain simultaneous recordings from several electrocardiographic leads to observe this phenomenon because the arrhythmia may periodically appear relatively monomorphic in any single lead. (2) The rate of the ventricular tachycardia can range from 150 to 280 bpm with an average rate between 200 and 240 bpm. Variations in the R-R interval between successive complexes are frequently observed. (3) Spontaneous terminations are common. (4) There is occa-

sional progression of this arrhythmia to a sustained ventricular tachyarrhythmia that often degenerates into ventricular fibrillation and therefore can result in sudden cardiac death.

The requirement of surface electrocardiographic abnormalities of repolarization—i.e., Q-T or Q-TU prolongation—for diagnosis of torsades de pointes remains controversial. Like the arrhythmia itself, the Q-T interval prolongation may be intermittent and in some patients seen only in relationship to a particular stress. The stress may be emotional or exertional, as in the case of the congenital long Q-T syndromes or following compensatory pauses due to ventricular ectopy in the patient with bradycardia-associated or "pause-dependent" long Q-T syndrome. Because of the variability of the Q-T (or Q-TU) interval and frequent absence of documentation of the classic electrocardiographic features of torsades de pointes, it is important to utilize a constellation of clinical and electrocardiographic findings for recognition of the underlying etiology and

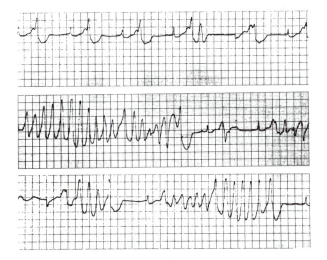

Figure 1 A polymorphic ventricular tachycardia with typical morphologic characteristics of torsades de pointes.

the clinical implications of this unique rhythm disturbance. Nevertheless, the identification of Q-T interval prolongation in the presence of polymorphic ventricular tachycardia generally provides a basis for the institution of appropriate therapeutic measures.

DETERMINATION OF THE Q-T INTERVAL

The Q-T interval should be an indicator of the time from earliest ventricular myocardial activation to its latest repolarization. However, total repolarization may be underestimated by the Q-T interval as small areas of delayed ventricular depolarization, and repolarization may not be observed on the surface electrocardiogram. Additionally, prolonged depolarization can result in Q-T interval prolongation in the absence of repolarization abnormalities. Despite these limitations and the inherent inaccuracy and nonreproducibility of the Q-T interval measurement, the Q-T and Q-Tc intervals can provide for identification of prolonged repolarization. The normal response for the Q-T interval is to shorten as heart rate increases, and therefore several mathematical relationships have been employed to normalize the Q-T interval for heart rate. A common formula proposed by Bazett results in a corrected Q-T (QTc) interval defined as the Q-T interval divided by the square root of the preceding R-R interval. Lepeschkin proposed upper limits for the Q-Tc interval as 0.39 sec for men and 0.41 sec for women. Many investigators utilize a value of 0.44 sec as the upper limit of normal value for both sexes. However, at rapid heart rates, the Q-T interval does not remain constant. The value for the square root of the R-R interval changes to a greater extent than does the Q-T interval itself. Therefore, the Q-Tc determination is not constant at rapid heart rates. An additional technical problem with Q-T interval determination is the frequent presence of U waves, particularly in patients who have experienced torsades de pointes. The etiology of this slow wave remains poorly defined. U waves may represent the result of afterdepolarizations. From a mechanistic point of view, this hypothesis is interesting and may explain many of the phenomena associated with the long Q-T syndromes.

CONDITIONS ASSOCIATED WITH Q-T PROLONGATION AND TORSADES DE POINTES

Polymorphic ventricular tachycardia with characteristics strongly suggestive of torsades de pointes has been observed in association with a host of clinical syndromes producing Q-T prolongation. An incomplete list of potential causes of Q-T interval prolongation that may result in torsades de pointes is

provided in Table 1. The classic approach to this disorder has been to classify patients based on whether the abnormalities of repolarization were acquired or congenital. Based on several clinical and electrocardiographic observations, Jackman has proposed that the long Q-T syndromes be divided primarily on the basis of whether the arrhythmia is "pause-dependent" or "adrenergic-dependent." Tachycardia initiation in patients with drug-facilitated QT prolongation, electrolyte imbalance, and dietary deficiencies is frequently preceded by a pause. Moreover, interventions that produce acceleration of the heart rate and prevention of pauses often result in control of this disorder.

Alternatively, several lines of evidence have implicated a significant role of the autonomic nervous system in the genesis of torsades de pointes, particularly in association with the congenital syndromes. Stressful events that result in enhanced sympathetic activity often trigger the arrhythmia in susceptible individuals. Furthermore, prevention of arrhythmia recurrence can be achieved by beta-blocking agents and/or unilateral left cervicothoracic sympathetic ganglionectomy. Central nervous system events and alteration of sympathetic tone can result in marked

Table 1 Conditions Associated with Q-T Interval Prolongation That May Result in Torsades de Pointes

1. Drugs and toxins
   Antiarrhythmic agents (see Table 2)
   Psychotropics
     Phenothiazines, tricyclics, tetracyclics
   Antibiotics
     Erythromycin, pentamidine,
     trimethoprim-sulfamethoxazole
   Vasodilators
     Prenylamine, lidoflazine, indoran
   Organophosphate insecticides
2. Electrolyte imbalance
   Hypokalemia, hypomagnesemia, ? hypocalcemia
3. Hormone-related
   Hypothyroidism, vasopressin
4. Severe bradycardia
   Sinus node dysfunction
   Conduction system disease
5. Starvation diets
   Liquid protein diet
6. Cardiac diseases
   Myocarditis
   Ischemia
   Mitral valve prolapse ?
7. Central nervous system disorders
   Subarachnoid hemorrhage
   Cerebral vascular occlusion
   Central nervous system tumors
   Intracranial trauma
   Central nervous system infections
8. Congenital syndromes
   Jervell and Lange-Nielsen syndrome
   Romano-Ward syndrome
   Sporadic
9. Autonomic imbalance or manipulation

abnormalities of the T wave and the Q-T interval. Additionally, pathologic evaluation has suggested the existence of a focal neuritis in the sinus node and the conduction tissue in some patients with a congenital form of this disorder. Thus, despite the fact that any individual patient may exhibit characteristics of both (or neither) pause and adrenergic-dependent long Q-T syndrome, this classification permits identification, allows for a rationale for therapy, and may provide an understanding of the underlying arrhythmogenic mechanisms.

PAUSE-DEPENDENT TORSADES DE POINTES

Despite the fact that antiarrhythmic agents may confer their clinical efficacy by causing prolongation of refractoriness, they also are the most common causes of torsades de pointes. Virtually every antiarrhythmic agent that prolongs refractoriness has been implicated as a cause of this arrhythmia (Table 2). Quinidine was the first antiarrhythmic agent known to be associated with the development of torsades de pointes and has been the most extensively evaluated. The reported incidence of quinidine-associated torsades de pointes ranges from 0.5 to 10 percent, with the most reasonable estimate being 2 percent from several large series. There appears to be an association between the baseline Q-T interval and the development of this ventricular arrhythmia. Individuals whose baseline Q-T interval approaches the upper limit of normal may be at an increased risk for the development of arrhythmia. There does not appear to be a dose-dependent relationship between drug level and development or frequency of torsades de pointes. In fact, quinidine levels are frequently found to be low or in the low normal range at the time of arrhythmia occurrence. This is not surprising, as in this setting torsades de pointes generally occurs soon after the institution of quinidine therapy. Approximately half of the patients who experience this arrhythmia do so within

the first several days to 1 week of therapy. In the remainder of patients, torsades de pointes may occur after taking quinidine, without complication, for weeks to years. In this latter circumstance, changes in quinidine dosage or preparation, discontinuation and reinstitution of therapy, and the administration of other medications have been implicated as the cause for arrhythmia precipitation.

Quinidine, like all class IA antiarrhythmia agents, is associated with prolongation of the Q-T interval. The T waves become wide, rounded, and low in amplitude. These changes may be most pronounced in the middle to lateral precordial leads. Additionally, prominent U waves may be seen that become part of and potentially obscure the termination of the T wave. Unfortunately, the Q-T interval itself is neither sensitive nor specific for predicting the occurrence of torsades de pointes. Attempts have been made to utilize a value of 0.60 sec for the uncorrected Q-T interval as a discriminator for future development of ventricular arrhythmias. Approximately half of the patients who develop torsades de pointes have a Q-T interval of less than this value. Additionally, there may only be minimal Q-T prolongation prior to the first episode of this arrhythmia. Recently, Kadish has described a significant difference in the response of the Q-Tc interval to exercise in patients who have had torsades de pointes after the administration of a class IA agent compared with a control population. A paradoxical increase in the Q-T interval was observed during exercise in patients who had suffered a spontaneous arrhythmic event. If this relationship is prospectively confirmed, exercise-induced prolongation of refractoriness may be a potential basis for the screening of patients considered to be at risk for the development of torsades de pointes.

It has often been suggested that T-wave morphology is more important than the actual Q-T interval in determining patients at risk for torsades de pointes. Development of an accentuated U wave or a bizarre T-U complex following a pause may be a

Table 2 Antiarrhythmic Drugs Causing Torsades de Pointes

Antiarrhythmic Classification	Electrophysiologic Effects	Antiarrhythmic Agents Implicated in Causing Torsades de Pointes
Class 1A	Moderate prolongation of refractoriness Moderate depression of conduction	Quinidine Procainamide Disopyramide
Class 1B	No or minimal prolongation of refractoriness Some depression of conduction, particularly in abnormal myocardium	Torsades de pointes not clearly demonstrated
Class 1C	Minimal prolongation of refractoriness Significant depression of conduction	Ventricular arrhythmias but torsades de pointes not clearly demonstrated
Class II	Beta-adrenergic antagonists	Only documented for sotalol (has class III properties)
Class III	Selective prolongation of refractoriness	Amiodarone (has class I and II effects) Sotalol
Class IV	Calcium-channel blocking agents	Only documented for bepridil (has class III properties)

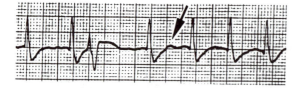

Figure 2 The postpause accentuation of repolarization abnormalities in a patient receiving amiodarone for atrial fibrillation. This patient subsequently developed torsades de pointes.

marker for the development of torsades de pointes (Figs. 2 and 3). Not only can sudden cardiac deceleration or a pause produce T and U wave abnormalities in patients with metabolic-related torsades de pointes, but a pause is invariably seen prior to the initiation of the ventricular tachyarrhythmia in this syndrome. The ventricular complex that follows the pause and results in tachycardia initiation produces a long cycle–short cycle sequence, and the pause itself is often the result of a prior ventricular premature complex. Thus, a short cycle–long cycle–short cycle sequence ensues, as shown in Fig. 4. The short interval that occurs as a consequence of the first complex has been termed the "pre-initiating" cycle by Roden. The pause that follows or the "initiating" cycle may provide the appropriate milieu for the generation of afterdepolarizations.

Early afterdepolarizations may explain several features of pause-dependent prolonged Q-T syndrome, including the development of the accentuated T-U complex following a pause, the dependency of a pause preceding the initiation of the tachyarrhythmia, the association of this arrhythmia with bradycardia, and finally a rationale for the response to specific therapeutic interventions. Early afterdepolarizations are interruptions of repolarization generally occurring at the time of the T wave during phase III of the action potential. They may terminate by returning the cell to resting membrane potential or result in one or more action potentials.

Characteristic of early depolarizations are their occurrence at slow heart rates or following long pauses. Additionally, with longer pauses, repetitive activity is more likely to ensue. Therefore, measures that increase the heart rate and prevent pauses such as ventricular pacing (often considered the primary modality of therapy) would be expected to be efficacious on this basis.

Cranfield and Aronson extended Roden's observations and suggested that not only does the first tachycardia complex potentially result from an early afterdepolarization but the premature complex that produces the pre-initiating cycle, and therefore the pause, may in and of itself have been the result of an early afterdepolarization. Perhaps it is for this reason that frequent ventricular ectopy and more specifically bigeminy may be warning signs of an impending event. However, the mechanism of this arrhythmia is far from completely understood. It is certainly possible that some other mechanism, more specifically reentry or the spontaneous depolarization of multiple automatic foci, could produce this rhythm disorder. Of note is the observation that initiation by programmed electrical stimulation (the hallmark of the reentrant arrhythmias) is not observed with any significant frequency in this disorder. However, this does not exclude the possibility of a reentrant mechanism in the maintenance of this arrhythmia after its initiation.

FACTORS PREDISPOSING TO TORSADES DE POINTES

Whether specific heart diseases or rhythm disturbances provide a predisposition for the generation of drug-associated torsades de pointes is unclear. It is not surprising that atrial fibrillation has frequently provided an appropriate milieu for this ventricular arrhythmia. Rapid changes in R-R intervals would allow for potential long cycle–short cycle sequences that are seen prior to the initiation of torsades de pointes of the pause-dependent variety. Termination of atrial fibrillation is often associated with a pause

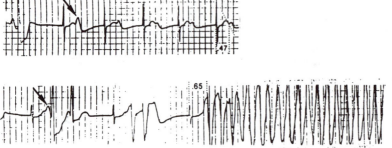

Figure 3 Shown in the upper panel is an example of postpause U-wave accentuation (*arrow*). This patient had been receiving disopyramide. The Q-T interval extrapolated from the downstroke of the T wave was calculated to be 470 msec. In the lower panel, ventricular tachycardia occurs after a pause that followed two extrasystoles. The first tachycardia complex occurring 650 msec after the last normal QRS complex may have arisen from a large U wave. (Modified from Jackman WM, Friday KJ, Anderson JL, et al. Prog Cardiovasc Dis 1988; 31:115–172, with permission.)

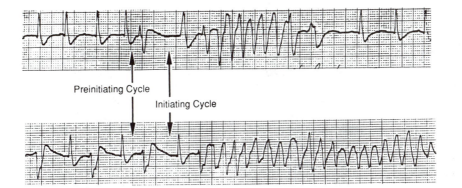

Figure 4 Shown in the upper and lower panel is an example of the short cycle–long cycle–short cycle sequence that may result in the initiation of drug-associated torsades de pointes. The patient was noted to have Q-T interval prolongation after the administration of 800 mg of amiodarone. The pause preceding the tachycardia or the "initiating cycle" is a result of a ventricular extrasystole. This same extrasystole also resulted in a short cycle or pre-initiating cycle. Both the unsustained run of ventricular tachycardia and the sustained episode seen in the lower panel (which ultimately degenerated to ventricular fibrillation) were initiated by an extrasystole following a pause. This apparent short cycle–long cycle–short cycle sequence preceding the onset of drug-associated torsades de pointes is common (see text for discussion).

prior to restoration of sinus rhythm. It has been noted that this is not an infrequent time for the occurrence of torsades de pointes. A correlate to this observation has been that after termination of torsades de pointes, patients who were treated with a class IA agent for atrial fibrillation were frequently noted to be in sinus rhythm. Digoxin is a frequent concomitant medication, particularly in patients with atrial dysrhythmias or left ventricular dysfunction. Therefore questions exist as to its potential contribution to the genesis of torsades de pointes. Generally, no significant evidence for digoxin toxicity or high digoxin levels has been found in these patients. There is also little or no evidence to implicate this cardiac glycoside as a cause of torsades de pointes in the absence of other medication.

Severe depletion of either potassium or magnesium has been associated with torsades de pointes. More important is the mild depletion of these electrolytes as the result of diuretic therapy. Mild depletion of these electrolytes may be the cause of the late occurrence torsades de pointes after the institution of antiarrhythmic therapy in patients who would otherwise have been asymptomatic and on stable doses of medication. Moreover, depressed left ventricular function may even by itself predispose to the development of drug-associated torsades de pointes. Diuretics, being a primary modality of therapy in this disorder, may compound the risk for arrhythmia genesis after institution of antiarrhythmic therapy. Therefore, administration of antiarrhythmic therapy to patients with atrial fibrillation and ventricular

dysfunction, as well as to patients with pretreatment evidence of marginal Q-T interval prolongation, should be performed judiciously. Continuous observation may be warranted in this patient population during the initial administration of antiarrhythmic agents that can result in abnormalities of repolarization.

ADRENERGIC-DEPENDENT LONG Q-T SYNDROME

Adrenergic-dependence is seen primarily in patients with a congenital form of the long Q-T syndrome. These congenital syndromes are associated with intermittent Q-T interval prolongation and ventricular arrhythmias typically first becoming manifest during childhood. The Jervell and Lange-Nielsen syndrome is of autosomal recessive inheritance and is associated with congenital deafness. The Romano-Ward syndrome is not associated with hearing loss and is transmitted in an autosomal dominant pattern. There is also a third form that is often referred to as "sporadic" and is not familial or associated with deafness.

Initiation of torsades de pointes in the adrenergic-dependent population is often produced by a stress that could result in catecholamine release, such as the ringing of an alarm clock, a loud startling noise, or extreme exertion. There is generally no pause seen prior to tachycardia initiation. The Q-T interval is typically only intermittently prolonged but often shows inappropriate shortening with exercise or administration of catecholamines. Programmed electrical stimulation generally fails to reproduce the clinical arrhythmia. Interestingly, however, Jackman has suggested that infusion of catecholamine will produce T-U wave abnormalities that can precipitate or precede paroxysms of torsades de pointes in susceptible patients. Patients with atypical forms of this syndrome have also been noted. These patients may be seen later in life with no family history of syncope or sudden cardiac death. Relatively normal Q-T and Q-Tc intervals are typically observed (Fig. 5).

Mitral valve prolapse appears to be a risk factor for the development of polymorphic ventricular arrhythmias. This may be particularly true for those patients who demonstrate the characteristic inferolateral ST-T wave abnormalities often associated with mitral valve prolapse. These patients may be part of the large spectrum of this disorder. Additionally, there are patients who display features of both pause-dependent and adrenergic-dependent long Q-T syndrome.

Intracranial processes, most notably subarachnoid hemorrhage but also cerebral vascular occlusions, intracranial bleeding, and central nervous system tumors, are associated with the production of marked T-wave abnormalities and infrequently with torsades de pointes. Manipulation of the sympathetic nervous system such as might occur with a radical neck dissection may also produce similar abnormalities of the T and U waves. Therefore, a complete neurologic evaluation is important in the assessment of patients with manifestations of the adrenergic-dependent long Q-T syndrome.

Polymorphic Ventricular Tachycardia in the Absence of Q-T Interval Prolongation

Myocardial infarction and/or ischemia is known to be associated with the generation of polymorphic ventricular tachycardia and ventricular fibrillation.

However, there are patients who exhibit paroxysms of polymorphic ventricular tachyarrhythmia that have features typical of torsades de pointes in the absence of significant Q-T interval prolongation. Frequently, these patients have underlying structural heart disease similar to that seen in patients with sustained monomorphic ventricular tachycardia. The polymorphic ventricular tachycardia observed in these patients can often be reproducibly initiated by programmed electrical stimulation and not infrequently suppressed by class IA antiarrhythmic agents. Conversely, initiation of polymorphic ventricular tachycardia by timed extrastimuli in the long Q-T syndromes is infrequent and not a reproducible event.

Electrocardiographically, the spontaneous arrhythmic episodes also differ from those seen with typical torsades de pointes. There is no dependency on a pause, on bradycardia, or on the pre-initiating cycle for tachycardia occurrence (Fig. 6). Additionally, there appears to be no postextrasystolic accentuation of T or U wave abnormalities.

THERAPY

Pause-Dependent or Acquired Q-T Interval Prolongation

Initial management of patients demonstrating paroxysms of torsades de pointes includes the correction of metabolic abnormalities and elimination of all medication that is typically associated with this arrhythmia. Evaluation of electrolyte abnormalities, particularly hypokalemia and hypomagnesemia, should be performed. Serum potassium level should ideally be raised to at least the 4.5 mEq per liter range. Hospitalization with continuous monitoring is required. Frequently, the paroxysm of torsades de pointes is self-limiting and requires no further intervention. If the patient develops hemodynamically compromising episodes of torsades de pointes or episodes that degenerate into ventricular fibrillation, recurrences are frequent and further intervention is necessary. Torsades de pointes is not in and of itself

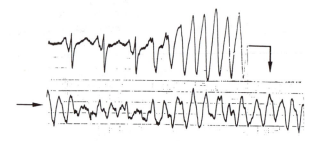

Figure 5 Torsades de pointes occurring in a 60-year-old man with no prior history of myocardial disease or drug administration. In addition, there was no family history of sudden death syndrome. Resting electrocardiograms obtained prior to and after this event revealed normal Q-T and Q-Tc intervals. Note that the onset of this arrhythmia is not associated with a pause (see text for discussion).

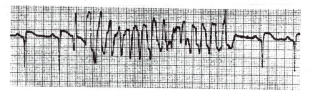

Figure 6 A spontaneous paroxysm of torsades de pointes occurring in a patient with coronary artery disease and a left ventricular aneurysm. A single ventricular depolarization after the second sinus complex initiated a typical paroxysm of torsades de pointes. (Modified from Horowitz LN, Greenspan AM, Spielman SR, et al. Circulation 1981; 63:1120. Reprinted by permission of The American Heart Association.)

a particularly difficult rhythm to terminate with direct current cardioversion if this is required.

Interventions that result in shortening of the Q-T interval generally prevent life-threatening recurrences of this form of torsades de pointes. Institution of pacing or use of isoproterenol to increase the heart rate to between 90 and 110 bpm has been considered the primary form of therapy of this disorder. Both atrial and ventricular pacing have been utilized in an attempt to achieve heart rate acceleration and the prevention of pauses. Maintaining a constant rapid ventricular response may be difficult with atrial pacing because of atrioventricular nodal Wenckebach or higher degrees of atrioventricular block. Although atropine may facilitate conduction through the atrioventricular node, it may also produce higher degrees of block if preexisting conduction abnormalities are present in the His-Purkinje system. Atrial premature complexes could additionally provide short then long cycle initiating sequences that may be a prerequisite for the development of this arrhythmia. Although ventricular pacing has the slight disadvantage of the potential initiation of ventricular tachyarrhythmias on insertion of a right ventricular catheter, once catheter position has been obtained, one is assured of a more stable catheter position, with the ability to increase heart rate and potentially suppress premature ventricular complexes and thereby prevent tachycardia initiation.

Isoproterenol generally results in shortening of the Q-T interval and suppression of recurrent episodes of torsades de pointes. Unfortunately, catecholamine infusion is not without a certain degree of risk in patients with coronary artery disease.

Magnesium sulfate has been utilized in doses of 1 to 2 g given intravenously over a few minutes, followed by the continuous infusion of 3 to 20 mg per minute if pacing is ineffective. Lidocaine and phenytoin have additionally been utilized with some success in the acute management of drug-associated torsades de pointes. Bretylium may antagonize the effect of quinidine and may be efficacious in torsades de pointes secondary to other antiarrhythmic agents despite its intrinsic capacity to prolong repolarization. Because of the limited utility and/or experience with the aforementioned antiarrhythmic agents in this disorder, one should probably reserve their use for situations in which more conventional therapy (pacing and isoproterenol) has been ineffective. Class IA antiarrhythmic agents should absolutely be avoided in the initial management of these patients because they generally result in arrhythmia aggravation.

Once the patient has been stabilized, the physician must again address the situation that prompted the institution of the agent felt to be associated with the generation of torsades de pointes. Concern exists as to whether or not there is cross-reactivity among antiarrhythmic agents within a particular class.

There have been some suggestions that patients who develop torsades de pointes on one class IA antiarrhythmic agent may be predisposed to developing this arrhythmia when given another class IA agent. If a class IB antiarrhythmic agent can be successfully employed, this should be a strong consideration. These agents have not been definitely linked to the generation of torsades de pointes. Little data are available as to the incidence of torsades de pointes with class IC antiarrhythmic agents. Unfortunately, these agents have their own inherent limitations because of their myocardial depressant effects and their significant risk of proarrhythmia. If psychotropic agents need to be utilized, haloperidol and other butyrophenones may be less arrhythmogenic than the phenothiazines and tricyclic antidepressant agents.

Adrenergic-Dependent or Congenital Q-T Syndromes

The administration of propranolol has been linked with a marked decrease in the mortality reported to be associated with the congenital long Q-T syndromes. Schwartz has suggested that a decrease in mortality from 73 to 6 percent may be found after institution of this form of therapy. The propranolol should be given in full beta-blocking doses, and patient compliance is extremely important. Left cervicothoracic stellate ganglionectomy may provide additional control for patients who have persistent recurrences despite adequate beta-blocking effect. Unfortunately, this often results in Horner's syndrome. A third potential modality of therapy appears to be chronic ventricular pacing. Eldar and associates successfully employed this form of therapy in a small population of patients with congenital Q-T prolongation syndrome who were either intolerant of more conventional forms of therapy or who had recurrent episodes of torsades de pointes despite other autonomic manipulations. The automatic implantable cardioverter defibrillator may be considered a potential therapeutic modality for patients who have had recurrence despite adequate beta-blockade or in whom the etiology of the arrhythmic event remains unclear. However, it would be unacceptable to implant the automatic implantable cardioverter defibrillator as the sole therapy in patients with frequent long paroxysms of hemodynamically tolerated tachycardia. The automatic implantable cardioverter defibrillator would deliver frequent and unnecessary discharges.

Polymorphic Ventricular Tachycardia Without Q-T Prolongation

Polymorphic ventricular tachycardia without Q-T interval prolongation or pause-dependent characteristics responds very differently from torsades de pointes associated with Q-T prolongation. Frequently, these arrhythmias can be controlled with conventional antiarrhythmic therapy, including the class I antiarrhythmic agents. Isoproterenol and rapid ventricular pacing should be avoided because they may aggravate the underlying disease process. An attempt should be made to define possible precipitating causes for this arrhythmia. Fixed coronary artery disease with coronary ischemia as well as the possibility of coronary artery spasm should be considered. In the absence of acute ischemia or other obvious causes such as a hypertrophic cardiomyopathy that could result in the generation of this arrhythmia, the patient may be approached in much the same way as those with a cardiac arrest or sustained ventricular tachycardia. If the arrhythmia can be initiated by programmed electrical stimulation in the baseline state and suppressed with antiarrhythmic therapy, this is perhaps the best therapeutic option. However, if arrhythmia suppression cannot be accomplished by antiarrhythmic therapy, an automatic implantable cardioverter defibrillator may be considered for patients who have had hemodynamically compromising episodes of this arrhythmia.

SUGGESTED READING

Bhandari AK, Shapiro WA, Morady F, et al. Electrophysiologic testing in patients with the long QT syndrome. Circulation 1985; 71:63–71.

Cranefield PF, Aronson RS. Torsades de pointes and other pause-induced ventricular tachycardias: The short-long-short sequence and early afterdepolarizations. PACE 1988; 11:670.

Dessertenne F. La tachycardie ventriculaire a deux foyers opposes variable. Arch Mal Coeur 1966; 59:263–272.

Eldar M, Griffin JC, Abbott JA, et al. Permanent cardiac pacing in patients with the long QT syndrome. J Am Coll Cardiol 1987; 10:600–607.

Horowitz LN, Greenspan AM, Spielman SR, et al. Torsades de pointes: Electrophysiologic studies in patients without transient pharmacologic or metabolic abnormalities. Circulation 1981; 63:1120.

Jackman WM, Friday KJ, Anderson JL, et al. The long QT syndromes: A critical review, new clinical observations and a unifying hypothesis. Prog Cardiovasc Dis 1988; 31:115–172.

Kadish AH, Weisman HF, Veltri EP, et al. Paradoxical effects of exercise on the QT interval in patients with polymorphic ventricular tachycardia receiving type Ia antiarrhythmic agents. Circulation 1990; 81:14–19.

Kay GN, Plumb VJ, Arciniegas JG, et al. Torsades de pointes: The long-short initiating sequence and other clinical features: Observations in 32 patients. J Am Coll Cardiol 1983; 2:806–817.

Keren A, Tzivoni D, Gavish D, et al. Etiology, warning signs and therapy of torsades de pointes. Circulation 1981; 64:1167.

Khan MM, Logan KR, McComb JM, et al. Management of recurrent ventricular tachyarrhythmias associated with Q-T prolongation. Am J Cardiol 1981; 47:130.

Nguyen PT, Scheinman MM, Seger J. Polymorphous ventricular tachycardia: Clinical characterization, therapy, and the QT interval. Circulation 1986; 74:340–349.

Roden DM, Woosley RL, Primm RK. Incidence and clinical features of the quinidine-associated long QT syndrome: Implications for patient care. Am Heart J 1986; 111:1088.

Schwartz PJ, Periti M, Malliana A. The long QT syndrome. Am Heart J 1975; 89:378–390.

Sclarovksy S, Strasberg B, Lewin RF, et al. Polymorphous ventricular tachycardia: Clinical features and treatment. Am J Cardiol 1979; 44:339.

Selzer A, Wray WH. Paroxysmal ventricular fibrillation occurring during treatment of chronic atrial arrhythmias. Circulation 1964; 30:17.

Smith WM, Gallagher JJ. "Les Torsades de pointes:" An unusual ventricular arrhythmia. Ann Intern Med 1980; 93:578–584.

Soffer J, Dreifus LS, Michelson EL. Polymorphous ventricular tachycardia associated with normal and long Q-T intervals. Am J Cardiol 1982; 49:2021.

Stratmann HG, Kennedy HL. Torsades de pointes associated with drugs and toxins: Recognition and management. Am Heart J 1987; 113:1470.

Tzivoni D, Banai S, Schuger C, et al. Treatment of torsades de pointes with magnesium sulfate. Circulation 1988; 77:392–397.

Waldo AL, Akhtar M, Brugada P, et al. The minimally appropriate electrophysiologic study for the initial assessment of patients with documented sustained monomorphic ventricular tachycardia. PACE 1985; 8:918.

ACCELERATED IDIOVENTRICULAR RHYTHM

STEVE Z. BINENBAUM, M.D. Ph.D.

Accelerated idioventricular rhythm (AIVR) has been known by various synonyms: isorhythmic ventricular tachycardia (VT), slow VT, nonparoxysmal VT, and AIVR. The last term, coined by Marriott some three decades ago, has taken a firm hold in the literature, and it is used here exclusively.

AIVR is a rhythm of ventricular origin with a rate of 50 to 100 beats per minute.

CLINICAL BACKGROUND

AIVR (Fig. 1) can be encountered in a variety of clinical situations in both health and disease (Table 1). It was initially recognized in the electrocardiogram mainly in the clinical setting of digitalis toxicity, where it has malignant potential (type II AIVR) and in acute inferior wall myocardial infarction, where it is considered benign (type I AIVR). With the introduction of Holter ambulatory long-term

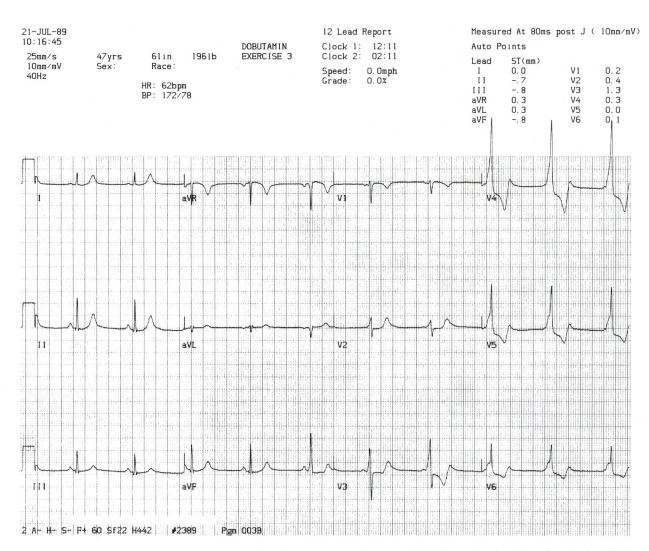

21-JUL-89
10:16:45

25mm/s   47yrs   61in   1961b   DOBUTAMIN   Clock 1:   12:11
10mm/mV   Sex: Race: EXERCISE 3   Clock 2:   02:11
40Hz
                             HR: 62bpm   Speed: 0.0mph
                             BP: 172/78   Grade: 0.0%

12 Lead Report

Measured At 80ms post J (10mm/mV)

Auto Points

Lead	ST(mm)		
I	0.0	V1	0.2
II	-.7	V2	0.4
III	-.8	V3	1.3
aVR	0.3	V4	0.3
aVL	0.3	V5	0.0
aVF	-.8	V6	0.1

Figure 1   Onset of AIVR. This 12-lead electrocardiogram shows the onset of AIVR. As the sinus rate slowed, the AIVR emerged. Note the fusion complexes (fifth through seventh).

electrocardiographic recordings, AIVR was noted in other settings as well. AIVR was reported in an asymptomatic healthy normal individual in whom the AIVR focus had all the properties of the cardiac pacemaker: automaticity, stability over a period of

Table 1   AIVR and Associated Clinical Conditions

Reperfusion (thrombolysis) 40–50%
Acute myocardial infarction, inferior 30%
Acute myocardial infarction, anterior 5%
High degree atrioventricular block
Digitalis toxicity (multifocal, multirates)
Pregnancy
Normal (very rare)
Rheumatic heart disease
Carotid sinus massage (rare, in normal sinus rhythm)
Exercise stress test (if severe coronary artery disease)
Post direct current shock ablation
Dobutamine infusion

months, autonomic innervation, and physiologic rate modulation. Holter recordings in hospitalized postinfarction patients also clearly documented the malignant potential of AIVR.

Two types of AIVR are recognized (Table 2): type I AIVR is common, has a benign natural history, and usually requires observation only. Type II AIVR is less common, has a high potential to degenerate into malignant arrhythmias, and like VT requires aggressive treatment.

Type I AIVR emerges gradually whenever the rate of the AIVR focus is greater than the underlying dominant rate (see Fig. 1). The transition from sinus rhythm to AIVR is usually smooth and gradual, with fusion complexes. The same is true for termination of AIVR whenever the rate of the AIVR focus is slower than the underlying dominant rate, with gradual transition and fusion complexes. Since the sinus and atrioventricular nodes are affected in infe-

Table 2 Characteristics of AIVR

Rate, beats per minute	50–100
QRS, complex msec	>120
Onset	Gradual
Onset time, type I AIVR	Late diastole
type II AIVR	Early diastole
Run, number of complexes	3–30
Offset	Gradual
Fusion complexes	Common
Hemodynamic compromise, type I	Usually no
type II	Yes
Prognosis, type I AIVR	Benign
type II AIVR	Serious
digitalis toxicity	Poor
Malignant potential, type I AIVR	Usually no
type II AIVR	Yes

a run of 3 to 30 monomorphic complexes at a constant frequency of between 50 and 100 beats per minute, which terminates spontaneously as the underlying supraventricular rhythm gradually re-emerges. Typically, fusion complexes (Fig. 2) are seen frequently. Because of the relatively slow rate and brief duration of the typical AIVR, there are usually no hemodynamic sequelae and the patient is asymptomatic. No specific treatment is required.

Type II AIVR has a natural history similar to that of sustained VT with abrupt (paroxysmal) onset in early diastole and a relatively high rate that is variable or fluctuating. It has a high conversion rate to more malignant arrhythmias.

rior wall myocardial infarction, AIVR was originally noted more frequently in this setting (30 percent). It is less frequently observed during anterior wall myocardial infarction (5 percent).

A typical type I AIVR is initiated by a late diastolic premature ventricular complex that introduces

AIVR: IDENTIFYING THE PERSON AT RISK

The most common clinical situation in which AIVR is encountered is during the first 48 hours after acute myocardial infarction—in 30 percent of patients with inferior infarction and in 5 percent of patients with anterior infarction. AIVR is frequently

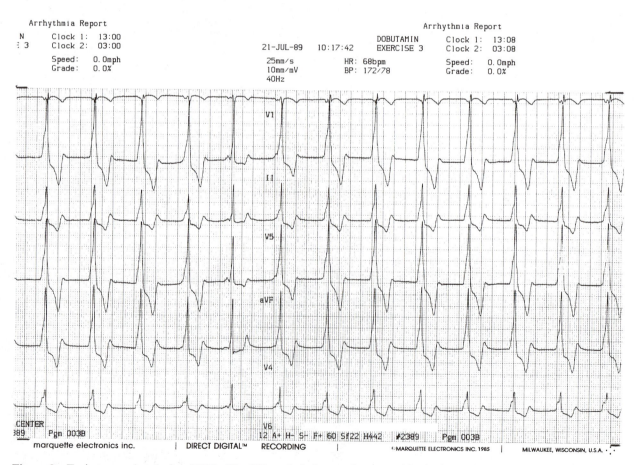

Figure 2 Fusion complex during AIVR. The fifth and sixth complexes on this rhythm strip are preceded by a P wave, and fusion is present.

Table 3 Therapy of AIVR

Treatment needed?	
type I AIVR	Usually no
type II AIVR	Yes
Malignant ventricular arrhythmia potential	
type I AIVR	Rare
type II AIVR	Yes
Oxygen, pH, potassium, calcium, magnesium	Correct
Rate slow (<70 beats per minute), hemodynamic compromise	Atropine
hemodynamic compromise	Pacing
Rate fast (70–120 beats per minute), hemodynamic compromise	Lidocaine, IA
Treatment guided by	Clinical, ECG Holter (rare)
Antiarrhythmic	
Short term	Usually no
Long term	Usually no
Pacing devices	Occasionally
Temporary pacemaker	Occasionally
Direct current cardioversion/defibrillation	Rare

seen (in 40 to 50 percent of patients) during thrombolysis within minutes of reperfusion.

Certain characteristics of AIVR suggest that it may possess significant potential to degenerate into malignant ventricular arrhythmias and therefore requires more aggressive treatment. When the initiating ventricular premature complex has a short coupling interval and the rate fluctuates widely, type II AIVR should be suspected and treatment should be instituted.

TREATMENT OF AIVR

Type I AIVR usually requires no specific treatment beyond correction of identified abnormalities of electrolytes, oxygen, and pH. However, if the patient is symptomatic, the treatment goal is to suppress the AIVR focus by a faster pacemaker. This can usually be accomplished by administration of intravenous atropine or occasionally by overdrive suppression utilizing a temporary pacemaker. The pacemaker should preferably be in the atrial position. See Table 3 regarding therapeutic choices.

Type II AIVR usually requires treatment because of its natural history of degeneration into malignant ventricular arrhythmias, e.g., VT, polymorphic VT, or ventricular fibrillation. The treatment of type II AIVR is identical to the treatment of VT (see the chapter *Sustained Ventricular Tachycardias*). Therapy should include intravenous lidocaine initially, and if this is ineffective, procainamide. Oral therapy may be required if the arrhythmia persists after discontinuation of the intravenous medication 48 to 72 hours after institution of therapy.

In the unusual event of failure to control type II AIVR effectively by the above regimen or spontaneous conversion of the AIVR to VT, the arrhythmia substrate must be fully defined by noninvasive studies and anatomically by cardiac catheterization. Subsequent invasive cardiac electrophysiologic study may define the optimal antiarrhythmic treatment utilizing antiarrhythmic drugs, devices, or surgery.

SUGGESTED READING

Bigger JT, Sahar DI. Clinical types of proarrhythmic response to antiarrhythmic drugs. Am J Cardiol 1987; 59, 5E–9E.

Cercek B, Lew AS, Laramee P, et al. Time course and characteristics of ventricular arrhythmias after reperfusion in acute myocardial infarction. Am J Cardiol 1987; 60, 214–218.

Gorgles APM, Vos MA, Letsch IS, et al. Usefulness of the accelerated idioventricular rhythm as a marker for myocardial necrosis and reperfusion during thrombolytic therapy in acute myocardial infarction. Am J Cardiol 1988; 61:231–235.

Panidis IP, Morganroth J. Sudden death in hospitalized patients: Cardiac rhythm disturbances detected by ambulatory ECG monitoring. J Am Coll Cardiol 1983; 2:798–805.

Talbot S, Greaves M. Association of ventricular extrasystole and ventricular tachycardia with idioventricular rhythm. Br Heart J 1976; 38:457–464.

Zipes DP. Specific arrhythmias: Diagnosis and treatment. In: Braunwald E, ed. Heart disease: A textbook of cardiovascular medicine. Philadelphia: WB Saunders, 1988:724–725.

VENTRICULAR ARRHYTHMIAS IN MITRAL VALVE PROLAPSE

ROBERT M. JERESATY, M.D.

Mitral valve prolapse (MVP) is defined as displacement of one or both leaflets of the mitral valve across the mitral annulus into the left atrium, as demonstrated by angiography, echocardiography, or pathologic studies. On auscultation, MVP is often manifested by a midsystolic click with or without a late systolic murmur or by a holosystolic murmur in its advanced form, the so-called *floppy mitral valve*. Barlow has recently reclassified this entity into billowing of leaflets, which is often evident echocardiographically and is often associated with a click, and a true prolapse, which is defined as a failure of apposition of leaflet edges, resulting in mitral insufficiency. I believe that the term prolapse has become generally accepted, and billowing may be an initial stage or a manifestation of the benign form of this disorder, whereas prolapse as defined by Barlow is a late stage or a manifestation of a severe form of the same disorder. Moreover, prolapse defined as displacement of an organ or part of an organ from its normal position may apply to the body of the leaflets or to their edge or both. Thus I believe that introducing "billowing" may be confusing, and I would favor continuing to use the term mitral valve prolapse in designating this common disorder of the mitral valve.

A syndrome consisting of auscultatory and echocardiographic evidence of MVP, nonspecific symptoms (e.g., chest pain, palpitations), electrocardiographic abnormalities, and arrhythmias has been recognized by many investigators. The existence of this syndrome has been questioned recently on the basis of the following: (1) in epidemiologic surveys, most individuals shown to have MVP have been asymptomatic, (2) symptoms and arrhythmias that have been reported in association with MVP are prevalent in the general population in the absence of MVP, (3) patients referred to tertiary centers could be selected for having unexplained symptoms in association with unrelated auscultatory or echocardiographic findings (selection bias), (4) the above-mentioned symptoms often prompt consideration and recognition of MVP (ascertainment bias). The relationship of arrhythmias to MVP is discussed later in this chapter. We have not heard the final word in this controversy, and further epidemiologic studies undoubtedly will shed light on this important issue. It is my contention that an etiologic relationship will be found between MVP and at least two of these findings, i.e., atypical chest pain and palpitations due to arrhythmias that have been grouped with MVP as a distinct syndrome.

CRITERIA FOR DIAGNOSIS

A nonejection click is the diagnostic auscultatory hallmark of MVP. M-mode echocardiography is diagnostic when, being two-dimensionally guided, it shows pronounced late systolic dipping. The two-dimensional echocardiographic criteria have recently been tightened, requiring prolapse of one or both leaflets in the parasternal long-axis view. Thickening and redundancy of the mitral leaflets on echocardiography reinforce the diagnosis by pointing to intrinsic involvement of the mitral valve rather than to a normal variant and represent important risk factors. Doppler echocardiography, preferably with color flow mapping, is helpful in the diagnosis and assessment of the severity of mitral regurgitation in MVP.

PREVALENCE OF VENTRICULAR ARRHYTHMIAS IN MVP

Most investigators in tertiary centers who have studied the prevalence of ventricular arrhythmias in MVP have concluded that they are more common in this syndrome than in the general population and that there was a causal relationship between this common valvular disorder and these common rhythm disorders. DeMaria and associates have reported a 58 percent prevalence of ventricular premature complexes in their MVP group as compared with 25 percent in "normal subjects" who were referred for evaluation of chest pain. The Framingham study, which was expected to provide an accurate determination of the true prevalence of arrhythmias in MVP as compared with the general population, unfortunately was flawed because it was based primarily on "loose" M-mode echocardiographic criteria with the probability of overdiagnosis of MVP in subjects who exhibited an unusually poor concordance between the commonly encountered echocardiographic findings leading to the diagnosis and the uncommonly encountered auscultatory characteristics in this series. The overdiagnosis of MVP by M-mode echocardiography in this study may have caused dilution of the MVP group by normal subjects with minor echocardiographic changes that probably represented a normal variant. Despite these shortcomings, the Framingham study found a higher prevalence of arrhythmias in the group with MVP than in the general population, but the excess of arrhythmias in those with MVP did not reach statistical significance. In a recent report on nonischemic ventricular tachycardia in 52 patients, 24 percent of the patients had MVP, but the causal relationship between MVP and ventricular tachycardia was dismissed by the authors as unconvincing because the tachycardia was felt to originate in the outflow tract of the right ventricle.

Ventricular premature complexes have frequently been detected in association with MVP, and a prevalence of 58 to 90 percent has been reported on Holter monitoring. In some patients, complex ventricular arrhythmias have been documented. Sustained ventricular tachycardia and fibrillation resulting in cardiac arrest have also been reported in a relatively small number of patients with MVP and are discussed under sudden death.

MECHANISM OF VENTRICULAR ARRHYTHMIAS IN MVP

Several theories have been proposed to explain the genesis of arrhythmias in MVP. Unfortunately, the results of electrophysiologic studies have been conflicting and have not been helpful in defining the nature of the ventricular arrhythmias that are encountered in this disorder. Excessive traction on the papillary muscle by the prolapsing leaflets has been postulated by some workers, including Barlow and the author. Another factor responsible for ventricular arrhythmias may be mechanical stimulation of the endocardium by the elongated chordae tendineae. Arrhythmias may also originate from endocardial friction lesions and their myocardial extensions, which are felt to result from friction of the chordae against the endocardium. The abnormally tense and redundant mitral leaflets that contain muscle fibers capable of developing diastolic depolarization may represent another source of arrhythmias. Triggered automaticity has been demonstrated in some cases. Prolongation of the Q-T interval has been found in a few but not in most MVP series. Some workers have attributed the ventricular arrhythmias in MVP to the mitral insufficiency that is often associated with the severe forms of the disorder. In the advanced forms, this theory is probably correct. However, complex ventricular arrhythmias, including life-threatening ones and some cases of ventricular fibrillation have been documented in MVP in the absence of mitral regurgitation or in the presence of hemodynamically insignificant mitral regurgitation. Further studies are clearly needed to elucidate the mechanism of arrhythmias in MVP. It is probable that patients with MVP and arrhythmias may represent an etiologically heterogenous group.

INDICATIONS FOR HOLTER MONITORING IN MVP

Holter monitoring is not recommended in all patients with MVP in view of the benign nature of the arrhythmias in this common disorder. The cost of the test is another factor mitigating against its routine use. Such monitoring should be carried out in patients complaining of distressing palpitations, presyncope, or syncope in order to confirm or exclude an arrhythmic etiology and with a view to treatment. For patients who experience symptoms daily, a continuous 24-hour ambulatory recording is sufficient for the diagnosis of arrhythmias and the relationship between symptoms and arrhythmias. However, many patients do not have daily symptoms, and in such cases, patient-activated intermittent recorders and trans-telephone electrocardiographic capability are most helpful in evaluation.

MANAGEMENT OF VENTRICULAR ARRHYTHMIAS IN MVP

Ventricular arrhythmias are probably common in MVP and yet their potential complications, such as syncope and sudden death, are rare occurrences. It is generally accepted that the prognostic significance of ventricular arrhythmias, particularly ventricular premature complexes, depends on the underlying cardiac disorder and the underlying left ventricular dysfunction. In the absence of severe mitral regurgitation, ventricular arrhythmias in MVP, particularly ventricular premature complexes, have the same benign outlook as in subjects with normal hearts. Thus, the generally benign nature of ventricular arrhythmias in MVP would not favor aggressive management, and even frequent or complex ventricular premature complexes do not require treatment in this disorder.

Antiarrhythmic therapy is recommended in the following patients (Table 1):

1. Patients with symptomatic and distressing ventricular arrhythmias, including frequent palpitations, dizziness, and particularly syncope, when these symptoms are shown to be attributable to arrhythmias by ambulatory monitoring.
2. Patients with a history of sustained ventricular tachycardia or ventricular fibrillation.
3. Patients with a family history of MVP and sudden death. In these patients, ventricular premature complexes, particularly the complex types, require aggressive management.

Table 1 Indications for Antiarrhythmic Therapy in Patients With Mitral Valve Prolapse

Markedly symptomatic and distressing ventricular arrhythmias
Sustained ventricular tachycardia or ventricular fibrillation
Family history of mitral valve prolapse and sudden death

These indications for antiarrhythmic therapy are uncommon, and the great majority of patients with MVP with arrhythmias do not require antiarrhythmic therapy because they are either asymptomatic or they have mild symptoms that are or are not related to arrhythmias. Moreover, the ventricular arrhythmias in MVP usually consist of benign ventricular premature complexes of slight to moderate frequency. Since most patients with MVP are young, the initiation of antiarrhythmic therapy implies exposure of these patients over long periods to the adverse effects of pharmacologic agents. Proarrhythmic effects of such agents are important considerations when initiating treatment in a generally benign cardiac disorder.

In the management of ventricular arrhythmias in MVP, particular attention should be given to the avoidance of stimulants, including caffeine, nicotine, and alcohol. This recommendation is predicated on the arrhythmogenic potential of these substances, particularly in the setting of a disorder such as MVP in which a hyperadrenergic state has been demonstrated by some investigators.

Of the antiarrhythmic agents, most experience has been accumulated with the beta blockers. In addition to their intrinsic antiarrhythmic properties, beta blockers may be particularly valuable in MVP because they may potentially lessen prolapse and may neutralize the hyperadrenergic state when present. Moreover, these agents may have a beneficial effect on the perception of cardiac "skipping," even in the absence of objective reduction of the underlying arrhythmias. They have been found effective in suppression or significant reduction of ventricular premature complexes in about 50 percent of treated patients.

Class IA (quinidine-like) antiarrhythmic drugs have been used alone or in combination with beta blockers. However, they should be used with caution in patients with MVP because they may worsen ventricular arrhythmias, possibly by causing a prolongation of the Q-T interval. Of the class IB (lidocaine-like) agents, mexiletine has been used in some patients with success. Phenytoin was found to be effective in the management of ventricular arrhythmias by Barlow. Tocainide, because of its hematologic and pulmonary complications, is now restricted to life-threatening ventricular arrhythmias and its use would not, therefore, be appropriate in most of the arrhythmias associated with MVP. Class IC drugs are quite effective in suppressing ventricular arrhythmias, which are not associated with structural heart disease and left ventricular dysfunction. Although a long experience has not been accumulated with their use in MVP, they would have been ideally suited for this disorder, which is usually associated with normal left ventricular function. Unfortunately, the restrictions recently imposed by the Food and Drug Administration (FDA) on the use of flecainide and encainide as the result of the Cardiac Arrhythmia Suppression Trial (CAST) make it impossible to continue their use, except in patients with life-threatening arrhythmias. Paradoxically, the proarrhythmic effect of these agents is particularly evident in patients with poor left ventricular function and sustained ventricular tachycardia, for which their use is reserved by the FDA. It is of interest that moricizine, a drug with class IA and IB properties that is not yet approved by the FDA and that did not increase mortality in the CAST trial, has been found by one group to be particularly effective in the suppression of ventricular arrhythmias in MVP. In 17 patients with MVP who had symptomatic complex ventricular arrhythmias, this drug was effective in suppressing 90 percent of ventricular premature complexes, 99 percent of unsustained runs of ventricular tachycardia, and all sustained runs of ventricular tachycardia, resulting in abolition of palpitations, dizziness, and syncopal episodes. It was well tolerated and had a low incidence of minor side effects.

The role of amiodarone has not been well established in MVP, and this drug should be reserved for the most complex and life-threatening arrhythmias. Sotalol has been recommended by Barlow for MVP, but further studies are needed to confirm its effectiveness and to evaluate its proarrhythmic propensity in this disorder.

A systematic approach to the management of life-threatening ventricular arrhythmias based on acute drug testing, Holter monitoring, and exercise testing is recommended when sustained ventricular tachycardia or ventricular fibrillation has been documented in association with MVP and in a selected group of patients with disabling, unsustained ventricular arrhythmias, particularly when they are associated with syncope or a family history of sudden death. The role of electrophysiologic studies in the management of ventricular arrhythmias in MVP has not yet been defined and should be reserved for the same group of patients who may be candidates for acute drug testing. The most effective method for the management of serious ventricular arrhythmias in MVP is awaiting the results of an ongoing study comparing invasive with noninvasive techniques.

Automatic burst extrastimulus pacemaker has been inserted in a few patients. An automatic implantable cardioverter defibrillator has been successfully used in patients with MVP who have sustained a cardiac arrest (see the chapter *Automatic Implantable Cardioverter Defibrillator*).

Mitral valve replacement was performed with excellent results in a few patients who had recurrent ventricular fibrillation despite aggressive antiarrhythmic therapy. These patients should now be considered candidates for an automatic implantable cardioverter defibrillator and, if significant mitral regurgitation is present, mitral valve repair should be performed at the operation to implant the device. To my knowledge, the effect of mitral valve replacement or repair by itself on the ventricular arrhythmias in MVP has not been reported. The role of the correction of the associated mitral insufficiency as opposed to the correction of the underlying MVP has not been elucidated.

SUDDEN DEATH IN MVP

Sudden death, the most feared complication of MVP, is fortunately a rare occurrence. To my knowledge, only 90 cases of sudden death have been reported. I am also aware of ten additional cases confirmed at necropsy that were reported to me and in whom MVP was the sole abnormality. A group of patients with MVP who were successfully resuscitated after ventricular fibrillation and tachycardia have been reported. Judging from cases of sudden death mentioned by medical audiences during discussions of MVP, it appears that a larger number of patients with sudden death go unreported.

In their pathologic studies, Davies and coworkers reported four cases of sudden death in MVP in the absence of severe mitral regurgitation, ischemic heart disease, or cardiomyopathy. These four cases were encountered in 5 years in material drawn from the coroner's office, compared with an annual average of 250 cases of sudden death due to ischemic heart disease. This suggests that 0.3 instances of sudden death might be expected among patients with MVP without mitral regurgitation for every 100 cases of sudden death due to coronary artery disease. As pointed out by Boudoulas and associates, selection bias may be at work with this estimate, since it is more likely that an autopsy will be performed in patients with MVP and sudden death than in patients with known coronary artery disease.

The rare occurrence of sudden death in MVP, a syndrome that affects 5 percent of the population, raises legitimate questions about the causal link between the syndrome and this dramatic complication, particularly since cases of sudden death of unknown etiology continue to be reported. In my opinion, a chance association between MVP and sudden death is most unlikely. If accepted as a complication of MVP, sudden death is so uncommon that it should not be mentioned to patients or their families for fear of creating undue anxiety and neurosis. The age of the patients who died suddenly ranges from 9 to 89; only five were 20 years of age or younger. Death occurred during physical stress in only four patients.

Sudden death is discussed here because its mechanism is generally thought to be arrhythmic. Ventricular fibrillation has been documented both in patients who have died suddenly and in those who were successfully resuscitated. Bradyarrhythmias have not been detected in the reported cases. In addition to the mechanisms of ventricular arrhythmias mentioned above, the relatively frequent occurrence of preexcitation in MVP offers a possible mechanism for sudden death: atrial flutter and fibrillation leading to ventricular fibrillation. Accessory pathways have been found at autopsy in two patients with MVP who died suddenly. Coronary embolism may be a rare mechanism of sudden death in MVP. Electrolyte abnormalities, particularly hypokalemia, and the antiarrhythmic drugs themselves may cause malignant arrhythmias terminating in ventricular fibrillation.

The typical patient with MVP who suffers a cardiac arrest is a middle-aged woman with history of syncope or presyncope who had a mitral regurgitant murmur and an abnormal electrocardiogram showing ST-T changes in the inferior and left precordial leads and multiple ventricular premature complexes. Left ventriculography has shown marked MVP in such patients. Thickening and redundancy of the mitral valve, as demonstrated by echocardiography, has recently been reported as another risk factor for sudden death. It would seem that patients who have MVP and a regurgitant murmur and/or a thickened mitral valve on echocardiography are at a higher risk of dying suddenly and of developing progressive mitral insufficiency with or without ruptured chordae tendineae and infective endocarditis than those with "silent" MVP, isolated clicks, and/or thin valve.

This profile of patients with MVP who died suddenly, particularly with reference to severity of prolapse and the findings of mitral regurgitation, has been confirmed by subsequent reports. However, others have reported sudden death in a few patients with minimal MVP at necropsy, in one patient with "silent" MVP, and in two patients with isolated clicks. The predictive value of this composite picture of MVP patients who have died suddenly has not been tested in a prospective fashion and, in view of the relatively rare occurrence of sudden death, this testing would require a large series of MVP patients and a long follow-up period. In any case, prudence dictates aggressive management of complex ventricular arrhythmias in patients with MVP, thickened mitral valve on echocardiography, mitral regurgitation on auscultation and on Doppler studies, and a history of syncope, particularly if there is a family history of sudden death related to MVP.

SUGGESTED READING

Barlow JB, Cheng TO. Mitral valve billowing and prolapse. In: Cheng TO, ed. The international textbook of cardiology. New York: Pergammon Press, 1986: pp 497–524.

Boudoulas H, Kligfield P, Wolley CF. Mitral valve prolapse: sudden death. In: Boudoulas H, Wooley CF, eds. Mitral valve prolapse and the mitral valve prolapse syndrome. Mount Kisco, NY: Futura, 1988.

Jeresaty RM. Mitral valve prolapse. New York: Raven Press, 1979.

Jeresaty RM. Mitral valve prolapse: An overview. J Cardiol 1988; 18 (Suppl 18):3–8. Guidelines for ambulatory electrocardiography. A report of the American College of Cardiology American Heart Association Task Force. J Am Coll Cardiol 1989; 13:249–260.

Kligfield P, Levy D, Devereux RB, et al. Arrhythmias and sudden death in mitral valve prolapse. Am Heart J 1987; 113:1298–1307.

Savage DD, Levy D, Garrison RJ, et al. Mitral valve prolapse in the general population. 3. Dysrhythmias: The Framingham Study. Am Heart J 1983; 106:582.

Schaal SF. Mitral valve prolapse: Cardiac arrhythmias and electrophysiological correlate. In: Boudoulas H, Wooley CF, eds. Mitral valve prolapse and the mitral valve prolapse syndrome. Mount Kisco, NY: Futura, 1988.

ARRHYTHMIAS IN HYPERTROPHIC CARDIOMYOPATHY

LAMEH FANANAPAZIR, M.D.
BARRY J. MARON, M.D.

Hypertrophic cardiomyopathy is a primary myocardial disease with a diverse clinical spectrum and natural history that includes patients who are subject to premature sudden cardiac death, often unheralded by prior symptoms, and those with progressive heart failure associated with ventricular enlargement and wall thinning.

Sudden death is the most unpredictable and devastating complication of hypertrophic cardiomyopathy and occurs most commonly in young patients (10 to 30 years of age). The etiology and determinants of sudden cardiac death and arrest in patients with hypertrophic cardiomyopathy have been debated, and a number of mechanisms have been proposed. Nevertheless, despite these efforts, the issue remains largely unresolved. Indeed, potential mechanisms that may be responsible for sudden death are complex and are probably not identical in all patients. To date, most investigators favor the concept that ventricular and supraventricular arrhythmias are significantly implicated. In this regard, most recently, substantial information has been assembled that relates electrophysiologic findings to cardiac symptoms and sudden death in this disease. Consequently, in this chapter we have summarized and integrated the available clinical, Holter, and electrophysiologic data that bear on the critical considerations of risk of sudden cardiac death and management of arrhythmias in patients with hypertrophic cardiomyopathy.

RISK EVALUATION OF THE PATIENT WITH HYPERTROPHIC CARDIOMYOPATHY

History and Clinical Examination

Initial evaluation includes determining whether the patient with hypertrophic cardiomyopathy has a clinical profile that increases the risk of sudden cardiac death: (1) young age; (2) "malignant" family history of premature (less than 50 years of age) sudden cardiac death (more than or equal to two first-degree relatives); and (3) previous cardiac arrest or syncope. A loud precordial systolic murmur (in the supine position) that increases in intensity with standing may indicate significant obstruction to left ventricular outflow. Clinical examination also aids in establishing the cardiac rhythm and presence or absence of cardiac failure.

Noninvasive and Invasive Studies

We discontinue all cardioactive drugs in the hospital for at least five half-lives prior to the noninvasive and invasive tests. We have found this policy to be safe and necessary for clinical, hemodynamic, and electrophysiologic evaluation of the patient with hypertrophic cardiomyopathy.

Twelve-Lead Electrocardiogram

The electrocardiogram is abnormal in more than 95 percent of patients with hypertrophic cardiomyopathy. In the young patient, it may be the first sign that a family member has the disease. Apart from establishing the rhythm, the electrocardiogram is scrutinized for evidence of preexcitation and atrioventricular conduction abnormalities. Left bundle branch block is more common than right bundle branch block in patients with hypertrophic cardiomyopathy. The importance of right bundle branch in patients with hypertrophic cardiomyopathy lies in the fact that they are likely to develop complete heart block and to require a permanent pacemaker following left ventricular myotomy and myectomy, because septal muscle resection itself often results in left bundle branch block.

Ambulatory Electrocardiographic Monitoring

Ventricular tachycardia is recorded in about 20 percent of patients with hypertrophic cardiomyopathy during 24- to 48-hour ambulatory monitoring. Characteristically, ventricular tachycardia in asymptomatic patients is unsustained and monomorphic, with a relatively slow rate and short runs (usually 3 to 15 beats; rarely more than 20 beats). Frequently, different morphologies and rates of monomorphic ventricular tachycardia are recorded during 24- to 48-hour Holter monitoring (Fig. 1). Occasionally, unsustained ventricular tachycardia is polymorphic (Fig. 2).

Data obtained from ambulatory electrocardiographic monitoring have focused attention on the potential importance of ventricular tachycardia as a mechanism for sudden death in patients with hypertrophic cardiomyopathy. Two centers have indepen-

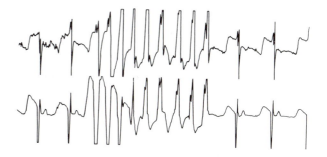

Figure 2   Unsustained polymorphic ventricular tachycardia recorded during 48-hour Holter monitoring in a hypertrophic cardiomyopathy patient who presented with syncope.

dently reported that even brief episodes of asymptomatic ventricular tachycardia on 24- or 48-hour ambulatory monitoring identify a subgroup of patients at higher risk for sudden death over the subsequent years. These studies were similar in design, evaluating patients in a cross-sectional fashion at one point in time with Holter monitoring and then assessing their longitudinal clinical condition after 3 to 4 years. In one of the studies, the single observation of three or more consecutive ventricular complexes at a rate of more than 100 per minute conferred an 8 percent risk of sudden death per year, compared with only a 1 percent risk in those patients without ventricular tachycardia (over a 3-year follow-up period). Additionally, left ventricular wall thickness and mass tend to be greater in patients with ventricular tachycardia. This finding implies a causal relationship between increased left ventricular mass, ventricular tachycardia, and risk of sudden death in patients with hypertrophic cardiomyopathy.

Nevertheless, it should be emphasized that the occurrence of ventricular tachycardia on Holter monitoring may be a marker for sudden death only in *some* patients with hypertrophic cardiomyopathy, because the vast majority of patients who have ventricular tachycardia during ambulatory monitoring are *not* subject to sudden cardiac death. In this context, only one-fifth of asymptomatic patients with hypertrophic cardiomyopathy who have ventricular tachycardia during ambulatory monitoring can be shown to have an arrhythmogenic left ventricular substrate at electrophysiologic study. Thus, empirical therapy based on the presence of ventricular tachycardia during ambulatory monitoring could result in unnecessary treatment with antiarrhythmic medications that have serious potential side effects. The value of ventricular tachycardia recorded during ambulatory monitoring as a marker of sudden cardiac death is further diminished by the fact that this arrhythmia occurs rarely in children and young adults less than 25 years of age, and several sudden

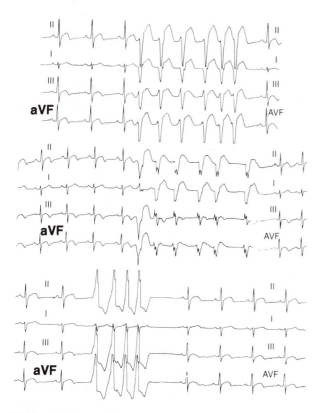

Figure 1   Unsustained ventricular tachycardia with different morphologies and rates recorded during 48-hour Holter monitoring in a patient with hypertrophic cardiomyopathy who presented with syncope and in whom a sustained polymorphic ventricular tachycardia was induced at electrophysiologic study.

deaths have been reported in children who were known to have had normal Holter recordings. Thus, unsustained ventricular tachycardia cannot be used as a marker for sudden death in an age group that is most at risk for this event, and consequently its greatest clinical utility may well be confined to the adult age group.

Echocardiography

Hypertrophic cardiomyopathy is defined by the echocardiographic demonstration of increased left ventricular wall thickness in the absence of another cardiac or systemic disease that may produce left ventricular hypertrophy. Echocardiography also establishes the following: (1) severity and distribution of left ventricular hypertrophy (patients with particularly marked left ventricular wall thickness may be at increased risk for sudden cardiac death); (2) severity of left ventricular outflow obstruction and suitability of the cardiac anatomy for ventricular septal myotomy-myectomy; (3) left atrial size (pertinent to the management of patients with atrial fibrillation); and (4) the likelihood that the patient has entered the dilating and thinning phase of the disease.

Exercise Test

We routinely perform treadmill (Bruce protocol) exercise tests in our patients with hypertrophic cardiomyopathy. These tests, although useful in documenting symptomatic deterioration and in the assessment of response to medication and surgery, have not proved to be of great value in identifying patients who are at risk for sudden cardiac death. Although it has been suggested that brachial arterial blood pressure responses during exercise may identify patients who are at risk for sudden cardiac death, we are skeptical of this claim. Most sudden cardiac arrest survivors and patients with syncope have normal blood pressure responses during exercise, and thus exercise-induced hypotension must be a relatively uncommon cause of these events in hypertrophic cardiomyopathy patients. Until we have evolved better methods of identifying patients at risk for sudden cardiac death, we advise patients with hypertrophic cardiomyopathy, including those with normal exercise tests, to avoid competitive sports.

We also perform repeat exercise tests following antiarrhythmic therapy, because in some patients, proarrhythmic drug effects may not be apparent during programmed stimulation; nevertheless, the patient may develop an exercise-induced ventricular arrhythmia.

Signal-Averaged Electrocardiography

Our preliminary experience with signal-averaged electrocardiography (see the chapter *Signal-Averaged Electrocardiography*) shows that late potentials are significantly associated with Holter documentation of ventricular tachycardia and inducibility of sustained ventricular arrhythmias. The sensitivity and specificity of this test in this regard are about 75 percent and 80 percent, respectively. Although we have not found that this test predicts efficacy of antiarrhythmic drugs, appearance of late potentials or increases in signal-averaged indices of late potentials may indicate a much greater ease of inducibility of arrhythmia, particularly during amiodarone therapy.

Cardiac Catheterization

At our institution, all symptomatic patients considered to be at high risk for sudden cardiac death undergo right- and left-sided heart hemodynamic studies. These studies include assessment of left ventricular outflow tract gradient under basal conditions and following provocative maneuvers (Valsalva maneuver, amyl nitrite inhalation, and isoproterenol infusion), biplane left ventriculograms, and coronary angiography. We define hemodynamically significant obstruction at rest as a basal left ventricular outflow tract gradient of higher than 30 mm Hg.

Detection of pulmonary hypertension and elevated left atrial pressures identifies those patients who may respond adversely to verapamil and in whom institution of this therapy is best carried out under inpatient observation. Patients with hypertrophic cardiomyopathy usually have normal epicardial vessels, but occasionally a patient with this disease may have coexisting coronary artery disease.

Two categories of patients with obstructive hypertrophic cardiomyopathy are referred for relief of left ventricular outflow tract obstruction (usually ventricular septal myotomy-myectomy): (1) patients in whom symptoms are refractory to or who can no longer tolerate medical treatment with diuretics, verapamil, or beta blockers; and (2) survivors of sudden cardiac arrest who are otherwise asymptomatic but who are candidates for the automatic implantable defibrillator and cardioverter. Thus, asymptomatic patients who do not have potentially lethal arrhythmias do not undergo surgery solely to relieve severe left ventricular outflow tract obstruction.

Electrophysiologic Study

Electrophysiologic studies have an established role in the diagnosis and management of sudden cardiac arrest, syncope, and arrhythmias in patients with cardiac disease states other than hypertrophic cardiomyopathy. Several authors have reported a variety of electrophysiologic findings in patients with hypertrophic cardiomyopathy, including induction of supraventricular and ventricular arrhythmias and conduction abnormalities. However, because these studies have involved small selected groups of patients, the clinical relevance of these findings and the role of electrophysiologic studies in patients with hypertrophic cardiomyopathy have remained controversial. Hypertrophic cardiomyopathy is a clinically heterogenous disease, and thus relatively large numbers of patients must be studied to evaluate the relation of abnormal electrophysiologic findings to various clinical presentations. We recently reported our findings in 155 patients with hypertrophic cardiomyopathy who underwent electrophysiologic studies. Consequently, these studies have become an integral part of our evaluation of these patients who have arrhythmias or who are considered at high risk for sudden cardiac death.

SAFETY CONSIDERATIONS

We have now performed more than 400 electrophysiologic studies in patients with hypertrophic cardiomyopathy without a fatality. The only serious complication has been a femoral arteriovenous fistula that required surgical repair. The following measures may have contributed to the safety of the electrophysiologic studies: (1) Routine assessment of the hemodynamic state of patients (severity of left ventricular outflow obstruction and filling pressures just prior to the electrophysiologic study) and correction of dehydration following the overnight fast by infusion of fluids, because hypovolemia frequently results in sinus tachycardia and aggravates the left ventricular outflow tract obstruction; (2) Sedation to reduce anxiety-related increases in catecholamine levels; (3) Affixing two self-adhesive R2 electrocardiogram/defibrillation pads (R2 Corporation) that are attached to two independent defibrillators (Physio-control, Lifepak 6s, Cardiac monitor). If an arrhythmia is induced that results in loss of consciousness, both defibrillators are charged simultaneously to 200 J for rapid sequential direct current shocks if the first shock fails to terminate the arrhythmia. Thereby the period of time that the hypertrophied myocardium suffers ischemia between shocks is reduced from more than 10 to less than 3 sec. This not only may increase the success of cardioversion but also may prevent intractable ventricular fibrillation from developing secondary to ischemic myocardial damage; and (4) Systemic pressure is monitored continuously through an arterial line, and an adequate interval is allowed to lapse between stimulation steps to allow the arterial pressure to normalize.

PROCEDURE

Three multiple electrode catheters are introduced through the femoral vein and positioned across the tricuspid valve in the high right atrium to record the His bundle electrogram, and also posi-tioned at the right ventricular apex. In patients with a clinical history of supraventricular tachycardia, a quadripolar catheter is also placed in the coronary sinus via a subclavian vein. The femoral artery is cannulated for continuous recording of the systemic arterial pressure and for left ventricular stimulation. Following programmed atrial stimulation, the high right atrial catheter is repositioned in the right ventricular outflow tract for programmed ventricular stimulation. Intracardiac electrograms are recorded simultaneously with surface leads I, II, and V_1, and V_6 on light-sensitive paper at 100 mm per second. Twelve-lead electrocardiograms are recorded during induced arrhythmia. The heart is stimulated with 2.0 msec pulses at twice the diastolic threshold. Atrial stimulation includes introduction of extrastimuli into sinus rhythm, and following a paced atrial drive at a cycle length of 600 msec, overdrive pacing at multiple cycle lengths, and incremental pacing. Ventricular stimulation protocol involves a stepwise increase in "aggressiveness," as follows: (1) insertion of one, two, and three premature stimuli during sinus rhythm at the right ventricular apex; (2) introduction of one and two premature stimuli after three paced ventricular drive cycle lengths of 600 msec, 500 msec, and 400 msec, first at the right ventricular apex and then at the right ventricular outflow tract; (3) introduction of three premature stimuli after the three paced ventricular drive cycle lengths at the right ventricular apex and right ventricular outflow tract; and (4) introduction of one, two, and three premature stimuli after the three paced ventricular drive cycle lengths at a left ventricular site. The endpoint of the stimulation protocol is myocardial refractoriness or induction of a sustained ventricular arrhythmia.

The following electrophysiologic variables are assessed: basic intervals (A-H, H-V, QRS, and Q-T), sinus node and corrected sinus node recovery times, sinoatrial conduction time, atrial effective and functional refractory periods, atrioventricular nodal effective and functional refractory period, Wenckebach's cycle length, maximal atrial rate with 1:1 atrioventricular conduction, ventricular refractory periods at the three ventricular paced cycle lengths determined at the three ventricular sites, the shortest premature extrastimulus intervals that did or did not result in induction of a sustained ventricular arrhythmia, and the type and hemodynamic consequences of any induced atrial and ventricular arrhythmias. If a sustained atrial or ventricular arrhythmia is induced, the programmed stimulation is repeated following an infusion of 10 mg per kilogram body weight of procainamide.

Standard definitions are used for atrioventricular nodal conduction and infranodal conduction. Other definitions used follow.

Unsustained Ventricular Tachycardia. Three to thirty consecutive ventricular complexes, at greater than or equal to 120 per minute and terminating spontaneously.

Sustained Ventricular Tachycardia. This is ventricular tachycardia of more than 30 complexes duration or requiring termination because of hemodynamic compromise. Ventricular tachycardia with continuous changing QRS morphology is termed polymorphic and one with uniform QRS complexes is termed monomorphic.

Ventricular Fibrillation. Ventricular fibrillation is a ventricular arrhythmia with no discernible discrete ventricular complexes identifiable on the surface 12-lead electrocardiogram and with continuous intracardiac ventricular electrical activity.

Sudden Cardiac Arrest. Sudden cardiac arrest is a history of a resuscitation attempt requiring direct current cardioversion within 2 hours of collapse.

ABNORMAL FINDINGS: SIGNIFICANCE AND MANAGEMENT

Sinus Node Disease

Sinus node disease is a common finding in patients with hypertrophic cardiomyopathy and often manifests itself as sinus bradycardia or pauses (Fig. 3), chronotropic incompetence during exercise, and/or excessive sensitivity to verapamil and beta-blocker therapy. Less commonly, hypertrophic cardiomyopathy patients with sinus node disease have inappropriately high sinus rates (unrelated to cardiac failure or any other apparent cause), which at rest and mild exertion may vary from 100 to 180 per minute. This latter group of patients derive considerable symptomatic relief from verapamil and beta-blocker therapy and do not tolerate discontinuation of these medications for more than a few days. Any studies planned in these patients must therefore be completed expeditiously.

At electrophysiologic testing, although only 7 percent of hypertrophic cardiomyopathy patients have prolonged sinus node recovery times (greater than 1,500 msec), two-thirds have abnormal sinoatrial conduction times (greater than 120 msec). In our study, all patients with symptomatic sinus node disease had markedly prolonged sinoatrial conduction times.

Atrioventricular Node and Infranodal Conduction Disease

Patients with hypertrophic cardiomyopathy are prone to heart block as well as rapid rates during supraventricular arrhythmias (Fig. 4).

In our series, of those patients who were in sinus rhythm and had never had a documented episode of heart block, 6 percent had delayed atrioventricular conduction abnormalities (Wenckebach's block developed at heart rates of less than 120 per minute). A similar number of patients were capable of rapid atrioventricular nodal conduction (heart rates of 200 to 280 per minute).

An abnormally prolonged infranodal conduction time (H-V interval longer than 55 msec) was present in 30 percent of the patients, and the H-V interval increases or infra-Hisian block develops

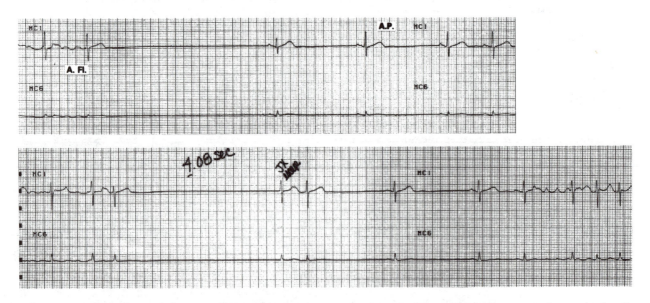

Figure 3 Sinus pauses in a hypertrophic cardiomyopathy who presented with recurrent syncope and an episode of sudden cardiac arrest. At electrophysiologic study, abnormal findings were a corrected sinus node recovery time of 600 msec, a sinoatrial conduction time of 320 msec, and an H-V interval of 80 msec. No atrial or ventricular arrhythmias were induced. The patient has been free of symptoms for 2 years following implantation of a dual-chamber pacing system.

Figure 4 Atrial fibrillation with rapid ventricular response (shortest R-R interval, 240 msec and mean rate, 222 beats per minute) in a hypertrophic cardiomyopathy patient who presented with frequent presyncopal episodes and who during decremental atrial pacing had a Wenckebach cycle length of 260 msec and a shortest 1:1 atrioventricular conduction cycle length of 270 msec.

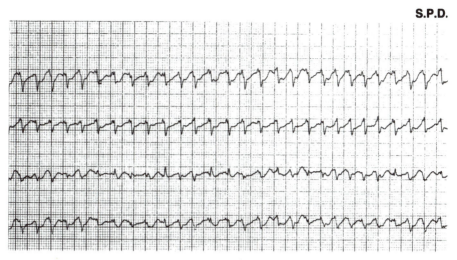

during atrial premature stimulation and/or atrial incremental pacing in 5 percent of the patients; these findings reflect the marked involvement of the ventricular septum in the disease process in patients with hypertrophic cardiomyopathy.

Verapamil, beta blockers, and antiarrhythmic drugs (frequently used in patients with hypertrophic cardiomyopathy) often aggravate sinus node dysfunction and atrioventricular nodal and infranodal conduction and consequently may precipitate catastrophic bradycardia or heart block. Patients identified by electrophysiologic tests as at risk of developing bradyarrhythmias may still be treated with these medications if deemed necessary, provided the patient receives a permanent pacemaker. In view of the frequent coexistence of sinus node disease and nodal and infranodal conduction abnormalities, our policy is to implant dual-chamber permanent pacing systems with rate-response capabilities.

Supraventricular Arrhythmias

Because of diastolic and systolic left ventricular dysfunction and a tendency to develop myocardial ischemia, hypertrophic cardiomyopathy patients have a poor tolerance for sudden onset of arrhythmias associated with rapid heart rates. The most common supraventricular arrhythmias in such patients are atrial fibrillation, atrial tachycardia, and atrioventricular reentrant tachycardia.

Progressive disease and dilation of the atria predispose to atrial fibrillation. Indeed, attempts to maintain sinus rhythm in those patients in whom the size of the left atrium is greater than 6 cm on echocardiography are usually unsuccessful. Atrial fibrillation can be a challenging arrhythmia to manage in hypertrophic cardiomyopathy; the rapid irregular ventricular response and loss of atrial transport mechanism during paroxysms of atrial fibrillation may result in acute hemodynamic collapse. Our pol-

icy is to utilize anticoagulants in all patients with paroxysmal or chronic atrial fibrillation in order to prevent systemic embolization. If the atria are only modestly enlarged or if atrial fibrillation is a recent complication, we attempt to control the arrhythmia with a combination of a class IA antiarrhythmic drug (quinidine or procainamide) and a beta blocker and/or verapamil therapy. If these medications fail to control symptomatic paroxysmal atrial fibrillation, we may prescribe amiodarone. Catheter ablation of the atrioventricular node is another reasonable alternative in patients whose disease is refractory to antiarrhythmic drug therapy.

Electrophysiologic studies are useful in this subgroup of patients for several reasons. First, induction of atrial fibrillation (this occurs in 11 percent of patients and most frequently in those patients with spontaneous arrhythmia) allows the hemodynamic consequences of the arrhythmia to be assessed. Second, patients with paroxysmal atrial fibrillation frequently have infranodal conduction disease and are much more likely to have inducible ventricular arrhythmias. These findings, which indicate the widespread nature of the disease in this subgroup of patients with hypertrophic cardiomyopathy, alert the clinician to the possibility that antiarrhythmic therapy directed at the atrial fibrillation may also produce heart block or aggravate ventricular arrhythmias.

Spontaneously occurring atrial tachycardia is not infrequently recorded during Holter monitoring and may be induced at electrophysiologic study in more than 20 percent of patients; the arrhythmia is often mapped to the right atrium and characteristically has a variable cycle length of 230 to 385 msec (mean 275 ± 35 msec).

There are reports of cardiac arrest in occasional patients with hypertrophic cardiomyopathy caused by accessory atrioventricular pathways. However, in our experience accessory atrioventricular pathways were present in only 7 out of 155 or 5 percent of patients who underwent electrophysiologic studies. Of these seven patients, three presented with palpitations, and one each with syncope, presyncope, and a malignant family history of sudden cardiac death. In one patient, orthodromic reciprocating tachycardia degenerated into atrial fibrillation complicated by profound hypotension. In all seven patients, the accessory pathway was single and situated in the posteroseptal region in four patients, the left posterior region in one patient, and the left lateral region in two. The accessory pathway was capable of antegrade and retrograde conduction in five patients and was concealed in two patients. The shortest preexcited R-R interval during induced atrial fibrillation was longer than 260 msec in the five patients showing antegrade conduction over the accessory pathway.

Dual atrioventricular nodal pathways were identified in three patients; in two patients this was of the common (slow-fast) variety, and in the remaining patient it was of the uncommon (fast-slow) variety. None of the three patients had spontaneous episodes of atrioventricular nodal tachycardia.

Ventricular Arrhythmias

Programmed ventricular stimulation resulted in induction of unsustained ventricular tachycardia in 22 out of 155 or 14 percent of patients. Unsustained ventricular tachycardia was polymorphic in 12 patients and monomorphic in 10 patients. Inducibility of unsustained ventricular tachycardia was unrelated to any particular clinical, Holter, or electrophysiologic findings. Therefore, we do not regard induction of brief episodes of this arrhythmia to be of any clinical significance.

Sustained ventricular arrhythmia was induced in 66 of 155 or 43 percent of patients. The arrhythmia was polymorphic (Fig. 5) ventricular tachycardia in 48 of 66 (73 percent), monomorphic (Fig. 6) in 16 of 66 (24 percent), and ventricular fibrillation in 2 of 66 (3 percent). In the remaining 57 percent of the patients, a significantly more aggressive stimula-

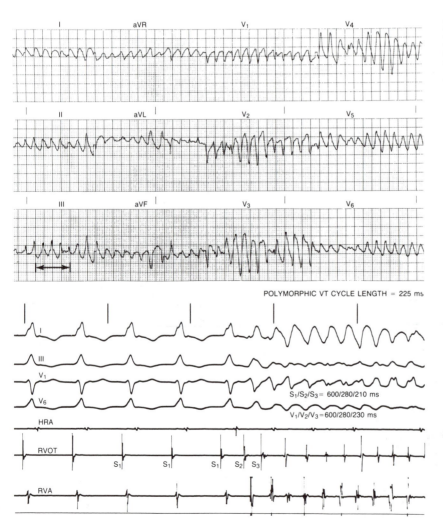

Figure 5 Induction of a sustained polymorphic ventricular tachycardia in a sudden cardiac arrest survivor with hypertrophic cardiomyopathy. The patient had no other abnormal electrophysiologic abnormality and no hemodynamic abnormality at cardiac catheterization.

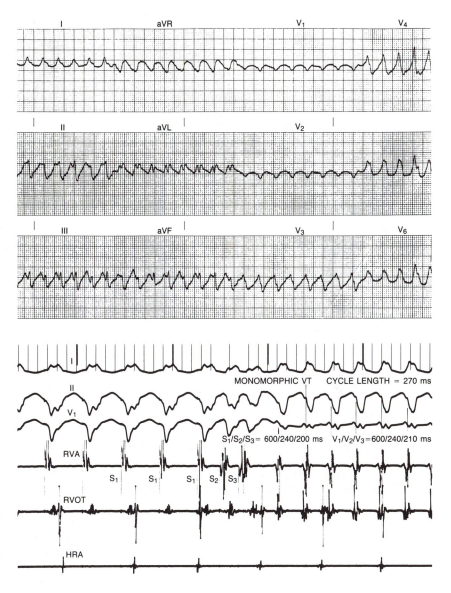

Figure 6 Induction of a sustained monomorphic ventricular tachycardia in a hypertrophic cardiomyopathy patient who presented with an episode of syncope.

tion protocol failed to induce a sustained ventricular arrhythmia (Fig. 7).

Sustained ventricular arrhythmia was induced from a right ventricular site in 51 of 66 patients but required a left ventricular site in 15 of 66. The cycle lengths of sustained polymorphic ventricular tachycardia (221 ± 26 msec) were significantly shorter (p < 0.025) than those of sustained monomorphic ventricular tachycardia (266 ± 59 msec). The rapid rates of both morphologies of ventricular tachycardia resulted in marked and prompt systemic arterial hypotension and loss of consciousness in 64 of 66 patients. In 31 patients, ventricular tachycardia degenerated into ventricular fibrillation within 11 ± 4 sec (range 4 to 37 sec) of induction. Overdrive ventricular pacing successfully terminated ventricular tachycardia in only two (3 percent) patients. Direct-

current cardioversion was successful (single direct current shock of 200 J) in 60 patients but required a second direct current shock (300 J) in the remaining five patients.

The prevalence of induced sustained ventricular arrhythmias was unaffected by age, previous cardiac surgery for left ventricular outflow obstruction, or resting or provocable left ventricular outflow tract obstruction. However, we did identify a strong association between inducibility of sustained ventricular arrhythmia and clinical presentation. Thus, a substantial proportion of patients selected for study because of prior cardiac arrest or syncope had inducible ventricular arrhythmia at electrophysiologic study; 77 percent of patients with cardiac arrest had sustained ventricular arrhythmia during programmed ventricular stimulation, as did 49 percent

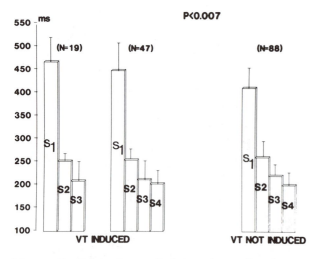

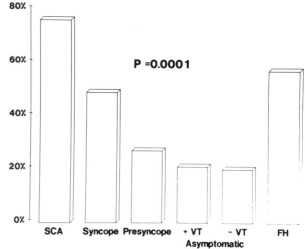

Figure 7 Comparison of "aggressiveness" of programmed ventricular stimulation (number of premature stimuli and prematurity intervals) that resulted in induction of sustained ventricular arrhythmia and that did not result in induction of a sustained ventricular arrhythmia.

Figure 8 Inducibility of sustained ventricular arrhythmia at electrophysiologic study in the various clinical presentations of subgroups of hypertrophic cardiomyopathy patients.

of patients with syncope. These prevalences of sustained ventricular arrhythmia are in contrast to only about 20 percent in asymptomatic patients (with ventricular tachycardia on Holter monitoring) and only 10 percent of patients with mild palpitations and no arrhythmias on Holter monitoring (Fig. 8). In each clinical category, recording of ventricular tachycardia during ambulatory monitoring was associated with inducibility of sustained ventricular tachycardia at electrophysiologic study (Fig. 9).

Because induction of sustained polymorphic ventricular tachycardia is considered by some

workers to be a nonspecific finding in other cardiac disease states, it has been suggested that to minimize induction of this arrhythmia, a conservative programmed ventricular stimulation protocol that involves no more than two premature stimuli should be adopted in patients with hypertrophic cardiomyopathy. The following points relate to the relevance of inducible sustained polymorphic ventricular tachycardia in hypertrophic cardiomyopathy patients and appropriateness of the stimulation protocol adopted and described by us: (1) a standard programmed ventricular stimulation protocol that was

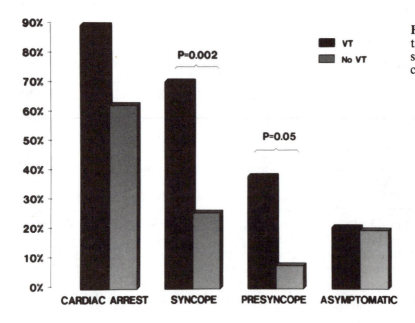

Figure 9 Relation of inducibility of ventricular tachycardia at electrophysiologic study to the presence of ventricular tachycardia during ambulatory monitoring.

not more aggressive than that employed for investigating other cardiac disease states resulted in the induction of sustained polymorphic ventricular tachycardia in a high number (32 percent) of our patients (polymorphic ventricular tachycardia accounted for 73 percent of sustained ventricular arrhythmias); (2) sustained polymorphic ventricular tachycardia was induced by a programmed ventricular stimulation protocol that was not more aggressive than that resulting in the induction of sustained monomorphic ventricular tachycardia; (3) the inducibility of sustained ventricular arrhythmia, including polymorphic ventricular tachycardia, was very significantly associated with a clinical presentation of sudden cardiac arrest and with syncope (see Figs. 8–10); and (4) the cumulative yield of the programmed ventricular stimulation, however, was significantly improved with three premature stimuli (Fig. 11); two-thirds of patients subject to cardiac death or syncope had inducible sustained ventricular tachycardia with this number of premature stimuli. The specificity of using three versus two premature stimuli also seems reasonable, because only 10 percent of those patients with mild palpitations and normal Holter recordings had an inducible sustained ventricular tachycardia with three premature stimuli (Fig. 11). In addition, although prior studies have shown that programmed ventricular stimulation protocols that involve the use of two to four premature stimuli may induce nonsustained ventricular arrhythmias in up to 40 percent of patients without structural heart disease, sustained ventricular ar-

rhythmias (including sustained polymorphic ventricular tachycardia) are rarely induced. These findings lead us to conclude that the induction of sustained polymorphic or monomorphic ventricular tachycardia by our programmed ventricular stimulation protocol is clinically relevant in patients with hypertrophic cardiomyopathy and reliably identifies an arrhythmogenic left ventricle.

Patients with hypertrophic cardiomyopathy occasionally have large fibrotic areas separating myocardial muscle bundles, conditions that favor large reentrant circuits and relatively slow monomorphic ventricular tachycardia. In many patients, however, the ventricles are diffusely diseased, with dispersed regions of fibrosis and myocardial fiber disarray. These substrates may support smaller reentrant circuits and permit the arrhythmia to change direction frequently, resulting in a rapid polymorphic ventricular tachycardia.

A further significant electrophysiologic finding has been that although in patients without an inducible sustained ventricular arrhythmia the effective refractory periods determined at the three ventricular sites were similar, in patients with an inducible sustained ventricular arrhythmia the left ventricular effective refractory periods were significantly (20 to 30 msec) shorter than the effective refractory periods measured at the two right ventricular sites (Fig. 12). These differences may reflect increased ventricular dispersion of refractoriness and may determine in part arrhythmia induction at a given site in preference to other sites.

Figure 10 Frequency with which different morphologic types of sustained ventricular arrhythmias are induced in the various presenting subgroups of hypertrophic cardiomyopathy.

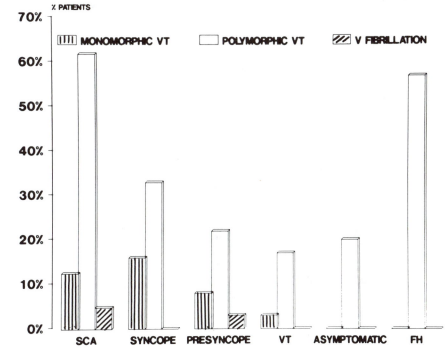

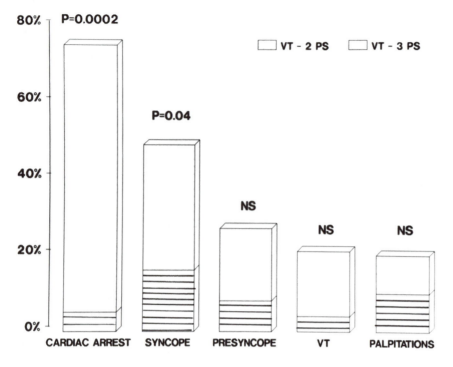

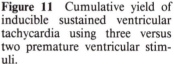

Figure 11 Cumulative yield of inducible sustained ventricular tachycardia using three versus two premature ventricular stimuli.

MANAGEMENT OF VENTRICULAR ARRHYTHMIAS

As part of an ongoing prospective study, we implant an automatic implantable cardioverter defibrillator in all hypertrophic cardiomyopathy patients who have survived an episode of sudden cardiac arrest and in whom a sustained ventricular arrhythmia is induced at electrophysiologic study (Table 1). All other patients who are considered to have an arrhythmogenic left ventricle receive the automatic implantable cardioverter defibrillator device only after they have failed to achieve satisfactory results with at least two antiarrhythmic drugs. Because antiarrhythmic drugs may precipitate heart block or may be proarrhythmic in patients with hypertrophic cardiomyopathy, we believe that the effects of these drugs should be tested by serial electrophysiologic studies once therapeutic blood or tissue levels are achieved. Not infrequently, management of sudden cardiac arrest survivors or patients with syncope requires implantation of an automatic

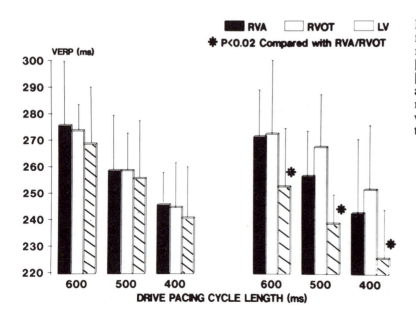

Figure 12 Comparison of ventricular effective refractory periods (VERP) determined at three sites (right ventricular apex [RVA], right ventricular outflow tract [RVOT], and left ventricular site [LV]) and at three drive pacing cycle lengths (600 msec, 500 msec, and 400 msec) in patients with and patients without inducible sustained ventricular arrhythmias.

Table 1 Management of Patients with Hypertrophic Cardiomyopathy

Clinical Subgroup	LVOT Obstruction	Electrophysiologic Study (EPS)	Therapy
Cardiac arrest	0	Bradycardia	PP
	0	VT	AICD
	+	Bradycardia	MM + PP
	+	VT	MM + AICD
Syncope/presyncope	0	Bradycardia	PP
	0	VT	AA → EPS → *AICD
	+	Bradycardia	MM + PP
	+	VT	MM → EPS → AA → *AICD
Asymptomatic VT with ≤2 PS	0	VT	AA → *AICD if induced
Malignant FH			
Marked LV hypertrophy	+	VT	MM → EPS → AA → * AICD (if induced with ≤2 PS)
Chest pain/dyspnea + Asymptomatic VT	+	VT	MM → EPS → AA → * AICD (if induced with ≤2 PS)

Abbreviations: AA = antiarrhythmic therapy; EPS = electrophysiologic study; VT = ventricular tachycardia; AICD = Automatic Implantable Cardioverter and Defibrillator; MM = myotomy and myectomy; FH = family history; LV = left ventricle; PS = premature stimuli; * = failed antiarrhythmic therapy.

cardioverter defibrillator device in addition to a permanent pacemaker and/or ventricular septal myotomy-myectomy.

SUGGESTED READING

Anderson KP, Stinson EB, Derby GC, et al. Vulnerability of patients with hypertrophic cardiomyopathy to ventricular arrhythmia induction in the operating room. Am J Cardiol 1983; 51:811–815.

Bjarnason I, Hardarson T, Jonsson S. Cardiac arrhythmias in hypertrophic cardiomyopathy. Br Heart J 1982; 48:198–203.

Brugada P, Abdollah H, Heddle B, Wellens HJJ. Results of a ventricular stimulation protocol using a maximum of 4 premature stimuli in patients without documented or suspected ventricular arrhythmias. J Am Coll Cardiol 1983; 52:1214–1218.

Brugada P, Green M, Abdollah H, Wellens HJJ. Significance of ventricular arrhythmias initiated by programmed ventricular stimulation: The importance of the type of ventricular arrhythmia induced and the number of premature stimuli required. Circulation 1984; 69:87–92.

Buxton AE, Waxman HL, Marchlinski FE, et al. Role of triple extra stimuli during electrophysiologic study of patients with documented sustained ventricular tachyarrhythmias. Circulation 1984; 69:532–540.

Canedo MI, Frank MJ, Abdulla AM. Rhythm disturbances in hypertrophic cardiomyopathy: Prevalence, relation to symptoms and management. Am J Cardiol 1980; 45:848–855.

Chmielewski CA, Riley RS, Mahendtan A, Most AS. Complete heart block as a cause of syncope in asymmetric septal hypertrophy. Am Heart J 1977; 93:91–93.

Fananapazir L, Tracy CM, Leon ML, et al. Electrophysiologic abnormalities in patients with hypertrophic cardiomyopathy: A consecutive analysis in 155 patients. Circulation 1989; 80:1259–1268.

Fidler GI, Tajik AJ, Weidman WH, et al. Idiopathic hypertrophic subaortic stenosis in the young. Am J Cardiol 1978; 42:793–799.

Frank MJ, Watkin LD, Prisant LM, et al. Potentially lethal arrhythmias and their management in hypertrophic cardiomyopathy. Am J Cardiol 1984; 53:1608–1613.

Glancy DL, O'Brien KP, Gold HK, Epstein SE. Atrial fibrillation in patients with idiopathic hypertrophic subaortic stenosis. Br Heart J 1970; 32:652–659.

Ingham RE, Mason JW, Rossen RM, Harrison DC. Electrophysiologic findings in patients with idiopathic hypertrophic subaortic stenosis. Am J Cardiol 1978; 41:811–816.

Joseph S, Balcon R, McDonald L. Syncope in hypertrophic obstructive cardiomyopathy due to asystole. Br Heart J 1972; 34:974–976.

Kowey PR, Eisenberg R, Engel TR. Sustained arrhythmias in hypertrophic obstructive cardiomyopathy. N Engl J Med 1984; 310:1566–1569.

Krikler DM, Davis MJ, Rowland E, et al. Sudden death in hypertrophic cardiomyopathy: Associated accessory atrioventricular pathways. Br Heart J 1980; 43:245–251.

Livelli FD, Bigger JT, Reiffel JA, et al. Response to programmed ventricular stimulation: Sensitivity, specificity and relation to heart disease. Am J Cardiol 1982; 50:452–458.

Louie EK, Maron BJ. Familial spontaneous complete heart block in hypertrophic cardiomyopathy. Br Heart J 1986; 55:469–474.

Mann DE, Luck JC, Griffin JC, et al. Induction of clinical ventricular tachycardia using programmed stimulation: Value of third and fourth extra stimuli. Am J Cardiol 1983; 52:50–61.

Maron BJ, Bonow RO, Cannon RO, et al. Hypertrophic cardiomyopathy: Interrelations of clinical manifestations, pathophysiology and therapy. N Engl J Med 1987; 316:780–789 and 1987; 316:844–852.

Maron BJ, Epstein SE. Hypertrophic cardiomyopathy: A discussion of nomenclature. Am J Cardiol 1979; 434:1242–1244.

Maron BJ, Henry WL, Clark CE, et al. Asymmetric septal hypertrophy in childhood. Circulation 1976; 3:9–19.

Maron BJ, Lipson LC, Roberts WC, et al. "Malignant" hypertrophic cardiomyopathy: Identification of a subgroup of families with unusually frequent premature deaths. Am J Cardiol 1978; 14:1133–1140.

Maron BJ, Roberts WC, Edwards JE, et al. Sudden death in patients with hypertrophic cardiomyopathy: Characterization of 26 patients without function limitation. Am J Cardiol 1978; 41:803–810.

Maron BJ, Roberts WC, Epstein SE. Sudden death in hypertrophic cardiomyopathy; A profile of 78 patients. Circulation 1982; 65:1388–1394.

Maron BJ, Savage DD, Wolfson JK, Epstein SE. Prognostic significance of 24 hour ambulatory monitoring in patients with hypertrophic cardiomyopathy: A prospective study. Am J Cardiol 1981; 48:252–257.

McKenna WJ, Chetty S, Oakley CM, Goodwin JF. Arrhythmia in hypertrophic cardiomyopathy: Exercise and 48-hour ambulatory electrocardiographic assessment with and without beta adrenergic blocking therapy. Am J Cardiol 1980; 45:1–5.

McKenna WJ, Deanfield J, Faruqui A, et al. Prognosis in hypertrophic cardiomyopathy: Role of age and clinical, electrocardiographic and hemodynamic features. Am J Cardiol 1981; 47:532–538.

McKenna WJ, England D, Doi YL, et al. Arrhythmia in hypertrophic cardiomyopathy. I: Influence on prognosis. Br Heart J 1981; 46:168–172.

McKenna WJ, Harris L, Deanfield J. Syncope in hypertrophic cardiomyopathy. Br Heart J 1982; 47:177–179.

McKenna JW, Krikler DM, Goodwin JF. Symposium on Cardiac Arrhythmias I: Arrhythmias in dilated and hypertrophic cardiomyopathy. Med Clin North Am 1984; 68:983–1000.

Morady F, DiCarlo L, Winston S, et al. A prospective comparison of triple extra stimuli and left ventricular tachycardia induction. Circulation 1984; 70:52–57.

Morady F, Shen E, Schwartz A, et al. Long-term follow-up of patients with recurrent unexplained syncope evaluated by electrophysiologic testing. J Am Coll Cardiol 1983; 2:1053–1056.

Morady F, Schienman MM, Hess DS, et al. Electrophysiologic testing in the management of survivors of out-of-hospital cardiac arrest. Am J Cardiol 1983; 51:85–89.

Nicod P, Polikar R, Peterson KL. Hypertrophic cardiomyopathy and sudden death. N Engl J Med 1988; 318:1255–1257.

Savage DD, Sedes SF, Maron BJ, et al. Prevalence of arrhythmias during 24-hour electrocardiographic monitoring and exercise testing in patients with obstructive and non-obstructive hypertrophic cardiomyopathy. Circulation 1979; 59:866–875.

Schiavone WA, Maoloney JD, Lever HM, et al. Electrophysiologic studies of patients with hypertrophic cardiomyopathy with syncope of undetermined etiology. PACE 1986; 9:476–481.

Stafford WJ, Trohman RG, Bilsker M, et al. Cardiac arrest in an adolescent with atrial fibrillation and hypertrophic cardiomyopathy. J Am Coll Cardiol 1986; 7:701–704.

Watson RM, Schwartz JL, Maron BJ, et al. Inducible polymorphic ventricular tachycardia and ventricular fibrillation in a subgroup of patients with hypertrophic cardiomyopathy at high risk for sudden death. J Am Coll Cardiol 1987; 10:761–774.

Wellens HJJ, Brugada P, Stevenson WG. Programmed electrical stimulation of the heart in patients with life-threatening ventricular arrhythmias: What is the significance of induced arrhythmias and what is the correct stimulation protocol? Circulation 1985; 72:1–7.

LONG Q-T SYNDROME

PETER J. SCHWARTZ, M.D.

The idiopathic long Q-T syndrome (LQTS) is a clinical disorder whose most characteristic manifestation is the occurrence of syncopal episodes, precipitated by physical or emotional stress, in a young individual with a prolonged Q-T interval on the surface electrocardiogram (Fig. 1). Most episodes of syncope or cardiac arrest are caused by torsades de pointes ventricular tachycardia. If these patients do not receive treatment, the syncopal episodes recur and eventually prove fatal in a large proportion of cases.

When an electrocardiographic screening of the family is performed, a prolongation of the Q-T interval can often be detected and a history of sudden unexpected death is frequently recorded. Two variants of LQTS have been described, one with congenital deafness and one with normal hearing. Although this is a familial disease, there are a significant number of cases without evidence of familial involvement.

The diagnosis is relatively simple in the presence of syncope associated with stressful events in a young person with a prolonged Q-T interval. However, there are often additional abnormalities that we have found diagnostically helpful, among them, the occurrence of T-wave alternans (Fig. 2) or bizarre configurations of the T wave, or specific alterations in the body surface mapping or in the movement of the posterior left ventricular wall as detected by echocardiography. In doubtful cases, the presence of two major criteria or of one major and two minor criteria (Table 1) is useful for a correct diagnosis.

The pathogenetic mechanisms of LQTS, the knowledge of which is essential in order to plan a rational therapy, are not yet completely understood despite considerable progress in this area. Two hypotheses receive serious consideration—the "sympathetic imbalance" and the "intracardiac abnormality" hypotheses. The sympathetic imbalance hypothesis suggests that the primary abnormality in LQTS is below-normal right-sided cardiac sympathetic activity; this would be accompanied by a reflex hyperactivity of left-sided cardiac sympathetic nerves. Essential to this concept is the notion that left-sided sympathetic nerves are quantitatively dominant at the ventricular level. The reproduction of most of the characteristic electrocardiographic manifestations of LQTS by ablation of the right stellate ganglion, which creates a sympathetic imbalance with left-sided dominance, strongly supports this hypothesis. The intracardiac abnormality hypothesis suggests the involvement of membrane potassium conductance. Indeed, prolongation of repolarization and increase in cardiac excitability would result following decreased potassium conductance. These effects can facilitate arrhythmia development, particularly in the presence of catecholamines. In both cases the sympathetic nervous system, acting mostly through the quantitatively dominant left stellate

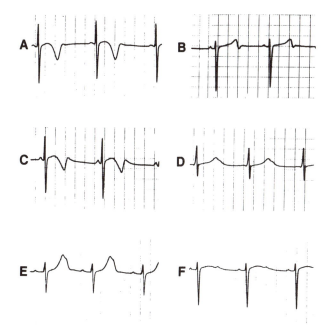

Figure 1 Examples of morphologic abnormalities in the ventricular repolarization of LQTS patients (lead V_3). *A*, A 13-year-old boy with deep negative T wave. *B*, A 10-year-old girl with diphasic (prevalently positive) T wave. *C*, An 11-year-old boy with diphasic (prevalently negative) T wave. *D*, A 19-year-old woman with notched T wave. *E*, A 46-year-old woman with peaked and notched T wave. *F*, A 16-year-old girl with a notch on the late portion of the T wave.

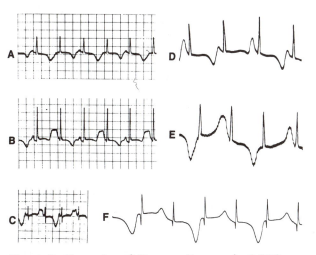

Figure 2 Examples of T-wave alternans in LQTS patients. *A* and *B*, A 9-year-old girl: alternation of T wave occurred during an unintentionally induced episode of fear. *C*, A 3-year-old boy. (Modified from Schwartz PJ, Malliani A. Am Heart J 1975;89:45–50.)

Table 1 Diagnostic Criteria for LQTS

Major	Minor
Prolonged Q-T interval (Q-Tc > 440 msec)	Congenital deafness
Stress-induced syncope	Episodes of T-wave alternans
Family members with LQTS	Low heart rate (in children)
	Abnormal ventricular repolarization

ganglion, would function as the trigger for malignant arrhythmias. This concept has played a key role in the development of a rational therapeutic strategy for LQTS.

As specified further on, proper therapy dramatically improves prognosis. Therefore, the knowledge of this uncommon but often lethal disease should be spread among general practitioners, pediatricians, and neurologists. Indeed, LQTS is often misdiagnosed as epilepsy or as hysterical faintings (because of syncope followed by convulsions in association with highly emotional states such as fear or anger), and patients therefore receive inappropriate therapy for long periods at the risk of their lives.

GENERAL PRINCIPLES OF THERAPY

The strong evidence for sympathetic activation as the trigger for the life-threatening arrhythmias of LQTS obviously suggests antiadrenergic interventions as the mainstay of therapy. Beta blockers are the obvious first choice, but favorable results also can be expected from the ablation of the left stellate ganglion, which represents a main relay station for cardiac sympathetic activity directed to the ventricles, the stimulation of which can often induce malignant arrhythmias.

Given the suggested relationship between triggered activity and the arrhythmias of LQTS, interventions that interfere with the possibility for early or delayed afterdepolarizations to reach threshold could be useful. Similarly, if cases of LQTS exist in which syncope is triggered by a further reduction in heart rate, cardiac pacing would be expected to be beneficial.

When dealing with an uncommon disease, difficulties arise in the assessment of the efficacy of any therapeutic intervention. Clearly, no single physician or medical center has sufficient data from which to extrapolate general conclusions. Since 1974, I have sought and received information from physicians around the world who were managing LQTS patients. The early data base was greatly enlarged by the institution in 1979, together with A. J. Moss and R. S. Crampton of the International Prospective Study for LQTS, with the goals of defining the natural history of LQTS and evaluating the efficacy of several therapies during a 20 to 25-year follow-up period. Up to December 1989, more than 2,500 individuals affected by LQTS and family members of LQTS patients have been enrolled. The bulk of the information that is received and continuously updated allows an assessment of the state of therapy for LQTS with a certain degree of confidence.

It makes no sense to discuss therapy without a solid frame of reference for the risk of death among untreated affected patients. Our repeated surveys in 1975 and in 1985 indicate consistently that mortality among untreated LQTS patients with syncopal episodes is close to 60 percent within approximately 10 years from onset of symptoms. It is also important to keep in mind that the majority of patients become symptomatic before or around age 15 years.

MANAGEMENT OF THE SYMPTOMATIC PATIENT

A symptomatic LQTS patient is defined as one who has experienced either syncope or cardiac arrest. All symptomatic patients must be treated. The occurrence of sudden death in middle-aged individuals who stopped therapy strongly suggests that treatment should be lifelong.

Data on several hundred symptomatic patients treated with beta blockers indicate that this treatment modality has efficacy, i.e., suppression of syncopal episodes, in 75 to 80 percent of patients. The mortality in those treated with beta blockers has consistently remained at the level of 6 percent. This is an impressive reduction when compared with the mortality figures for untreated individuals and confirms the critical role of sympathetic activity in the development of the lethal arrhythmias in LQTS. The protective effect of beta blockade may be somewhat overestimated, because approximately 20 percent of such patients continued to have syncopal episodes and underwent additional antiadrenergic therapy with high thoracic left sympathectomy.

Data are now available for 80 patients who were treated with left sympathectomy and show an 8 percent mortality during an average follow-up of almost 6 years. It is interesting to note that, independent of positive effect on survival, the majority of patients had only a partial reduction of the Q-T interval, which remained prolonged, and approximately 30 percent had one more syncopal episode, usually in the first few months after surgery. To the best of my knowledge, these figures include all the patients who underwent this type of treatment, including a small series of patients in whom less favorable results have been reported. After surgery, the majority of patients continue to take beta blockers, usually at a lower dose of that proved ineffective by the continuation

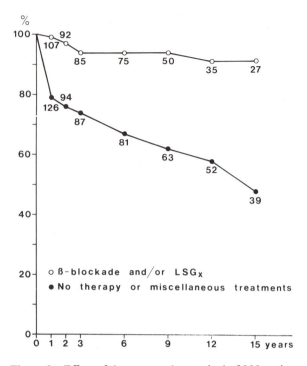

Figure 3 Effect of therapy on the survival of 233 patients affected by idiopathic LQTS after the first syncopal episode. The protective effect of beta-adrenergic blockade and of left stellectomy (LSG$_x$) is evident. The mortality 3-years after the first syncope episode is 6 percent in the group treated with antiadrenergic interventions and 26 percent in the group treated differently or not treated. Fifteen years after the first syncope episode, the respective mortality rates are 9 percent and 53 percent. (From Schwartz PJ, Locati E. Eur Heart J 1985;6:103D–114D; with permission.)

of cardiac events; there is no evidence that this is a sound or necessary policy, and it is probably implemented more for the clinician's own psychological assurance than for rational reasons. Indeed, patients in whom beta blockers have been stopped do very well, and some of them engage in competitive sports. Considering that almost all the patients operated on were not protected by full-dose beta blockade and that they should therefore be viewed as at even higher risk than the usual LQTS patients, these results appear to be extremely satisfactory. Indeed, for the overall population, using the combined pharmacologic and/or surgical antiadrenergic therapy, mortality has now been reduced to approximately 3 to 4 percent; this is a dramatic change from the 60 percent for untreated patients, and was the direct consequence of the understanding of the mechanisms involved in the initiation of the life-threatening arrhythmias. The protection afforded by sympathectomy to patients who had been unsuccessfully treated with beta blockers suggests, but does not prove, the presence of an alpha-adrenergic–mediated arrhythmogenic mechanism.

One typical feature of LQTS is an unusually low heart rate. Not surprisingly, cardiac pacing has occasionally been employed in the management of LQTS. At variance with the initial observations, a relatively recent report suggests that cardiac pacing may be effective in preventing syncope in selected patients. Cardiac pacing can be used when full-dose beta blockade cannot be administered because of excessively low heart rate, and it is indicated whenever there is electrocardiographic evidence that the syncopal episodes are bradycardia-dependent and that the torsades de pointes is preceded by a further slowing in heart rate.

The possible involvement of afterdepolarizations in the origin of the arrhythmias of LQTS has suggested the use of calcium entry blockers. Although a few instances of clinical success have been observed, the information available remains too limited for valid generalization. Despite these limitations, the use of calcium entry blockers may be considered when the most effective therapies fail.

In two LQTS patients, autotransplant has been attempted. The rationale for such a complex intervention is greatly weakened by two pathophysiologic considerations. First, after complete postganglionic denervation, denervation supersensitivity is present, and the deleterious effects of catecholamines in these hearts are likely to be exaggerated. Second, within 9 to 12 months, reinnervation is likely to occur, probably with further regional inhomogeneities. Such an event is not anticipated with high thoracic left sympathectomy because the main synapses are also removed.

Another consideration in management is the automatic implantable cardiac defibrillator. When a patient continues to have syncope despite full-dose beta blockade and high thoracic left sympathectomy, the implantable defibrillator represents a rational approach to providing a failsafe system while unconventional therapies are being evaluated. However, it must be kept in mind that the implantable defibrillator does not prevent malignant arrhythmias, and that LQTS is characterized by relatively frequent episodes of ventricular tachycardia-fibrillation occurring in young individuals. To use a mode of treatment that is bound to result in frequent cardioversions in a child or teenager, with the attendant negative psychological effects, is not justified when the two most effective therapies have not yet been properly employed.

Once a type of therapy has been decided upon, there is a question of the dosage or, in the case of surgery, of the extent and the technique.

The most frequently used beta blocker for the management of LQTS is propranolol. Our policy has been that of starting with 2 mg per kilogram per day and then of increasing up to 3 mg per kilogram per day if one episode of syncope recurs; this dosage is subdivided into three daily administrations. There is growing and positive experience with nadolol, which can be given once or twice daily, although there is less certainty about the necessary doses for children. We use between 40 and 160 mg per day. Other beta blockers, particularly atenolol, have been used but with definitely less success; indeed, relatively many of the few deaths in LQTS patients that occurred while they were on therapy with beta blockers occurred in individuals treated with atenolol.

The surgical therapy also requires some qualification. High thoracic left sympathectomy is often but incorrectly referred to as "left stellectomy." This distinction is not semantic and has important practical implications. To arrive at the same degree of denervation achieved in animals with the ablation of one stellate ganglion, in humans it is necessary to remove the first four to five thoracic ganglia. On the other hand, there is no need to remove the cephalic portion of the left stellate ganglion; in this way, the Horner syndrome is almost always avoided. The technique used in Milan (by Ruberti) involves a small incision at the base of the neck followed by an extrapleural approach; this avoids the need for a thoracotomy and results in a minor surgical procedure usually requiring 25 to 30 minutes. The main drawback to this approach is that the surgeon has to work in a small, deep hole; this requires a precise knowledge of the anatomy in the different layers and extensive experience with this technique, without which the fourth and fifth thoracic ganglia become almost impossible to reach. If this type of experience is lacking, we suggest the traditional approach which, although requiring a thoracotomy, allows good visualization of the sympathetic chain and minimizes the chances for error. When the stellate ganglion is exposed, before proceeding to its section, we always perform a pharmacologic blockade by infiltration with lidocaine in order to avoid an "injury current" that would release an inordinate amount of norepinephrine. This surgery has only two mild sequelae: one is the disappearance of sweating in the right hand, which becomes warmer and dryer, and the other is a modest lowering of the left upper eyelid, which after a few weeks is minimal.

MANAGEMENT OF THE ASYMPTOMATIC PATIENT

The single most difficult question when dealing with a patient affected by LQTS is what to do with his or her siblings who have a prolonged Q-T interval but have never had syncopal episodes, the so-called "asymptomatic LQTS patients." Approximately 20 percent of such patients will become symptomatic, i.e., will have syncope or cardiac arrest. As the diagnosis has already been made, they should immediately be placed on beta blockers therapy if they survive. Therefore, the key issue is to know the risk of dying during the *first* event. Although the International Prospective Study will eventually provide this information, we do not yet know the incidence of death during the first attack in LQTS with certainty; my own rough personal estimate is an incidence in the range of 3 to 5 per 1,000 patients.

This situation poses serious questions for clinical management that may also have medicolegal implications. Accordingly, it is not realistically possible to dictate an ideal therapeutic approach until the actual risk is quantified, and I will limit myself to a discussion of my current policy.

The decision is made more difficult by the fact that if therapy is deemed necessary, it will have to be continued for the duration of the patient's life or for several decades at least. A lifelong medical treatment is bound to generate significant negative psychological effects; if treatment is not really necessary (this is probably true for 99 percent of these individuals), this may be an almost unacceptable price to pay. Conversely, even if the risk is numerically limited, what is at stake is the patient's life. The decision of whether to treat or not to treat should not be the responsibility of the physician alone. I always discuss the options extensively with the parents or with the patient if he or she is an adult; only after careful exposition of current knowledge of the condition and the therapy do I indicate my personal position.

I suggest treatment of asymptomatic LQTS patients in five conditions only. For those with congenital deafness, because of the demonstrated increased risk of a cardiac event in this subgroup; for neonates and during the first year of life, because of enhanced risk during the first few months of life of a lethal event that would then be labeled as sudden infant death syndrome or crib death; for siblings of children affected by LQTS who died suddenly because of the obvious emotional situation present in the family; for those patients who are unlikely, for whatever reason, to take oral medication regularly and continuously as is necessary with LQTS; and whenever there is manifest anxiety or an explicit request for treatment after a thorough explanation and discussion with the family. In the remaining situations, after having instructed family members in cardiopulmonary resuscitation and particularly in the importance and efficacy of thump-version, I favor a conservative approach. In this choice I feel supported by the large percentage of family members with prolonged Q-T intervals who remain asymptomatic for their entire lives, by the fact that the overwhelming majority of patients survive the first syncope episode, and by the significantly better quality of life achieved in the absence of lifelong daily medications. In this always difficult choice, I am supported by a system that does not encourage medicolegal litigation and that allows me to make purely medical choices considering only what, to the best of my knowledge, is in the best interest of the patient.

SUGGESTED READING

Cranefield PF, Aronson RS. Cardiac arrhythmias: The role of triggered activity and other mechanisms. Mount Kisco, NY: Futura, 1988:553–579.

Moss AJ, Schwartz PJ, Crampton RS, et al. The long QT syndrome: A prospective international study. Circulation 1985; 71:17–21.

Schwartz PJ. The rationale and the role of left stellectomy for the prevention of malignant arrhythmias. Ann NY Acad Sci 1984; 427:199–221.

Schwartz PJ. The idiopathic long QT syndrome: Progress and questions. Am Heart J 1985; 109:399–411.

Schwartz PJ, Locati E, Priori SG, Zaza A. The idiopathic long QT syndrome. In: Zipes DP, Jalife J, eds. Cardiac electrophysiology. From cell to bedside. Philadelphia: WB Saunders, 1990: 779–797.

Schwartz PJ, Periti M, Malliani A. The long QT syndrome. Am Heart J 1975; 89:378–390.

ARRHYTHMOGENIC RIGHT VENTRICULAR DYSPLASIA

FRANK I. MARCUS, M.D.
LIONEL FAITELSON, M.D.
WILLIAM SCOTT, M.D.

Arrhythmogenic right ventricular dysplasia (ARVD) is an unusual disease in which ventricular arrhythmias are associated with a predominantly right-sided cardiomyopathy.

HISTORICAL ASPECTS

In 1905, William Osler described a heart with "parchment-like" thinning of both auricles and ventricles, the right side more dilated than the left, in the absence of any abnormality or obstruction of the coronary arteries. This heart belonged to a man in his 40s who died suddenly while walking uphill. In 1952, Uhl described a 7-month-old girl who had severe right-sided congestive heart failure and marked thinning of the right ventricular wall. Since then there have been numerous case reports of patients with localized or diffuse myocardial contraction abnormalities of the right ventricle associated with ventricular arrhythmias. In adults, pathologic examination usually does not show the translucent, parchment-like myocardium; rather the myocardium is largely replaced by fatty tissue, and the thickness of the right ventricular wall may not be diminished. Fontaine and colleagues in France described these patients as having right ventricular dysplasia. The relationship between right ventricular dysplasia and "parchment" heart as described by Osler and by Uhl is not clear. It is possible that the marked thinning of the right ventricle that may involve a large portion of the myocardium is an extreme form of right ventricular dysplasia. The extensive right ventricular involvement may result in congestive heart failure during early infancy. Patients with right ventricular dysplasia may have a lesser degree of involvement of the right ventricle, allowing them to reach adult life. It is also possible that Uhl's anomaly and right ventricular dysplasia represent distinct and different pathologic entities.

ETIOLOGY AND PATHOGENESIS

The cause of ARVD is not known. The familial occurrence of ARVD in nine families led Nava and colleagues to conclude that the disease may be a genetic condition with autosomal dominance and variable expression and penetrance. However, most patients with this condition do not have a familial history of sudden death or arrhythmias. The ventricular arrhythmias are usually not symptomatic until patients are in their teens or older. This raises the possibility that some patients with ARVD may inherit the predisposition to progressive right ventricular myocardial degeneration that is the substrate for reentrant ventricular arrhythmias. It has been speculated that ventricular arrhythmias associated with this condition may be aggravated by regular participation in athletics. Many patients with ARVD either are competitive athletes or participate in athletics regularly. Exercise may cause an increase in the dilation of the right ventricle that would enhance the predisposition to ventricular arrhythmias.

It is also possible that some patients with the sporadic form of this condition may have had infectious myocarditis predominantly affecting the right ventricle. With degeneration of some myocardial fibers, the substrate for ventricular arrhythmias develops. This sequence has been documented in case reports.

CLINICAL PRESENTATION

Patients with ARVD may become aware of their condition by the incidental finding of cardiac enlargement on routine chest x-ray film, by the appearance of ventricular ectopy on routine electrocardiogram, or by the onset of symptomatic arrhythmias. Patients with ARVD described in the literature during the 1960s and 1970s commonly presented with transient or sustained ventricular tachycardia. Recently, it has been recognized that this condition may be an important cause of sudden unexpected death in younger individuals. In a postmortem study from northern Italy, 20 percent of 60 patients under the age of 35 years who died suddenly and unexpectedly and who were examined after death had histologic findings consistent with ARVD. In five patients, sudden death was the first manifestation of cardiac disease. A large proportion of the deaths (10 of 12) occurred during physical exertion. Several of the larger series of patients with right ventricular dysplasia included patients who were resuscitated from ventricular fibrillation, this being their initial clinical presentation. The incidence of right ventricular dysplasia as a cause of arrhythmic death in younger individuals may now be better assessed since ARVD has become well recognized.

One should suspect the presence of right ventricular dysplasia as a cause of ventricular arrhythmias or syncope in a patient who has no apparent heart disease. The suspicion is heightened if the patient is a male, since this condition is more prevalent in men. The ventricular ectopy usually arises from the right ventricular free wall and has a left bundle branch block configuration. The QRS axis during ventricular tachycardia is between −90 and +120 degrees.

An extreme rightward direction of the QRS axis during ventricular tachycardia is uncommon. Adult patients with right ventricular dysplasia who have ventricular tachycardia usually have abnormal T-wave inversion in the right precordial leads (Fig. 1). The extent of the precordial T-wave inversion has been correlated with the degree of right ventricular enlargement. At the end of the QRS complex, especially in leads V_1 to V_3, a sharp spike in the S-T segment may be seen (Fig. 2). This has been termed the postexcitation or epsilon wave and probably represents delayed depolarization of some parts of the right ventricle.

Physical examination is not diagnostic. Careful inspection of the precordium may show asymmetry with prominence of the left precordium, indicating that considerable right ventricular enlargement occurred during early childhood. A fourth heart sound may be heard as well as a third heart sound. The chest x-ray film showed cardiac enlargement in 16 of 22 patients described by Marcus and coworkers. The configuration of the heart was globular.

Confirmation of the diagnosis of right ventricular dysplasia consists of establishing that the right ventricle is abnormal by noninvasive means, including echocardiography and radionuclide angiography, or by invasive testing, including right ventricular angiography and/or myocardial biopsy. The difficulty of confirming this diagnosis can be appreciated if it is considered that the overall size and function of

the right ventricle may be normal and that the only clue to confirm the diagnosis of ARVD may be the finding of localized wall motion abnormalities in the right ventricle, a chamber that normally has an irregular and complex configuration.

ECHOCARDIOGRAPHIC EVALUATION OF ARVD

Earlier studies using echocardiography relied on the ratio of right ventricular–left ventricular diameter for diagnostic purposes. Although it is difficult to measure the absolute diameter of the right ventricle, Manyari and associates showed that a right ventricular–left ventricular *end-systolic* volume ratio greater than 1.5 had a sensitivity of 86 percent and a specificity of 97 percent in a group of patients suspected of having right ventricular dysplasia. A right ventricular–left-ventricular *end-diastolic* volume ratio greater than 1.8 had a sensitivity of 100 percent and a specificity of 97 percent. Recently a standardized approach to the examination of the right ventricle was proposed by Foale and coworkers. The right ventricle was examined by two-dimensional (2-D) echocardiography in an ordered series of transducer locations and orientations. Diastolic measurements were made of the right ventricular inflow tract, outflow tract, and right ventricular body, and a range of normal values for cavity size

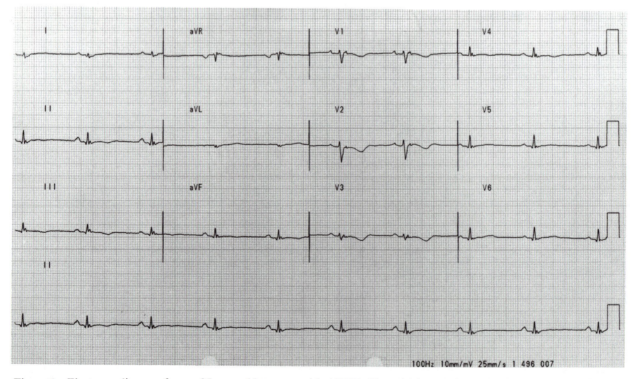

100Hz 10mm/mV 25mm/s 1 496 007

Figure 1 Electrocardiogram from a 25-year-old woman with ARVD. Note the inverted T waves in leads V_1 through V_4.

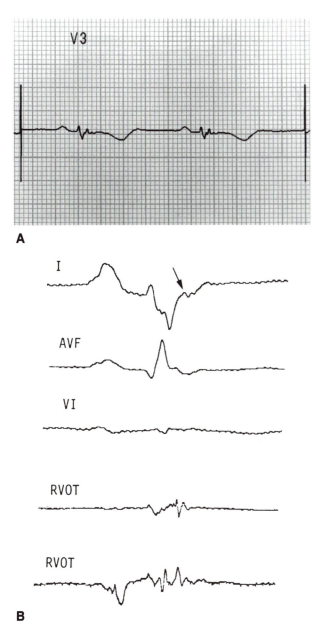

A

B

Figure 2 *A*, Enlargement of V₃ lead from the same electrocardiogram as in Figure 1. Observe the sharp spikes appearing at the end of the QRS complex. These are epsilon waves. *B*, Tracings obtained during an electrophysiologic study in the same patient. The bottom tracing is from the two distal catheter poles (1 and 2) in the right ventricular outflow tract (RVOT). The tracing immediately above is from the middle poles (2 and 3) of the same quadripolar catheter. Note that the late fractionated potentials in the RVOT correspond to the epsilon wave (*arrow*) in lead I.

and right ventricular wall thickness was established. Additional criteria for the echocardiographic diagnosis of right ventricular dysplasia are right ventricular contraction abnormalities, which may be segmental. It should be evident that an adequate 2-D examination to detect right ventricular dysplasia re-

quires special attention to detail and a thorough evaluation of the various portions of the right ventricle. Using these detailed measurements and analyses, echocardiographic examination appears to be quite sensitive for the diagnosis of right ventricular dysplasia. However, this technique is not specific for this condition. Other abnormalities that may be confused with right ventricular dysplasia by echocardiography include ischemic heart disease, tricuspid regurgitation, and pulmonary heart disease. Difficulty in assessment of the precise sensitivity and specificity of echocardiographic examination for the diagnosis of right ventricular dysplasia is due to lack of an accepted gold standard for comparison. When the clinician requests echocardiographic evaluation of a patient with suspected right ventricular dysplasia, the echocardiographer needs to perform a thorough study focusing on the dimensions as well as the presence of right ventricular contraction abnormalities in multiple chamber planes. Some of the patients may have an abnormality confined only to one segment. A "routine study" is likely to lack sensitivity for this diagnosis.

Radioisotopic diagnosis of right ventricular dysplasia has utilized evaluation of right ventricular ejection fraction at rest and/or with exercise, semiquantitative assessment of right ventricular wall motion abnormalities, or right ventricle–left ventricle ratio. One difficulty in utilizing specific values for identifying decreased right ventricular function is that different normal values for right ventricular ejection fraction at rest are reported ranging from 43 ± 6 percent to 67 ± 5 percent. Biplane cineangiography right ventricular ejection fraction is greater than 60 percent in normals. Although it is not clear why the "normal" scintigraphic right ventricular ejection fraction is as much as 20 percent lower than that assessed by angiographic criteria, it is difficult to extrapolate data from the literature and apply it to different laboratories. Also, until recently quantitative assessment of regional wall motion has not been possible. Manyari and coworkers assessed the value of radionuclide cardiac scintigraphy for the diagnosis of right ventricular dysplasia in 14 patients with this condition compared with 30 patients who did not have this condition, determined by cardiac catheterization and right ventricular angiography. Using the multigated blood pool method at rest and exercise for both right ventricular and left ventricular assessment, they determined that the normal right ventricular ejection fraction at rest was 49 ± 6 percent; with exercise it increased to 60 ± 5 percent. Segmental right ventricular function was evaluated using a visual method. End diastolic and systolic right ventricular–left ventricular volumes were calculated as the ratios between the normalized right ventricular–left ventricular counts in the end-diastolic and end-systolic frames, respectively. All patients with right ventricular dysplasia were identified by a scintigraphic right ventricular ejection fraction of less than 50 percent during exercise, a right ventricular wall motion abnormality during exercise, or a right ventricular–left ventricular end-diastolic volume ratio greater than 1.8. These variables had 100 percent sensitivity and a negative predictive value of 100 percent. For these three variables the specificity was 90 percent, 97 percent, and 97 percent, respectively, and positive predictive values were 81 percent, 93 percent, and 93 percent. All patients with right ventricular dysplasia who had cardiac scintigraphy did not increase their right ventricular ejection fraction by more than 6 percent.

All cardiac scintigraphic findings of right ventricular dysplasia except for wall motion abnormalities indicate poor right ventricular function and can be seen with a generalized cardiomyopathy. Marked decrease in right ventricular function in the presence of normal or nearly normal left ventricular function in a patient with ventricular tachycardia of left bundle branch block configuration is consistent with this diagnosis. It should be mentioned that wall motion abnormalities seen at rest should be confirmed during exercise, since apparent hypokinesis at rest may not be present with exercise. The high sensitivity and specificity and the predictive accuracy reported by Manyari for the diagnosis of right ventricular dysplasia need to be confirmed utilizing quantitative assessment of right ventricular function.

OTHER NONINVASIVE TECHNIQUES

Magnetic resonance imaging of the heart may play an important role in the diagnosis of right ventricular dysplasia. This technique provides anatomic information regarding the size of the right ventricle, right ventricular wall thickness, and the presence of fatty replacement of myocardial tissue. Fatty tissue yields a bright image compared with myocardial muscle. By this means, it should be possible to delineate not only the presence of right ventricular dysplasia but also to document the extent of the pathologic process.

RIGHT VENTRICULAR ANGIOGRAPHY

Right ventricular angiography is considered the gold standard in the diagnosis of an increase in size or abnormality of wall motion in patients suspected of having right ventricular dysplasia. Assessing enlargement of the right ventricle is difficult because of its complex geometric shape. Right ventricular volume can be assessed accurately using computer techniques and Simpson's rule. A method described by Ferlinz is simpler and is based on the model of the right ventricle as a pyramid with a triangular base. The accuracy of this model has been verified by

correlation with casts from human hearts. Biplane angiography is performed in the 30-degree right anterior oblique and 60-degree left anterior oblique views, although only the right anterior oblique view is necessary. It is important to obtain excellent opacification of the right ventricle by the use of a Berman balloon catheter placed in the midportion of the right ventricular inflow tract. A test injection of 10 ml of saline is given. If ventricular ectopy is triggered, the catheter is withdrawn until a nonarrhythmic location is found.

Angiographic findings of right ventricular dysplasia include parietal fissuring of the right ventricular wall distal to the moderator band, stagnation of contrast agent in the inferior wall persisting until opacification of the left ventricle, irregular opacification of the right ventricular infundibulum, and increased right ventricular volume. None of these findings has absolute sensitivity or specificity; however, localized akinetic or dyskinetic bulges appear to be the most specific finding. An additional concern regarding the reliability of right ventricular angiography is the observation that assessment of right ventricular dimensions, contractility, and regional wall motion may vary among observers.

MYOCARDIAL BIOPSY AND HISTOPATHOLOGY

The diagnosis of ARVD by endomyocardial biopsy lacks sensitivity because the typical pathologic changes described below are present in the right ventricular free wall and may not be seen in the right ventricular septum, the usual site of endomyocardial biopsy.

Histopathology

The pathologic hallmark of right ventricular dysplasia is a large amount of fatty tissue in the right ventricular myocardium and a paucity of myocardial fibers. In a typical case the right ventricular myocardium is 1-mm thick in comparison with the normal myocardial thickness of 3 to 4 mm. The muscle fibers, although hypertrophied, are well preserved in the subendocardial region. In the media, the muscle myofibrils interdigitate between fat and fibrotic tissue, and a large number of arterioles may be present. These may be of larger diameter than is expected in normal cardiac adipose tissue. The arterioles may be normal or may show medial proliferation. There may be patchy areas of subendocardial fibrosis. This pathologic picture may be caused by degeneration of myocardial fibers with replacement by fat. The abnormalities described in the right ventricle are not uniformly present. They are mainly located in those areas that have been termed "the triangle of dysplasia," that is, the infundibulum, the apex, and the diaphragmatic zone located below the tricuspid valve.

The left ventricle may be involved in the pathologic process but the histologic appearance is different from that of the right ventricle in that there may be large amounts of fibrous tissue. Recently electron microscopic examination of the right ventricle in this condition has shown abnormal intercalated disks in both right and left ventricles. These disks are attenuated and flattened with a decrease in Z-band material. The specificity of this finding for ARVD has not been clearly established.

MEDICAL THERAPY

There has not been a systematic evaluation of antiarrhythmic drug therapy in ARVD. It appears that amiodarone alone or in conjunction with class I antiarrhythmic drugs is the most effective regimen in preventing recurrent sustained ventricular tachycardia. It should be stressed that a wide variety of antiarrhythmic drugs alone or in combination have been found to be effective in preventing ventricular tachycardia recurrence or in slowing the ventricular rate. Membrane-active drugs in combination with a beta-adrenergic blocking drug are especially effective in preventing recurrent ventricular tachycardia that is induced by exercise.

INTRACARDIAC ABLATION

Patients whose recurrence of ventricular arrhythmias cannot be prevented by antiarrhythmic drugs are candidates for attempted ablation with direct current (DC) energy. Fontaine as well as others have reported successful control of ventricular arrhythmias in the majority of patients with ARVD in whom this therapy has been tried. This procedure may have to be repeated two or more times to achieve satisfactory results, defined as elimination of recurrent ventricular tachycardia or modification of the rate of the arrhythmia so that it is sufficiently slow and/or self-terminating in order to permit the patient a normal lifestyle. Ablation may result in freedom from symptomatic arrhythmias without the need for antiarrhythmic drugs, but many patients require continuation of antiarrhythmic drugs in order to control the arrhythmia. There has been concern that DC ablation may be particularly hazardous because of the possibility of right ventricular rupture caused by thinning of the right ventricular free wall in some patients with this condition. Of the 30 reported patients with ARVD who have had this procedure, there have been no deaths attributable to right ventricular rupture. However, two patients died of cardiogenic shock during the procedure. It is advisable not to use DC energies greater than 250

joules with any one shock. It may be safer to use the catheter tip as the cathode, since there is less barotrauma during DC ablation than if the catheter is the anode. An adhesive thoracic posterior electrode is usually used as the anode.

SURGICAL TREATMENT

Two surgical procedures have been used to treat patients with ARVD who have ventricular tachycardia that is refractory to medical therapy. The procedure first described is that of simple ventriculotomy and was performed by Guiraudon and colleagues in 12 patients between 1971 and 1983. During open-chest surgery ventricular tachycardia was induced, and the earliest electrical activation during ventricular tachycardia was identified. Several ventricular incisions were made in this region. The ventriculotomy procedure was successful in preventing recurrent ventricular tachycardia in most patients, but at least 3 of 15 patients have had late recurrence of ventricular tachycardia. The recurrences are understandable because this condition is not limited to one region of the right ventricle, and recurrences from other locations of diseased ventricle can be expected.

Another surgical procedure is that of disconnecting the right ventricle, thus isolating ventricular tachycardia or fibrillation to the right ventricle. This procedure is predicated on the hypothesis that the right ventricle is not needed to maintain adequate left ventricular hemodynamic function. The safety and hemodynamic consequences of this procedure were first studied in dogs, after which Guiraudon performed total disconnection of the right ventricular free wall in five patients. One patient died at surgery of malignant hyperthermia, one died 4 years later of congestive heart failure, and the other three have been free of recurrent ventricular tachycardia. However, the long-term outlook is guarded because of marked right ventricular dilatation. This raises the possibility that gradual right ventricular failure may be an inevitable outcome of this procedure. Since there is no ideal surgical procedure for these patients, cardiac transplantation has been considered for the rare patient with right ventricular dysplasia who has recurrent incapacitating ventricular tachycardia or ventricular fibrillation despite medical treatment, including attempts at right ventricular ablation.

LONG-TERM OUTLOOK FOR PATIENTS WITH RIGHT VENTRICULAR DYSPLASIA

In general, patients with right ventricular dysplasia have a prognosis considerably better than patients with sustained ventricular tachycardia of left ventricular origin. This observation is probably related to better hemodynamic tolerance of ventricular tachycardia because of good left ventricular function with less likelihood of degeneration to ventricular fibrillation. Patients with right ventricular dysplasia who present with or who have recurrent syncope seem to have a worse long-term outlook than those who do not have this symptom. It would appear that if ventricular tachycardia can be prevented or if ventricular tachycardia recurs at a rate that is well tolerated, sudden cardiac death is uncommon.

SUGGESTED READING

Blomstrom-Lundqvist C. Thesis: The syndrome of arrhythmogenic right ventricular dysplasia—diagnostic and prognostic implications. Goteborg, Sweden, 1987.

Daubert C, Descaves C, Foulgoc JL, et al. Critical analysis of cineangiographic criteria for diagnosis of arrhythmogenic right ventricular dysplasia. Am Heart J 1988; 115:448–459.

Ferlinz J. Right ventricular function in adult cardiovascular disease. Prog Cardiovasc Dis 1982; 25:225–267.

Foale RA, Nihoyannopoulos P, Ribeiro P, et al. Right ventricular abnormalities in ventricular tachycardia of right ventricular origin: Relation to electrophysiological abnormalities. Br Heart J 1986; 56:45–54.

Fontaine G, Fontaliran F, Linares-Cruz E, et al. The arrhythmogenic right ventricle. In: Iwa T, Fontaine G, eds. Cardiac arrhythmias: Recent progress in investigation and management. The Hague: Elsevier Science Pub, 1988:189.

Fontaine G, Guiraudon G, Frank R, et al. Stimulation studies and epicardial mapping in ventricular tachycardia: Study of

mechanisms and selection for surgery. In: Kulbertus HE, ed. Reentrant arrhythmias. Lancaster: MTP Publications, 1977:334.

Hasumi M, Sekiguchi M, Hiroe M, et al. Endomyocardial biopsy approach to patients with ventricular tachycardia with special reference to arrhythmogenic right ventricular dysplasia. Jpn Circ J 1987; 51:242–249.

Jones DL, Guiraudon GM, Klein GJ. Total disconnection of the right ventricular free wall: Physiological consequences in the dog. Am Heart J 1984; 107:1169–1177.

Leclercq JF, Chouty F, Cauchemez B, et al. Results of electrical fulguration in arrhythmogenic right ventricular disease. Am J Cardiol 1988; 62:220–224.

Manyari DE, Duff HJ, Kostuk WJ, et al. Usefulness of noninvasive studies for diagnosis of right ventricular dysplasia. Am J Cardiol 1986; 57:1147–1153.

Marcus FI, Fontaine GH, Guiraudon G, et al. Right ventricular dysplasia: A report of 24 adult cases. Circulation 1982; 65:384–398.

Nava A, Thiene G, Canciani B, et al. Familial occurrence of right ventricular dysplasia: A study involving nine families. J Am Coll Cardiol 1988; 12:1222–1228.

Rizzon P, Breithardt G, Chiddo A, eds. Arrhythmogenic right ventricle. Eur Heart J 1989; 10(Suppl 10):81–106.

Segall HN. Parchment heart (Osler). Am Heart J 1950; 40:948–950.

Sugrue DD, Edwards WD, Olney BA. Histologic abnormalities of the left ventricle in a patient with arrhythmogenic right ventricular dysplasia. Heart Vessels 1985; 1:179–181.

Thiene G, Nava A, Corrado D, et al. Right ventricular cardiomyopathy and sudden death in young people. N Engl J Med 1988; 318:129–133.

Uhl HS. A previously undescribed congenital malformation of the heart: Almost total absence of the myocardium of the right ventricle. Bull Johns Hopkins Hosp 1972; 91:197–209.

EXERCISE AND CATECHOLAMINE-INDUCED VENTRICULAR ARRHYTHMIAS

ROSS J. SIMPSON, JR, M.D.
ALAN WOELFEL, M.D.
JAMES R. FOSTER, M.D.

In 1932, Wilson described a 31-year-old American farmer admitted to the University of Michigan Hospital for evaluation of a 7-year history of exercise-induced palpitations, breathlessness, and syncope. His past medical history was unremarkable for any record of rheumatic or coronary heart disease, and physical examination and chest x-ray films did not reveal any obvious cardiac abnormalities. An electrocardiogram showed T-wave inversions in leads II and III and isolated premature ventricular complexes. Exercise testing induced six consecutive premature complexes on one occasion and a 25-

minute monomorphic, ventricular tachycardia at a rate of 200 bpm on another occasion. Treatment with quinidine improved his symptoms, but he died suddenly several months following hospital discharge.

Since this original description of exercise-induced ventricular tachycardia, we have learned much about the diagnosis, mechanism, and treatment of most forms of ventricular tachycardia. However, ventricular tachycardia induced by exercise or by catecholamines remains a poorly understood form. The absence of an effective taxonomy for the diverse ventricular arrhythmias induced by exercise contributes to the confusion surrounding these arrhythmias. Exercise- and catecholamine-induced arrhythmias are a diverse group of arrhythmias occurring by means of a variety of physiologic mechanisms. Multiple types of ventricular arrhythmias, including frequent or complex ventricular ectopy and ventricular fibrillation, may all occur in susceptible patients during exercise or intense emotional stress. Wilson's patient represents a classic presentation for exercise-induced ventricular tachycardia. However, in modern practice, exercise-induced ventricular tachyarrhythmias may be seen in isolation or in combination with ventricular arrhythmias occurring at times of low catecholamine stimulation. The components of exercise and catecholamine stimulation that may precipitate arrhythmias in these patients may include increased heart rate, segmental myocardial ischemia in patients with critical stenosis of a major coronary artery, and direct effects of catecholamines on electrical properties of dysfunctional cardiac fibers.

In this section, we present our personal taxonomy of these diverse arrhythmias and our personal approach to diagnostic testing and treatment of patients with exercise- or catecholamine-induced arrhythmias.

FREQUENT OR COMPLEX VENTRICULAR ECTOPY

Frequent or complex ventricular ectopy during or immediately following exercise is a common occurrence in both asymptomatic populations screened by treadmill exercise tests and in patients undergoing diagnostic testing for suspected coronary artery disease. These arrhythmias are variable in their induction with exercise, and serial exercise testing often fails to reproduce them reliably. Approximately 7 percent of asymptomatic, apparently healthy adults will develop ventricular ectopy of up to nine ventricular complexes in any 1-minute interval during exercise or up to three consecutive ventricular premature complexes on a single exercise test. The prevalence of these ventricular arrhythmias appears to increase with a person's age and is more common in men than in women. However, over short-term follow-up these arrhythmias do not increase the risk to the patient of myocardial infarction, development of angina pectoris, syncope, or sudden death.

Similar results are seen in patients suspected of having ischemic heart disease. In these patients, exercise-induced frequent ventricular couplets or ventricular tachycardia of three or more consecutive complexes during exercise testing is most likely in patients with abnormal left ventricular function or extensive coronary artery disease. These arrhythmias may carry a worse 3-year survival risk to patients. However, they do not appear to add independent risk over that predicted from the extent of coronary artery disease, the ejection fraction, and myocardial contraction abnormalities noted at cardiac catheterization. Thus, these arrhythmias are probably markers for left ventricular dysfunction or high-grade coronary artery obstruction.

For this reason, in patients who do not have symptoms referable to their arrhythmia, we often recommend against specific therapy or diagnostic testing aimed at treating frequent ventricular ectopy, pairs, or triplets of premature ventricular complexes. Rather, we direct our efforts at uncovering and optimizing treatment for underlying ischemic heart disease, left ventricular dysfunction, systemic hypertension, and left ventricular hypertrophy. In addition, we review the patient's medications for drugs that may potentiate arrhythmias.

Repeat exercise testing following therapy is often prudent, since a second test may reveal a more sustained, symptomatic tachyarrhythmia. However, since the reproducibility of these arrhythmias is often poor, the efficacy of any therapy cannot be judged by serial exercise testing. If frequent ectopy reoccurs during exercise despite optimal treatment for ischemia, electrolyte abnormalities, and left ventricular function, and if proarrhythmic effects of antiarrhythmic drugs have been excluded as a cause of the arrhythmia, additional therapy for the arrhythmia is not prescribed.

VENTRICULAR FIBRILLATION, TORSADES DE POINTES, AND POLYMORPHIC VENTRICULAR TACHYCARDIA

Fortunately, these life-threatening ventricular arrhythmias are rare during exercise testing. The cause of these arrhythmias is varied; they may be due to myocardial ischemia provoked by exercise or congenital or to acquired ventricular repolarization abnormalities. In patients with ischemia, ventricular fibrillation is often preceded by hypotension or failure of systolic blood pressure to increase appropriately during exercise. In these patients, severe three-vessel coronary disease or obstruction of the main left coronary artery is often found at cardiac catheterization. In patients with repolarization abnormalities, the Q-T interval may be long at rest or may not shorten appropriately with exercise. Antiarrhythmic drugs such as quinidine as well as other drugs may cause such repolarization abnormalities.

In patients in whom antiarrhythmic drugs, electrolyte abnormalities, or other causes of repolarization abnormalities cannot be implicated, aggressive diagnostic testing to identify myocardial ischemia as the cause of the arrhythmias is recommended. If myocardial ischemia is present, it should be aggressively treated with coronary artery bypass surgery. Coronary angioplasty is usually not recommended because the 25 to 30 percent early restenosis rate may place these patients at risk of recurrent, possibly fatal arrhythmia. Pharmacologic anti-ischemic therapy is probably too unreliable in view of the potentially fatal outcomes of unsuccessful treatment. Repeat and usually serial exercise testing following surgery to document consistent absence of the arrhythmia, as well as to demonstrate control of ischemia, is also mandatory because of the life-threatening nature of the rhythm disturbance.

The advisability of preoperative electrophysiologic study depends on the status of left ventricular function. If the patient does not have a segmental contraction abnormality on ventriculography, induction of a clinically relevant ventricular arrhythmia is unlikely. However, preoperative electrophysiologic testing is recommended when a discrete wall motion abnormality or aneurysm is present, because such patients may be susceptible to ventricular arrhythmias in the absence of acute ischemia. Induction of a clinically important ventricular tachyarrhythmia may modify the surgical procedure to include aneurysmectomy, electrophysiologic mapping, cryoablation, or application of epicardial patches for subsequent implantation of an automatic defibrillator.

SUSTAINED MONOMORPHIC VENTRICULAR TACHYCARDIA

As with Wilson's patient, this arrhythmia may be the sole or initial manifestation of a cardiac abnormality. It may also occur in patients with previously known organic heart disease including coronary artery disease, cardiomyopathy, sarcodosis, or valvular heart disease. Some patients have cardiac disease at autopsy that is not diagnosed clinically. However, it rarely occurs as a consequence of acute ischemia. A minority of these patients may also have ventricular tachycardia at rest or at times of minimal sympathetic stimulation.

The pathophysiologic basis for the arrhythmia is varied. The rhythm appears to be due to abnormal sensitivity of the heart to increased catecholamines during exercise, since patients do not have abnormally high resting or exercise-induced serum norepinephrine levels. Catecholamines may induce delayed afterdepolarizations or enhance abnormal automaticity in diseased cardiac fibers. Afterdepolarizations are strongly suspected of causing many of these arrhythmias, since arrhythmia induction may be provoked by isoproterenol as well as exercise, and the rhythm responds both to beta-blocking drugs and calcium-channel blocking drugs.

One common form of exercise-induced ventricular tachycardia is repetitive monomorphic tachycardia. Patients with this arrhythmia tend to be young or in their middle years of life with no identifiable disease. Ventricular tachycardia tends to occur in multiple, nonsustained paroxysms of uniform morphology. A left bundle branch block configuration with either a normal or a right axis is common. Although repetitive monomorphic ventricular tachycardia may occur in some patients at rest and at times of low catecholamine stimulation, it most

often manifests during exercise or immediately after stopping exercise. This rhythm is generally well tolerated by the patient and generally breaks spontaneously as adrenergic tone subsides. The prognosis appears to be excellent, and treatment appears to be necessary only for relief of symptoms. Treatment with verapamil or beta blocking drugs is generally efficacious for arrhythmias occurring at rest and arrhythmias provoked by exercise.

Our approach to the management of patients with exercise-induced ventricular tachycardia depends on whether the rhythm appears in isolation, i.e., in the absence of ventricular tachycardia not brought on by exercise or catecholamines, and whether there is present obvious organic heart disease or a cardiac myocardial contraction abnormality. A history of symptoms not associated with exercise, a history of angina, myocardial infarction, sustained or nonsustained ventricular tachycardia noted on Holter monitor or cardiac contraction abnormalities often prompt electrophysiologic testing. If electrophysiologic testing induces a clinically important arrhythmia, treatment based on the electrophysiologic study is undertaken. However, arrhythmias induced by electrophysiologic testing and those arrhythmias induced by exercise or catecholamine infusion may be two distinct arrhythmias, and additional treatment of the latter arrhythmia based on serial exercise testing or isuprel infusion may be necessary.

Management

Prior to treating exercise-induced ventricular tachycardia, the reproducibility of arrhythmia induction must be determined. In 60 to 70 percent of patients, this arrhythmia is reproducible on serial exercise testing. Serial exercise testing is appropriate and safe, since cardiac arrest and the need for resuscitation are rare in the absence of severe, acute ischemia. If the rhythm cannot be reproduced on two consecutive exercise tests, induction is attempted by infusion of isoproterenol. Isoproterenol is infused at a rate of 1 μg per minute with an increase in infusion rate by 1 μg per minute every 3 minutes. The infusion is stopped when the rhythm is reproduced, side effects limit the infusion, or an infusion rate of 5 μg per minute is achieved. Isoproterenol infusion is often less efficient in reproducing symptomatic exercise-induced ventricular arrhythmias than exercise. However, it serves as a useful adjunct to diagnostic testing, particularly if the induction of the arrhythmia is variable on serial exercise testing.

In patients with reproducible exercise-induced ventricular tachycardia, beta blockade prevents recurrent episodes in most patients. In many of these patients success correlates with preventing achievement of the sinus rate during maximal exercise associated with induction of tachycardia. It is essential to exercise these patients to maximum capacity, since submaximal exercise may be misleading by failing to reveal continued susceptibility to ventricular tachycardia.

The dose of beta-blocking drug necessary to control the arrhythmia varies but may be as high as 400 mg per day of propranolol or its equivalent. Efficacy as well as side effects of a high-dose beta-blocking drug should be assessed by serial exercise testing. Verapamil may also be effective in controlling exercise-induced ventricular tachycardia, particularly repetitive monomorphic ventricular tachycardia. Except in this latter arrhythmia, verapamil may be slightly less effective than beta-blocking drugs in controlling exercise-induced ventricular tachycardia. However, fewer side effects of verapamil and its ability to preserve exercise capacity make this drug an inviting alternative in patients without a history of syncope or with contraindications to or serious side effects from beta-blocking drugs. Patients without detectable heart disease are also more likely to respond to verapamil. Dosages of verapamil to control the arrhythmia may be as high as 320 mg every 8 hours.

Exercise- and catecholamine-induced ventricular arrhythmias comprise a variety of arrhythmias occurring by a variety of pathophysiologic mechanisms. Therapy should be aimed at precisely defining the type of rhythm disturbance being treated, defining its reproducibility and assessing the presence and extent of underlying heart disease. Severe myocardial ischemia may cause relatively low grades of ventricular ectopy and, rarely, ventricular fibrillation. In these cases, therapy should be directed at the ischemia, not primarily at the arrhythmia. In contrast, monomorphic ventricular tachycardia induced by exercise is rarely caused by acute ischemia, although it may occur in patients with chronic coronary disease. Many patients with exercise-induced or monomorphic ventricular tachycardia have no detectable heart disease, in which case the prognosis may be good. The best therapy for exercise-induced monomorphic ventricular tachycardia appears to involve use of a beta blocking drug or verapamil. However, even in these patients, the underlying mechanism of the tachycardia is variable and other ventricular rhythms may be present along with serious organic heart disease. It is essential to undertake diagnostic testing to define the type of underlying organic heart disease, to perform serial exercise testing and possibly electrophysiologic study to establish reproducibility of the ventricular tachycardia, and to document arrhythmia control with therapy.

SUGGESTED READING

Busby MJ, Shefrin EA, Fleg JL. Prevalence and long-term significance of exercise-induced frequent or repetitive ventricular ectopic beats in apparently healthy volunteers. J Am Coll Cardiol 1989; 14:1659–1665.

Califf RM, McKinnis RA, McNeer JF, et al. Prognostic value of ventricular arrhythmias associated with treadmill exercise testing in patients studied with cardiac catheterization for suspected ischemic heart disease. J Am Coll Cardiol 1983; 2:1060–1067.

Hong RA, Bhandari AK, McKay CR, et al. Life-threatening ventricular tachycardia and fibrillation induced by painless myocardial ischemia during exercise testing. JAMA 1987; 257:1937–1940.

Rasmussen K, Lunde PI, Lie M. Coronary bypass surgery in exercise-induced ventricular tachycardia. Eur Heart J 1987; 8:444–448.

Sokoloff NM, Spielman SR, Greenspan AM, et al. Plasma norepinephrine in exercise-induced ventricular tachycardia. J Am Coll Cardiol 1986; 8:11–17.

Wilson FN, Wishart SW, McLeod AG, Barker PS. A clinical type of paroxysmal tachycardia of ventricular origin in which paroxysms are induced by exertion. Am Heart J 1932; 8:155–169.

Woelfel A, Foster JR, Simpson RJ Jr, Gettes LS. Reproducibility and treatment of exercise-induced ventricular tachycardia. Am J Cardiol 1984; 53:751–756.

Woelfel A, Foster JR, McAllister RG, et al. Efficacy of verapamil in exercise-induced ventricular tachycardia. Am J Cardiol 1985; 56:292–297.

VENTRICULAR ARRHYTHMIAS IN PEDIATRIC PATIENTS WITH AND WITHOUT CONGENITAL HEART DISEASE

VICTORIA L. VETTER, M.D.

Although ventricular arrhythmias have been considered uncommon in children, such patients are no longer unusual in the practice of pediatric cardiology. The increase in the incidence of ventricular arrhythmias in some of these patients is only apparent and is related to increased surveillance with newer monitoring techniques, including in-hospital monitoring, long-term ambulatory monitoring, and transtelephonic monitoring. The use of provocative tests, such as exercise stress testing or electrophysiologic studies, also has increased the identification of these patients. On the other hand, there has been a real increase in ventricular arrhythmias because of longer survival of patients with congenital or acquired heart defects as a result of recent medical and surgical advances, especially in the field of congenital heart surgery.

Ventricular arrhythmias include ventricular premature complexes (VPCs)—otherwise known as ventricular extrasystoles or ventricular premature beats (VPBs)—ventricular tachycardia, ventricular fibrillation, and accelerated ventricular rhythms.

Management of children with ventricular arrhythmias requires correct diagnosis, awareness of the manifestations of these arrhythmias, an understanding of the associated conditions, and knowledge of appropriate therapy.

ELECTROCARDIOGRAPHIC DIAGNOSIS

The surface electrocardiographic criteria for diagnosis of VPCs in children include (1) prematurity of the QRS complex (more than 80 msec earlier than expected), (2) prolonged duration of the QRS complex (80 msec or longer in an infant and more than 90 msec after 3 years of age), (3) abnormal QRS complex configuration, (4) abnormal ST-T wave direction, usually opposite that of the sinus complex, (5) absence of a normal P wave preceding the QRS complex at an appropriate interval, (6) fusion complexes, and (7) no premature atrial complex or P wave preceding the premature complex.

VPCs must be differentiated from aberrantly conducted atrial premature complexes. In pediatrics, aberrant atrial premature complexes are most commonly conducted with a right bundle branch block pattern and VPCs have a left bundle branch block pattern, although this is not a constant occurrence. VPCs must also be differentiated from junctional premature complexes, which are rare, and from intermittent preexcitation, which is not uncommon in the pediatric population.

Ventricular tachycardia also must be differentiated from all other forms of wide QRS tachycardias, including (1) supraventricular tachycardia with bundle branch aberrancy, (2) antidromic supraventricular tachycardia using accessory atrioventricular connections, (3) atrial flutter or fibrillation with rapid conduction over an accessory atrioventricular connection, and (4) supraventricular tachycardia utilizing a nodoventricular connection. Although some studies suggest that these forms of wide complex tachycardia are more common than ventricular tachycardia, this has not been our experience (Fig. 1).

The following electrocardiographic associations and criteria have been considered necessary for a diagnosis of ventricular tachycardia (VT), but an electrophysiologic study may be necessary to rule out other forms of wide QRS complex tachycardias in certain situations.

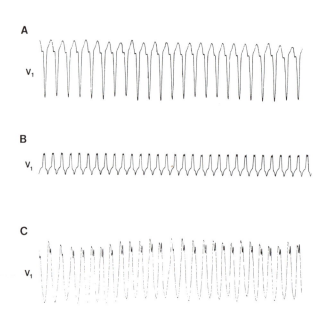

Figure 1 Electrocardiographic lead V_1 during tachycardia in three patients. *A* is from a patient with VT. Note the left bundle branch block pattern. *B* is an electrocardiogram from an infant with antidromic supraventricular tachycardia using an accessory atrioventricular connection. *C* is an electrocardiogram from a 10-year-old boy with Wolff-Parkinson-White syndrome during atrial fibrillation. Definitive diagnosis of the origin of the arrhythmia in any of these patients could not be made from the surface electrocardiogram alone.

1. VT consists of three or more consecutive ventricular complexes.
2. VT rates are generally faster than 120 beats per minute and may exceed 300 beats per minute.
3. Left bundle branch block is the most common morphology, but right bundle branch block pattern or both may be seen. Left bundle branch block pattern is unusual in supraventricular tachycardia in the absence of the Wolff-Parkinson-White syndrome.
4. Atrioventricular dissociation is suggestive of VT, although many children with VT have 1:1 retrograde ventriculoatrial conduction.
5. Fusion beats are suggestive of VT.
6. VT morphology similar to that of isolated PVCs is suggestive of VT.
7. Sustained VT is defined as more than 30 seconds' duration or less if it results in hemodynamic collapse.

Figure 2 shows a typical electrocardiogram in a child with VT.

Careful measurement of the corrected Q-T (Q-Tc) interval is essential to the evaluation of the patient with a ventricular arrhythmia. The Q-Tc should be measured in an area of the electrocardio-

gram free of VPCs and is considered to be the longest interval in any lead. Normal values for children are considered to be less than 0.45 second.

An accelerated ventricular rhythm is a rhythm originating from the ventricle with all the characteristics of VT but with a rate that is only slightly more rapid than the underlying sinus rhythm, usually less than 120 beats per minute (Fig. 3). These patients generally require no therapy but should be followed because an occasional patient will have acceleration of his or her VT to a much higher rate and develop symptoms.

CLINICAL MANIFESTATIONS OF VENTRICULAR TACHYCARDIA

Symptoms of VT in pediatric patients include dyspnea, chest or abdominal pain, dizziness, palpitations, syncope, or cardiac arrest. Most patients who have VT and heart disease have symptoms, compared with only one-third of those who have VT without heart disease. The type and degree of symptoms also appear to be rate-related, with symptoms being most common in patients with rates of 150 beats per minute or greater. However, slower rates do not always imply a good prognosis.

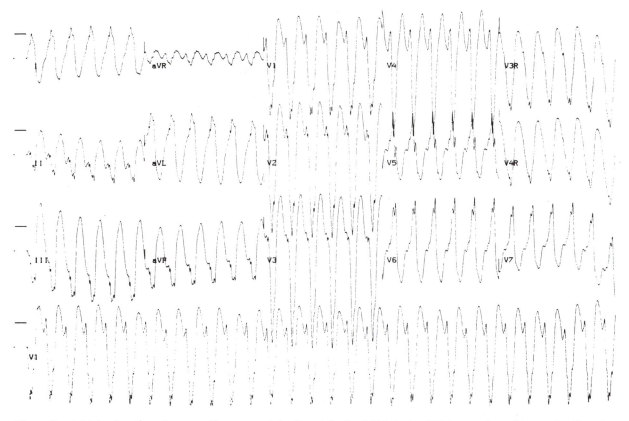

Figure 2   A 15-lead resting electrocardiogram and rhythm strip (lead V_1) during VT in a patient after repair of tetralogy of Fallot. Note the left bundle branch block pattern.

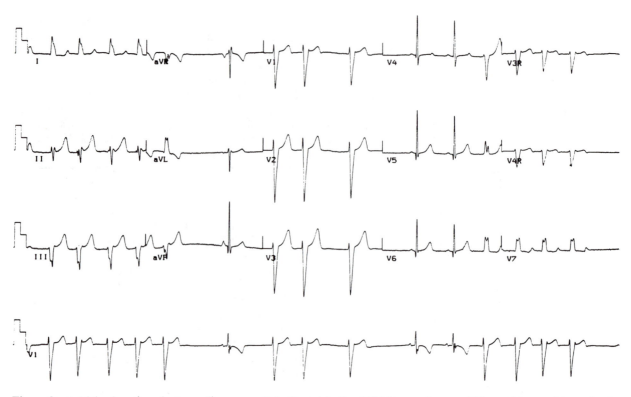

Figure 3 A 15-lead resting electrocardiogram and rhythm strip (lead V_1) from a 3-year-old boy with repetitive episodes of accelerated ventricular rhythm. The ventricular rate is irregular and slightly faster than the sinus rate.

PROGNOSIS

Reviews of VT in children have reported a relatively high incidence of death of 10 to 47 percent. The higher incidence occurs in patients with associated heart disease. Sudden death has been reported in patients with "normal" hearts at an incidence of 6 to 8 percent.

ASSOCIATED CONDITIONS

Causes of Acute Ventricular Tachycardia

The causes of acute VT that is not associated with congenital heart defects are shown in Table 1. These include metabolic and electrolyte derangements such as hypoxia, acidosis, and hypokalemia or hyperkalemia. Other common acute associations of acute VT in pediatrics are those seen with infectious processes such as myocarditis or pericarditis. Trauma, either occurring at the time of thoracic surgery or blunt cardiac trauma, may be associated with ventricular arrhythmias. Coronary abnormalities, including aneurysms associated with Kawasaki's disease with resultant myocardial ischemia or infarction, may result in ventricular arrhythmias. One of the more common associations occurs with the use of general anesthesia (especially halothane) and various other drugs (especially antiarrhythmic

agents). The remaining unexplained acute associations are termed idiopathic.

The treatment of these conditions includes the primary treatment of the underlying disorder with supportive therapy of the patient during the VT. If the ventricular arrhythmia is causing hemodynamic compromise, cardioversion or acute medical therapy such as intravenous lidocaine or other pharmacologic agents to suppress it may be necessary until the underlying condition is corrected (Table 2).

Table 1 Causes of Acute Ventricular Arrhythmias in Children

Metabolic	*Infectious*
Hypoxia	Myocarditis
Acidosis	Pericarditis
Hypoglycemia	Rheumatic fever
Hypocalcemia	
Hypo- or hyperkalemia	*Drugs*
	General anesthetics
Trauma	Antiarrhythmics
Blunt: cardiac contusion	Caffeine
Thoracic surgery	Nicotine
Cardiac catheters	Sympathomimetics
	Tricyclic antidepressants
Myocardial Ischemia	Digoxin
Abnormal coronaries	
Congenital	*Idiopathic*
Kawasaki's disease	
Hyperlipidemia	

Table 2 Drugs Used to Treat Acute Ventricular Tachycardia

Drug	Intravenous Dosage	Acute Level	Complications or Side Effects
Lidocaine	1 mg/kg bolus every 5–15 min Infusion: 10–15 μg/kg/min	1.5–6.0 mg/L	Hypotension Bradycardia Drowsiness Seizures Coma
Propranolol	0.1 mg/kg over 5 min q6h		Bradycardia Hypotension Hypoglycemia
Procainamide	15 mg/kg over 30–45 min 5 mg/kg over 5–10 min Infusion: 20–100 μg/kg/min	4–10 mg/L N-acetylated procainamide 4–8 mg/L	Bradycardia Proarrhythmia VT ventricular fibrillation Atrioventricular block Hypotension
Phenytoin	3–5 mg/kg over 5 min	10–20 μg/ml	Local burning Hypotension
Bretylium	5 mg/kg bolus Give every 15 min Infusion: 5–10 mg/kg over 10 min q6h		Hypotension Bradycardia Increased ventricular arrhythmias

Causes of Chronic Ventricular Tachycardia

The causes of chronic VT that is not associated with congenital heart diseases are shown in Table 3. These include the categories of acquired heart disease such as rheumatic fever, Kawasaki's disease, collagen vascular diseases, and Lyme disease. Other large categories that are discussed in greater detail here include myocarditis, cardiomyopathies, and tumors.

Primary arrhythmias, including the congenital long Q-T syndrome, congenital complete atrioventricular block, and other forms of familial VT, are being recognized with increasing frequency. Antiarrhythmic drugs and other pharmacologic agents that may produce ventricular arrhythmias are shown in Table 4.

Treatment of these patients should be directed toward the primary disease. Isolated single VPCs do not require therapy, but patients with conditions that may be progressive, such as myocarditis, should be monitored and followed carefully. Patients with symptoms from their arrhythmia or hemodynamic compromise should be treated according to their clinical situation. The most commonly used drugs for chronic VT in children are shown in Table 5. It is important to be certain that treatment is necessary because many of these agents have significant deleterious side effects, as indicated.

Most commonly with chronic VT no association is found, and the VT in these patients is labeled idiopathic.

Table 3 Causes of Chronic Ventricular Arrhythmias in Children

Congenital Heart Disease
Tetralogy of Fallot, VSD, CAVC (postoperative)
Complex congenital heart disease
  (pre- and postoperative)
Mitral valve prolapse
Aortic stenosis and insufficiency
Ebstein's anomaly

Cardiomyopathies
Hypertrophic
  Right ventricular dysplasia
  Postmyocarditis
  End-stage congenital heart disease
  Connective tissue disease
    SLE, Marfan's syndrome
  Muscular dystrophy
  Friedreich's ataxia

Acquired Heart Disease
Rheumatic heart disease
Kawasaki's disease

Tumors and Infiltrates
Rhabdomyoma
Hemosiderosis
  Thalassemia
  Sickle cell
Oncocytic cardiomyopathy
Leukemia

VSD = ventricular septal defect, CAVC = complete atrioventricular canal, SLE = systemic lupus erythematosus.

Table 4 Drugs Associated with Q-T
Interval Prolongation

Antiarrhythmic agents
Quinidine
Procainamide
Encainide
Flecainide
Amiodarone
Sotalol
Phenothiazines
Tricyclic antidepressants
Lithium carbonate
Organophosphates
Anthracyclines

IDIOPATHIC VENTRICULAR ARRHYTHMIAS

Although VPCs occur in normal children, this phenomenon occurs much less commonly than in adults. VPCs are infrequent in neonates but their incidence gradually increases with age, with ambulatory monitoring revealing a 26 percent incidence in healthy boys aged 10 to 13 years. When VPCs are seen in healthy newborns, they generally resolve by 12 weeks of age and usually require no treatment once the presence of a normal heart and the absence of symptoms are confirmed. These early ventricular arrhythmias probably relate to developmental fac-

Table 5 Drugs Used to Treat Chronic Ventricular Tachycardia in Children

Drug	Oral Dosage	Levels	Complications or Side Effects	
Propranolol	0.25– 4 mg/kg q6h	50–100 μg/L	CNS:	Dizziness
Nadolol	0.5–1 mg/kg q12h	0.03–0.13 μg/ml		Depression
				Weakness, fatigue
				Memory loss
				Insomnia
			GI:	Nausea
				Vomiting
				Abdominal pain
				Diarrhea
			Other:	Bronchospasm
				Hypoglycemia
			CV:	Hypotension
				Bradycardia
				Increased atrioventricular block
				Congestive heart failure
Procainamide	20–100 mg/kg/day q4–6h	4–10 mg/L N-acetylated procainamide 4–8 mg/L	CNS:	Dizziness Weakness
			GI:	Anorexia
				Nausea and vomiting
				Abdominal pain
				Diarrhea
			Other:	Lupus-like syndrome
			CV:	Proarrhythmia
				Hypotension
				Atrioventricular block
Quinidine	20–60 mg/kg/day q6–8h	2–5 mg/L	CNS:	Disturbed vision
				Headache
				Dizziness
			GI:	Nausea, vomiting
				Diarrhea
				Abdominal pain
			CV:	Proarrhythmia
				Hypotension
				Atrioventricular block
				Increased digoxin levels
Flecainide	50–150 mg/m²/day q12h	0.2–1.0 mg/L	CNS:	Dizziness
				Visual disturbance
				Headache
				Tremor
			GI:	Nausea, vomiting
				Abdominal pain
			Other:	Fatigue, dyspnea
			CV:	Proarrhythmia
				Atrioventricular block, sinus bradycardia
				Hypotension
				Increased congestive heart failure

continued

Table 5 Drugs Used to Treat Chronic Ventricular Tachycardia in Children *(Continued)*

Drug	Oral Dosage	Levels	Complications or Side Effects	
Mexiletine	2–4 mg/kg/dose q8h	2.0 mg/L	CNS:	Dizziness Tremor Insomnia Coordination problems
			CV:	Hypotension Bradycardia
			GI:	Nausea, vomiting
Phenytoin	2–4 mg/kg q12h	10–20 mg/L	CNS:	Nystagmus Ataxia, dizziness Mental confusion
			GI:	Nausea Vomiting
			Other:	Rash Gingival hyperplasia Hirsutism
Amiodarone	Loading: 10–20 mg/kg/day Maintenance: 5–10 mg/kg/day		CNS:	Fatigue Tremor Coordination
			GI:	Nausea, vomiting Anorexia Abdominal pain Constipation
			CV:	Proarrhythmia Atrioventricular block Sinus bradycardia Congestive heart failure Increases digoxin and quinidine levels

CNS = central nervous system, GI = gastrointestinal system, CV = cardiovascular system.

tors associated with the autonomic nervous system. These apparently benign arrhythmias frequently resolve in older children as well and may be related to transient or exogenous factors, including mild viral myocarditis or excessive intake of caffeine or sympathomimetic drugs, including cold and asthma medications.

There have been a number of reviews and reports of children with idiopathic VT and presumably normal hearts. These are children who are not known to have heart disease, but up to 60 to 70 percent present with symptoms, including palpitations, chest pain, abdominal pain, and presyncope or syncope. It is generally thought that these patients all have a favorable prognosis, but a mortality of up to 13 percent has been reported. Recent reports have demonstrated that many patients considered to have normal hearts may have subclinical cardiac abnormalities consisting of various forms of cardiomyopathy or myocarditis. Endomyocardial biopsy may reveal unexpected abnormalities. This is also the case with right ventricular angiograms, which show the typical signs of a hypokinetic right ventricle consistent with arrhythmogenic right ventricular dysplasia. Elevations of end-diastolic pressure, increased ventricular volumes, or regional wall motion abnormalities may be noted at cardiac catheterization in 60 to 70 percent of patients with idiopathic ventricular

tachycardia. Likewise, a decreased shortening fraction may be found on echocardiographic assessment. Thus, VT may be the first manifestation of a cardiomyopathy.

Management of Patients with Idiopathic Ventricular Tachycardia

All patients, symptomatic and asymptomatic, who present with sustained VT at rates greater than 150 beats per minute should have a complete evaluation to rule out the presence of abnormalities of the heart. Patients with lower rates who have symptoms or any abnormal studies should have a complete evaluation as well. The physical examination may reveal evidence of a previously undiagnosed murmur consistent with mitral valve prolapse or an extra heart sound consistent with a myopathic state. In addition, these patients should have an electrocardiogram, a chest x-ray study, an echocardiogram, an exercise stress test, and cardiac catheterization, including angiographic and electrophysiologic study. Although we have not employed routine endomyocardial biopsy, recent studies suggest a high positive return from this study.

Patients with normal hearts according to these evaluations and with no symptoms, no VT induced by exercise, and rates of less than 150 beats per minute are not generally treated at our institution. Most patients who remain consistently at elevated rates over several months to years eventually develop a myopathic picture and require treatment; therefore, careful follow-up is needed in patients who are not treated initially. Intermittent short episodes of VT are generally well tolerated and may not require treatment. Another interesting group is composed of those patients with complex ventricular arrhythmias and unsustained VT that account for up to 30 to 50 percent of the patient's rhythm. A typical electrocardiographic rhythm strip of such a patient is shown in Figure 4. Many of these patients have subclinical abnormalities caused by a cardiomyopathy that may be discovered only at cardiac catheterization. Treatment often improves the patient's general state of health, increasing exercise tolerance and decreasing fatigue, which the patient may have accepted as a normal state previously. Patients with abnormal hearts, symptoms, or exercise-induced VT (especially with rates significantly higher than the underlying sinus rate would be expected to be) are generally treated at our institution. The most commonly used drugs are shown in Table 5.

CHRONIC VENTRICULAR TACHYCARDIA ASSOCIATED WITH CONGENITAL HEART DISEASE

The most common congenital heart defect that has been associated with ventricular arrhythmias is tetralogy of Fallot. Sudden death is reported to occur in 2 to 5 percent of patients after repair of tetralogy of Fallot. Previously, death had been attributed to conduction disturbances, but more recent data have indicated that VT is more likely to be responsible for this sudden death. When VPCs are noted on the resting, stress, or ambulatory electrocardiogram, an incidence of sudden death of 30 to 38 percent has been noted. More recently, the electrophysiologic study has been used to induce VT in these patients in an attempt to identify and pretreat those at greatest risk for sudden death. The VT associated with patients with tetralogy of Fallot can be reproducibly initiated and terminated during electrophysiologic study (Fig. 5). Although it appears likely that this arrhythmia results from a reentrant mechanism, there has been some suggestion that triggered automaticity may be responsible. The site of origin of this VT is most commonly the right ventricular outflow tract, but some patients may have the VT localized to the ventricular septum near the site of the ventricular septal defect closure. Although there is some disagreement, abnormal hemodynamics after repair, including abnormal right ventricular function, elevated right ventricular systolic or diastolic pressure, or severe pulmonary insufficiency, may predispose patients to the development of VT.

Management and Treatment

These patients should have yearly 24-hour ambulatory monitoring and an exercise stress test between 8 and 12 years of age, at the time of symptoms, or before participation in vigorous physical

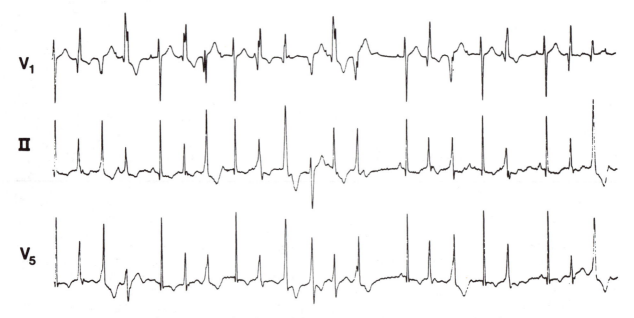

Figure 4 Electrocardiographic rhythm strip with leads V_1, II, and V_5 in an adolescent girl with complex ventricular arrhythmia consisting of multiform premature ventricular complexes and nonsustained VT representing 30 to 40 percent of the total rhythm on 24-hour ambulatory monitoring. Cardiac catheterization revealed evidence of subclinical cardiomyopathy.

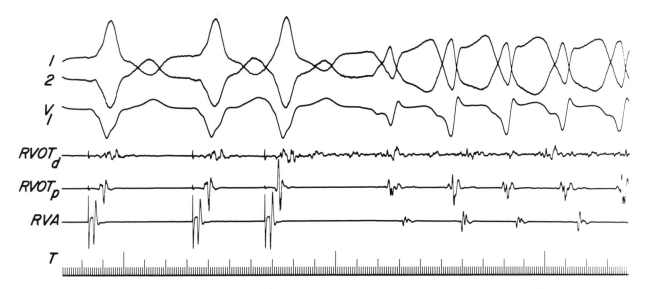

Figure 5 VT induction in a patient after repair of tetralogy of Fallot. Electrocardiographic leads 1, 2, and V_1 are shown with intracardiac electrograms from the distal right ventricular outflow tract ($RVOT_d$), proximal RVOT ($RVOT_p$), and RV apex (RVA), along with 10-msec time lines (T). A single ventricular extrastimulus, introduced after the eighth paced complex (second complex from the left), resulted in initiation of VT. Continuous electrical activity was noted during the VT in the distal RVOT. (Reprinted from Horowitz LN, Vetter VL, Harken A, Josephson ME: Electrophysiologic characteristics of sustained ventricular tachycardia occurring after repair of tetralogy of Fallot. Am J Cardiol 1980; 46:446–452; with permission.)

activities or competitive team sports. If more than 10 VPCs per hour are noted on ambulatory monitoring, we suggest exercise stress testing at that time. We also recommend that an electrophysiologic study be performed at the time of the postoperative catheterization or in patients with more than 10 VPCs per hour in any hour, couplets, complex, or multiform VPCs, unsustained or sustained VT, symptoms, or ventricular ectopy on exercise testing. Since ventricular arrhythmias may be progressive, a negative electrophysiologic or other study in previous years may not indicate the patient's current status. A patient with new findings or symptoms may need repeat studies.

We reserve treatment for those patients with sustained VT or symptomatic unsustained VT, especially if it is exercise-related and associated with abnormal hemodynamics. The presence of VPCs or couplets in the absence of symptoms in a patient with a good repair and the failure to induce VT in the electrophysiology laboratory would result in our following the patient closely without treatment.

The initial drug that we currently use in these patients is mexiletine. In patients with inducible VT in the laboratory, we use the electrophysiologic drug study to guide our therapy. Ambulatory monitoring with an end point of resolution of complex ventricular ectopy such as unsustained VT but not of all VPCs or couplets would also be used along with exercise stress testing in those patients whose ar-

rhythmia was exacerbated by exercise. Additional drugs that have been successfully used in these patients with tetralogy of Fallot include propranolol or other beta blockers such as nadolol, class IA agents such as procainamide, and amiodarone. Phenytoin, which was the drug of choice in the 1970s, does not seem to be any more effective than the lidocaine derivatives and has a much higher incidence of side effects, especially in adolescents. In patients in whom mexiletine, propranolol (or other beta blockers), or class I agents are not successful, we strongly consider surgical ablation, which has been quite effective in this group of postoperative patients.

OTHER FORMS OF CONGENITAL HEART DISEASE

Ventricular arrhythmias have been noted both before and after surgery in association with other congenital heart lesions, including Ebstein's anomaly of the tricuspid valve, aortic stenosis and insufficiency, D-transposition of the great arteries, ventricular septal defects, and atrioventricular canal defects. These arrhythmias may be related to long-standing pressure or volume overload, fibrosis, residual defects, scarring after surgery, or incomplete myocardial preservation at the time of the surgical correction.

Patients with congenital coronary artery anomalies are known to be at risk for sudden death presumed secondary to ventricular arrhythmias. As many as 15 percent of young athletes who die suddenly have been found to have had anomalous origin of the left coronary artery from the right sinus of Valsalva, with the left coronary artery passing between the aorta and pulmonary artery, where it may be compressed. This lesion should be considered in patients who present with VT, especially if the VT occurs on exertion. Diagnosis is made by coronary angiography.

Treatment

These arrhythmias should be treated according to the clinical status and symptoms produced, as outlined in the section on tetralogy of Fallot.

MITRAL VALVE PROLAPSE

Although there are reports of sudden death in children and adolescents with mitral valve prolapse, this is much less common than the 1.4 percent incidence cited in adults. Ambulatory monitoring and exercise stress testing have revealed ventricular arrhythmias in up to 46 percent of children with mitral valve prolapse. One-fourth of these arrhythmias were considered life-threatening.

Management and Treatment

We recommend at least one 24-hour ambulatory monitor when the patient presents and repeat studies at the time of appearance of any symptoms. If the symptoms are fleeting, transtelephonic monitors with a continuous-loop memory may be the only way to obtain a recording of the arrhythmia. For any patient with symptoms, including chest pain, palpitations, presyncope, or syncope, we perform an exercise stress test. Patients with sustained rapid VT or significant symptoms such as syncope should have an electrophysiologic study. Patients with sustained VT, symptomatic unsustained VT, or symptomatic complex VPCs should be treated. If the arrhythmia is exacerbated by exercise, we generally treat these children. Propranolol or nadolol has been our drug of choice. Because many of these patients have prolonged Q-T intervals, we do not recommend the use of class I agents.

MYOCARDITIS

Most series concerning sudden death in children include cases of acute myocarditis as an important etiology, with 5 to 6 percent of sudden unexpected deaths in children being attributable to this associa-

tion. The sudden death is thought to be related to the occurrence of ventricular arrhythmias, particularly VT and ventricular fibrillation. Some of these patients develop complete heart block and alternate between the ventricular arrhythmias and the heart block. Because these patients are often hemodynamically compromised without tachycardia, profound collapse may accompany the onset of VT. Aggressive management is necessary, with cardioversion, lidocaine, and other pharmacologic agents as needed (see Table 2). Complete heart block with slow rates should be treated immediately with temporary pacing. Pharmacologic agents, such as isoproterenol, may be used temporarily but increase the risk of VT in these patients. Although this form of heart block usually resolves, permanent pacing may be necessary in those patients with persistent heart block.

CARDIOMYOPATHIES

Hypertrophic Cardiomyopathy

There is a high incidence of sudden death (up to 30 percent) in children with idiopathic hypertrophic subaortic stenosis or hypertrophic cardiomyopathy. This sudden death is frequently exercise-related and is presumed to be secondary to ventricular arrhythmias. A family history of sudden death or ventricular arrhythmias on 24-hour ambulatory monitors may identify a high-risk population, although some studies have shown no association between the previous presence of ventricular arrhythmias and sudden death. The presenting event in many patients is sudden death associated with exercise.

Dilated Cardiomyopathy

Dilated cardiomyopathies are associated with ventricular arrhythmias and sudden death. These cardiomyopathies may be associated with generalized myopathies, such as Duchenne muscular dystrophy and Friedreich's ataxia, or with metabolic abnormalities, especially of fatty acid metabolism. Other secondary forms of dilated cardiomyopathies include those associated with hemoglobinopathies producing hemosiderosis, such as thalassemia and sickle cell disease. Many patients with dilated cardiomyopathies have evidence of a preceding episode of myocarditis. Those with no identifiable cause are classified as idiopathic, although many of these probably have metabolic abnormalities still to be identified.

Management and Treatment

Ambulatory monitoring and exercise stress testing are the most helpful tests for identifying patients in this group who are experiencing ventricular arrhythmias. Because many of these patients are severely limited in their exercise capabilities, ambulatory monitoring may be the only method of documenting arrhythmias. There are no data to indicate whether suppression of ventricular arrhythmia in these patients prolongs life. Our current management includes the treatment of any symptomatic arrhythmias and suppression of sustained ventricular tachycardia. Because the limited cardiac function may prohibit use of beta blockers, class I agents are generally the drugs of choice. These patients must be carefully monitored in the hospital to look for the presence of proarrhythmic effects of these drugs as well as a decrease in cardiac function. In some patients, an increase in digoxin dosage improves cardiac function and decreases the ventricular arrhythmia. This should be accomplished with careful monitoring. Amiodarone has been used successfully in this group.

RIGHT VENTRICULAR DYSPLASIA

An unusual form of cardiomyopathy known as arrhythmogenic right ventricular dysplasia may be the cause of VT in some children who are thought to have normal hearts. The diagnosis is made by right ventricular angiography, which shows localized areas of hypokinesis in the infundibulum, free wall, or right ventricular apex. This may accompany right ventricular dilation and decreased contractility, but at times the abnormal hypokinetic areas may be an isolated finding. The VT always has a left bundle branch block pattern. Surgical therapy may be curative if medical therapy is unsuccessful.

TUMORS

For several years, there has been a known association of ventricular arrhythmias and cardiac rhabdomyomas. More recently, Garson described an incessant form of VT seen in infants and young children that was secondary to myocardial hamartomas and could be treated successfully with surgery. A more diffuse infiltrative type of disease known as histiocytoid or oncocytic cardiomyopathy of infancy is known to manifest as incessant VT in infancy and is usually fatal. Our experience with a small group of young patients with incessant or refractory VT indicates that in some VT may be controlled with aggressive medical management, including combination drug therapy. This has included amiodarone or a combination of amiodarone and procainamide. These tumors may regress with time, similar to the regression of rhabdomyomas, and antiarrhythmic therapy may be discontinued after a few years.

CONGENITAL LONG Q-T SYNDROME

Two hereditary syndromes associated with ventricular arrhythmias and sudden death manifest with prolongation of the Q-T interval and have been described in children. These include the syndrome of Jervell and Lange-Nielsen associated with congenital deafness and the Romano-Ward syndrome without deafness. These disorders are associated with a very high mortality (73 percent) in untreated patients. The sudden death is secondary to malignant ventricular arrhythmias, including torsades de pointes and ventricular fibrillation. Figure 6 is an example of an electrocardiogram in a patient with torsades de pointes and congenital long Q-T syndrome. A primary myocardial abnormality involving potassium channels and an imbalance of the sympathetic nervous system or oversensitivity of the ventricular myocardium to the sympathetic nervous system has been implicated in the etiology of the syndrome. The diagnosis should be entertained in any patient with stress- or exercise-related syncope or ventricular arrhythmia. In addition to the prolonged Q-T interval, the electrocardiogram may show prominent U waves, particularly in the midprecordial leads, or bizarre T-wave patterns, as shown in Figure 7. T-wave alternans is said to be diagnostic of this disorder. In addition, many patients have marked sinus arrhythmia or sinus bradycardia.

Diagnosis

Diagnosis is made by a careful history, both of the individual's episodes and a complete family history looking for sudden unexplained death, syncopal episodes in family members, unusual seizure disorders, or hearing deficits. Careful evaluation of the electrocardiogram and 24-hour ambulatory monitoring may reveal a prolonged Q-Tc interval. Several measurements should be made at different heart rates to determine the longest Q-Tc interval. These patients should have an exercise stress test, which may reveal a prolongation of the Q-Tc interval with exercise. It has been stated that electrophysiologic studies are not indicated in these patients, but we have found that a prolongation of the Q-Tc interval with atrial pacing may be helpful in diagnosing those cases with borderline prolongation of the Q-T interval on the resting electrocardiogram. Another helpful provocative test is the infusion of isoproterenol, which produces a prolongation of the Q-T interval, changes in the T-wave configuration or an increased prominence of the U wave, and the development of ventricular arrhythmias in patients who have the long Q-T syndrome.

Treatment

Treatment consists of the use of beta blockers. We have used propranolol and nadolol successfully.

A

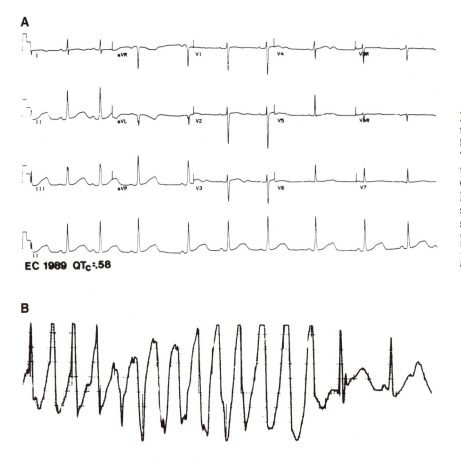

EC 1989 QT$_c$:.58

Figure 6 *A* 15-lead resting electrocardiogram in a 10-year-old boy with recurrent syncope. The T wave revealed a notched pattern, especially in lead II. The Q-Tc interval is markedly prolonged at 0.58 sec. *B,* Rhythm strip in the same patient during a syncopal episode revealing the pattern of torsades de pointes. Note the change in amplitude and polarity of the R wave.

B

We do not recommend the use of longer acting beta blockers that may be given once daily because the levels may decrease significantly during sleep or in the early morning hours when the patient may be at greatest risk. If beta-blocker therapy is not successful, left stellate ganglionectomy has been shown to be effective in certain patients. We prefer to use other drugs rather than surgery initially and have chosen mexiletine as our second-line drug in recent

patients. Phenytoin or phenobarbital may be useful in some patients, but they are not well tolerated by adolescents. In patients with persistent ventricular arrhythmias or in whom persistent bradycardia limits the use of beta blockers in adequate doses, a permanent pacemaker has been used. The rate is set approximately 10 to 15 percent higher than the patient's intrinsic rate and is used to control the heart rate even during exercise. Atrial pacing is preferred,

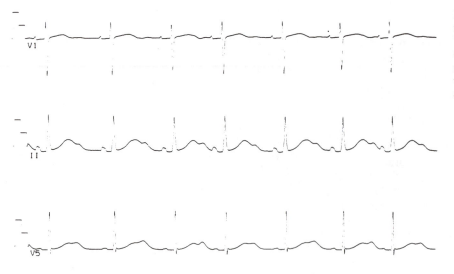

Figure 7 Rhythm strip of electrocardiographic leads V$_1$, II, and V$_5$ revealing the typical prolonged Q-Tc interval to 0.55 sec and bizarre T waves seen in patients with congenital long Q-T syndrome.

although we have used ventricular pacing as well. In resistant cases, implantation of an automatic internal defibrillator is indicated.

OTHER ASSOCIATED CONDITIONS

Ventricular arrhythmias have been associated with several other conditions, including congenital complete heart block, sick sinus syndrome, and complete postoperative atrioventricular block. These patients should be routinely monitored to look for the development of ventricular arrhythmias. Exercise stress testing may also be used as a provocative test to identify the presence of significant arrhythmias. Patients with these slow heart rates who are having ventricular arrhythmias should have their rates increased with implantation of a permanent pacing system.

INVESTIGATION OF THE PATIENT WITH VENTRICULAR ARRHYTHMIAS

The use of 24-hour ambulatory monitoring and transtelephonic monitoring has been discussed in the preceding individual sections. Exercise stress testing has been shown to be an effective method of evaluating VT. In most symptomatic patients, exercise increases the ventricular arrhythmia, whereas in most asymptomatic patients it suppresses the arrhythmia. Suppression of VPCs has been considered a sign of benignity but should not be used as the only

criterion, as serious arrhythmias may be suppressed by exercise. Electrophysiologic studies are a special consideration and are discussed in greater detail below.

Electrophysiologic Testing

The specific indications for performance of electrophysiologic studies in children with ventricular tachycardia include (1) diagnosis in a patient with wide QRS complex tachycardia, (2) sustained VT in a patient with a VT rate of more than 150 beats per minute, (3) unsustained VT or complex VPCs in a patient with an abnormal heart, (4) suspected VT in the setting of an abnormal heart or in the presence of syncope or cardiac arrest of unknown etiology, (5) determination of appropriate medical treatment in patients with inducible VT, and (6) characterization of the VT in terms of mechanism and location.

Since VT and complex ventricular arrhythmias are uncommon in patients with normal hearts, the electrophysiologic study should be performed in conjunction with cardiac catheterization and angiography to look for potential anatomic or organic causes of the VT, such as coronary artery anomalies, tumors, or subclinical cardiomyopathies.

The electrophysiologic study protocol used in the evaluation of VT is shown in Table 6.

Intracardiac recordings during VT show the absence of His bundle deflections consistently preceding ventricular depolarizations and atrial capture normalizing the QRS complex. One of the most

---

Table 6 Protocol for Electrophysiologic Study of Ventricular Tachycardia

Basal Measurements:
　SCL, AH, HV, Q-RV apex
　Duration of fragmented electrograms
　Late potentials
　Endocardial activation map in sinus rhythm

Evaluation of Sinus, Atrial, and Atrioventricular Nodal Function

Evaluation of Ventricular Refractoriness:
　Ventricular refractory periods at two or more cycle lengths and at two or more sites (right ventricular apex, right ventricular
　　outflow tract, left ventricle when indicated)
　Determination of dispersion of ventricular refractoriness

VT Induction:
　Rapid ventricular pacing
　Single, double, triple ventricular stimulation at two or more cycle lengths at two or more sites
　Isoproterenol ± stimulation

Characterization of VT and Termination:
　Confirmation of diagnosis of VT
　VT cycle length
　Site of origin (earliest activation)
　Termination of VT
　　Response to VT to prematures and rapid ventricular pacing
　　Lidocaine
　　Cardioversion

Drug Studies:
　Drug success at preventing VT initiation

significant differences between children and adults is the difference in the mechanisms that are apparently producing the tachycardia. Over 90 percent of adults have inducible VT in the electrophysiology laboratory, which is presumed to indicate a reentrant mechanism. In contrast, only 30 to 50 percent of children have inducible or reentrant VT. It is not clear whether failure to induce VT in these children definitely indicates an automatic mechanism or is an indication that their tachycardia is just more difficult to induce.

Most of these ventricular tachycardias in children with normal hearts have a left bundle branch block morphology, originate in the right ventricle, and are not inducible. The majority of patients with VT after repair of tetralogy of Fallot have inducible VT.

SUGGESTED READING

Deal BJ, Scott MM, Scagliotti D, et al. Ventricular tachycardia in a young population without overt heart disease. Circulation 1986; 73:1111–1118.

Dungan WT, Garson A Jr, Gillette PC. Arrhythmogenic right ventricular dysplasia: A cause of ventricular tachycardia in children with apparently normal hearts. Am Heart J 1981; 102:745–750.

Dunnigan A, Pierpont ME, Smith SA, et al. Cardiac and skeletal myopathy associated with cardiac dysrhythmias. Am J Cardiol 1984; 53:731–737.

Fulton DR, Kyung JC, Burton ST. Ventricular tachycardia in children without heart disease. Am J Cardiol 1985; 55:1328–1331.

Garson A Jr. Evaluation and treatment of chronic ventricular dysrhythmias in the young. CVR & R 1981; 2:1164–1196.

Gillette PC. Ventricular arrhythmias. In: Roberts NK, Gelbrand H, eds. Cardiac arrhythmias in the neonate, infant, and child. New York: Appleton-Century-Crofts; 1977:195.

Garson A Jr. Ventricular dysrhythmias. In: Gillette PC, Garson A Jr, eds. Pediatric cardiac dysrhythmias. New York: Grune & Stratton; 1981:295.

Garson A Jr, Gillette PC, Titus JL, et al. Surgical treatment of ventricular tachycardia in infants. N Engl J Med 1984; 310:1443–1445.

Garson A Jr, Moak JP, Friedman RA, et al. Surgical treatment of arrhythmias in children. Cardiol Clin 1989; 7:319–329.

Garson A Jr, Porter CJ, Gillette PC, McNamara DG. Induction of ventricular tachycardia during electrophysiologic study after repair of tetralogy of Fallot. J Am Coll Cardiol 1983; 1:1493–1502.

Gaum WE, Biancaniello T, Kaplan S. Accelerated ventricular rhythm in childhood. Am J Cardiol 1979; 43:162–164.

Hesslein PS. Ventricular arrhythmias. In: Liebman J, Plonsey R, Rudy Y, eds. Pediatric and fundamental electrocardiography. The Hague: Martinus Nijhoff, 1987:241.

Horowitz LN. Sudden death in children and adolescents. In: Morganroth J, ed. Sudden cardiac death. New York: Grune & Stratton, 1985:33.

Horowitz LN, Vetter VL, Harken AH, Josephson ME. Electrophysiologic characteristics of sustained ventricular tachycardia occurring after repair of tetralogy of Fallot. Am J Cardiol 1980; 46:446–452.

Kavey REW, Blackman MS, Sondheimer HM, Byrum CJ. Ventricular arrhythmias and mitral valve prolapse in childhood. J Pediatr 1984; 105:885–890.

McKenna WJ, England D, Doi YL, et al. Arrhythmia in hypertrophic cardiomyopathy I: Influence on prognosis. Br Heart J 1981; 46:168–172.

McKenna WJ, Franklin RCG, Nihoyannopoulos P, et al. Arrhythmia and prognosis in infants, children and adolescents with hypertrophic cardiomyopathy. J Am Coll Cardiol 1988; 11:147–153.

Moak JP, Smith RT, Garson A Jr. Newer antiarrhythmic drugs in children. Am Heart J 1986; 113:179–185.

Moss AJ, Schwartz PJ, Crampton RS, et al. The long QT syndrome: A prospective international study. Circulation 1985; 1:17–21.

Ott DA, Garson A, Cooley DA, McNamara DG. Definitive operation for refractory cardiac tachyarrhythmias in children. J Thorac Cardiovasc Surg 1985; 90:681–689.

Pederson DH, Zipes DP, Foster PR, Troup PJ. Ventricular tachycardia and ventricular fibrillation in a young population. Circulation 1979; 60:988–997.

Rocchini AP, Chun PO, Dick MD. Ventricular tachycardia in children. Am J Cardiol 1981; 47:1091–1097.

Schwartz PJ. Idiopathic long QT syndrome: Progress and questions. Am Heart J 1985; 109:399–411.

Stevens DC, Schreiner RL, Hurwitz RA, Gresham EL. Fetal and neonatal ventricular arrhythmia. Pediatrics 1979; 63:771–777.

Strain JE, Grose RM, Factor SM, Fisher JD. Results of endomyocardial biopsy in patients with spontaneous ventricular tachycardia but without apparent structural heart disease. Circulation 1983; 68:1171–1181.

Vetter VL. Management of arrhythmias in children—unusual features. In: Dreifus LS, ed. Cardiac arrhythmias: Electrophysiologic techniques and management. Philadelphia: FA Davis, 1985:329.

Vetter VL, Horowitz LN. Electrophysiologic residua and sequelae of surgery for congenital heart defects. Am J Cardiol 1982; 50:588–604.

Vetter VL, Horowitz LN. Postoperative pediatric electrocardiographic and electrophysiologic sequelae. In: Liebman J, Plonsey R, Rudy Y, eds. Pediatric and fundamental electrocardiography. The Hague: Martinus Nijhoff, 1987:187.

Vetter VL, Josephson ME, Horowitz LN. Idiopathic recurrent sustained ventricular tachycardia in children and adolescents. Am J Cardiol 1981; 47:315–322.

WIDE QRS COMPLEX TACHYCARDIA

CHARLES R. WEBB, M.D.

Wide QRS complex tachycardia is an emergency commonly seen in the emergency room or in hospitalized patients, many of whom have underlying cardiovascular disease. Appropriate recording, documentation, and assessment are essential if the patient is hemodynamically stable because the arrhythmia is likely to recur, but perhaps never again under medical supervision. The initial electrocardiographic recording during the acute event facilitates appropriate in-hospital evaluation and long-term outpatient management. Termination of the tachycardia without adequate documentation can result in uncertainty of diagnosis and inappropriate hospital admission or discharge and can confound the chronic management plan.

DEFINITION

Wide QRS complex tachycardia may be defined as a cardiac arrhythmia having a rate greater than 100 complexes per minute (or an R-R cycle length of less than 600 msec) and a QRS complex duration greater than 120 msec in any lead on a standardized 12-lead electrocardiogram. For *descriptive* purposes, the QRS morphology during tachycardia is assigned a bundle branch block pattern (left or right or normal). A *right bundle branch block pattern* is assigned if the QRS complex is predominantly positive in lead V_1; prominent terminal negative S waves in leads I and V_5 or V_6 are supportive findings. A *left bundle branch block pattern* is assigned when the intrinsicoid deflection is delayed in the lateral electrocardiographic leads (I, and V_5 or V_6); usually V_1 is predominantly negative. The tachycardia may be further characterized by the predominant or mean QRS axis during the tachycardia as normal axis (0 < axis < 90 degrees), left axis deviation (< 0 degrees), or right axis deviation (> 90 degrees).

A wide QRS complex tachycardia may be the result of a supraventricular tachycardia with aberrant conduction or a ventricular tachycardia. Obviously then, the prognosis and therapy require an appropriate diagnosis. The distinction may be immediately obvious but is often problematic.

APPROACH TO THE PATIENT

The patient must be transported to an environment equipped with a continuous cardiac monitor with recording capability, a 12-lead electrocardiogram machine, cardiorespiratory resuscitative drugs and equipment, and knowledgeable personnel. A defibrillator must be available in case cardioversion is required for emergency termination of a life-threatening arrhythmia.

DIFFERENTIAL DIAGNOSIS

The differential diagnosis of a regular wide complex tachycardia includes the following conditions:

1. Supraventricular tachycardia with a functional bundle branch block
2. Supraventricular tachycardia with a preexistent bundle branch block
3. Supraventricular tachycardia with antegrade atrioventricular conduction over an accessory atrioventricular pathway (antedromic SVT)
4. Ventricular tachycardia.

Age, heart rate, blood pressure, level of consciousness, duration, or presence or absence of heart disease is not an accurate predictor of the tachycardia mechanism. Ventricular tachycardia is the most common mechanism of wide QRS complex tachycardia at any age. In patients with a history of myocardial infarction particularly, it is prudent to assume that the tachycardia is ventricular until proved otherwise, but these patients also frequently have supraventricular arrhythmia. Some patients have both.

Occasionally patients with very fast tachycardia are alert and conversational despite rapid ventricular tachycardia and underlying ventricular dysfunction. Presumably this results from an optimal balance of a low cardiac output and adequate peripheral vasoregulation to maintain cerebral perfusion.

A heart rate of 150 complexes per minute is suggestive of atrial flutter with 2:1 heart block. However, there is no particular heart rate that excludes ventricular tachycardia or supraventricular tachycardia. Either mechanism may present as very fast or relatively slow. Patients who present with a history of recurrence of tachycardia spanning 2 or more years usually have supraventricular tachycardia. In the elderly, a relatively slow supraventricular tachycardia may result in hypotension and near-syncope due to impaired cerebrovascular autoregulation, partial vascular occlusion, impaired myocardial performance, inadequate peripheral vasomotor responses, dehydration, or drugs.

Electrocardiographic Techniques

Wide QRS tachycardia can be difficult to evaluate; however, certain electrocardiographic criteria have been shown to be helpful in separating supraventricular from ventricular tachycardia. Atrioventricular dissociation is virtually diagnostic for ventricular tachycardia, but atrioventricular association may occur in either supraventricular or ventricular tachycardia. A single-lead electrocardiographic monitoring strip is diagnostic of ventricular tachycardia *when the QRS and P wave morphologies are distinct and atrioventricular dissociation is apparent.* Since wide QRS complexes are usually tall as well as wide, it is often difficult to discern the smaller P waves on emergency or bedside monitoring equipment because they are buried within the QRS complex or a broad T wave. A fortuitously timed sinus complex may capture the ventricle, resulting in occasional ventricular *capture complexes* that are narrow and look like sinus complexes (because they are) during the tachycardia. Such sinus complexes, which occur later in electrical diastole, may result in ventricular *fusion complexes* that are a morphologic hybrid of sinus and tachycardia QRS complexes. The presence of this phenomenon is not completely specific, as premature junctional, fascicular, or ventricular complexes may also fuse with tachycardia complexes.

Recording three or more electrocardiographic leads simultaneously allows comparison of barely perceptible P waves in several leads and may clarify the presence or absence of any temporal relationship to the QRS complexes. If there is a 1:1 relationship with normal P waves preceding each QRS complex, sinus rhythm or another atrial rhythm is present. If there is atrioventricular dissociation, i.e., atrial and ventricular activity are independent, then ventricular tachycardia is diagnosed. If there is a 1:1 relationship with inverted P waves following each QRS complex, either ventricular tachycardia with retrograde conduction or supraventricular tachycardia may be present.

A standard 12-lead electrocardiogram should be recorded during tachycardia whenever possible because it provides a better "fingerprint" of the arrhythmia. The likelihood of detecting P waves is greater. Furthermore, the QRS morphology may be useful to discriminate tachycardia of supraventricular or ventricular origin. A QRS width greater than 140 to 160 msec is highly suggestive of a ventricular tachycardia. Marked leftward deviation of the mean QRS vector is also highly correlated with ventricular tachycardia. Capture and fusion complexes, although diagnostic of ventricular tachycardia, are relatively uncommon. A "concordant pattern" of precordial complexes is said to occur when all leads in V_1 to V_6 are entirely upright or entirely inverted. This is also highly suggestive of ventricular tachycardia but not common. Be aware that in the presence of antegrade conduction over an accessory atrioventricular pathway, the ventricle is activated ectopically, and such supraventricular tachycardia cannot be distinguished from ventricular tachycardia by surface electrocardiography. Furthermore, the presence of delta waves in the resting electrocardiogram by no means excludes the possibility of ventricular tachycardia.

If the mechanism of the arrhythmia remains unclear, positioning of chest leads one interspace higher or lower or on the back (nearer to the left atrium) may reveal P waves. When noninvasive methods are not diagnostic and if the patient is stable, a "pill electrode" may be swallowed into the esophagus during the tachycardia in order to record an electrogram at the level of the left atrium. Otherwise a temporary pacing wire may be passed through a nasogastric tube.

The most reliable method of detection of atrial activity during tachycardia is to record the right intraatrial electrogram by inserting a temporary pacing wire transvenously with fluoroscopic guidance or a balloon-tipped electrode catheter with electrocardiographic monitoring while the proximal portion of the lead is connected to lead V_1. A quadripolar catheter allows simultaneous recording and pacing.

In addition to passive recording, a pacing lead allows other diagnostic and therapeutic interventions. Atrial pacing at rates exceeding the tachycardia rate can artificially produce the phenomena of atrial capture and fusion complexes with transient normalization or near-normalization of the QRS complexes. The latter method may also allow for termination of the tachycardia by pacing in the atrium. Theoretically, atropine or isoproterenol, by enhancing atrioventricular nodal conduction, may facilitate capture and fusion complexes but clinically could cause degeneration of the tachycardia to ventricular fibrillation. Many supraventricular tachycardias can be terminated by atrial entrainment, but this is not absolutely diagnostic, as relatively slow ventricular tachycardias may also be terminated by impulses conducted across the atrioventricular node. If the tachycardia is ventricular in origin, the electrode catheter may be advanced across the tricuspid valve to the right ventricular apex to provide a stable position from which to attempt to entrain and terminate ventricular tachycardia.

ROLE OF CAROTID SINUS MASSAGE

Carotid sinus massage may slow or terminate atrioventricular nodal or atrioventricular reentrant supraventricular tachycardia. It may result in atrioventricular nodal block and dissociate the ventricles from the atria during supraventricular tachycardias that originate in the atrium or high within the atrioventricular node (sinus node reentry, intraatrial reentry, atrial flutter or fibrillation, or automatic atrial tachycardia). P waves may become apparent, and a functional (rate-dependent) bundle branch block may resolve. Some cardiologists feel that the right carotid sinus has a greater effect on the sinus node and the left on the atrioventricular node.

ROLE OF PHARMACOLOGIC MANEUVERS

Pharmacologic maneuvers may be of diagnostic value. Intravenous lidocaine is uniquely effective for ventricular tachycardia; it has no efficacy for termination of atrial tachycardias. It may occasionally interrupt conduction over an accessory atrioventricular pathway.

Intravenous propranolol, verapamil, diltiazem, or digitalis glycosides slow atrioventricular nodal conduction. Hence a tachycardia whose mechanism depends on antegrade or retrograde atrioventricular nodal conduction will become slower and more tolerable. If intermittent atrioventricular nodal block is produced, the tachycardia will terminate.

Digitalis glycosides are least likely to exacerbate hypotension and are preferred if there is evidence of heart failure. The disadvantage is the slow onset of action, even when administered intravenously, which makes them undesirable if the patient's condition is deteriorating rapidly.

Calcium channel antagonists (verapamil or diltiazem) and beta-adrenergic blockers (propranolol) are contraindicated if the patient is hypotensive or has evidence of heart failure. However, if there is no evidence of fluid overload or heart failure, it is valuable to administer about 200 ml of normal saline (0.9 percent aqueous sodium chloride) intravenously to achieve an adequate intravascular volume and decrease baroreceptor drive for tachycardia. This often corrects hypotension, relieves anxiety, slows the supraventricular tachycardia rate, and occasionally allows spontaneous resolution of the tachycardia. If the patient's blood pressure is restored to normal, calcium antagonists or beta-adrenergic blockers may be safely given with an effect similar to that of the digitalis glycosides but more rapid in onset and easier to titrate.

Adenosine when administered intravenously blocks atrioventricular nodal conduction rapidly. Since it is metabolized rapidly in plasma and human tissues, its duration of action is very brief (about 5 minutes). The advantage is rapid termination of supraventricular tachycardia, brief duration of hypotension or other side effects such as facial flushing, and the potential for early discharge of the patient from the acute care setting.

A new ultra–short-acting beta-adrenergic blocking agent, esmolol, also offers the opportunity of observing a brief effect on atrioventricular nodal conduction and termination of supraventricular tachycardia while minimizing any residual side effect.

If the patient has a wide complex tachycardia and has a history of the Wolff-Parkinson-White syndrome, or delta waves on the electrocardiogram in sinus rhythm, or is young without underlying cardiovascular disease, tachycardia mediated by conduction over an accessory atrioventricular pathway must be considered. If an atrioventricular nodal blocking agent is administered and atrial fibrillation ensues, rapid conduction over the accessory pathway can be catastrophic and even degenerate to ventricular fibrillation requiring cardioversion. In such patients, intravenous procainamide is the agent of choice because it may effectively block the accessory pathway and thereby slow or terminate atrioventricular reentry or atrial fibrillation or flutter. Procainamide is also effective for termination of ventricular tachycardia.

RETROSPECTIVE ASSESSMENT

Frequently, the cardiologist is consulted after the tachycardia is terminated and the only clinical recording is a 12-lead electrocardiogram. A variety of guidelines have been published to help determine the mechanism of the tachycardia based on the QRS complex morphology (Table 1). Comparison with the resting electrocardiogram in sinus rhythm is helpful. If the patient has aberrant conduction with a wide QRS complex morphology in sinus rhythm, aberration will be present during supraventricular tachycardia. If the QRS morphology is similar during sinus rhythm and tachycardia, the origin of the tachycardia is supraventricular.

ELECTROPHYSIOLOGIC STUDIES

The diagnosis can be made electrophysiologically if the patient is stable enough for safe transport to the laboratory during the arrhythmia in order to allow insertion of a catheter across the tricuspid valve to record a His bundle electrogram. Otherwise the tachycardia may be electively induced in the laboratory. A *supraventricular tachycardia* is recog-

Table 1 Electrocardiographic Criteria that Favor A Diagnosis of Ventricular Tachycardia

Atrioventricular dissociation
Ventriculoatrial block
QRS duration >140 msec with right bundle branch block
QRS duration >160 msec with left bundle branch block
Positive QRS concordance
Extreme left axis deviation (axis <−90 degrees to ± 180 degrees)
Left bundle branch block with right axis deviation
Different QRS pattern during tachycardia compared with a
  baseline electrocardiogram in patients with preexisting
  bundle branch block

nized electrophysiologically by the presence of a His bundle potential preceding each QRS complex with an HV interval equal to or exceeding that recorded when the patient is in sinus rhythm. In contrast, during *ventricular tachycardia*, the HV interval, if a His bundle potential is recorded, is shorter than normal. More commonly, the His bundle potential is buried within the QRS complex during ventricular tachycardia and cannot be discerned even on a recording from a catheter that is properly positioned to record the His bundle electrogram. This phenomenon may also be observed during antegrade conduction over an accessory atrioventricular pathway (preexcitation syndrome) during atrial tachycardia, or during antidromic atrioventricular reentrant supraventricular tachycardia.

Each patient with sustained ventricular tachycardia should undergo a diagnostic cardiac catheterization and coronary angiography to look for correctable anatomic causes. Cardiac electrophysiologic studies should be performed in the following circumstances:

1. If no correctable precipitating etiology is found
2. If the mechanism of the tachycardia is uncertain
3. If the tachycardia is known or suspected to be ventricular tachycardia
4. Whenever the tachycardia is associated with hemodynamic compromise, cardiac arrest, or requires cardioversion
5. If the tachycardia is recurrent despite attempts at medical management.

The goal is to prevent recurrence. Formal electrophysiologic testing should determine the integrity of sinus node function, the conduction system, and the inducibility of the tachycardia. Serial antiarrhythmic drug and/or device testing is performed to determine the best method for each patient to prevent or rapidly terminate the tachycardia. Noninducibility of the tachycardia when the patient is on drug therapy is the gold standard of electrophysiologic testing. However, for tachycardias that are relatively refractory to drug therapy, conversion to nonsustained tachycardia or substantial slowing of the tachycardia rate with alleviation of hemodynamic compromise and symptoms has been reported to give satisfactory long-term results with flecainide or amiodarone.

ANTITACHYCARDIA PACING AND DEVICES

Antitachycardia devices are usually reserved for patients whose disease is refractory or intolerant to electrophysiologically guided drug therapy. The type of antitachycardia device is determined by the mechanism of the tachycardia and associated symptoms. If the patient remains alert and the tachycardia is reproducibly and reliably terminated by pacing, an antitachycardia pacemaker may be considered. If the tachycardia is hemodynamically unstable, an automatic implantable cardioverter defibrillator (AICD) is indicated. For ventricular tachycardia, even if it is well tolerated, the possibility of acceleration by attempted antitachycardia pacing requires that a backup AICD also be implanted. However, if tachycardia recurs frequently and the patient remains awake during tachycardia, a combination of antiarrhythmic drug therapy or antitachycardia pacing with an implantable defibrillator (see the chapter *Automatic Implantable Cardioverter Defibrillator*) is necessary to minimize the patient's discomfort.

SURGICAL APPROACHES

In selected patients with monomorphic ventricular tachycardia, particularly with coronary artery disease and a discrete chronic infarction scar or aneurysm, endocardial resection or catheter ablation, which is still investigational, is effective. Resection of an accessory pathway in the Wolff-Parkinson-White syndrome is first-line therapy for patients with life-threatening arrhythmias (such as atrial flutter or fibrillation with rapid conduction) or drug refractoriness or intolerance. Posterior paraseptal accessory atrioventricular connections have also been successfully ablated by a transvenous catheter.

SUGGESTED READING

Akhtar M, Shenasa M, Jazayeri M, et al. Wide QRS tachycardia: Reappraisal of a common clinical problem. Ann Intern Med 1988; 109:905–912.

Morady F, Baerman JM, DiCarlo LA Jr: A prevalent misconception regarding wide-complex tachycardias. JAMA 1985; 254:2790–2792.

Pick A, Langendorf R. Differentiation of supraventricular and ventricular tachycardia. Prog Cardiovasc Dis 1960; 2:391–407.

Wellens HJJ, Bar FW, Vanagt EJ, et al. The differentiation between ventricular tachycardia and supraventricular tachycardia with aberrant conduction: The value of the 12-lead electrocardiogram. In: Wellens HJJ, Kulbertus HE, eds. What's new in electrocardiography. The Hague: Martinus Nijhoff Publishers, 1981:184.

VI BRADYARRHYTHMIAS

SINUS NODE DYSFUNCTION: SINUS BRADYARRHYTHMIAS AND THE BRADY-TACHY SYNDROME

JAMES A. REIFFEL, M.D.

DEFINITION

Sinus node dysfunction may be defined as any abnormality in sinus node function, a definition that does not mandate the presence of symptoms. Traditionally, sinus node dysfunction has been recognized by undue or inappropriate sinus bradycardia, by periods of sinoatrial exit block or sinoatrial arrest, or by alternating sinus bradycardia and atrial tachyarrhythmias (so-called brady-tachy syndrome) (Figs. 1 to 3). Although both inappropriate sinus tachycardia and sinus node reentry might also fit this definition of sinus node dysfunction, clinically only the bradyarrhythmic manifestations have been considered when one recognizes the sick sinus syndrome. Neither etiology nor pathology is important regarding the definition (although both may be important in regard to prognosis and treatment).

PRESENTATION

Clinically, patients and physicians are most concerned with sinus node dysfunction when it is symptomatic.

In the setting of symptomatic sinus node dysfunction, symptom production can take several forms. With abrupt sinoatrial exit block, sinoatrial arrest, or marked sinus bradycardia, symptoms result from the inappropriate and prolonged pause (see Fig. 1). Such symptoms usually represent cerebral hypoperfusion, e.g., syncope and presyncopal lightheadedness. With inappropriate but less severe sinus bradycardia, symptoms take other forms. For symptomatic sinus bradycardia at rest, the associated symptoms may be fatigue, lethargy, or subtle central nervous system signs such as personality changes. For inappropriately slow sinus rates with activity, in which the sinus rate increases from its resting value (which may be normal) but not to a rate adequate or appropriate for the level of activity (called chronotropic incompetence), the symptoms are those of inadequate cardiac output—typically, exertional fatigue and/or dyspnea. Rarely, with marked sinus bradycardia and its associated increase in ventricular filling (and often end-diastolic pressure), dyspnea at rest and/or angina may result. However, this is truly infrequent in my experience. None of the above symptoms in and of themselves are specific for sinus node dysfunction. Thus, evaluation of the patient at hand requires both detection of the abnormal rhythm and determination of its relationship to the symptoms present.

In the brady-tachy syndrome (see Fig. 3), symptoms may result from either the tachycardia or the bradycardic phase. The symptoms in the tachycardia phase depend upon the nature of the tachycardia (atrial fibrillation, atrial flutter, paroxysmal supraventricular tachycardia), its rate, regularity, and atrioventricular relationship, and the presence or absence of underlying heart disease. Thus, they may include palpitations, dizziness, chest discomfort, dyspnea, and diaphoresis. Generally the tachycardia causes overdrive suppression of the sinus node (unless there is coexisting sinus node entrance block), which results in a prolonged pause or undue sinus bradycardia at the termination of the tachycardia. This may also be symptomatic.

MECHANISTIC IMPLICATIONS

Asymptomatic sinus node dysfunction is important only insofar as it may be of prognostic value and insofar as it may have an impact on the therapy of any associated disease. For the former reason, etiology is important. In my experience, sinus node dysfunction due to parasympathetic predominance or sensitivity is more common in the young than in the elderly and often lessens with time. This, however, is

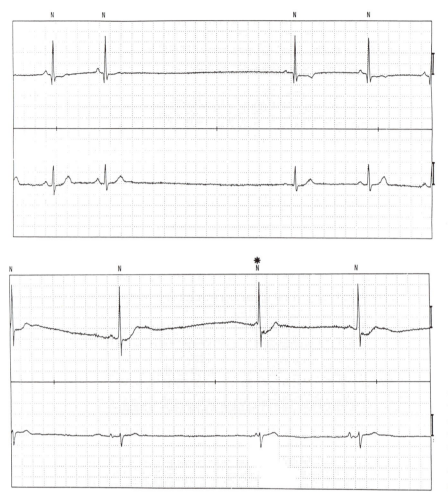

Figure 1 Holter recordings from a patient with sinoatrial arrest (top two simultaneous tracings) and a patient with marked sinus bradycardia (bottom two simultaneous tracings). Note in the tracings from the first patient that the long pause is not a multiple of the sinus cycle length, thus distinguishing sinoatrial arrest from sinoatrial exit block (in which case the long pause would have been a multiple of the basic sinus cycle length). Note in the tracings from the second patient that the third QRS complex is a junctional escape complex (marked with an asterisk), which occurred simultaneously with the inscription of the sinus P wave. The "N" labels above each set of Holter leads indicate a normal QRS complex with an associated sinus P wave and are automatically placed over each QRS complex in our Holter system. In subsequent figures, the "N" is replaced by an "S" when the beat is an atrial premature complex.

not uniformly the case. Parasympathetically mediated sinus node dysfunction, whether symptomatic or asymptomatic, can develop later in life — often in association with esophageal dysfunction, urinary tract dysfunction, carotid artery disease, and gastrointestinal tract disorders — and therefore it can be a factor in swallowing syncope, micturition syncope, and the hypersensitive carotid sinus syndrome (see the chapter *Hypersensitive Carotid Sinus Syndrome*). In contrast, intrinsic sinus node dysfunction is more common in the elderly. Intrinsic sinus node dysfunction, whether symptomatic or asymptomatic, may be part of diffuse conduction system dysfunction and/or may be associated with disease in the surrounding atrium. Such diseases may be ischemic, metabolic, inflammatory, or infiltrative (such as amyloidosis). Often, however, primary degeneration is the problem. In the brady-tachy syndrome, which I believe is more common in patients with intrinsic disease than in patients with parasympathetic dysfunction, there is often (but not always) an associated alteration in atrial size and/or histology. In the brady-tachy syndrome, there is also a significant incidence of pulmonary and systemic emboli, and symptoms from this are frequent enough that anticoagulation therapy of patients with the brady-tachy syndrome should be recommended.

PHARMACOLOGIC DENERVATION

Intrinsic and extrinsic (parasympathetically mediated) sinus node dysfunction can be distinguished by the response to atropine or pharmacologic denervation with atropine and propranolol. The inability to achieve a sinus rate of more than 90 beats per minute following atropine (given as 1-mg intravenous doses every 3 minutes until successive doses fail to cause a further increase in rate) is an easy means of confirming intrinsic disease in the office setting. However, caution needs to be used in the elderly and in patients with glaucoma, chronic obstructive pulmonary disease, prostatic hypertrophy, or other conditions in which atropine may be contraindicated.

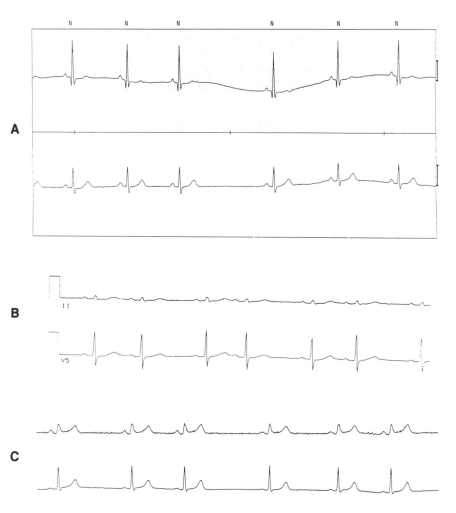

Figure 2 Three examples of sinoatrial Wenckebach type of sinoatrial exit block. The top two leads (*A*) are from a Holter recording. Note that the cycles preceding the pause were progressively shortening and the cycles following the pause again showed progressive shortening. The middle set of two leads (*B*) is from a patient with 3:2 sinoatrial Wenckebach block, and the bottom two leads (*C*) are from a patient with variable 4:3 and 3:2 sinoatrial Wenckebach block. These were both noted on routine electrocardiograms.

PHARMACOLOGIC CAUSES

Sinus node dysfunction may also result from pharmacologic agents. Such dysfunction, which may present as sinus bradycardia, sinoatrial arrest, sinoatrial exit block, and/or chronotropic incompetence, is more apt to occur when these agents are given to patients with latent sinus node dysfunction than when the patient's predrug sinus node function is truly normal. The most frequently offending agents include beta-adrenergic blocking drugs, calcium antagonists, sympatholytic antihypertensives, digitalis (infrequently), lithium carbonate, and all antiarrhythmic agents. Among the latter, amiodarone is particularly potent in this respect, whereas the class IB agents (lidocaine, mexiletine, and tocainide) are rare offenders.

ASSOCIATED FINDINGS

Because sinus node dysfunction is often associated with disease elsewhere in the conduction system, certain abnormalities aside from sinus bradycardia, sinoatrial arrest, and sinoatrial exit block should raise suspicion of this disorder. These include atrioventricular nodal dysfunction (such as atrial fibrillation with a slow ventricular response in the absence of drugs), "lone" atrial fibrillation, and failure to restore sinus rhythm with cardioversion. Therefore, when drugs are used to treat atrial fibrillation, these clues suggesting underlying sinus node dysfunction should be kept in mind. The presence of latent sinus node dysfunction may influence drug risk, drug choice, and consideration of pacemaker implantation prior to drug initiation.

DIAGNOSTIC ASSESSMENT

Since sinus node dysfunction is an electrocardiographic entity, whether symptomatic or asymptomatic, the diagnosis must utilize electrocardiographic techniques. These may be invasive or noninvasive, but the latter are always utilized first.

Although the standard 12-lead electrocardio-

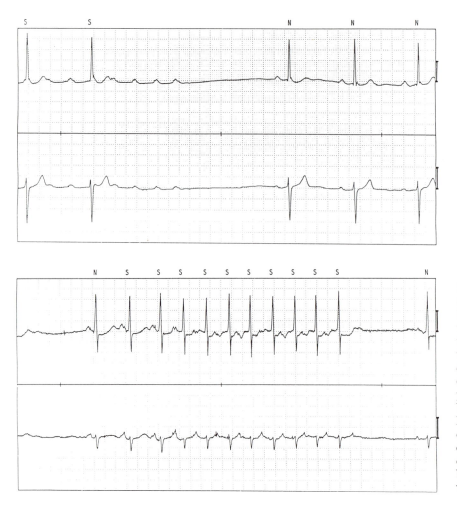

Figure 3 Two sets of Holter recordings from patients with the brady-tachy syndrome. Note in the first patient (top two leads) that the strip shows the termination of a burst of atrial tachycardia with variable atrioventricular conduction, followed by a sinus pause and then modest sinus bradycardia. The lower set of leads is from another patient, this one having sinus bradycardia recorded both before and after each of his short but symptomatic bursts of paroxysmal supraventricular tachycardia.

gram may establish the diagnosis, this is rarely the case. It is most useful in patients with persistent bradycardia or in those whose symptoms are sufficiently protracted so as to allow the patient to reach a medical facility before they terminate. Most often, symptoms of sinus node dysfunction are transient and intermittent; thus, more protracted ambulatory recordings are usually needed. The standard 24-hour Holter monitor recording is most useful in patients with daily or almost daily symptoms. It is also useful as a quantitative aid in patients who have asymptomatic sinus node dysfunction detected on a routine electrocardiogram. Analysis of Holter recordings, however, requires reference to an accurate time-, activity-, and symptom-annotated diary as well as a knowledge of normal heart rate variation. During sleep, for example, sinus bradycardia is expected and may reach low heart rates in the 30s and 40s (BPM) in normal individuals. Thus such rates do not always indicate sinus node dysfunction. Rates in the 30s during the daytime awake hours, however, would usually be considered abnormal (Fig. 4).

In most symptomatic patients, intermittent recorders are probably more useful. These may be continuous loop recorders that record and store the electrocardiogram only when the patient triggers the device during a symptomatic event, or transtelephonic recorders. The continuous loop recorders typically save 30 seconds or more of the electrocardiogram prior to the trigger as well as 30 seconds or more of electrocardiogram following the trigger. Transtelephonic recorders allow the patient to send a realtime electrocardiogram or an electrocardiogram previously recorded during a symptomatic period transtelephonically. Some devices can now be used in both of these ways.

In patients whose symptoms may be caused by chronotropic incompetence, a standard exercise tolerance test should be performed. Analysis should include heart rate response as well as the typical examination of ischemic alterations or ectopy. It should be noted, however, that regardless of the means by which the electrocardiogram is obtained, it must be closely examined. Blocked atrial premature

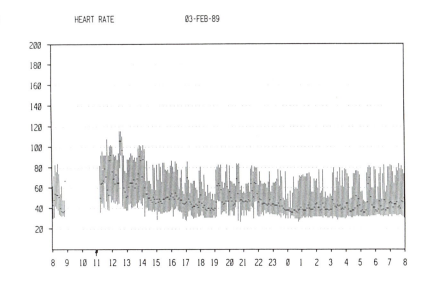

Figure 4 A heart rate plot from a 24-hour Holter recording. Note that the sinus bradycardia with rates in the 30s was present not only during sleep (which was midnight to 8:00 AM) but during waking hours as well. This patient was symptomatic and was treated with pacemaker implantation.

complexes, which may mimic sinus pauses (Fig. 5), must be recognized, as they are neither pathologic nor indications to initiate the treatment modalities utilized in the sick sinus syndrome (see further on).

In patients whose symptoms are not captured by noninvasive monitoring—usually because of their brevity and/or infrequency—invasive diagnostic tests are useful. Invasive electrophysiologic (EP) studies of sinus node function are also useful for quantitative analysis of asymptomatic sinus node dysfunction and serially as a guide to the effects of pharmacologic agents (see the chapter *Electrophysiologic Techniques*). Invasive EP techniques use electrogram recording and/or programmed stimulation to initiate a symptomatic period and/or to quantitate some parameter of sinus node function. Right atrial pacing, for example, may mimic or initiate a tachyarrhythmia, and both the length of the

pause and the time to restore normal sinus rhythm after its termination can be examined. Characteristics of sinoatrial conduction and sinus node refractoriness can also be assessed. When a symptomatic event is initiated, the diagnosis is established. When sinoatrial automaticity or conduction is quantitated, the likelihood that sinus node dysfunction may account for currently intermittent symptoms and the likelihood of subsequent symptom development can be ascertained. Patients with sinus bradycardia and normal or borderline EP findings rarely have symptoms caused by sinus node dysfunction and rarely develop them in 2 to 5 years of follow-up. The converse is also true.

EP studies can also be utilized to guide drug therapy. If one is concerned about the safety of an agent in its relation to sinus node function, EP measurements can be taken before and after its adminis-

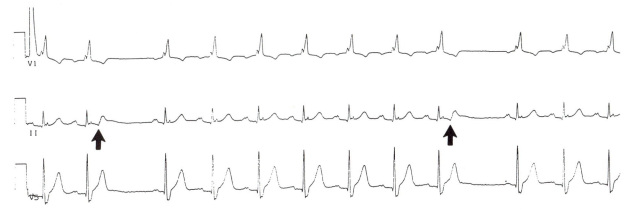

Figure 5 A 3-lead rhythm strip that superficially seems to show brief sinus pauses. Close examination of the second and ninth T waves, however, shows the presence of blocked atrial premature complexes at the junction of the S-T segment and the T-wave upstroke (*arrows*). Thus, these are not sinus pauses but rather an appropriate resetting of the sinus node following the atrial premature complexes that conducted retrogradely into a normal sinus node.

tration. When the agent is available in an intravenous form, both assessments can be made in one study. If no significant changes occur, the agent can usually be used safely with regard to the sinus node. Conversely, if significant changes are detected, an alternative agent should be chosen or a pacemaker should be implanted prior to its use. In such patients, an alternative approach is to start the drug at a low dose under monitored conditions and/or with a temporary pacemaker in place and gradually increase the dose under observation. This is a much more time-consuming and more costly process for the patient because of the hospital time involved.

In patients with the brady-tachy syndrome, serial EP studies can be used to judge antiarrhythmic efficacy in the tachycardia phase and to judge safety regarding the bradycardic phase. If the tachyarrhythmia is inducible prior to the drug tested but is no longer inducible after drug administration, the drug will usually be effective therapeutically in the chronic state.

TREATMENT

Treatment of patients with sinus node dysfunction is only necessary in those with symptoms (Fig. 6). The treatment choice only infrequently depends upon etiology. To some extent, it depends on the nature of the symptoms.

Since the treatment of tachyarrhythmias is covered elsewhere in this book, I will not discuss them here. Suffice it to say that since digitalis appears to worsen sinus node function only infrequently and has typically shortened the pause following atrial pacing in most studies, I usually try it first when treating tachycardias in the brady-tachy syndrome.

When sinus node dysfunction is pharmacologically induced, treatment should consist of removing the offending agent if possible. Thus, for example, a vasodilating antihypertensive agent may be tried in lieu of clonidine, or mexiletine may be tried in place of flecainide. Occasionally, in fact, hydralazine has been used even in normotensive patients to improve sinus node function in symptomatic patients because of its reflexly induced increase in sympathetic tone. When the offending agent cannot be eliminated, pacemaker implantation is usually necessary.

Similarly, when sinus node dysfunction is attributable to other reversible factors, such as metabolic derangements (e.g., hypothyroidism, acidosis, electrolyte disorders), the underlying disorder should be corrected and evidence for sinus node dysfunction reassessed.

When the underlying disorder is likely to be transient, only transient therapy may be needed. For example, sinus node dysfunction may be seen in the acute phase of any acute myocardial infarction and in the initial hospital phases of inferior or lateral myocardial infarctions. However, chronic symptomatic sick sinus syndrome following these events is not typical. Thus, the presence of symptomatic sinus node dysfunction early after an acute myocardial infarction should not prompt permanent pacemaker implantation; rather, belladonna administration or temporary pacemaker insertion should be utilized, and sinus node function should be reassessed during the convalescent or late hospital phase. One additional comment about post–myocardial infarction sinus node dysfunction is needed. In some patients, particularly in the early postmyocardial infarction phases, sinus bradycardia is asymptomatic but is associated with escape ventricular ectopy. As this ectopy may trigger serious ventricular tachyarrhythmias, temporary pacing may be needed to prevent the bradycardia, even though the sinus node dysfunction itself is asymptomatic. In this circumstance, all antiarrhythmic drugs may be dangerous without a temporary pacer because they may provoke much more serious sinus node dysfunction.

In patients with parasympathetically mediated ("extrinsic") sinus node dysfunction, a search for and correction of the initiating disorder may be the only treatment needed. For example, if a gastrointestinal or genitourinary disorder is the trigger, if it is treatable, its resolution may be associated with resolution of the sinus node dysfunction. In clinical practice, however, these patterns of sinus node dysfunction are seen infrequently. Similarly, the hypersensitive carotid sinus may be denervated as an alternative to pacemaker implantation, or chronic belladonna administration may be employed when the associated bradycardia requires treatment. In some patients, symptomatic parasympathetically mediated sinus node dysfunction can be efficiently treated with chronic belladonna alkaloid administra-

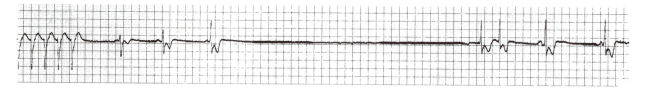

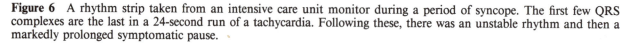

Figure 6 A rhythm strip taken from an intensive care unit monitor during a period of syncope. The first few QRS complexes are the last in a 24-second run of a tachycardia. Following these, there was an unstable rhythm and then a markedly prolonged symptomatic pause.

tion (e.g., atropine, propantheline, tincture of belladonna). In most patients, however, the parasympatholytic and/or central nervous system side effects limit the feasibility of this approach. Most elderly patients, for example, cannot tolerate significant doses of these agents because they often precipitate side effects of lethargy and confusion and/or symptoms of prostatism or constipation. Thus, I have found this approach to be most feasible in young patients. It may also be most appropriate in such patients, as many in their teens and early twenties "outgrow" their sinus node dysfunction as they get older. If the only symptoms are associated with chronotropic incompetence, alkaloids may be given as needed just prior to activity.

PACEMAKER CONSIDERATIONS

Unfortunately, most patients with sinus node dysfunction who are encountered in clinical practice do not fall into the above categories. They are often middle-aged or elderly individuals with chronic dysfunction of the sinus node due to aging-related degeneration of the sinus node and often other components of the cardiac conduction system; ischemic damage; or inflammatory, infiltrative, or other disorders. Since the dysfunction, once symptomatic, is permanent, its treatment must likewise be permanent. Such treatment, except as noted above, requires permanent pacemaker implantation. Pacemaker implantation will not be challenged by third-party insurance carriers when the device is implanted for a bradyarrhythmia that has been documented to be associated with symptoms (using the diagnostic techniques discussed above) or when the symptom is unmonitored but no alternative for the symptom other than a severe bradyarrhythmia has been found with a detailed work-up. Pacemaker implantation is also not usually challenged if the degree of bradycardia is severe enough to pose a danger to the patient (sinus rate less than 30 beats per minute or pauses of less than 3 seconds) or if it is needed to support some form of pharmacologic therapy that cannot be stopped and for which no alternative exists. This is most frequently encountered in patients with the brady-tachy syndrome and in patients with angina, hypertension, or congestive heart failure. Again, however, I emphasize that asymptomatic sinus node dysfunction does not require or justify permanent pacemaker insertion.

Once the decision to implant a pacemaker has been made, the physician must decide what type of pacemaker to implant. In general, I have found the following approach to be useful in patients with sinus node dysfunction:

1. In patients with infrequent and transient episodes of sinoatrial arrest or exit block, marked sinus bradycardia, or posttachycardia pauses, a VVI unit

with a relatively slow rate (50 beats per minute) is all the patient needs.

2. In patients with persistent sinus bradycardia at rest but chronotropic competence with activity, an AAI, VVI, or DVI unit with a rate of 70 to 80 beats per minute is usually adequate. AAI should be used when atrioventricular conduction is normal, VVI or DVI when atrioventricular conduction is impaired. DVI is preferable to VVI when atrioventricular synchrony must be maintained because of underlying hemodynamic considerations (impaired left ventricular contractility or compliance) or when ventriculoatrial conduction is intact and avoidance of the "pacemaker syndrome" is necessary.

3. The advent of DDD pacing has made DVI outmoded for most patients with atrioventricular block and normal sinus node function, as DDD pacing not only allows pacing to prevent a symptomatic bradycardia but also allows a physiologic increase in ventricular rate with maintenance of atrioventricular synchrony with activity. In patients with sinus node dysfunction, however, the DDD unit loses some of its advantage over the DVI unit. In patients with sinus node dysfunction and chronotropic incompetence, for example, DDD pacing does not physiologically increase the ventricular rate, since the sinus rate that triggers ventricular pacing is no longer appropriate in these patients. Thus, in patients with symptomatic chronotropic incompetence, non–P wave triggered rate-responsive pacers may be better choices. Such pacers utilize chest wall muscle activity, respiratory rate, thoracic impedance, temperature, Q-T interval, catecholamine effects, and other physiologic sensors to trigger a graded increase in pacing rate with activity. There can be VVIR or DDDR units. In patients with sinus node dysfunction but preserved chronotropic competence, DDD units are not appropriate unless an atrioventricular conduction disorder exists.

4. Additional considerations in the choice between DVI and DDD pacing are encountered in patients with brady-tachy syndrome. Since DVI pacing is associated with asynchronous atrial stimulation, there is a risk of precipitating the patient's atrial tachyarrhythmia with such devices. Assessment of this risk can be made by preimplant EP study. Additionally, in patients with the brady-tachy syndrome, the presence of an atrial tachyarrhythmia may trigger an inappropriately rapid ventricular rate if a DDD unit is implanted. Thus, the upper tracking rate chosen must be limited (thus also limiting chronotropic competence) or the DDD unit should be avoided altogether. Again, a preimplant EP study that shows drug efficacy against the tachycardia will be helpful in designing therapy, as the ideal combination of drug plus optimal device may be chosen.

Supported in part by USPHS Grant RR00645.

SUGGESTED READING

Bigger JT Jr, Reiffel JA. Sick sinus syndrome. Ann Rev Med 1979; 30:91–118.

Bigger JT Jr, Reiffel JA, Coromilas J. Ambulatory electrocardiography. In: Platia E, ed. Non-pharmacologic management of cardiac arrhythmias. Philadelphia: JB Lippincott, 1986:36.

Jordan JL, Yamaguchi I, Mandel WJ. Studies on the mechanism of sinus node dysfunction in the sick sinus syndrome. Circulation 1978; 57:217–223.

Karagueuzian HS, Jordan JL, Sugi K, et al. Appropriate diagnostic studies for sinus node dysfunction. PACE 1985; 8:242–254.

Reiffel JA. Electrophysiologic evaluation of sinus node function. Cardiol Clin 1986; 4:401–416.

Reiffel JA. Clinical electrophysiology of the sinus node. In: Mazgalev T, Dreifus LS, Michelson EL, eds. Electrophysiology of the sino-atrial and atrioventricular nodes: Integrative physiologic, morphologic, autonomic, and pharmacologic aspects. New York: Alan R. Liss, 1988:239.

Reiffel JA, Ferrick K, Zimmerman J, Bigger JT Jr. Electrophysiologic studies of the sinus node and atria. Cardiovas Clin 1985; 16:37–59.

Reiffel JA, Spotnitz HM. Pacemakers, pacemaker mediated tachycardias, and antitachycardia pacemakers. In: Vlay S, ed. Manual of cardiac arrhythmias. Boston: Little Brown, 1987:358.

HYPERSENSITIVE CAROTID SINUS SYNDROME

STEPHEN C. HAMMILL, M.D.
BERNARD J. GERSH, M.B., Ch.B., D.Phil.

The syndrome of syncope or near-syncope in association with a hypersensitive carotid sinus reflex has been known since the time of Galen and has been studied extensively in both animals and humans. The clinician must distinguish between the hypersensitive carotid sinus reflex, which occurs commonly, and carotid sinus syncope, which occurs less frequently. The hypersensitive carotid sinus reflex is defined as cardiac asystole lasting 3 seconds or more or a decrease in systolic blood pressure of 50 mm Hg or more in response to digital stimulation of the carotid sinus. The hypersensitive carotid sinus reflex rarely occurs in the first two decades of life. The incidence then increases with age, to 25 to 30 percent in men over 50 years old; men are affected twice as often as women. The reflex usually is evoked more easily by stimulation of the right than the left sinus, and it may be present bilaterally. In contrast, carotid sinus syncope, the less common condition, occurs in 5 to 20 percent of persons with a hypersensitive reflex.

The cardiovascular response to digital stimulation of the carotid sinus is divided into two types: (1) the cardioinhibitory type with bradycardia or asystole, with or without systemic hypotension; and (2) the vasodepressor type with hypotension independent of changes in heart rate. The cardioinhibitory type occurs in approximately 60 percent of patients, the vasodepressor type occurs in 10 percent of patients, and a mixed type occurs in 30 percent of patients. A primary cerebral type was described; however, this now is believed not to exist. It is considered to be attributable to an impairment of consciousness with carotid sinus massage, as a result of decreased cerebral blood flow in a patient with preexisting occlusive cerebral vascular disease.

The carotid sinus baroreceptors are located in the adventitia of a small dilatation of the internal carotid artery, just above the bifurcation of the common carotid artery. They consist of extensively branched and myelinated nerve endings. Impulses from the carotid sinus ascend in the glossopharyngeal and vagus nerves to the sensory nucleus of the vagus and the vasomotor centers. An increase in tension within the carotid sinus activates the dorsal motor nucleus of the vagus (cardioinhibitory center) and inhibits tonic discharge from the vasomotor center, with concomitant slowing of the heart rate and decrease in blood pressure.

In some patients with cardioinhibitory carotid sinus hypersensitivity, there may be increased sensitivity to vagal stimulation at the interface between the efferent vagal limb and the heart. A hypersensitive carotid sinus response in such patients may reflect hypervagotonia. The carotid sinus is unusually susceptible to the development of atheroma, which may account for the increasing incidence of carotid sinus hypersensitivity with aging. The majority of patients have no obvious abnormality in the region of the carotid sinus; however, certain patients have enlarged cervical lymph nodes, local tumors, aneurysmal dilation of the internal carotid artery, and atherosclerotic changes in the carotid bifurcation or common carotid arteries. Others have had prior neck surgery and radiation therapy.

CLINICAL PRESENTATION

Patients with carotid sinus syncope complain of lightheadedness, blurring of vision, a feeling of general weakness, near-syncope, and syncope. At times, the loss of consciousness can be of sudden onset, immediately preceded or accompanied by pallor, coldness of the skin, and deep respiration. During the syncopal episode the patient usually is motionless and limp but occasionally, when cardiac asystole is prolonged, a tonic spasm of the body and a few clonic jerks of the limbs and face can be seen. Unconsciousness is usually brief, and the sensorium is quickly restored. The sensorium begins clearing soon after the patient is placed in the prone position. To produce syncope, cardiac asystole must last from 5 to 15 seconds. Electrocardiographic abnormalities include sinoatrial slowing, atrial conduction defects, prolongation of the P-R interval, atrioventricular block, sinoatrial arrest, junctional escape, complete asystole, and ventricular ectopic complexes.

The vasodepressor type of carotid sinus hypersensitivity occurs less frequently. Patients with this syndrome present with clinical symptoms similar to those of the cardioinhibitory type, except that the syncope does not occur in the recumbent position. The symptoms tend to last longer because the blood pressure may not recover to its normal level for several minutes. Palpation of a peripheral artery or electrocardiographic recording during an episode of vasodepressor carotid sinus syncope will document no or only minor slowing of the sinus rate despite symptomatic hypotension.

VASODEPRESSOR SYNCOPE IN PATIENTS WITHOUT CAROTID SINUS HYPERSENSITIVITY

Recent reports have described the use of beta-adrenergic receptor stimulation with isoproterenol in association with upright tilting to induce vasodepressor syncope in patients with a clinical history consistent with this disorder but with otherwise normal cardiac and neurologic findings including electrophysiologic testing and carotid sinus massage. This response is believed to be due to stimulation of C fibers in the left ventricle after vigorous contraction of the left ventricle around an empty cavity. This is the postulated mechanism of vasodepressor syncope in such patients, and a suggested treatment has been beta-adrenergic receptor blockade with propranolol or metoprolol.

It has not yet been established whether this reflex has any association with the vasodepressor component in patients with carotid sinus hypersensitivity. However, a common mechanism may exist, and the successful use of alpha-adrenergic receptor stimulation with ephedrine and beta-adrenergic receptor blockade with metoprolol has been reported in a patient with carotid sinus syncope.

METHOD OF CAROTID SINUS STIMULATION

Initially, the physician should check for satisfactory pulsation of the carotid and temporal arteries and auscultate the carotid vessels for bruits. If carotid artery obstruction is suspected or there is a history of cerebrovascular disease, the test should not be performed. The patient is placed in the supine position; significant head rotation is avoided, and the head is kept in a neutral position between flexion and extension. The examiner's fingers feel gently for the fusiform carotid sinus or the area of greatest arterial pulsation in front of the sternomastoid muscle at the upper border of the thyroid cartilage. The right and left sinuses are firmly massaged sequentially for 5 seconds each, and 30 seconds should elapse between tests of the two sides. This test should be done with electrocardiographic and blood pressure monitoring. If no abnormalities are identified, the procedure should be repeated with the patient in an upright position, either sitting or on a tilt-table. Repeating the test in the upright position helps to identify patients who have vasodepressor carotid sinus hypersensitivity and in whom there is little change in heart rate but significant decrease in blood pressure. The hypotension often is less pronounced in the supine position, and the vasodepressor response may not be detected. For the examiner to be certain that the patient's syncope is related to carotid sinus hypersensitivity, carotid sinus massage should produce a significant cardioinhibitory or vasodepressor response (Fig. 1) with associated symptoms that duplicate the patient's spontaneous symptoms of near syncope or syncope.

APPROACH TO THE PATIENT WITH SYNCOPE PRESUMED DUE TO CAROTID SINUS HYPERSENSITIVITY

Testing to rule out other causes of syncope generally is not required in the unusual patient who has a classic history of carotid sinus hypersensitivity—i.e., syncope occurring after extrinsic pressure on the carotid sinus—or has obvious anatomic abnormalities in the region of the carotid sinus. Unfortunately, the majority of patients with syncope compatible

Figure 1 Example of electrocardiographic tracing during carotid sinus massage (*dark line above tracing*) producing sinus arrest with junctional escape beats.

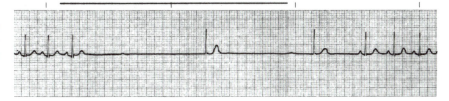

with carotid sinus hypersensitivity do not have the classic history. Instead, they present with syncope whose cause is unclear after careful history taking, physical examination, review of the electrocardiogram, and routine blood tests. During the physical examination, carotid sinus massage should be performed only in the absence of any physical signs or history to suggest cerebrovascular disease. The patient's electrocardiogram and blood pressure should be recorded during the carotid sinus massage in the supine and then the upright (or sitting) position (as described above). Carotid sinus hypersensitivity should be diagnosed as the cause of the patient's syncope only if carotid sinus massage produces asystole or hypotension and reproduces the clinical syndrome.

Role of Electrophysiologic Testing

It often is difficult to establish firmly that a patient's syncope is caused by carotid sinus hypersensitivity because this finding is common in older patients who also have other cardiovascular abnormalities that could account for syncope. In a patient with syncope in whom carotid sinus hypersensitivity is believed to be the cause, electrophysiologic testing may be used to exclude other cardiogenic causes of syncope, such as intermittent complete heart block or ventricular tachycardia.

Once other causes of syncope have been excluded, carotid sinus massage can be performed in the electrophysiology laboratory with the patient in the upright position. Use of a tilt-table helps to separate the cardioinhibitory from the vasodepressor components of carotid sinus hypersensitivity. If the patient exhibits asystole and hypotension in response to carotid sinus massage, atrioventricular sequential pacing should be performed and carotid sinus massage should be repeated. A persistent decrease in blood pressure despite the maintenance of a normal heart rate and atrioventricular synchrony establishes the diagnosis of a vasodepressor component.

Electrophysiologic testing also can help to determine the optimal pacing mode if pacing is considered for treatment. The presence of the pacemaker syndrome associated with ventricular pacing and the likelihood that pacing will relieve the patient's symptoms can be assessed. This is helpful information in patients with a significant vasodepressor component to their carotid sinus hypersensitivity since in these patients the symptoms will not be completely alleviated by permanent pacing, and pharmacologic or mechanical therapy is usually required to prevent vasodepression. Thus, patients with a mixed carotid sinus hypersensitivity can be forewarned that pacing may not entirely relieve their near-syncope or syncope.

Carotid sinus hypersensitivity may not always be a reproducible finding. In some cases, the patient may have a history consistent with carotid sinus syncope but no abnormality during carotid sinus massage in an office examination. Then, at the time of electrophysiologic testing, carotid sinus massage results in asystole or hypotension and reproduces their clinical syncope. Variations in autonomic tone and intravascular fluid status are assumed to be the cause of this inconsistency.

Treatment

Patients who have had only a single episode of syncope believed to be due to carotid sinus hypersensitivity often have no recurrences (Table 1). All that is required is an explanation of the abnormality, avoidance of known precipitating factors (such as tight neckwear, stretching the skin during shaving, or looking over the shoulder when driving backward), and careful follow-up. Other forms of treatment that can be reserved for patients who have recurrent episodes of syncope include discontinuation of medications known to cause vasodilation or hypovolemia (diuretics, nitrates), use of support stockings, pharmacologic agents, permanent pacing, and surgery (Table 2). The selection of therapy is based on the relative influences of the cardioinhibitory and vaso-

Table 1 Treatment and Follow-Up in 53 Patients With Symptomatic Carotid Sinus Hypersensitivity*

	No Treatment	Anticholinergic Drug	Pacemaker
Number of patients	11	19	23
Cardioinhibitory carotid sinus hypersensitivity	77%	90%	83%
Mixed carotid sinus hypersensitivity	23%	10%	17%
		Follow-up	
Duration (mean)	39 mo	41 mo	23 mo
Syncope	27%	21%	9%
Near-syncope	9%	0	22%
Asymptomatic	64%	79%	69%

*Data from Sugrue DD, Gersh BJ, Holmes DR Jr, et al. Symptomatic "isolated" carotid sinus hypersensitivity: Natural history and results of treatment with anticholinergic drugs or pacemaker. J Am Coll Cardiol 1986; 7:158–162.

Table 2 Treatment of Carotid Sinus Syncope

Cardioinhibitory Component
  Anticholinergic drugs
  Permanent pacing
    Ventricular (absence of pacemaker syndrome)
    Dual-chamber
Vasodepressor Component
  Elasticized body garment
  High-salt diet
  Fluorohydrocortisone
  Ephedrine

depressor components on the patient's carotid sinus syncope.

Cardioinhibitory Carotid Sinus Hypersensitivity. Patients with pure cardioinhibitory carotid sinus hypersensitivity can be treated with anticholinergic therapy or permanent pacing. Anticholinergic therapy is achieved with propantheline bromide in doses ranging from 7.5 mg three times daily to 15 mg four times daily. Anticholinergic therapy may be limited by side effects including dry mouth, blurred vision, urinary difficulties, and constipation. This form of therapy is contraindicated in patients known to have glaucoma. In the elderly, ocular pressure should be assessed before anticholinergic therapy is begun.

Permanent pacing is the other standard form of treatment for patients with cardioinhibitory carotid sinus hypersensitivity. Atrial pacing is not recommended because many patients have atrioventricular conduction defects in addition to sinus node dysfunction at the time of carotid sinus syncope. Ventricular pacing is effective but should be avoided when there is evidence of ventriculoatrial conduction, which indicates that the patient is at increased risk of pacemaker syndrome. We usually implant a dual-chamber pacing system to avoid pacemaker syndrome.

Vasodepressor Carotid Sinus Hypersensitivity. The vasodepressor component can be treated mechanically with elastic stockings that go up to the thigh or waist, fluid expansion with a high-salt diet or fluorohydrocortisone, or a vasoconstrictor medi-

cation such as ephedrine. Patients who have frequent syncope and near-syncope from the vasodepressor component of carotid sinus hypersensitivity may have a satisfactory clinical response to the use of elastic stockings. Patients who have infrequent syncope often find the stockings difficult to wear long term. These patients may elect to try a pharmacologic course; the most commonly used medication at this time is ephedrine, usually at 25 mg three or four times daily. Adverse reactions to ephedrine include nervousness, difficulty in sleeping, and palpitations. A trial of a beta-blocking agent may be worthwhile, but there are no systematic studies to support or refute this approach.

Severe carotid sinus syncope that fails to respond adequately to the above measures may require surgical denervation of the carotid sinus or transection of the glossopharyngeal nerve and upper rootlets of the vagus nerve at their exit from the brainstem. The number of reported cases of surgical therapy is too small to warrant conclusions regarding benefit. Carotid sinus irradiation has not proved to be a useful therapy.

SUGGESTED READING

Almquist A, Gornick C, Benson W Jr, et al. Carotid sinus hypersensitivity: Evaluation of the vasodepressor component. Circulation 1985; 71:927–936.

Madigan NP, Flaker GC, Curtis JJ, et al. Carotid sinus hypersensitivity: Beneficial effects of dual-chamber pacing. Am J Cardiol 1984; 53:1034–1040.

Nelson SD, Kou WH, De Buitleir M, et al. Value of programmed ventricular stimulation in presumed carotid sinus syndrome. Am J Cardiol 1987; 60:1073–1077.

Stryjer D, Friedensohn A, Schlesinger Z. Ventricular pacing as the preferable mode for long-term pacing in patients with carotid sinus syncope of the cardioinhibitory type. PACE 1986; 9:705–709.

Sugrue DD, Gersh BJ, Holmes DR Jr, et al. Symptomatic "isolated" carotid sinus hypersensitivity: Natural history and results of treatment with anticholinergic drugs or pacemaker. J Am Coll Cardiol 1986; 7:158–162.

Thomas JE, Hammill SC. Carotid sinus syncope. In: Brandenburg RO, Fuster V, Giuliani ER, McGoon DC, eds. Cardiology: Fundamentals and practice. Chicago: Year Book Medical Publishers, 1987:693.

Waxman MB, Yao L, Cameron DA, et al. Isoproterenol induction of vasodepressor-type reaction in vasodepressor-prone persons. Am J Cardiol 1989; 63:58–65.

INTRAVENTRICULAR CONDUCTION DISTURBANCES AND ATRIOVENTRICULAR BLOCK

AGUSTIN CASTELLANOS, M.D.
PEDRO FERNANDEZ, M.D.
ROBERT J. MYERBURG, M.D.

Knowledge of the treatment of symptomatic atrioventricular (AV) conduction disturbances must be based on an understanding of the various intraventricular blocks that sometimes precede (and may even be responsible for) them.

INTRAVENTRICULAR BLOCK

So much has been written about the conduction disturbances presented in Table 1 that only certain specific points will be emphasized here. Foremost among them is the fact that although working criteria have been proposed for the diagnosis of intraventricular block (imposed by the need to interpret routine clinical electrocardiograms), it can be argued that the sensitivity and specificity of these criteria still require independent confirmation. The newer techniques of endocardial and epicardial mapping and phase imaging appear to be promising in this regard.

The following points are noteworthy:

1. Left anterior fascicular block is only one of the many processes capable of producing abnormal left axis deviation.

2. In contrast to left anterior fascicular block, left posterior fascicular block is rarely diagnosed. It is possible to do so when, in the presence of "complete" right bundle branch block, there is extreme right axis deviation ($\geq$ 120 degrees) occurring in the absence of right ventricular hypertrophy, pulmonary disease, abnormal (anatomic) heart position, and extensive high lateral wall myocardial infarction.

3. Although several criteria have been proposed for the identification of left septal (middle) fascicular block, this conduction disturbance is exceptionally well diagnosed in routine electrocardiographic interpretation.

4. The so-called "incomplete" right bundle branch block is simply an electrocardiographic pattern which, in addition to being caused by a conduction delay through a right bundle branch of normal length, can be due to conduction disturbances in a stretched right bundle branch or in one or more of the peripheral fascicles of the right bundle, that is, in the outflow tract or dysplastic right ventricular tissues.

5. Nonspecific intraventricular conduction defects with QRS complex duration longer than 120 msec may be generalized (as in hyperkalemia or after administration of certain antiarrhythmic medications) as well as localized (focal). Localized defects occur, not infrequently, inside an acutely ischemic area or around a chronically fibrotic or infarcted region (periinfarction block).

In general, the clinical importance of the corresponding patterns relates to which ones can be precursors of symptomatic AV block, as is discussed subsequently.

ATRIOVENTRICULAR BLOCK

An all-inclusive universal classification of these conduction disturbances is lacking. The one shown in Table 2 is presented mainly for didactic reasons.

Table 1 Intraventricular Conduction Defects

Left anterior fascicular block
Left posterior fascicular block
Left (middle) septal fascicular block
Right bundle branch block
   Complete
   Incomplete
Left bundle branch block
   Complete
   Incomplete
Nonspecific intraventricular block
   Localized (focal): periinfarction, intrainjury
   Generalized: hyperkalemic, drug-induced, diffuse
      fibrosis-induced
Combinations of the above

Table 2 Atrioventricular Blocks

Rate-Independent

First degree
Second degree
   Type I (Wenckebach periods)
   Type II (Mobitz)
   Alternating Wenckebach periods
Reverse alternating Wenckebach periods
High degree or advanced
Complete
   Chronic
   Temporary or paroxysmal

Rate-Dependent

Tachycardia-dependent
Bradycardia-dependent

Rate-Associated

Vagal block at the AV node
   Pseudo-Wenckebach
   Pseudo-Mobitz or pseudo–bradycardia dependent

RATE-INDEPENDENT BLOCKS

The fundamental electrocardiographic features of these conduction disturbances during *stable* sinus rhythm have been described many times. Emphasis should be placed on the fact that the classic description refers to instances in which the sinus rate does not show marked variations. A persistently perfectly regular sinus rate is an illusion. Hence, for practical purposes, the regularity of the rate will be considered to apply only to the (given) moment at which the AV block appears.

1. First-degree AV block is characterized by prolongation of the P-R interval.

2. It is customary to classify second-degree AV block occurring during "regular" sinus rhythm as type I (Wenckebach periods) or type II (Mobitz). However, during rapid ectopic atrial rhythms (atrial tachycardias, atrial flutter, or rapid atrial stimulation), it is not uncommon to observe the so-called alternate Wenckebach periods. These are episodes of 2:1 AV block during which there is a progressive prolongation of the P-R interval of conducted beats, terminating in a greater degree of block (2:1 or 3:1). In addition, recently, reversed alternating Wenckebach periods have been discussed. These are episodes of 2:1 AV block (emerging from runs of 3:2 block), but with the P-R interval of the conducted beats showing a gradual decrease until terminating in a lesser degree of AV block.

3. Although Wenckebach phenomena can occur in any part of the heart, most take place within the AV node. On the other hand, the majority of type II Mobitz blocks are infra-AV nodal phenomena occurring in patients with bundle branch, bifascicular, or trifascicular blocks. We prefer to categorize them according to how they start. Characteristically, their onset is not heralded by any marked (or insignificant) increase in the preceding P-R intervals. Moreover, they can lead to one or multiple blocked P waves. Mobitz type II blocks with varying ratios are not seen more often in the United States because pacemakers are implanted in patients almost as soon as they are identified.

RATE-DEPENDENT AV BLOCKS

The more frequent tachycardia-dependent AV blocks appear (usually in patients with wide QRS complexes) when the rates increase above (or cycle lengths decrease below) a critical value. The latter does not necessarily have to be in the tachycardia (greater than 100 per minute) range; it must simply be a value that is specific only for a point and moment in time. These conduction disturbances may appear to be rate-independent when the preblock rates are very close to the critical value. Usually they are best diagnosed when there are abrupt changes in cycle lengths.

On the other hand, bradycardia-dependent AV blocks are rare. As the name suggests, they appear (in patients with wide QRS complexes) when the rates decrease below the critical value. Mechanically, their occurrence is dependent on the decrease in rate, that is, on an increase in the cycle length; if these parameters are unchanged, the conduction disturbance cannot occur.

AV BLOCKS ASSOCIATED WITH BUT NOT DEPENDENT ON A DECREASE IN SINUS RATES

These conduction disturbances are not rare. They are seen during Holter monitoring in ambulatory patients or in patients with acute inferior myocardial infarction. Classically, they coexist with narrow QRS complexes and are accompanied by a gradual decrease in the P-P intervals until one or two (rarely more) P waves are blocked. The P-R interval immediately preceding the blocked P wave may show an appreciable increment (pseudo or atypical Wenckebach), or it may appear to be unchanged (pseudo-Mobitz or pseudo–bradycardia-dependent AV block). This relates to the underlying electrogenetic mechanism: enhanced vagal effects, greater on the AV node than on the sinus node. Because of such differential vagal action, there is a gradual decrease in sinus rate (owing to lesser effects on the sinus node). The more intense vagal effects on the AV node may be gradual when the blocked P wave is preceded by progressive P-R interval prolongation, but if they are abrupt, the preceding P-R intervals are constant. In contrast to bradycardia-dependent AV block (in which if there is no bradycardia, there is no block), here the bradycardia is an associated (but not essential) phenomenon, since the (AV nodal) block can still appear when the atrial rate is kept constant by atrial pacing.

PAROXYSMAL AV BLOCK

This term has been used in reference to episodes of 1:1 AV conduction interrupted by the occurrence of a sudden, unexpected block of several P waves, generally leading to symptoms (Fig. 1). According to its mode of onset, Mobitz type II block as well as tachycardia- and bradycardia-dependent blocks can occur paroxysmally. Because these blocks are infra-AV nodal, usually occurring at the bundle branches, the preceding (conducted) QRS complexes are wide. Rarely, when they are due exclusively to His bundle lesions, the corresponding ventricular complexes are narrow (see Fig. 1).

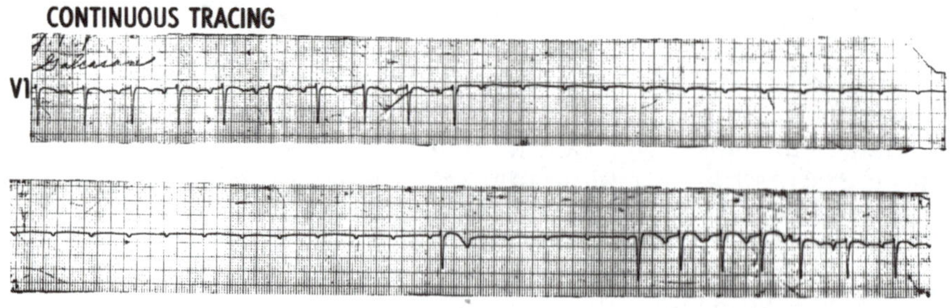

CONTINUOUS TRACING

Figure 1 Paroxysmal AV (or transient complete) block in a patient with intra-Hisian block. Note the absence of idioventricular escapes as well as reinitiation of 1:1 conduction toward the end of the lower strip.

Because paroxysmal AV block is preceded by long periods of sinus rhythm with 1:1 AV conduction, the supraventricular impulses constantly reaching the ventricles keep the potential escape "foci" (idioventricular centers) in a state of overdrive suppression. Consequently, when the block occurs, it takes some time for the idioventricular centers to become active and to "warm up" (see Fig. 1). Depending on the time required for this to occur, the patient develops symptoms, including simple dizziness, presyncope, syncope, or typical Adams-Stokes attacks.

Because the idioventricular rhythms eventually are activated in most cases, the majority of patients developing paroxysmal block do not die (see Fig. 1). This explains why paroxysmal (or chronic, if the latter becomes established) AV block is not a frequent cause of sudden death. However, prior to the introduction of implantable pacemakers, some patients with persistently symptomatic chronic or paroxysmal AV block did die (Fig. 2). For example, in 1971, Bellet, following a review of the available literature, stated that prior to the initiation of large-scale long-term pacing, 50 to 60 percent of subjects who suffered a first Adams-Stokes attack died within a year, most often from a subsequent attack. These patients were prone to recurrent episodes.

TREATMENT OF AV BLOCK CAUSED BY CHRONIC CONDUCTION SYSTEM DISEASE

Although as stated earlier most patients do not die from the first clinical manifestation of AV block not caused by acute ischemia or infarction, pacemakers are implanted to abolish symptoms that can interfere with a good quality of life and even to prevent episodes leading to accidents capable of causing neurologic and orthopedic complications.

IDENTIFICATION OF PATIENTS PRONE TO DEVELOPING SYMPTOMATIC AV BLOCK

Already in the 1960s, it was observed that if preblock electrocardiograms were available in patients with symptomatic nonischemic complete (chronic or paroxysmal) AV block, most showed left bundle branch block or the combination of right bundle branch block usually with left anterior and rarely left posterior fascicular block (the so-called bifascicular blocks).

Coupled with the introduction and widespread use of the techniques of recording the intracardiac potentials from the His bundle, this observation led several groups to perform prospective studies to evaluate the natural history of bundle branch and trifascicular blocks as well as to identify possible markers for the development of advanced types of AV conduction disturbances before their occurrence.

In the final report of their prospective study, McAnulty and coworkers discussed 554 patients with chronic bifascicular and trifascicular block followed for an average of 42.4 months. Advanced AV block was documented in 19 patients at an average of 24 months after entry into the study. The cumulative incidence of AV block at 5 years was 4.9 percent (a rate of approximately 1 percent per year). Seventeen patients were successfully treated with implanted pacemakers. However, two patients died:

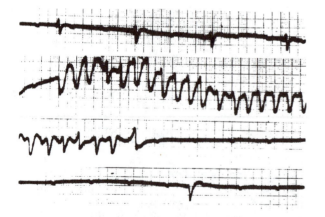

Figure 2 Strips obtained in 1954 showing death in a patient with chronic complete AV block due to primary conduction system disease who had recurrent syncopal attacks. The ventricular tachycardia was a bradycardia-related arrhythmia that caused overdrive suppression of all idioventricular pacemakers. (Courtesy of Dr. Luis Azan.)

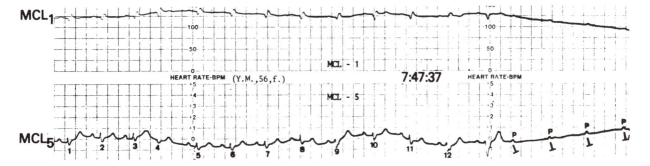

Figure 3 Holter recording obtained at the onset of paroxysmal AV block and of syncope (7:47:37) in a patient with primary conduction system disease. (From Medina-Ravell V, Rodriguez-Salas L, Castellanos A, Myerburg RJ. Death due to paroxysmal atrioventricular block during ambulatory electrocardiographic monitoring. PACE 1989; 12:65–69, with permission.)

one before a device could be inserted, and one because of failure of a temporary pacemaker. Overall, there were 67 (47 percent) sudden deaths in this group of patients, in whom the predictors of death were coronary artery disease and increasing age.

The series of Scheinman and associates included 401 patients followed for a mean of around 36 months. Atrioventricular block developed in 19 patients, 12 of whom had H-V intervals of 70 msec or longer. These authors concluded that *prophylactic*

pacing was of no value for relief of symptoms or prolongation of life. Yet these authors considered an H-V interval greater than 100 msec and/or atrial pacing–induced infranodal block as a possible indicator of the development of spontaneous AV block.

Although intentional drug-induced (with ajmaline or procainamide) first-, second- or high-degree AV block may suggest a limited His-Purkinje reserve, the available data do not lead to definite recommendations for prophylactic pacemaker im-

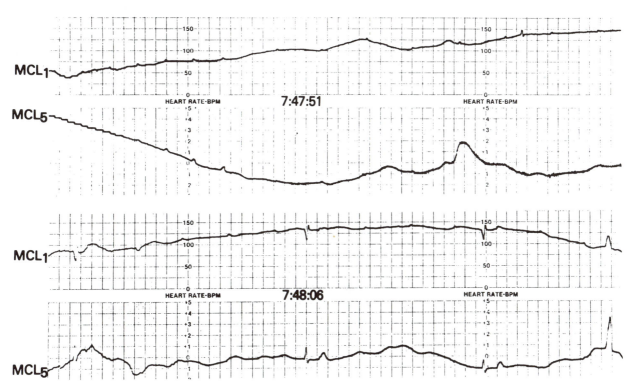

Figure 4 Same patient as in Figure 3. Holter recording obtained up to 29 seconds later showing very slow idioventricular escapes. (From Medina-Ravell V, Rodriguez-Salas L, Castellanos A, Myerburg RJ. Death due to paroxysmal atrioventricular block during ambulatory electrocardiographic monitoring. PACE 1989; 12:65–69, with permission.)

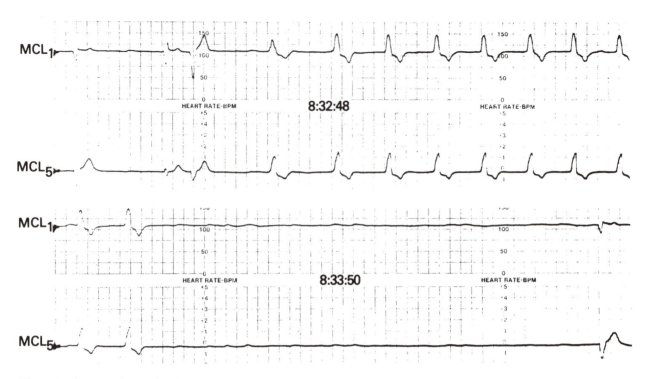

Figure 5 Same patient as in Figures 3 and 4. Holter recording showing that complete AV block persisted until cessation of all cardiac electrical activity, which took place 47 minutes after the onset of AV block. Most likely, this patient would have lived if cardiopulmonary resuscitation could have been started on time. (From Medina-Ravell V, Rodriguez-Salas L, Castellanos A, Myerburg RJ. Death due to paroxysmal atrioventricular block during ambulatory electrocardiographic monitoring. PACE 1989; 12:65–69, with permission.)

plantation based on pharmacologic challenge maneuvers. This especially applies to class IC drugs, which, in our experience, can induce infranodal block even in young patients studied for Wolff-Parkinson-White arrhythmias.

Considering these prospective studies, it can be asked why patients with complete AV block (paroxysmal or chronic) occasionally died before the introduction of implantable pacemakers. Patients usually do not succumb to the first (or even second or third) Adams-Stokes attack. Therefore, in those surviving the initial episodes, there is usually enough time for a pacemaker to be inserted. Most likely either AV conduction is spontaneously reestablished by itself (when AV block is paroxysmal, as in Fig. 1) or life-supporting idioventricular rhythms appear spontaneously after variable periods of ventricular standstill (owing to their awakening from overdrive suppression). Otherwise promptly instituted cardiopulmonary resuscitation can prove quite successful. In the absence of any of these events, death may occur (Figs. 3–5), but such a complication is extremely unusual at present in the United States.

Supported in part by a research grant from the National Heart, Lung, and Blood Institute (Grant No. HL-28130).

SUGGESTED READING

Bellet S. Clinical disorders of the heart beat. Philadelphia: Lea & Febiger, 1971:406–407.

Castellanos A, Pina IL, Zaman L, Myerburg RJ. Recent advances in the diagnosis of fascicular block. Cardiol Clin 1987; 5:469–488.

McAnulty JH, Rahimtoola SH, Murphy E, et al. Natural history of "high risk" bundle branch block. Final report of a prospective study. N Engl J Med 1982; 307:137–145.

Medina-Ravell V, Rodriguez-Salas L, Castellanos A, Myerburg RJ. Death due to paroxysmal atrioventricular block during ambulatory electrocardiographic monitoring. PACE 1989; 12:65–69.

Scheinman MM, Peters RW, Forady F, et al. Electrophysiologic studies in patients with bundle branch block. PACE 1983; 6:1157–1165.

Young ML, Gelband H, Castellanos A, Wolff GS. Reverse alternating Wenckebach periodicity. Am J Cardiol 1987; 60:90–94.

Zaman L, Moleiro F, Rozanski JJ, et al. Multiple electrophysiologic manifestations and clinical implications of vagally-mediated AV block. Am Heart J 1983; 106:92–99.

VII ARRHYTHMIAS IN SPECIFIC CLINICAL SITUATIONS

PREGNANCY

JAN RICHARD WEBER, M.D.

The referral of a pregnant patient to a cardiologist or internist for evaluation and treatment of palpitations or documented arrhythmias is not uncommon. There are several reasons for this.

First, pregnancy often provides the expectant mother with a greater frequency of physician contact than that experienced prior to the initiation of routine prenatal care. A variety of asymptomatic arrhythmias thereby may become apparent that might otherwise have gone unnoticed.

Second, even in the otherwise normal individual, the extreme physiologic demands placed upon the heart by pregnancy reduce cardiac reserve and tend to emphasize the hemodynamic consequences of any rhythm disturbance. Therefore, patients with preexisting arrhythmias who were entirely asymptomatic may be converted into symptomatic patients who fear not only for their own well-being but also for the well-being of their unborn child.

Third, for women with a variety of congenital and acquired heart diseases, advances in medical and surgical techniques have allowed increasing numbers to reach maturity and have children, whereas in earlier generations, childbearing would not have been considered, even if survival were possible. Because of the hemodynamic complexities of such patients and because of the arrhythmias that often accompany these conditions, the cardiologist is frequently asked for advice in management.

One common cause of "palpitations" experienced by pregnant individuals can be characterized as a "cardiac awareness" associated with the increased heart rate that normally accompanies the pregnant state. On average, the maternal resting heart rate increases by 10 beats per minute, and significant increases in cardiac output occur. Many pregnant individuals simply become aware of their hyperdynamic state, and it is not uncommon for the fear-provoking symptoms they experience to represent nothing more than sinus tachycardia that has been potentiated by the anxiety caused by this awareness. Reassurance about the normalcy of this phenomenon is generally the only treatment necessary once serious rhythm disturbances have been excluded.

Atrial, junctional, and ventricular premature complexes may also be experienced during pregnancy, just as they are in the nonpregnant state. Innocent ventricular bigeminy and trigeminy also occur with relative frequency. Unless they are subjectively disturbing, treatment of such arrhythmias is rarely necessary. Once again, reassurance may be all that is required. Malignant arrhythmias during the course of normal gestation are rare.

However, the stresses associated with pregnancy may induce arrhythmias that may also represent the first manifestation of underlying organic heart disease. In such individuals, arrhythmias may take on a much greater importance, and thorough investigation to exclude such underlying organic diseases must be undertaken. A new arrhythmia developing in the presence of organic heart disease may increase the already great hemodynamic burden of pregnancy and further restrict cardiac reserve, with a potential for catastrophic consequences.

EVALUATION OF THE PREGNANT PATIENT WITH ARRHYTHMIAS

A thorough physical examination with particular emphasis on the cardiovascular system is essential in any patient experiencing new-onset arrhythmias during pregnancy. The routine electrocardiogram may be useful if the premature complexes occur at the time the electrocardiogram is being performed, and useful clues may be provided by the discovery of conduction disturbances, evidence of myocardial infarction or pericarditis, or patterns suggestive of a variety of congenital anomalies. However, a 24-hour Holter monitor is required to delineate the nature, frequency, and severity of the arrhythmia being experienced.

When symptoms occur only rarely, a transtelephonic monitoring device may be necessary for identification of their cause. Unlike the routine for the 24-hour Holter monitor, the patient may be allowed to carry a transtelephonic device for several weeks at a time, recording cardiac rhythm only at the times palpitations or symptoms are present, and then transmitting the data via telephone at a later, more convenient time.

Cardiac ultrasonographic examination, including echocardiography and Doppler evaluation of cardiac flow, is an extremely important tool for evaluation of cardiac anatomy and function. In particular, congenital heart disease, valvular disease, pericardial disease, and ventricular dysfunction can be easily identified utilizing this technique. The test is harmless and noninvasive, and there is no risk of radiation to contend with, as is the case with roentgenograms or nuclear scanning.

Evaluation should also include appropriate tests to exclude underlying pulmonary, metabolic, and endocrine disorders, all of which may contribute to the development of rhythm disturbances.

TYPES OF RHYTHM DISTURBANCES

There is nothing unique about pregnancy that creates rhythm disturbances that are not experienced in nonpregnant individuals; arrhythmias in pregnant patients are identical to those seen in the general population. However, because of the decrease in P-R interval associated with pregnancy, second-degree heart block of the Wenckebach variety may be somewhat less common in the pregnant woman. Conversely, the threshold for reentrant supraventricular tachycardia, a common arrhythmia among normal young women, appears to be significantly higher during pregnancy, making its occurrence somewhat less frequent than in the nonpregnant population.

Acute onset of atrial fibrillation or atrial flutter should raise the suspicion of hyperthyroidism or pulmonary embolus. Additionally, patients should be questioned about the use of stimulants, including caffeine, amphetamines, cannabis, cocaine and its derivatives, and other toxins such as alcohol. Patients with these arrhythmias should undergo echocardiographic-Doppler evaluation to exclude rheumatic mitral valvular disease, mitral insufficiency, atrial septal defect (especially ostium secundum defects), and Ebstein's anomaly.

Paroxysmal supraventricular tachycardia is also a common arrhythmia experienced by women of childbearing age. Supraventricular arrhythmias with rapid ventricular response, such as those seen in the Wolff-Parkinson-White syndrome, should be re-garded as medical emergencies in view of the frequent development of congestive heart failure in the pregnant individual during such episodes.

When sustained runs of ventricular tachycardia or frequent multiform ventricular premature complexes are encountered, the physician should immediately become concerned about the possibility of peripartum cardiomyopathy. Once again, echocardiography may be the only test required to confirm this diagnosis. Nuclear scans should be avoided to prevent unnecessary radiation exposure.

ANTIARRHYTHMIC THERAPY

All pregnant individuals should be encouraged to eliminate the use of alcohol, cigarettes, caffeine, nonprescribed medications, and other potentially arrhythmogenic substances. When endocrine or other metabolic abnormalities exist, arrhythmias can often be corrected without specific antiarrhythmic therapy by appropriately controlling the underlying pathologic process. However, on occasion, antiarrhythmic agents are required to maintain patient comfort and safety. A general principle of antiarrhythmic therapy in pregnant individuals is to use the lowest effective dose possible. The need for antiarrhythmic therapy should be reassessed periodically during the course of pregnancy, and if the indication for an antiarrhythmic agent no longer appears to be present, a trial of discontinuation of therapy should be attempted.

As a matter of principle, no drug deemed nonessential to maternal well-being should be given at any time during pregnancy, but it is particularly important to minimize or avoid drug administration during the first trimester, during which time fetal development is most likely to be adversely affected. It must be remembered that any medication given to a pregnant individual is actually being given to two patients simultaneously, both the woman and the fetus. Thus, the effects of these medications must be considered with regard to both. Additionally, the effect a medication might have on uteroplacental blood flow and uterine muscle tone must also be considered.

Fortunately, most currently available antiarrhythmic agents can be considered applicable to the pregnant individual and can be administered with relative safety. Many of the currently available agents that have been in widespread use for many years have been well studied and can be considered safe with regard to fetal well-being. As a rule, it is best to avoid newer agents about which less information is available, unless failure of conventional therapy warrants their use.

One of the oldest agents available is digitalis, which has been widely used without any apparent toxicity to the fetus. Because of the increase in glomerular filtration rate and relative hypervolemia of the pregnant patient, dose requirements of digitalis during therapy may be two or three times those of a nonpregnant individual. Although digitalis freely crosses the placental barrier and fetal cardiac contractility has been shown to be increased with the use of this agent, it has not demonstrated any teratogenic or arrhythmogenic effects on the fetus. Digitalis may actually have a beneficial effect on contractility of the myometrium and may account for the shorter labors often experienced by women taking this medication.

Beta blockers have also been in use for many years, and it is clear that both cardioselective and noncardioselective beta blockers cross the placenta. Neither type of beta blocker has exhibited any adverse effect on fetal development. Beta blockers have little effect on the unstressed heart rate of the fetus because of the absence of significant beta-adrenergic control in the developing fetus. Neonates born of mothers treated with beta blockers do not manifest significant cardiac effects of beta blockade; however, there may nevertheless be sufficient quantities of beta-antagonists in the neonate as well as in the developing fetus that acute fetal stress response might be blunted. Thus, beta blockers cannot be considered totally harmless in situations that might predispose to fetal distress. Occasional reports of transient fetal abnormalities in offspring of patients being treated with beta blockers have included neonatal hypoglycemia, respiratory depression, hyperbilirubinemia, and polycythemia. Beta blockers may also be excreted in breast milk and have the potential for decreasing neonatal heart rate and respiratory function. Although these possibilities should be considered, clinically significant reactions to beta blockers in the fetus and the neonate are relatively uncommon.

In patients with supraventricular arrhythmias that are unresponsive to digitalis or beta blockade, verapamil may be considered. Kline and Repke reported the successful cardioversion of a digitalized hyperthyroid pregnant patient utilizing verapamil with continuous monitoring of fetal heart rhythm during cardioversion. No untoward effects on the fetus were observed, and it was therefore suggested that verapamil is safe and effective in this setting.

The treatment of ventricular arrhythmia has included a wide variety of antiarrhythmic agents, including quinidine, procainamide, lidocaine, phenytoin, mexiletine, and even amiodarone.

Quinidine has been effective and relatively safe, but there have been reports of induction of premature labor during therapy. In reality, this drug is only a mild stimulant of uterine contractions and does not appear to exert any significant effect until labor has actually begun spontaneously. Untoward effects on the fetus have not been reported.

The safe use of procainamide has also been described, but the significant reduction in blood pressure associated with the intravenous form of procainamide suggests that this agent should be used with extreme caution when given parenterally.

Lidocaine is extremely effective in controlling ventricular ectopy in the pregnant patient, but because of potential central nervous system blunting, both in the mother and in the fetus, the minimal effective dosage should be employed. Withdrawal of the medication should be completed as quickly as safely possible.

Phenytoin has been associated with a number of congenital anomalies, including congenital heart defects, craniofacial malformations, and mental and growth retardation. These anomalies may be present in as many as 6 percent of neonates who were exposed to phenytoin during development. Thus, alternative medications should be employed whenever possible.

The use of amiodarone in a pregnant patient has also been reported, with the child being healthy at birth and with no apparent thyroid abnormalities or corneal deposits. Growth and development after delivery were not affected in spite of high concentrations of amiodarone in maternal milk. However, limited information about the effect of amiodarone on fetal and neonatal growth and development suggest that the use of this medication in pregnant patients should be limited as much as possible.

Information about the effects of mexiletine during pregnancy is limited, and routine use of this medication should be avoided until further data are available.

Congenital complete heart block in the mother does not as a rule affect the outcome of pregnancy. If it is asymptomatic, no specific intervention may be required; however, symptomatic pregnant women with complete heart block can be managed effectively by utilizing artificial pacemakers. To limit radiation exposure, insertion of permanent pacemakers may be performed utilizing two-dimensional echocardiography rather than fluoroscopy. In doing so, radiation risks to the fetus can be minimized, with fluoroscopy used only to confirm accurate final placement of pacemaker leads.

In rare instances electrical cardioversion of refractory cases of supraventricular tachycardia may be required. Several such cases have been reported, often requiring repeated direct current shock to maintain a normal sinus rhythm. No apparent ill effects on the fetus have been demonstrated.

SUGGESTED READING

Brinkman CR, Woods JR. Effects of cardiovascular drugs during pregnancy. Cardiovasc Med 1976; I:231.

Godal M, Kervancioglu C, Oral D, et al. Permanent pacemaker implantation in a pregnant woman with the guidance of ECG

and two-dimensional echocardiography. PACE 1987;
10:543–545.

Kline V, Repke JT. Supraventricular tachycardia in pregnancy:
Cardioversion with verapamil. J Obstet Gynecol 1984;
63:16S–18S.

Rotmensch HH, Elkayam U, Frishman W. Antiarrhythmic drugs
during pregnancy. Ann Intern Med 1983; 98:487–497.

Strunge P, Frandsen J, Andreasen F. Amiodarone during pregnancy. Eur Heart J 1988; 9:106–109.

Szekely P, Julian DG. Heart disease in pregnancy. Curr Probl
Cardiol 1979; 4:1–74.

Szekely P, Snaith L. Heart disease in pregnancy. Edinburgh:
Churchill-Livingstone, 1974.

MANAGEMENT OF ARRHYTHMIAS IN ATHLETES

JAN RICHARD WEBER, M.D.

The demands made on the cardiovascular system by individuals participating in athletic activities
go far beyond those of the average individual. Because of these demands, abnormalities of cardiac
function, including arrhythmias, may become more
readily apparent, and their consequences may take
on greater significance. Similarly, medications used
to treat arrhythmias in athletes have greater demand
placed upon them, as they must be able to afford
protection at much higher levels of cardiac stimulation and must do so without producing any significant adverse effects on athletic performance. Thus,
just as athletes are judged by higher standards than
the average population, so, too, the effectiveness of
antiarrhythmic agents in these individuals must be
subjected to higher levels of scrutiny than when used
in more sedentary individuals.

Not uncommonly, well-trained athletes become
aware of palpitations and seek the advice of a physician to determine whether therapy is warranted. Palpitations may occur during exertion, immediately
following exercise, or while at rest. Concern about
such arrhythmias tends to heighten in the period of
time that immediately follows the demise of an un-
fortunate young athlete who experiences sudden
death during or immediately after athletic competition. These events characteristically attract a great
deal of media attention, and athletes who may have
been ignoring their palpitations then step forward
for evaluation because of heightened levels of anxiety. Asymptomatic arrhythmias may be identified
by coaches, trainers, team physicians, or family physicians during routine evaluation.

For the most part, the arrhythmias that produce
palpitations are found to be benign. The vast majority of them are due to isolated atrial or ventricular
premature complexes and pose no threat. However,
occasionally, such palpitations are indicative of
more complex and serious rhythm disturbances and
may also provide clues to the presence of significant
structural or functional cardiac disease.

EVALUATION OF THE ATHLETE WITH PALPITATIONS

The history and physical examination provide
important information regarding the etiology and
significance of rhythm disturbances. The patient
should be questioned about caffeine consumption,
alcohol use, and drug abuse. Sleep habits may also
be important, and a detailed assessment of the individual's exercise schedule may be useful to determine whether chronic fatigue or overtraining may be
contributing to rhythm abnormalities. Peculiar dietary habits or the use of vitamin and "health food"
supplements may also play a role in the genesis of
rhythm disturbances, and the use of anabolic
steroids should also be determined. Individuals
should also be questioned regarding their use of
minor stimulants, such as decongestants, which may
be mildly arrhythmogenic. The family history may
be noteworthy, particularly when syncope or sudden
death has occurred in a close relative. Recent unexpected weight loss may be an indicator of thyroid
dysfunction, and other symptoms of hyperthyroidism should be investigated.

The physical examination may reveal the presence of structural cardiac disease. A holosystolic or
late systolic murmur at the apex or the presence of a
midsystolic click may indicate the presence of mitral
valve prolapse. A systolic murmur at the lower left
sternal border that increases with Valsalva's maneuver or with mild exertion may indicate the presence
of hypertrophic obstructive cardiomyopathy. A thyroid nodule or hyperreflexia may be useful in assessing the presence of hyperthyroidism.

Blood chemistries generally have little value, but
when electrolyte or thyroid problems are suspected,
electrolyte levels should be evaluated and thyroid
function tests should be performed.

Most commonly, the routine electrocardiogram
(ECG) provides little information regarding rhythm
disturbances in athletes. Arrhythmias are not likely

to be seen, as their occurrence is generally sporadic and often exercise-related. Additionally, the presence of an ectopic complex on the ECG cannot be construed as the sole cause for an individual's symptoms, and rarely can the investigation cease after an isolated atrial or ventricular premature complex is identified. However, the ECG may indicate the presence of congenital long Q-T syndrome, conduction disturbances, or hypertrophic cardiomyopathy.

It is important to remember that the ECG of a well-trained athlete may appear to be quite abnormal if the usual standards are employed. The ECG of the athlete not uncommonly shows sinus bradycardia, profound sinus arrhythmia, and first-degree atrioventricular block. Second-degree block of the Wenckebach type is also not uncommon. Left and right atrial abnormalities may be present, and the QRS complex voltages are much higher than average. ST-T wave abnormalities and T-wave inversions are frequently seen. Thus, it is not reasonable to judge the ECG of the athlete by standards that are commonly employed when evaluating the more average individual.

The echocardiogram should be employed in the evaluation of individuals in whom hypertrophic cardiomyopathy, mitral valve prolapse, or other structural cardiac diseases are suspected. Once again, it is important to remember that the appearance of the athlete's heart on echocardiogram may be different from that of the average individual. Four-chamber cardiac enlargement is not uncommon, and a mild degree of left ventricular hypertrophy is to be expected. The presence of mild left ventricular enlargement and bradycardia often gives the appearance of diffuse mild to moderate left ventricular dysfunction, but they are actually indicators of a highly efficient myocardium with increased stroke volume.

The most important tools in assessing arrhythmias in athletes are the Holter monitor and the exercise test. A Holter monitor should be worn by the athlete during activities of daily living and, if possible, should also be worn during the specific type of physical activity that is associated with the symptoms being experienced by that individual. Thus, runners should be encouraged to run while wearing the Holter monitor; weight lifters should be asked to lift weights according to their usual routine while being monitored, and cyclists should be encouraged to ride at near peak exertion during the monitored interval. Obviously, sports such as gymnastics and swimming require substitute activities, but the sporting event of the individual should be approximated as closely as possible while he or she is wearing the Holter monitor to determine the type of arrhythmia being experienced. This is also true in assessing the effectiveness of any therapy that might later be initiated.

For arrhythmias that appear to be triggered by activity, treadmill exercise tests may also be useful.

In addition to its use in detecting myocardial ischemia, the stress test provides a safe environment for identifying significant rhythm disturbances in a setting where acute medical intervention is possible if warranted. It is important to note that the ST-T segment response to exercise may be abnormal in a well-trained athlete and may result in a false-positive test that incorrectly suggests the presence of atherosclerotic heart disease.

Rarely, cardiac catheterization is necessary to exclude the possibility of life-threatening cardiovascular disease, and in individuals in whom unexplained syncope has occurred, electrophysiologic testing may also be warranted to exclude the possibility of ventricular tachycardia or reciprocating tachycardia.

TYPES OF ARRHYTHMIAS

Most commonly, the palpitations experienced by athletes are indicators of the presence of isolated atrial or ventricular premature complexes. After identification of these arrhythmias, patient education and reassurance may be the only treatment necessary, and generally thereafter the individual will simply ignore these palpitations when they occur. Occasional individuals will, however, require treatment even in the presence of benign arrhythmias if their symptoms are bothersome enough to interfere with their sense of well-being. In such individuals, the risks versus benefits of therapy should be thoroughly discussed, and careful documentation of this discussion should be entered in the medical record.

Supraventricular Arrhythmias

Supraventricular tachycardia is not infrequently found in young individuals, and athletes are no exception. Paroxysmal atrial fibrillation, atrial flutter, and atrioventricular nodal reentrant tachycardia are not uncommon. Vagotonic maneuvers such as carotid sinus massage, Valsalva's maneuver, and immersion of the face in water to trigger the diving reflex may be effective ways of terminating such episodes. Exercise testing often confirms the presence of these arrhythmias. If relatively rare and well tolerated, these arrhythmias may be managed by the use of these vagotonic maneuvers, but occasionally pharmacologic therapy is required. Intermittent use of beta blockers or verapamil may provide adequate treatment for episodes that fail to respond. For particularly stubborn episodes, intravenous verapamil, intravenous beta blockers, and most recently adenosine have been utilized to abort the acute attack.

If attacks become more frequent or more hemodynamically significant, chronic therapy may be required. For the athlete, in whom performance is of great importance, digoxin should be used as first-line therapy in view of its lack of negative inotropy. Verapamil or alternatively diltiazem may also be effective but is likely to be less well tolerated. Beta blockers, although effective, more significantly interfere with athletic performance and are, therefore, not likely to be well accepted by the athlete. If used, a cardioselective beta blocker should be employed, as these agents seem to produce less exercise-induced fatigue. Class IA antiarrhythmic agents may also be necessary, with procainamide or quinidine being used first. Disopyramide is somewhat less well tolerated but may also be utilized if the other class IA agents are ineffective or not accepted. If atrial arrhythmias are severe and refractory enough to warrant consideration of amiodarone, discontinuation of athletic involvement may need to be considered, particularly if arrhythmia occurrence appears to be directly related to physical exertion.

Treatment of chronic atrial fibrillation in the athlete should follow standard guidelines, with oral digoxin being used as first-line therapy. If rate control is not obtained, the addition of cardioselective beta blockade may be required. Thereafter, conversion with quinidine may be necessary. If atrial fibrillation persists, 2 weeks of warfarin therapy followed by electrical cardioversion may be required. Thereafter, maintenance therapy with digoxin and if necessary quinidine should be continued. Evaluation of the effectiveness of the treatment regimen then requires stress testing and Holter monitoring during athletic activities that are representative of the individual's usual form of competition.

Atrioventricular reciprocating tachycardias, such as those seen in the Wolff-Parkinson-White syndrome, may also be encountered in athletes. Once recognized, the evaluation of reciprocating tachycardia in the athlete should follow the routine utilized for nonathletic individuals. Selection of an antiarrhythmic agent is largely dependent on the nature of the reentrant circuit, and choice of antiarrhythmic therapy may be somewhat limited, with any detrimental effect that these agents have on athletic competition becoming of secondary importance. In individuals with reciprocating tachycardia who have experienced syncope, competitive athletic activity should be avoided until it can be ascertained from exercise testing and Holter monitoring that the condition has been properly controlled. Frequent ongoing testing may be required to assure effective control and safety, but in instances where syncope has occurred and complete arrhythmia control cannot be assured, cessation of athletic activity should be recommended. Once again, the importance of documenting such a recommendation in the record must be emphasized, particularly when it's suspected that such a recommendation is likely to be ignored.

Ventricular Arrhythmias

In the athlete with known or suspected rhythm disturbances, the Holter monitor may reveal the presence of ventricular ectopy. Many individuals are acutely aware of even benign ventricular ectopy, to the point where their lifestyle and sense of well-being are negatively affected. Reassurance, along with lifestyle changes including reduction in caffeine and alcohol intake, is often effective and should certainly be attempted prior to the consideration of antiarrhythmic medications. When substances such as marijuana, cocaine, and other stimulants are suspected, the individual should be strongly encouraged to eliminate their use.

In individuals in whom no such factors are apparent and reassurance is inadequate, medical therapy may be required. The athlete should be apprised of the potential negative effects of the use of medications, including the possibility of a proarrhythmic effect, and if therapy is still considered to be essential, the medications chosen should be selected according to potential effectiveness as well as to minimize a negative effect on athletic performance. When arrhythmias appear to be related to catecholamine sensitivity as indicated by an increase in ectopy during exercise, low doses of beta blockers may be an effective form of therapy. As with supraventricular arrhythmias, cardioselective beta blockers such as metoprolol or atenolol should be considered first. Adequate arrhythmia control may be achieved without detectable effects on exercise performance in many individuals. Thereafter, class IA agents, which include quinidine, procainamide, and disopyramide, may need to be considered, either alone or in combination with a low dose of a cardioselective beta blocker. The class IA agents have little effect on exercise performance and may be quite effective. Class IC agents, such as flecainide and encainide, although better tolerated than the class IA agents, should be avoided until further information regarding their demonstrated proarrhythmic effect is available. Tocainide and mexiletine may be considered if class IA agents are not effective but in general they are not well tolerated by athletes because of their gastrointestinal and neurologic side effects.

Often after a trial of medical therapy the athlete who has demonstrated only benign arrhythmias will become more responsive to reassurance and more accepting of lifestyle changes rather than be subjected to the side effects produced by these medications.

Whether the patient is symptomatic or asymptomatic, high-grade ventricular arrhythmias, particularly ventricular tachycardia, require medical intervention. As always, athletes with high-grade ventricular arrhythmias should be thoroughly examined to exclude the possibility of congenital or organic heart disease. In particular, mitral valve prolapse, hypertrophic obstructive cardiomyopathy, dilated cardiomyopathy, and coronary artery disease should be excluded. Exercise testing and echocardiography should be considered essential. Individuals found to have evidence for coronary artery disease should be subjected to cardiac catheterization. Hypertrophic cardiomyopathy in conjunction with high-grade ventricular ectopy carries an ominous prognosis (see the chapter *Arrhythmias Associated with Hypertrophic Cardiomyopathy*), and competitive athletic activity should be discouraged in individuals with this combination.

In athletes who have not experienced syncope or near syncope and in whom ventricular tachycardia has not been documented, beta-blocker therapy may be highly effective in eliminating exercise-induced rhythm disturbances. Once again, class IA and IB agents may be necessary, either alone or in combination with beta-blocker therapy.

When ventricular tachycardia has been documented, and in patients who have experienced syncope or near syncope in whom an arrhythmia has been suspected, electrophysiologic testing is necessary. When inducible ventricular tachycardia is found, the athlete should be strongly discouraged from further competitive athletic performance, regardless of whether arrhythmia control is subsequently demonstrated by Holter monitoring and electrophysiologic testing. Cardiac catheterization in such individuals should be considered an essential part of the evaluation.

For athletes who continue their athletic competition in spite of recommendations to the contrary, attempts to maximize arrhythmia control include continued arrhythmia surveillance, including Holter monitoring and frequent exercise testing. Documentation of all recommendations should be thorough, and when appropriate, these recommendations should be communicated to family members and members of the athlete's coaching staff.

Ideally, every athlete should be screened for potential causes of sudden death before being allowed to participate in competitive sports. However, such screening, which would include a thorough history and physical examination, electrocardiogram, echo-Doppler evaluation, Holter monitor, and stress test, would be prohibitively expensive (about $2,000 per athlete). Most insurance plans do not allow for routine screening in asymptomatic individuals, and therefore these expenses would be out of pocket or would need to be paid for by the team sponsor. Happily, however, life-threatening rhythm disturbances and other cardiac diseases are quite rare among young athletes, and when family and personal history, physical examination, and twelve-lead ECGs are unrevealing, no further testing appears to be warranted in most cases.

SUGGESTED READING

Anderson JL. Criteria for selection of oral drug therapy in chronic ventricular arrhythmia. Mod Med 1989; 55:48–66.

Cantwell JD, Daugherty DT. Arrhythmias in athletes. Your Patient and Fitness. 1989; 3:12–19.

Cantwell JD, Wilson KE, Thomas RJ. Hypertrophic cardiomyopathy: Treatment and exercise recommendations. Your Patient and Fitness 1989; 2:20–22.

Cooksey JD, Reilly P, Brown S, et al. Exercise training and plasma catecholamines in patients with ischemic heart disease. Am J Cardiol 1978; 42:372–379.

Dreifus LS. Anti-arrhythmic drug selection in supraventricular tachyarrhythmias. Mod Med 1988; 56:82–98.

Epstein SE, Maron BJ. Sudden death and the competitive athlete: Perspectives on pre-participation screening studies. J Am Coll Cardiol 1986; 7:220–230.

Frank MJ, Watkins LO, Prisant LM, et al. Potentially lethal arrhythmias and their management in hypertrophic cardiomyopathy. Am J Cardiol 1984; 53:1608–1613.

Huston TP, Puffer JC, Rodney WM. The athletic heart syndrome. N Engl J Med 1985; 313:24–32.

Manolis AS, Estes NA III. Supraventricular tachycardia. Mechanisms and therapy. Arch Intern Med 1987; 147:1706–1716.

McLeod AA, Kraus WE, Williams RS. Effects of beta I-selective and non-selective beta-adrenoceptor blockade during exercise conditioning in healthy adults. Am Cardiol 1974; 53:1656–1661.

Siscovick DS, Weiss, NS, Fletcher RH, Lasky T. The incidence of primary cardiac arrest during vigorous exercise. N Engl J Med 1984; 311:874–880.

Wellens HJ, Brugada P, Penn OC. The management of pre-excitation syndromes. JAMA 1987; 257:2325–2333.

Wilmore JH. Exercise testing, training and beta-adrenergic blockade. Physician Sports Med 1988; 16:45–52.

Wolfelee Hiatt WR, Brammell HL, Carry MR, et al. Effects of selective and non-selective beta adrenergic blockade on mechanisms of exercise conditioning. Circulation 1986; 74:664–674.

ANESTHESIA AND SURGERY

ISAAC WIENER, M.D.

Up to 60 percent of patients undergoing general anesthesia and surgery manifest abnormalities of cardiac rhythm, but serious arrhythmias, i.e., those requiring treatment, are uncommon (0.9 percent). Arrhythmias are more common in patients with organic heart disease undergoing prolonged operation and can be an important sign of metabolic, respiratory, or anesthetic problems that require immediate attention. Cooperation between the cardiologist and the anesthesiologist is essential in the perioperative management of these patients.

FACTORS CONTRIBUTING TO ARRHYTHMIAS

Anesthetic Agents

Some anesthetic agents have a propensity to elicit ventricular arrhythmias, possibly through a central nervous system mechanism. This effect is greatest with cyclopropane and trichloroethylene, agents that are no longer widely used. Proarrhythmic effects are less pronounced with halogenated hydrocarbons (e.g., halothane, enflurane, and isoflurane) and have not been noted with nitrous oxide. However, in high concentrations all of these drugs may depress left ventricular function.

Intravenous narcotics, including morphine, meperidine, and fentanyl, have little proarrhythmic effect. Fentanyl is particularly useful in patients with severe left ventricular dysfunction because it has minimal hemodynamic effects.

Anesthetic Agents and Catecholamines

Halogenated hydrocarbons have been well documented to potentiate markedly the arrhythmogenic effects of catecholamines. The precise mechanism of this interaction is not well understood but may relate to the anesthetic's effect of decreasing threshold, whereas catecholamines increase phase 4 depolarization. Inhalational agents also influence slow channel inward current. Of inhalational agents currently used, halothane results in the greatest sensitization to catecholamines. Enflurane, which demonstrates an intermediate degree of sensitization, has a nonlinear catecholamine dose-response curve that makes prediction of the response to a given dose of catecholamine unreliable. Isoflurane results in the least sensitization and is the anesthetic agent most commonly used in patients with coronary artery disease.

Adrenergic agents vary in their proarrhythmic effects in the face of hydrocarbons. Epinephrine, norepinephrine, and dopamine frequently produce arrhythmias, whereas ephedrine, methoxamine, and phenylephrine rarely do. Cocaine and aminophylline influence catecholamine metabolism and may be arrhythmogenic.

Halogenated hydrocarbons should be avoided if it appears that a catecholamine infusion may be necessary. Alternatively, adrenergic agents that are not proarrhythmic should be used. When local epinephrine is used for hemostasis, the dosage should be carefully controlled. If inhaled catecholamines are used, selective agents should be employed.

Anesthetic Agents and Muscle Relaxants

In patients receiving many general anesthetics, succinylcholine results in a generalized autonomic stimulation that can cause arrhythmia, including sinus arrest and supraventricular and ventricular arrhythmias. These arrhythmias are particularly common with multiple injections of succinylcholine, suggesting sensitization. Succinylcholine-induced bradyarrhythmias may be prevented by atropine premedication. Pancuronium may be associated with sinus tachycardia, particularly when used in combination with isoflurane. Dimethyl tubocurarine and the newer, short-acting nondepolarizing agents, atracurium and vecuronium, generally do not produce cardiac arrhythmias.

Anesthetic Agents and Respiratory Derangements

Both hypoxia and respiratory acidosis, particularly when combined with anesthetic agents, can cause cardiac arrhythmias. These may be mediated by catecholamine release, possibly on a central nervous system basis. Cardiac arrhythmias may be an important marker of inadequate ventilation.

Electrolyte Abnormalities

Abnormalities of electrolyte concentration, particularly hypokalemia and hypomagnesemia, are potent contributors to arrhythmias. Serum measurements may not accurately reflect intracellular deficits. Potassium and magnesium levels should be checked and electrolyte supplementation considered in all patients with perioperative arrhythmias.

Temperature

Even moderate hypothermia can result in a decreased ventricular fibrillation threshold. Treatments for arrhythmias will not be successful unless warming is performed. Hyperthermia results in catecholamine release and exacerbation of arrhythmias.

Reflexes

Intubation, traction on ocular muscles, and traction on intraabdominal structures may result in parasympathetic or sympathetic stimulation, either of which may cause arrhythmias. These arrhythmias do not appear to be of major significance and can be avoided by skilled intubation, attention to surgical technique, and adequate ventilation.

Myocardial Ischemia and Infarction

New arrhythmias that develop perioperatively may be an indicator of myocardial ischemia or infarction. A decrease in oxygen supply produced by hypoxia or hypotension or an increase in oxygen demand caused by hypertension or tachycardia may result in ischemia. Ischemic events should be suspected in all patients with underlying atherosclerotic cardiovascular disease who develop new arrhythmias. Although confirmatory electrocardiographic findings are helpful, their absence does not exclude possible ischemia or infarction. Relief of ischemia whenever possible with intravenous nitrates or beta blockers should be attempted. Many feel that intravenous nitroglycerin should be used routinely in patients with coronary artery disease.

PREOPERATIVE EVALUATION

Careful preoperative evaluation and stabilization are essential to reduce perioperative arrhythmias. Increased operative risk has been associated with acute myocardial infarction within 3 to 6 months of surgery, severe congestive heart failure, severe arrhythmias, major intraabdominal or intrathoracic operations, prolonged procedures, and intraoperative hypotension. Goldman and coworkers have identified a variety of factors associated with severe cardiac complications: preoperative third heart sound, jugular venous distention, myocardial infarction in the preceding 6 months, more than five premature ventricular contractions per minute, rhythm other than sinus or premature atrial beats, age over 70 years, intraperitoneal, intrathoracic, or aortic operations, emergency operation, significant valvular or aortic stenosis, and poor general medical condition. Particular attention should be directed to any recent change in status (e.g., change in anginal pattern or increase in chronic heart failure). In patients with any of these risk factors and in other patients suspected of having underlying heart disease, a thorough noninvasive study of the patient's cardiac status is extremely helpful.

Patients with suspected ischemic heart disease should undergo stress thallium testing or dipyridamole-thallium testing for those who cannot exercise. Any patient who demonstrates ischemia should undergo coronary arteriography, with consideration given to revascularization for those with large areas of myocardium at risk. Although there are no controlled studies of such an aggressive approach, observational studies suggest a major reduction in perioperative infarction when such patients are identified.

Patients with suspected left ventricular dysfunction should have an echocardiogram or radionuclide wall motion study. Patients with significant left ventricular dysfunction should be considered for right-sided heart catheterization. In patients with uncompensated congestive heart failure, right-sided heart catheterization may be done several days preoperatively to allow optimization of diuretic, inotropic, and afterload reducing therapy. These patients should be continued on their medications throughout the operative period. In patients with stable or no clinical congestive heart failure, the right-sided heart catheterization is still very helpful for monitoring intraoperative fluid shifts and detecting problems early. In these stable patients, the Swan-Ganz catheter is best inserted in the operating room immediately prior to the procedure.

Chronic arrhythmias should be stabilized. Any symptoms suggestive of arrhythmia, e.g., recurrent syncope, should be satisfactorily evaluated preoperatively. Documentation of chronic asymptomatic benign or potentially malignant ventricular arrhythmias that are not treated will prevent concern when these arrhythmias are noted intraoperatively. There is no evidence that these arrhythmias require aggressive preoperative suppression.

For patients with symptomatic malignant arrhythmias, antiarrhythmic therapy should be continued up to the time of surgery. For patients at high risk, intravenous medication can be utilized during the procedure and oral medication resumed when feeding starts. In patients taking amiodarone, the long half-life of the drug allows continued protection during the operation. However, there are reports of precipitation of lung toxicity by inhalational anesthetics in patients on amiodarone therapy. Patients on amiodarone should be carefully evaluated for any signs of lung toxicity preoperatively and followed closely postoperatively.

Certain patients at high risk of intraoperative supraventricular arrhythmias (e.g., elderly patients undergoing pulmonary surgery, patients with mild to moderate valvular disease, and patients with prior supraventricular arrhythmias) can be identified. Preoperative digitalization should be considered in these patients.

TREATMENT OF ARRHYTHMIAS

Supraventricular Arrhythmias

Slow supraventricular arrhythmias, including atrial premature complexes, atrioventricular junctional rhythm, and wandering atrial pacemaker are the most common arrhythmias seen during administration of anesthesia. These arrhythmias are benign and do not require therapy.

Rapid supraventricular arrhythmias, supraventricular tachycardia, and atrial fibrillation should be treated as in a nonsurgical setting, with the goal of prompt control of rate. Intravenous verapamil, 5 to 10 mg over 2 minutes, is generally the agent of choice for rapid control of these arrhythmias, but esmolol and procainamide may be useful in specific cases (see Section III, *Supraventricular Tachyarrhythmias*). If a supraventricular arrhythmia results in marked hypotension or pulmonary congestion, cardioversion should be performed, followed by a search for precipitating causes and subsequent institution of drug therapy.

Ventricular Arrhythmias

Premature ventricular complexes are the second most common arrhythmia seen during anesthesia. Familiarity with the patient's history will avoid undue concern over chronic benign arrhythmias. New-onset ventricular arrhythmias should be considered a sign of serious derangement until proved otherwise. A thorough evaluation of anesthetic management, ventilation, and electrolytes should be undertaken. If no precipitating cause can be identified, specific antiarrhythmic therapy can be considered. For sustained ventricular arrhythmia, intravenous lidocaine is the drug of choice, and intravenous procainamide the second drug of choice. Cardioversion should be performed for arrhythmias associated with hemodynamic deterioration or those that do not respond promptly to medical therapy.

There are few data on which to base the recommendation for treatment of new ventricular arrhythmias without hemodynamic consequences. The temptation to suppress all ventricular premature complexes should be avoided. Concern that new arrhythmias may represent ischemia or infarction may be warranted in patients with known atherosclerotic cardiovascular disease. For this reason, suppression of frequent ventricular premature complexes, couplets, and runs of ventricular tachycardia appears reasonable.

Bradyarrhythmias

Most patients with bradyarrhythmias that require pacemakers during surgery (e.g., complete heart block, Mobitz II second-degree atrioventricular block, severe sinus node dysfunction) have functioning permanent pacemakers. However, an occasional patient with chronic bradycardia or atrioventricular nodal block that is asymptomatic

and has not required a permanent pacemaker but who manifests persistent slow rates may benefit from a temporary pacemaker. Patients with bifascicular block have a low incidence of progression to heart block during surgery and do not require pacemakers.

Symptomatic bradyarrhythmias, not related to a precipitating cause, generally respond to atropine. Isoproterenol should be required only rarely.

Pacemakers and the Automatic Implantable Cardioverter Defibrillator

An electrocautery used within a few inches of a pacemaker may damage the pacemaker or induce current in the lead, causing ventricular fibrillation or a myocardial burn and exit block. An electrocautery used within 1 to 2 feet of the pacemaker may inhibit a demand pacemaker. This latter problem is minimized if the pacemaker is bipolar and if the plate of the cautery is placed as far from the pacemaker as possible. If the cautery must be used within 12 to 24 inches of the pacemaker, the pacemaker should be programmed to an asynchronous mode. The practice of converting the pacemaker to a fixed rate by placing a magnet over it should be abandoned. With newer units, the use of the magnet together with the electrocautery may result in phantom programming. In some DDD pacemakers, programming to the asynchronous mode may also not be foolproof. The electrocautery has been recorded to induce inappropriate pacemaker end of life characteristics.

Similarly, the sensing circuits of the automatic implantable cardioverter defibrillator may be triggered by an electrocautery. The automatic implantable cardioverter defibrillator should be inactivated if an electrocautery will be used in its vicinity.

I wish to thank Drs. Ara Tilkian and Irwin Reich for their helpful comments.

SUGGESTED READING

Davis R. Etiology and treatment of perioperative cardiac dysrhythmias. In: Kaplan J, ed. Cardiac anesthesia. Orlando: Grune & Stratton, 1987.

Goldman L, Caldera D, Nussbaum S, et al. Multifactoral index of cardiac risk and noncardiac surgical procedures. N Engl J Med 1977; 297:845–850.

Katz RL, Bigger JT. Cardiac arrhythmias during anesthesia and operation. Anesthesiology 1970; 33:193–213.

Logan R, Kaplan J. The cardiac patient and noncardiac surgery. Curr Probl Cardiol 1982; 7:

Wells P, Kaplan J. Optimal management of patients with ischemic heart disease for noncardiac surgery by complementary anesthesiologist and cardiologist interaction. Am Heart J 1981; 102:1029–1037.

CARDIOMYOPATHY AND CONGESTIVE HEART FAILURE

MARIELL JESSUP, M.D.
SUSAN C. BROZENA, M.D.

A contemporary definition of congestive heart failure (CHF) has been proposed by Cohn: heart failure represents a syndrome in which cardiac dysfunction is associated with a reduced exercise tolerance, a high incidence of ventricular arrhythmias, and a shortened life expectancy. This syndrome is responsible for the death of nearly 400,000 patients each year, either as a result of progressive left ventricular failure and subsequent cardiogenic shock or sudden cardiac death.

The great majority of patients in the United States develop CHF secondary to an underlying dilated cardiomyopathy, primarily resulting from complications of coronary artery disease (ischemic cardiomyopathy) or idiopathic in origin. Miscellaneous causes of CHF include infiltrative diseases of the myocardium (e.g., amyloidosis), myocarditis, complications of valvular malfunction, toxic cardiomyopathies (e.g., following doxorubicin therapy or chronic alcoholism), other extracardiac abnormalities (e.g., pericardial constriction, severe anemia, primary pulmonary or systemic hypertension), and hypertrophic cardiomyopathy. This final etiologic category is discussed in the chapter *Arrhythmias in Hypertrophic Cardiomyopathy* and will not be considered further.

A number of important pharmacologic advances have enabled physicians to effect a significant improvement in both exercise capacity and overall survival in patients with chronic CHF. However, the prognostic and therapeutic implications of the frequent occurrence of complex and recurrent ventricular arrhythmias in these same patients are, as yet, unclear. We will focus on the management of the ventricular arrhythmias coexistent with CHF.

CONTROVERSY, NOT CONSENSUS

The major reason the management of ventricular arrhythmias in the setting of CHF continues to be so problematic is the lack of multicenter, controlled studies to address the issues that result from the following facts.

Fact I. Symptomatic congestive heart failure is a highly lethal disease with an estimated annual mortality rate of 15 to 50 percent. Despite these grim statistics, there is no unanimity as to the important determinants of survival in this population. A review of over a score of investigations published in the last decade reveals a measurement of left ventricular ejection fraction to be the only common denominator useful in predicting mortality in the CHF patient.

Fact II. Patients with dilated cardiomyopathy have a very high incidence of frequent and complex ventricular premature complexes, and over half have unsustained ventricular tachycardia, which, with few exceptions, is entirely asymptomatic.

Fact III. A significant portion of patients with dilated cardiomyopathy suffer sudden cardiac death. However, divergent reports on the proportion of sudden deaths that occur range from a low of 4 percent to a high of 86 percent. This is undoubtedly due, in part, to the absence of a standardized definition for the sudden death syndrome. Our own bias is that very few patients with severe CHF die an *unexpected* sudden death but more often succumb in the clinical setting of rapidly deteriorating cardiac failure. Nevertheless, this distinction is rarely addressed in most publications.

With these facts as our foundation, further areas of controversy emerge. There has, in general, been little emphasis placed on the separation of the patient with chronic left ventricular dysfunction from the one with left ventricular failure following an acute myocardial infarction with respect to an analysis of their ventricular arrhythmias. Few attempts have been made to analyze the pattern of ventricular ectopy or to apply a standardized arrhythmia classification to the CHF population. There has been no consensus regarding the *relationship* of any observed ventricular arrhythmia to the incidence of sudden death or to cardiac deaths in general. It is not even clear which arrhythmias are most dangerous for the patient with dilated cardiomyopathy. Indeed, some observations have suggested that sudden death in this group is secondary to profound bradyarrhythmias, often preceded by acute ischemia. Finally, empirical use of antiarrhythmic drug therapy in the CHF population results in a particularly high incidence of life-threatening, proarrhythmic events. Strategies useful to negotiate this maze of uncertainty, therefore, can claim no other scientific basis than that gained from clinical experience.

TREAT THE UNDERLYING CARDIOMYOPATHY

To begin on a more certain note, the management of symptomatic CHF is fairly straightforward. Most physicians would agree on the clinical utility of instituting diuretics and vasodilators, as the patient's symptoms require. The angiotensin-converting enzyme inhibitors are preferable as the vasodilators of choice to be added to diuretic therapy in all but the mildest cases of CHF. This group of drugs has been shown unequivocally to enhance aerobic capacity and prolong patient survival. Moreover, their use tends to preserve potassium homeostasis and probably decreases generalized sympathetic nervous system stimulation. Oral nitrate therapy can also be effective, particularly in the patient with coronary artery disease. Diuretics need to be titrated aggressively to keep the patient free from edema, ascites, or nocturnal orthopnea. The benefit of digitalis is becoming increasingly less controversial in this population, and we initiate digitalis therapy when moderate CHF ensues. All patients in atrial fibrillation and with left ventricular thrombi or severe congestive symptoms should be chronically given anticoagulation therapy. The elimination of dietary salt is encouraged, as is a moderation of physical and mental stress. Crucial to the use of the above drugs are diligent and periodic laboratory studies to exclude hypokalemia, hypomagnesemia, and digitalis toxicity. It is our practice to measure serum potassium concentration within several days after a change in a maintenance diuretic dosage.

Often, a patient with decompensated CHF will exhibit prolonged episodes of unsustained ventricular tachycardia or other forms of frequent ventricular ectopy, whereas associated symptoms may be masked. Fortunately, the majority of patients experience resolution of both their congestive symptoms and the alarmingly high number of ventricular premature complexes when appropriate anti–heart failure therapy is established.

SEARCHING FOR CORRECTABLE CAUSES

An investigation into the etiology of the cardiac dysfunction should be coincident with the start of treatment. Specifically, in almost every case of new-onset CHF, cardiac catheterization with coronary visualization should be performed to exclude significant coronary disease. Obtaining an endomyocardial biopsy at the same time involves little additional risk for the patient. This approach serves to detect treatable causes of the cardiomyopathy—most important, reversible ischemia. The patient's symptoms and ventricular ectopy may improve remarkably after administration of appropriate antianginal medications, coronary angioplasty, or bypass grafting procedures. Likewise, documentation of a resectable ventricular aneurysm at the time of catheterization paves the way for another, very beneficial surgical procedure that may alleviate CHF and/or ventricular arrhythmias.

In our experience, it is uncommon to find evidence of acute myocarditis by means of endomyocardial biopsy. Nevertheless, ventricular arrhythmias that occur in the setting of proven myocarditis should be aggressively suppressed, similar to that in patients with acute myocardial infarctions. The underlying pathophysiology (acute myocardial damage) for the two disease states probably has the same

implications for the development of malignant ventricular arrhythmias. Similarly, women in the peripartum period with acute CHF should be carefully monitored for the development of arrhythmias. Our tendency is to avoid giving digitalis in patients with acute myocarditis or acute peripartum cardiomyopathy because of their predisposition to experience both atrial and ventricular arrhythmias.

Infiltrative diseases of the myocardium are most often complicated by conduction disease, bradycardia, or heart block. Thus, once this diagnosis is made for a particular patient, a more frequent analysis of his or her electrocardiogram is appropriate. Not uncommonly, these patients present with an inappropriately slow heart rate for their degree of CHF decompensation. We have found activity-responsive pacemakers to be quite effective in this group of patients.

The medical therapy of CHF may be altered once the presence of significant coronary obstruction is established. Moreover, many investigators believe that the association of complex ventricular arrhythmias with ischemic cardiomyopathy carries a higher mortality rate than that associated with idiopathic cardiomyopathy. In addition, some studies have indicated that the predictive value of electrophysiologic studies may be different for the two most common forms of cardiomyopathy. Finally, any patient with unsustained ventricular tachycardia, ischemic cardiomyopathy, and a myocardial infarction within 3 months of the recognition of CHF, irrespective of symptoms, should be regarded differently from the patient with asymptomatic arrhythmia and chronic cardiomyopathy. The risk of sudden death is more than threefold greater in the first 6 months after a myocardial infarction. Consequently, we have a much lower threshold to seek an appropriate antiarrhythmic agent for the postinfarction patient.

SYMPTOMATIC OR ASYMPTOMATIC

The large majority of patients do reasonably well once medical therapy has been optimized, and their most troubling symptom is easy fatigability. This being the case, no further therapy is directed toward their asymptomatic ventricular arrhythmias. Indeed, we do not routinely obtain a 24-hour ambulatory electrocardiogram (Holter) on these patients, because the results of the recordings can be alarming. Thus, a patient with no episodes of palpitations, syncope, or dizziness (nonorthostatic) is managed only with respect to his or her symptoms of heart failure. This approach has not resulted in an unexpected number of sudden deaths or in an accelerated mortality from all causes in our patient population.

However, once the patient complains of palpitations or, more obviously, suffers a syncopal episode, a more assertive course is warranted. Again, the first step is to exclude active ischemia or electrolyte abnormalities. In the patient with frequent ventricular ectopy and associated palpitations, a trial of drug therapy is instituted during continuous electrocardiographic monitoring in the hospital. We usually start with procainamide and use mexiletine as a second choice. In our experience, quinidine is poorly tolerated by many patients with CHF, and tocainide is only slightly less well tolerated.

We generally undertake electrophysiologic testing as an initial step in patients presenting with syncope or sudden death. This is primarily because their overall poor cardiac condition makes any subsequent syncopal episodes all the more life-threatening. Likewise, multiple drug failures in the electrophysiologic laboratory that result in the necessity of cardioversion are poorly tolerated by the patient with severe CHF. Thus, when rapid ventricular tachycardia is induced in the laboratory, another decision must be made.

SYMPTOMATIC VENTRICULAR TACHYCARDIA

Therapy for the patient with an inducible ventricular arrhythmia is guided primarily by our expectation of that patient's overall survival. For example, in a patient with an ischemic cardiomyopathy and a left ventricular ejection fraction over 20 percent, either electrophysiologically guided therapy or an implantable defibrillator will very likely prolong life by avoiding sudden death. Conversely, in a patient with idiopathic cardiomyopathy, a left ventricular ejection fraction under 10 percent and New York Heart Association class IV symptoms, surgery for the placement of the defibrillator alone may be lethal. Moreover, the device will probably not enhance the patient's survival. In such a patient, if one or two initial drugs fail in the laboratory, we move quickly to amiodarone therapy.

The patient awaiting cardiac transplantation is yet another problem. Certainly, if an effective drug can be found easily in the electrophysiology laboratory, oral therapy is initiated. The usual case is that most drugs either are unsuitable for the end-stage cardiomyopathic patient or are not effective. However, the placement of a defibrillator exposes the patient to a higher risk of bleeding and infection at the time of transplantation. For this reason, we prefer amiodarone therapy in this population as well. The use of amiodarone, however, is not without its complications. Our concern has been focused on the hepatic effects of the drug in patients who,

after transplant, are placed on potentially hepatotoxic immunosuppressives. Unsuspected pulmonary toxicity from amiodarone would also be devastating in a patient awaiting a cardiac donor.

Most difficult of all, perhaps, is the patient with syncope, frequent ventricular ectopy, and no inducible arrhythmias in the laboratory. We have usually chosen to initiate an oral antiarrhythmic agent that significantly suppresses the ventricular arrhythmias observed by telemetry. Not uncommonly, this method of action is unsuccessful and amiodarone is, once again, our most frequently employed agent.

WHEN CONGESTIVE HEART FAILURE WORSENS

A common clinical situation occurs when a stable patient develops progressive cardiac dysfunction and becomes increasingly symptomatic. Potent intravenous inotropes, such as dopamine, dobutamine, or amrinone, are frequently employed. Now the patient, who may already have had many episodes of unsustained ventricular tachycardia, is under the constant observation by the staff of an intensive care unit. Ventricular arrhythmias almost always intensify in a deteriorating patient and can be extremely alarming to even the most experienced health professional.

In these cases, it is expeditious to begin an intravenous antiarrhythmic agent, usually lidocaine. Maintenance of serum electrolyte, magnesium, and therapeutic digitalis levels are of continued importance, as is adequate oxygenation. Our experience is that all of the inotropes are proarrhythmic in some patients, and prophylaxis of arrhythmia during acute decompensation is warranted. Once the patient is stabilized, a reassessment of the symptoms and the degree of ventricular ectopy can be done.

SUGGESTED READING

Anderson KP, Freedman RA, Mason JW. Sudden death in idiopathic dilated cardiomyopathy. Ann Intern Med 1987; 107:104–106.

Bigger JT Jr, ed. A symposium: Management of ventricular arrhythmias in patients with congestive heart failure. Am J Cardiol 1986; 57:1B–41B.

Dunica S, Coumel P. Incidence and mechanisms of sudden death in patients with left ventricular dysfunction. Heart Failure 1986; 1:244–255.

Francis GS. Should asymptomatic ventricular arrhythmias in patients with congestive heart failure be treated with antiarrhythmic drugs? J Am Coll Cardiol 1988; 12:274–283.

Podrid PJ, Lampert S, Graboys TB, et al. Aggravation of arrhythmia by antiarrhythmic drugs—incidence and predictors. Am J Cardiol 1987; 59:38E–44E.

CARDIAC CATHETERIZATION AND CORONARY ANGIOPLASTY

FREDRIC GEREWITZ, M.D.
WILLIAM J. UNTEREKER, M.D.

The technique of cardiac catheterization was introduced almost 60 years ago and has since then undergone many modifications and refinements. Selective angiography, which was initiated by Sones in 1959, set the stage for the development of coronary angioplasty in the 1970s.

These invasive procedures require the insertion and manipulation of catheters in the heart and the coronary arteries as well as the injection of contrast medium into these structures. It has long been recognized that the introduction of catheters and contrast media may lead to the development of various arrhythmias and electrocardiographic changes. The questions this chapter addresses are (1) what are these events, (2) how are they induced, and (3) how can one effectively and safely manage them?

RADIOCONTRAST MEDIA

A great deal of research has been devoted to the properties and effects of radiocontrast media. Historically, ionic media were developed first, followed by the relatively recent appearance of low osmolar ionic and nonionic agents.

Ionic media, available for clinical use since the late 1920s, have been associated with many physiologic alterations (Table 1). These effects (and others) are believed to account for the hemodynamic, hematologic, and electrophysiologic changes seen clinically.

The electrocardiographic and rhythm disturbances associated with contrast media are described below. Certain properties appear to be of critical importance: the osmolarity, sodium concentration, and calcium chelating properties of the agent employed.

Various electrophysiologic alterations have been described in relation to contrast media, including (1) prolongation of the action potential (as a function of the sodium concentration), (2) inactivation of fast sodium channels and conduction slowing, (3) fractionation of electrograms, suggesting dysynchronous myocardial activation, and (4) temporal dispersion of repolarization.

In general, the effects of nonionic media on the cardiac conduction system are much less pronounced than for ionic media. Hemodynamic changes and adverse reactions are also reduced with nonionic agents. However, because these agents are much more expensive (about 20 times the cost of ionic agents), it may be difficult to justify using them in all patients. At present we use nonionic contrast media in patients who are (or may readily become) hemodynamically unstable and in those individuals who have previously demonstrated a severe adverse systemic reaction to an ionic agent.

ELECTROCARDIOGRAPHIC CHANGES

It is routine to monitor three electrocardiographic leads continuously and to have the capacity to record six leads during cardiac catheterization. Following selective angiography, it is common to observe a variety of electrocardiographic alterations (Table 2). These changes tend to appear almost immediately, to last from 10 to 30 seconds, and to resolve within 2 minutes. Although the etiology of these electrocardiographic alterations is not understood, it is known that the presence of calcium-binding agents in contrast medium exacerbates these changes. Addition of calcium to conventional agents or the use of nonionic media reduces the magnitude of the changes. Although we routinely wait for at least partial resolution of such changes between injections, rarely is it necessary to see complete normalization before proceeding.

Table 1 Physiologic and Biochemical Effects of Ionic Contrast Media

Local hypocalcemia
Inhibition of acetylcholinesterase activity
Histamine release
Release of atrial natriuretic factor
Stimulation of fibrinolysis
Shifts in plasma volume secondary to hyperosmolarity of the contrast medium
Direct toxic effects of iodide on cells

Table 2 Electrocardiographic Alterations Associated with Coronary Angiography

Decrease in P-wave amplitude
Prolongation of the P-R interval
Shift in the QRS axis (rightward with right coronary artery injection and leftward with left coronary artery injection)
Increase in the QRS complex amplitude
Shift in the S-T and T wave vectors opposite to that of the QRS complex
Increase in the T-wave amplitude
Prolongation of the Q-T and Q-Tc intervals
Development of U waves
Slowing of the heart rate

Two particular electrocardiographic patterns warrant special mention. A marked prolongation of the Q-T interval may predispose the patient to the development of ventricular arrhythmias. It is prudent to permit the Q-T interval to return to baseline between coronary injections.

An occasional patient also develops a transient bundle branch block secondary to manipulation of a catheter: right bundle branch block during right-sided heart catheterization due to catheter-induced trauma to the right bundle, or more rarely left bundle branch block during left-sided heart catheterization due to catheter-induced trauma to the left bundle, which lies adjacent to the noncoronary cusp of the aortic valve. These events do not ordinarily require the insertion of a temporary transvenous pacemaker. Likewise, the existence of a chronic right bundle branch block does not necessitate the placement of a pacemaker. However, a prophylactic pacemaker should be inserted prior to right-sided heart catheterization in a patient who has a preexisting left bundle branch block.

BRADYARRHYTHMIAS

Sinus bradycardia is probably the most commonly induced arrhythmia during cardiac catheterization. Occasionally, sinus arrest or second-degree atrioventricular block may occur; first-degree atrioventricular block is rather common. The effect is most profound during the 5 to 20 seconds following injection and resolves within about 1 minute.

Sinus slowing follows selective right coronary artery injection in the majority of cases. This is probably because the right coronary artery most often supplies the inferior wall of the left ventricle. The mechanisms involved include activation of cholinergic neuroreflexes as well as direct effects of contrast media on the sinoatrial and atrioventricular nodes. Vagal reflexes, stimulated via chemoreceptors and possibly mechanoreceptors, produce bradycardia and hypotension (the Bezold-Jarisch reflex). This response is essentially abolished by the administration of atropine. However, evidence suggests that at least part of the slowing response is due to a direct tissue effect, including local pressure in the sinoatrial nodal artery and possibly inhibition of both slow and fast ionic channels in the sinoatrial and atrioventricular nodes. Although local hypoxemia secondary to injection of contrast medium is postulated as a mechanism for sinus bradycardia, standard contrast medium has a PO_2 similar to that of blood.

Sinus slowing may also occur after injection of the left coronary artery. This bradycardia, which appears to be almost exclusively mediated by reflexes, may be as profound as with right coronary artery injection. Atropine effectively prevents this occurrence.

Hyperosmolarity is the major regulator of this neuroreflex, with a minimal contribution from viscosity, organic iodide composition, cation content, addition of calcium, or rate of injection. Consequently, those contrast agents with lower osmolarity, such as the nonionic media and sodium methylglucamine ioxaglate, tend to create less bradycardia.

Many laboratories premedicate with atropine (0.01 mg per kilogram intramuscularly) for patients with no contraindication to its use. This may be supplemented by intravenous atropine during the procedure. Caution must be applied in those patients with unstable angina, whose resulting tachycardia may be deleterious. In the patient who demonstrates recurrent severe bradycardia despite the use of atropine, a temporary pacemaker is inserted. However, the need for this is rare.

Having the patient cough when bradycardia occurs is also useful. This creates a functional systole that may be repeated approximately once each second, often maintaining a cardiac output until the sinus rate recovers or a pacemaker is inserted.

TACHYARRHYTHMIAS

Supraventricular

Supraventricular tachyarrhythmias are generally confined to sinus tachycardia and atrial fibrillation or flutter. Sinus tachycardia most commonly occurs because of (1) anxiety, (2) premedication with atropine, (3) acute hemodynamic instability, and (4) severe cardiopulmonary disease. Since hemodynamic measurements, cineangiographic quality, and patient safety may be compromised by sinus tachycardia (or any tachycardia, for that matter), efforts must be made to reduce the heart rate prior to catheterization.

We routinely premedicate patients with diazepam (5 to 10 mg orally) and with diphenhydramine (25 to 50 mg orally or intravenously). This may be supplemented with intravenous diazepam or midazolam if the patient is still anxious upon arrival at the catheterization laboratory.

In patients who have severe unstable angina, valvular heart disease, or a marked tachycardia at the time of initial evaluation, atropine (about 0.01 mg per kilogram) is avoided as a premedication.

The patient who has tachycardia because of acute and/or severe disease must be optimally managed prior to catheterization. The catheterization laboratory is not the place to "tune up" the patient. However, for the patient who develops tachycardia during the procedure, intravenous propranolol (1 to 3 mg by slow intravenous injection) may be effective and may be used safely in this setting of close hemodynamic monitoring.

Atrial fibrillation (or flutter) uncommonly develops during catheterization. Although it may be induced by selective coronary injection, most often it is produced by mechanical stimulation of the right atrium with a stiff catheter (e.g., Cournand). Increased right atrial pressure also predisposes to the development of atrial premature complexes and atrial fibrillation. Balloon flotation catheters are less likely to induce atrial premature complexes and are used in the majority of patients in our laboratory. If atrial fibrillation develops during the catheterization, appropriate rate control may be achieved acutely using intravenous propranolol or verapamil. Intravenous procainamide (1 g intravenously over 20 minutes) may then be considered to restore sinus rhythm, especially in patients with severe disease and hemodynamic instability. Ordinarily, atrial fibrillation spontaneously converts without medication if the rhythm has not been a problem clinically.

Ventricular

Ventricular tachycardia is relatively uncommon during cardiac catheterization. It generally occurs in patients who have the appropriate substrate, such as a left ventricular aneurysm or right ventricular dysplasia. The arrhythmia may be initiated by radiocontrast injection, but more often it is the result of catheter manipulation. The form that develops in the presence of ischemia is usually polymorphic and is often a prelude to frank ventricular fibrillation.

If the patient is hemodynamically stable, various measures including coughing, administration of an intravenous antiarrhythmic agent, and rapid ventricular pacing with a temporary pacemaker may be attempted. If the arrhythmia persists, we sedate and electrically cardiovert the conscious patient; an anesthetist or anesthesiologist is present during this time. An unconscious patient is defibrillated immediately using the synchronous mode, as cardiopulmonary resuscitation is being initiated.

The most feared arrhythmic complication during cardiac catheterization is ventricular fibrillation, which has a reported incidence of 0.1 to 1.3 percent. As with sinus bradycardia, the onset is usually 5 to 20 seconds after a coronary injection. Many studies have investigated this problem, from which certain tentative conclusions may be drawn.

The implicated mechanisms include catheter manipulation, coronary injections, and ischemia. Ventricular fibrillation occurs most often with selective injection of the right coronary artery. The reasons for this are unknown. In addition, the injection of saphenous vein bypass grafts has a comparatively high incidence of ventricular fibrillation, again for unclear reasons.

Ventricular fibrillation appears to develop either spontaneously (initiated by a ventricular premature complex) or following sinus bradycardia with Q-T interval prolongation (again initiated by a ventricular premature complex). It has also been observed that low sodium concentrations and the presence of calcium-chelating agents in contrast media reduce the fibrillatory threshold. The addition of calcium to standard ionic media reduces the incidence of ventricular fibrillation.

These observations, as well as those described previously, support a role for both reentrant and automatic foci in the development of ventricular fibrillation. There is also evidence to suggest that delayed afterdepolarizations may be important in this process. We know that this problem is enhanced by acute ischemia. A favorite aphorism of Gruentzig was "ischemia plus dye equals fibrillation," and no experienced angiographer will disagree.

In order to reduce the risk of developing ventricular fibrillation, we avoid injecting into a coronary artery when the pressure tracing shows "ventricularization" or damping. We also avoid injections into small arteries (most frequently the conus branch of the right coronary artery), especially if contrast agent persists in the artery after an initial test. If damping cannot be avoided, we are careful to decannulate immediately after each injection and to pause before recannulating. Downsizing to a smaller catheter may also be useful in this situation. Last, if the contrast agent clears poorly or there is marked Q-T interval prolongation, we wait for resolution of such signs before performing another injection. The use of nonionic contrast media is associated with a lower incidence of ventricular fibrillation (especially if some sodium is present in the formulation), and it may be used for the patient who has had evidence of recent and recurrent ischemia. Prophylactic lidocaine should also be considered in such individuals.

When ventricular fibrillation does occur, the patient should be instructed to cough for as long as consciousness persists. The first operator should initiate chest compressions while the circulating nurse prepares to defibrillate. A defibrillator with a high-energy output is preferable. The patient should then be fully evaluated before a decision is made as to whether or not to continue the study. If resuscitation is prompt, the procedure may be completed.

PERCUTANEOUS TRANSLUMINAL CORONARY ANGIOPLASTY

The preceding discussion applies equally to percutaneous transluminal coronary angioplasty. It is important to remember that the patient will develop ischemia upon balloon inflation, increasing the likelihood of ventricular fibrillation and possibly severe bradycardia.

In patients who undergo percutaneous transluminal coronary angioplasty of a stenotic right coronary artery, we uniformly place a right-sided heart catheter that has pacing capabilities in the pulmonary artery. These include the Zucker and Myler catheters as well as a Swan-Ganz catheter with a pacing port. Our preference is the Baim-Turi catheter, which permits monitoring of the pulmonary artery pressures coupled with the advantages of a flotation catheter that can be rapidly withdrawn from the pulmonary artery to the right ventricular apex. As discussed previously, the presence of a chronic left bundle branch block is another indication for pacing capability any time a catheter is used to cross the tricuspid valve.

It is important to minimize the amount of contrast material used and to avoid test injections immediately after dilation of the artery while ischemia persists. If ischemia is prolonged because of spasm,

thrombus, or dissection, prophylactic lidocaine should be considered.

SUGGESTED READING

Coskey RL, Magidson O. Electrocardiographic response to selective coronary arteriography. Br Heart J 1967; 29:512.

Diagnostic Imaging (Suppl) 1987; 9:2.

Hanley PC, Holmes DR Jr, Julsrud PR, Smith HC. Use of conventional and newer radiographic contrast agents in cardiac angiography. Prog Cardiovasc Dis 1986; 28:435.

Murdock DK, Euler DE, Becker DM, et al. Ventricular fibrillation during coronary angiography: An analysis of mechanisms. Am Heart J 1985; 109:265.

ACUTE MYOCARDIAL INFARCTION

MARIUS SHARON, M.D.
LEONARD N. HOROWITZ, M.D.

PATHOPHYSIOLOGY OF TACHYARRHYTHMIAS

Acute myocardial infarction (MI) is caused predominantly by an acute occlusion of a severely narrowed atherosclerotic coronary artery by an evolving thrombus. The onset of acute ischemia is accompanied by significant changes in the electrophysiologic properties of the myocardial cells.

There is an abrupt reduction in transmembrane resting potential, amplitude, and duration of action potential. As the ischemic changes progress, the ischemic cells depolarize to resting potentials of less than −60 mV, and they become inexcitable. However, as they progress from the normal state to an inexcitable, quiet state, the cells pass through a range of reduced excitability, upstroke velocity, and time of repolarization. These events occur in areas of ischemic myocardium, presenting a variety of degrees from the center of ischemia to the border zone adjacent to nonischemic myocardium. Thus, the two key elements of reentrant tachyarrhythmias are created —slow conduction and unidirectional block.

Dispersion of Recovery and Fragmentation

Acute ischemia causes differences in refractoriness between ischemic and nonischemic zones within the ventricular myocardium, among clusters

of unequally injured cells. Acute ischemia shortens the effective refractory period of the Purkinje fibers and of the ischemic myocardial cells, whereas that of the adjacent normal cells remains unchanged. Studies have demonstrated that myocardial cells with prolonged refractory periods function as barriers in the way of the electrical current, which then travels through alternative, open pathways encircling the refractory barrier. In the ischemic myocardium, especially in the border zone, islets of injured cells are interspersed with normal tissue, and the conduction of the electrical impulse becomes so fragmented and slow that it intermittently spans diastole. The disparity in recovery time creates conditions for local unidirectional block, facilitating reentrant electrical activity. The delayed electrical impulse is then able to reactivate excitable tissue, initiating a reentrant circuit to produce ventricular tachycardia (VT). This irregular, low-amplitude, fragmented electrical activity can also create multiple fronts of activation with different conduction velocities leading to multiple desynchronized reentry circuits spreading in different directions, ultimately causing ventricular fibrillation (VF).

Abnormal Automaticity

The property of automaticity or spontaneous (phase 4) depolarization is normally present in the sinus node, atrioventricular (AV) node, His-Purkinje fibers, and specialized atrial fibers. Ischemically injured Purkinje cells demonstrate enhanced automaticity. The increased automaticity appears to play a role in the later stages of the ischemia (24 to 48 hours). It is usually represented by sustained or unsustained ventricular tachycardia, at slower rates than acute ischemic reentry tachycardia, and by accelerated idioventricular rhythms. It is less sensitive to lidocaine, and its clinical and prognostic importance in acute MI is questionable.

Afterdepolarizations

Delayed afterdepolarizations are low-amplitude potentials occurring after full repolarization of the myocardial fiber. Afterdepolarizations may trigger another afterdepolarization or full depolarization and cause a self-perpetuating response. The tachycardia initiated by afterdepolarizations is also called triggered activity, and it has been suggested that this mechanism rather than enhanced automaticity may be a major basis for the tachyarrhythmias occurring in the subacute later stages (24 to 72 hours) of acute MI.

PATHOPHYSIOLOGY OF BRADYARRHYTHMIAS

The bradyarrhythmias are represented by sinus and AV node dysfunction, including sinus bradycardia, sinus exit block, sinus arrest, and various degrees of AV block and intraventricular conduction defects. These arrhythmias and conduction disturbances are caused by ischemia of the various parts of the specialized conduction system and/or by imbalance of the autonomic nervous system. Ischemia of the pacemaker and specialized conduction tissue may be responsible for temporary or permanent loss of function. Autonomic imbalance causes only temporary dysfunction. Enhanced vagal tone is encountered early during acute MI, especially inferior wall MI. The bradycardia and hypotension that develop early in inferoposterior MI are due to the von Bezold-Jarisch reflex mediated through vagal discharge and respond to intravenous atropine. The occlusion of the right coronary artery and/or increased vagal tone may depress the sinus node, the AV node, and the AV conduction. Therefore, sinus bradycardia is often associated with a slow junctional escape rhythm or with various degrees of AV block. Bradycardia that develops or persists later than 12 hours after the onset of inferior MI (in the absence of negative chronotropic drugs) is caused by ischemia owing to the occlusion of the proximal right coronary artery and is generally insensitive to atropine. AV nodal block—first-degree, second-degree Mobitz I (Wenckebach), and high-degree or complete heart block—in the absence of sinus bradycardia is usually caused by occlusion of the right coronary artery below the sinus nodal branch but can also be enhanced by vagal discharge.

Intraventricular Conduction Defects

Ischemia of the conduction system below the AV node, in the His-Purkinje system, can cause bundle branch and fascicular blocks. It is usually associated with anterior wall MI and caused by occlusion of the left anterior descending coronary artery. When the occlusion is very proximal, the myocardial mass affected is large, with septal infarction, and in addition to peripheral bundle branch block, the conduction through the lower His bundle and proximal bundle branches may be affected.

ARRHYTHMIAS IN EARLY PHASE OF ACUTE MYOCARDIAL INFARCTION

Bradyarrhythmias

Sinus Bradycardia

Bradycardia is the most common arrhythmia in the first hours of acute MI varying between 25 and 40 percent of all patients seen. About three-quarters of all cases occur in the first hour after the onset of symptoms and are caused chiefly by increased vagal tone. Sinus bradycardia is the predominant early bradyarrhythmia present in about 25 to 30 percent of all acute cases of MI. Sinus bradycardia is generally well tolerated. However, it may be accompanied by junctional escape rhythm or various degrees of AV block. Atropine 0.5 to 1 mg given intravenously is usually effective in accelerating the sinus rate and improving the AV conduction. Intravenous atropine is indicated as initial therapy for symptomatic bradycardia (weakness, dizziness, syncope, and congestive heart failure). Care must be taken when administering atropine in this setting because sinus tachycardia may occur and cause increased ischemia.

AV Nodal Block

Ischemia or increased vagal tone can slow conduction through the AV node and cause first-degree, second-degree (Mobitz I), and complete AV block. It can depress the pacemaker activity with resulting slow junctional escape rhythm (below 55 beats per minute) during sinus bradycardia, sinus arrest, or complete AV block. In the absence of previous bundle branch block, the QRS complex in junctional rhythm and during AV block is of normal duration (narrow). When AV block has a 2:1 pattern, it may be confused with Mobitz II second-degree block; however, the association with inferior MI and a narrow QRS complex can help to diagnose Mobitz I correctly. Therefore, AV nodal dysfunction is usually transient.

Why Treat Bradyarrhythmias?

Sinus node dysfunction and disorders of AV conduction are usually well tolerated. However, almost one-half of the patients with bradycardia develop hypotension. Although the product of low heart rate and blood pressure may reduce the myocardial oxygen consumption, it also reduces the cardiac output significantly in patients with substantial infarcts, who may not be able to increase their stroke volume. Also, hypotension can substantially decrease coronary perfusion. There are conflicting reports regarding the prognostic significance of bradycardia and acute MI. Although some reports show good prognosis, others describe increased frequency of ventricular ectopic activity, including VT and VF.

Treatment

No treatment is necessary if the cardiac output is adequate, as demonstrated by good perfusion of the extremities and urine output, absence of pulmonary rales and other signs of congestive heart failure, and impairment of the mental status. If treatment is indicated, start with intravenous atropine 0.5 mg, which can be repeated up to five times over $2\frac{1}{2}$ hours. In our opinion, if 1.5 mg of cumulative doses of atropine fail to raise the heart rate, then atropine will not work and a temporary pacemaker should be considered (see the chapter *Temporary Pacemakers*). Caution should be employed with atropine because the resultant tachycardia may induce malignant ventricular arrhythmias. High doses of atropine commonly cause urinary retention and can produce flushing of the skin, dry mucosa, and mydriasis. Since bradyarrhythmias in early acute MI are usually self-limited, it may be acceptable to apply an external (transthoracic) pacemaker if the patient tolerates the energy level required to pace the heart and is not pacemaker-dependent. Isoproterenol can also be used, but briefly, as a bridge to pacemaker insertion in severe bradycardia. Prepared as a 0.1 mg per deciliter solution, it is started at 0.5 μg per minute and titrated to the desired heart rate response. Isoproterenol, a beta-adrenergic agonist, is a dangerous drug that can cause sinus tachycardia, systemic hypotension, and ventricular tachyarrhythmias and increase myocardial oxygen consumption. Most patients with symptomatic bradycardias that require a temporary pacemaker do well with a demand ventricular pacemaker. A minority of patients, those with large infarcts or with associated right ventricular infarction, need an AV sequential pacemaker to ensure the atrial mechanical participation to the cardiac output, without which the patient remains hypotensive and oliguric despite an adequate ventricular rate.

Tachyarrhythmias

Sinus Tachycardia

About 30 percent of patients with acute MI present with sinus tachycardia or hypertension or both, and another 10 percent can be unmasked by blocking the vagal overactivity with atropine. It is known that acute MI is accompanied by an immediate rise in plasma catecholamines. The release of

catecholamines is enhanced by pain, anxiety, and left ventricular failure. Catecholamines increase the temporal dispersion of repolarization, facilitating a reentrant tachyarrhythmia. They also enhance automaticity of ischemic Purkinje fibers and facilitate the propagation of slow calcium-mediated currents. They lower the threshold of VF.

Patients with sinus tachycardia occurring in the first hours of acute MI, as opposed to the late onset of persistent type, do not have a poor prognosis. The oxygen consumption, however, is increased. These patients are excellent candidates for beta-adrenergic blocking agents, started either intravenously or orally. If the heart rate and blood pressure were lowered initially by morphine sulfate, beta blockers can be started orally. Beta-adrenergic blockers have been demonstrated to influence positively both short-term and long-term prognosis. They reduce myocardial oxygen consumption and alleviate ischemia.

The drugs shown to have beneficial effects are the nonselective agents propranolol and timolol and the beta-1 selective metoprolol. The starting doses are 1 to 2 mg slowly intravenously for propranolol, followed by 80 to 240 mg per day, and 5 to 15 mg slowly intravenously for metoprolol, followed by 100 to 200 mg per day. Caution must be employed with beta-blocking agents. They can cause bradycardia, hypotension, AV nodal conduction delays, and in patients with large myocardial infarctions, congestive heart failure and cardiogenic shock.

Supraventricular tachycardias are present infrequently in acute MI, usually in the subacute phase. More frequently, atrial fibrillation accompanies the onset of MI. This group of arrhythmias is discussed later.

Ventricular Arrhythmias

Ventricular premature complexes (VPCs) are almost the rule in acute MI, with a reported incidence of 75 to 95 percent of cases. Complex VPCs were regarded in the past as precursors of VF, and suppression with antiarrhythmic drugs was advocated. However, recent evidence shows that only about half of the cases of VF are preceded by "warning arrhythmias"—frequent, multiform, consecutive, or early coupled VPCs (R on T phenomenon). In our experience, the indication for suppression of VPCs is the occurrence of long periods of ventricular bigeminy with a short coupling interval. In this case, the effective cardiac output is significantly lowered.

Ventricular Tachycardia

Unsustained VT in acute MI is reported with a frequency of 10 to 40 percent. The higher incidences include salvos (three to five consecutive VPCs). VT in early acute MI has the same significance of VPCs, expressing increased irritability of the ischemic myocardium. There is no correlation with the extent of MI and the prognosis is regarded as benign. It should be noted, however, that VF is often initiated by a rapidly degenerating VT. Unsustained VT need not be treated unless it is very frequent. Intravenous lidocaine is the drug of choice. Procainamide can be used if lidocaine is ineffective.

Ventricular Fibrillation

About 20 to 50 percent of all acute MI patients die suddenly before reaching the hospital, the majority because of VF. VF is defined as primary or secondary, according to the timing and associated clinical features. Primary VF occurs early in the course of MI (usually within 12 hours) without prior evidence of congestive heart failure. Secondary VF is associated with left ventricular failure and occurs relatively late, during the subacute phase of MI (usually after 24 hours). The incidence of primary VF is highest in the first hour after the onset of symptoms and decreases exponentially thereafter. About 70 percent of all episodes occur within 4 hours, 85 percent in 8 hours, and over 90 percent in 12 hours. Primary VF rarely occurs after 24 hours, unless recurrent ischemia develops. The incidence of VF in coronary care units varies from 4 to 18 percent, depending on the population studied and the average time delay between the onset of MI and admission to the coronary care unit. In a prospective study of mobile coronary care units in which one-third of the patients were seen within 30 minutes and 60 percent within 1 hour after the onset of symptoms, the incidence of VF was almost 30 percent. Controversies abound regarding the prognosis of primary VF and the need for prophylactic antiarrhythmic therapy. Most studies reveal a benign in-hospital prognosis when prompt defibrillation and cardiopulmonary resuscitation are possible. Others show increased hospital mortality for patients with primary VF.

Treatment

The treatment of VF is electrical direct current defibrillation applied as soon as possible utilizing energy of 200 to 360 joules. Cardiopulmonary resuscitation and lidocaine prophylaxis should be instituted concomitantly, but no other measure is more urgent than electrical countershock. If the first discharge interrupts the arrhythmia, lidocaine (1.5 mg per kilogram of body weight) should be administered intravenously and a 4 mg per minute infusion should be started. If VF recurs, additional electrical shock should be administered at a previous energy level and an additional lidocaine bolus of 1 mg per kilogram should be given intravenously at 5 to 10 minutes after the first bolus. If the arrhythmia is not

interrupted, a maximal energy defibrillatory shock should follow the first one, and the correct position of the paddles should be ensured.

If VF recurs, bretylium 500 mg should be delivered as an intravenous bolus, and it can be repeated once. If this fails, procainamide, 1 g, loaded slowly intravenously at maximum 50 mg per minute, should be delivered after defibrillation. In a few stubborn cases with multiple recurrent VF episodes, after these three drugs have been used sequentially and failed, combinations of these agents can be employed. Intravenous amiodarone can be administered as a 5 to 10 mg per kilogram bolus followed by a 40 to 50 mg per hour infusion. It has been shown to be effective in such refractory cases (see the chapter *Amiodarone*).

Repeated countershocks are necessary until the acute phase of ischemia subsides. Interventions to reduce ischemia may also be beneficial in controlling the arrhythmias. Intravenous beta blockers, nitroglycerin, and calcium antagonists may be antiarrhythmic in this setting.

Prophylactic Therapy for VF

The prognostic significance of in-hospital primary VF is controversial. Early studies reported higher mortality rates of acute MI patients with primary VF than of patients without VF, and so does a recent report from the Gruppo Italiano per lo Studio della Streptochinasi nell'Infarcto Miocardico (GISSI) study. Other studies, including the Multicenter Investigation of the Limitation of Infarct Size (MILIS), did not find a significant adverse effect of primary VF on mortality.

Reviewing the studies of intravenous lidocaine prophylaxis, it becomes apparent that judicious use of the drug, employing adequate loading and maintenance doses, and selective use in the relatively younger age groups (patients in their 50s or early 60s) and in patients without congestive heart failure probably reduces the incidence of primary VF. We favor the use of prophylactic lidocaine in acute MI for several reasons: (1) the incidence of recurrent VF is high (up to 30 percent) in patients with primary VF and repeated electrical defibrillations can add to myocardial damage; (2) even in an adequately equipped and trained emergency room or coronary care unit, it is preferable to prevent syncope and cardiovascular collapse that occur with VF, even if the survival advantage is equivocal; (3) the risks of lidocaine administration are low. The drug is well tolerated hemodynamically, except in extreme cases of intoxication. Most side effects are mild and include dizziness, slurred speech, paresthesias, and rarely delirium. These are related to the plasma level, which can be readily checked and the dose corrected. Since "warning" or "premonitory" ventricular arrhythmias do not predict VF, it makes sense to treat most patients with proven or suspected acute MI prophylactically.

Who Should Not Be Treated?

There are no absolute contraindications to lidocaine. However, in the following groups of patients, the risks may be greater than the benefits:

1. Elderly patients (over 70 years of age) are less likely to develop primary VF and are more likely to suffer toxic side effects.
2. Patients with uncompensated left ventricular failure have large infarcts in which secondary VF occurs; this does not respond as well to lidocaine, and decreased hepatic clearance of the drug with subsequent accumulation and toxicity occurs.
3. Patients with high-degree AV block due to ischemia of the His-Purkinje system and who develop bradycardia with a slow ventricular escape rhythm should not be treated with lidocaine. Lidocaine can abolish the automaticity of the Purkinje fibers and suppress the escape focus, leading to asystole. These patients have a high risk of developing VT or VF, but the treatment is temporary artificial ventricular pacing. With a well-functioning pacemaker in place, lidocaine may be administered if necessary.

In order to ensure prophylactic efficacy, lidocaine should be loaded with 1.5 mg per kilogram of body weight and a 2 to 4 mg per minute infusion (depending on body weight) should be started concomitantly. Because of rapid distribution within the body, additional boluses of 1 mg per kilogram at 10 and 20 minutes' delay should be given. Blood levels should be monitored and maintained between 2.5 and 5 μg per milliliter and the infusion rate adjusted accordingly. If asymptomatic unsustained ventricular arrhythmia breaks through in spite of adequate lidocaine blood levels, the drug should not be discontinued unless recurrent sustained VT or VF occurs. If this happens, procainamide is the second drug of choice. The loading dose is 1 g over 10 to 15 minutes, followed by a 4 mg per minute infusion. Caution must be employed with procainamide treatment because it can cause significant hypotension, excessive widening of the QRS complex, and Q-T prolongation, which can lead to torsades de pointes. The plasma level of procainamide should be 4 to 10 μg per milliliter. The plasma concentration of *N*-acetyl procainamide, an active metabolite of procainamide, should also be monitored, as it is responsible for much of the toxicity of procainamide.

ARRHYTHMIAS IN THE LATE PHASE OF MYOCARDIAL INFARCTION

Bradyarrhythmias

Sinus bradycardia occurring more than 6 hours after the onset of acute MI is usually caused by sinus node ischemia. It is often transitory, not accompanied by hypotension, and, if the rate is very low, the underlying junctional escape rhythm is adequate for maintaining cardiac output. Atropine is usually ineffective. Treatment becomes necessary only if the patient is symptomatic. Temporary transvenous atrial or ventricular pacing is usually sufficient. If the patient's hemodynamic stability is dependent on atrial "kick," AV sequential pacing is indicated. If the arrhythmia persists throughout the hospital period, a permanent pacemaker is required.

Conduction Abnormalities

Late development of first-degree AV block occurs with administration of digitalis glycosides, beta-adrenergic blockers, calcium antagonists, or as a conduction delay below the bundle of His in the presence of anterior MI. In this case, it is usually associated with widening of the QRS complex as a result of intraventricular conduction delay. First-degree AV block per se is not associated with increased mortality or hemodynamic impairment and does not need to be treated. However, in the presence of bilateral bundle branch block or a new fascicular block, it is associated with an increased risk of complete AV block and should tilt the balance in favor of placing a temporary ventricular pacemaker.

Second-degree AV block in this stage usually represents severe AV conduction defects in the His-Purkinje system (Mobitz II). It is rare in acute MI and is almost always associated with anterior infarction and a wide QRS complex, and it often reflects trifascicular block. Second-degree type II AV block is a marker of impending complete failure of the AV conduction, which often occurs abruptly with development of complete AV block and asystole. It is an absolute indication for immediate temporary ventricular pacemaker insertion.

Third-degree or complete AV block may occur suddenly, although it is usually preceded by Mobitz II second-degree AV block and intraventricular conduction defect. It is almost always associated with anterior infarction. The site of the block is infranodal, and the underlying rhythm is either an unstable, slow ventricular escape or, frequently, ventricular asystole. Temporary transvenous ventricular pacing is required on an emergency basis. Second-degree Mobitz II and third-degree AV block associated with bundle branch or intraventricular block develop in a group of patients with predominantly anterior MI who have an extremely high mortality rate. Although insertion of temporary transvenous ventricular pacemakers is indicated, permanent pacemaker insertion in these patients is debatable on the grounds that it does not reduce the short-term or the long-term mortality.

Prophylactic Pacemaker Insertion in Acute Myocardial Infarction

Bradycardias and conduction defects that are either symptomatic or potentially dangerous are approached according to their time of onset and the location of the block. Patients with early bradycardias or blocks associated with inferior MI have a much better prognosis than the late developing ones, which are associated with anterior MI. The early blocks are predominantly transient, whereas a substantial number of the late developing blocks are persistent. This concept guides the approach to pacemaker insertion in terms of appropriateness, timing, urgency, and the need for permanent pacing (Table 1).

New onset of infranodal conduction abnormalities indicates ischemia, infarction, and the potential for progression to complete heart block and sudden death. Patients who are admitted to the hospital with acute MI and bundle branch block may have developed the abnormality acutely prior to admission, or it may have predated the infarction. Isolated bundle branch block carries a low risk of progression to complete heart block and death. Bifascicular bundle branch block carries a higher risk of complete heart block (10 to 18 percent) and death, regardless of time of onset. A combination of old and new bundle branch block carries a very high risk of death (15 to 30 percent). Most of the life-threatening conduction abnormalities are associated with large infarcts and a poor prognosis because of pump failure. Thus most studies dealing with a small number of patients have been unable to demonstrate the benefit from temporary pacemaker insertion. However, in about 10 percent of these patients, the prognosis improves as a result of prophylactic pacemaker insertion. In addition, using modern transvenous balloon flotation electrodes and sterile technique, it is possible to introduce transvenous pacemakers without significant complications.

The necessity for permanent pacemaker insertion has been debated. Patients with the indications summarized in Table 1 have arguably greater risks of sudden death, and the long-term prognosis for these patients and the efficacy of the permanent pacemakers are uncertain. Most cases of sudden death are ultimately caused by VT or VF. Even so, an unknown number of patients with bundle branch block develop severe bradycardia or asystole complicated terminally by malignant tachyarrhythmias. Since there is only a small risk involving pacemaker

Table 1 Indications for Pacing After Acute Myocardial Infarction

Conduction Abnormalities	Temporary Pacing	Permanent Pacing
Sinus bradycardia	Yes, if symptomatic, slow ventricular rate unresponsive to atropine	Only if persistent, symptomatic, slow junctional rhythm
First-degree AV block	No	No
Second-degree AV block (Mobitz I)	Yes, if symptomatic, slow ventricular rate unresponsive to atropine	Rarely, if persistent
Second-degree AV block (Mobitz II)	Yes	Yes
Third-degree AV block, Intranodal	Yes, if symptomatic, slow ventricular rate unresponsive to atropine	Yes, if persistent
Infranodal (wide QRS complex)	Yes	Yes
Old or new bundle branch block	No	No
Bifascicular bundle branch block	Yes	Yes
First-degree AV block with bundle branch block	Yes	Yes
Long Q-T interval and polymorphic VT	Yes	No

insertion in most cases of transient second-degree AV block in anterior infarction, the pacemaker insertion seems prudent.

Supraventricular Tachycardias

Atrial premature complexes are common in acute MI. Atrial premature complexes may suggest distention of the atria owing to high left ventricular end-diastolic pressure, mitral regurgitation, or atrial irritability owing to ischemia, infarction, or pericarditis. They are innocuous, per se, do not affect cardiac output or prognosis, and do not require treatment. Paroxysmal supraventricular tachycardia occurs in up to 5 percent of acute MI patients and frequently recurs, with rates of 150 to 220 beats per minute. When sustained or frequently recurrent, it increases the myocardial oxygen consumption and impairs the ventricular performance by reducing the diastolic filling time. Supraventricular tachycardias are associated with decreased cardiac output and increased mortality.

Treatment

Augmentation of the vagal tone by carotid sinus compression, sustained Valsalva maneuver, or cold stimulus to the eyes (application of an ice bag) can help differentiate sinus tachycardia from paroxysmal supraventricular tachycardia, nonparoxysmal junctional tachycardia, or atrial flutter; it can also terminate the episode. A similar effect can be obtained by intravenous administration of 10 mg of edrophonium. Therapy is aimed at slowing the ventricular rate by potentiating the vagal tone and delaying the conduction through the AV node. Digoxin is helpful and has been used routinely for this purpose, but its effect is delayed. Verapamil, cautiously infused intravenously at 1 mg per minute, can be effective immediately. Verapamil, however, can cause hypotension, especially in acute MI if rapidly delivered owing to its negative inotropic effect and vasodilatory characteristics. Patients with a rapid ventricular rate and hypotension should be cardioverted electrically with relatively low energy levels starting at 50 joules.

Atrial flutter and atrial fibrillation are encountered in patients with left ventricular failure, atrial ischemia or infarction, pericarditis, or pulmonary emboli. Atrial flutter is an arrhythmia with regular atrial rates of 260 to 340 beats per minute and ventricular rates of 130 to 170 beats per minute due to 2:1 AV block. It occurs rarely in acute MI. Atrial fibrillation is common in acute MI, occurring in 10 to 15 percent of cases. The same principles guide the treatment of atrial flutter and atrial fibrillation. Initial rate control can usually be achieved with slow intravenous administration of verapamil, usually 5 to 15 mg followed by a verapamil drip at 5 to 10 mg per hour until therapeutic loading with either intravenous digoxin or oral verapamil is accomplished. For hemodynamically compromised patients or those with refractory arrhythmias with fast ventricular rates, direct current cardioversion is required.

Atrial fibrillation is particularly refractory to treatment or recurrent if the underlying cause has not been corrected. Apart from treating the underlying causes, therapy should be aimed at suppressing atrial premature complexes. Quinidine has been effective either alone or in combination with an AV node depressant such as verapamil or digoxin. Therapy is started with 600 to 800 mg daily and can be increased to 1,000 to 1,600 mg per day for maintenance. Although it is an effective drug when adequate plasma concentrations are maintained (3 to 6 μg per milliliter), quinidine has side effects such as diarrhea, nausea and vomiting, and immunogenic

thrombocytopenic purpura. There is a rare idiosyncratic reaction resulting in severe prolongation of the Q-T segment facilitating a type of polymorphic VT called torsades de pointes (see the chapter *Proarrhythmia*). When sustained, this arrhythmia causes syncope and is a precursor of VF and cardiac arrest. Caution must be employed in the combined therapy of quinidine and digoxin. Quinidine decreases the renal clearance of digoxin, and unmonitored therapy can lead to digitalis intoxication. Procainamide can also be used in therapy of atrial arrhythmias.

Ventricular Tachyarrhythmias

VPCs are associated with an increased risk of death after MI. However, suppression of the VPCs does not result in a proven prognostic benefit. Late onset of frequent VPCs must be investigated for the possibility of ongoing or recurrent ischemia.

Accelerated idioventricular rhythm is sometimes called "slow VT," with rates of 60 to 100 beats per minute. Most of the episodes are unsustained, self-limited, and occur in the first 48 hours. About half of them occur during sinus rate, which is slower than the ventricular rate, and they are intermittently overdriven by the speeding sinus rhythm. This arrhythmia is probably caused by increased automaticity in the Purkinje fibers and usually does not affect prognosis. It can, however, be associated with development of rapid VT.

Ventricular tachycardia occurring after 24 hours from the onset of MI can be unsustained or sustained. When unsustained VT is frequent and symptomatic, treatment is indicated. Sustained VT in the late phase can be associated with recurrent ischemia, but more often it is the result of a healed transmural infarction with left ventricular dysfunction and development of reentrant sustained monomorphic VT with rates of 140 to 250 beats per minute. This arrhythmia is associated with high (40 to 50 percent) mortality.

The management of an episode of sustained VT depends on the hemodynamic impact of the arrhythmia, which is a function of the ventricular rate and underlying functional state of the left ventricle. If the patient has stable blood pressure and is only moderately symptomatic, intravenous antiarrhythmic therapy should be initiated with lidocaine, 1.5 mg per kilogram, followed by one to two additional boluses of 1 mg per kilogram at 10-minute intervals. If conversion to sinus rhythm occurs, the patient should be placed on intravenous lidocaine infusion (4 mg per minute), and the rate of infusion should be adjusted to plasma levels of 2.5 to 5 μg per milliliter or less if significant side effects occur. If lidocaine does not convert the VT to sinus rhythm within 3 to 5 minutes from the last bolus, a trial of procainamide should be started at 50 mg per minute in a bolus of up to 1 g. Blood pressure should be monitored closely because of the hypotensive effect of procainamide. Following conversion of VT, an intravenous maintenance infusion of procainamide should be instituted at 4 mg per minute and plasma levels kept at 4 to 10 μg per milliliter. If both drugs fail, electrical cardioversion should be performed after pretreatment with intravenous sedatives or hypnotics. Equipment for cardiopulmonary resuscitation should be available, as respiratory depression or profound hypotension may develop. Synchronized direct current cardioversion should be started at low energy levels, as low as 25 to 50 joules. In marginally stable patients, one trial of synchronized direct current shock at 100 joules should be done and, if this is unsuccessful, 200 to 360 joules should be used.

Ventricular Fibrillation

Late-onset or secondary VF represents about 20 percent of all episodes of this arrhythmia in acute MI. It is predominantly associated with large Q-wave infarcts with secondary left ventricular failure. It occurs after 24 hours from the onset of acute MI, and the majority occur after 48 hours. The in-hospital mortality rate of patients with secondary VF is between 50 and 80 percent. In a subgroup of patients, late VF may be caused by an acute ischemic event or by extension of the infarct. Most cases occur as part of the gradual hemodynamic deterioration of patients with large MI. The treatment of VF has been described previously. Patients who have been successfully defibrillated may be placed on intravenous prophylactic therapy until correction of the hemodynamic and metabolic abnormalities and of the hypoxia is achieved. Intravenous prophylaxis with lidocaine or procainamide is not very effective. Aggressive management, e.g., coronary angiography and revascularization, may be offered to a small, stable subgroup of patients.

SUGGESTED READING

Hindman MC, Wagner GS, JaRo M, et al. The clinical significance of bundle branch block complicating acute myocardial infarction. 1. Clinical characteristics, hospital mortality, and one-year follow-up. Circulation 1978; 58:679.

Hindman MC, Wagner GS, JaRo M, et al. The clinical significance of bundle branch block complicating acute myocardial infarction. 2. Indications for temporary and permanent pacemaker insertion. Circulation 1978; 58:689.

Hjalmarson A. Early intervention with a beta-blocking drug after acute myocardial infarction. Am J Cardiol 1984; 54:11E–13E.

Lie KI, Wellens HJ, van Capelle FJ, et al. Lidocaine in the prevention of primary ventricular fibrillation: A double-blind, randomized study of 212 consecutive patients. N Engl J Med 1974; 291:1325–1326.

Partridge JF, Webb SW, Adgey AA. Arrhythmias in the first hours of acute myocardial infarction. Prog Cardiovasc Dis 1981; 23:265–278.

ENDOCRINE DISEASE

SALLY G. BEER, M.D.
LEONARD N. HOROWITZ, M.D.

When treating patients with endocrine disorders, one must be vigilant for changes in cardiac function and rhythm disturbances. It is important to understand the interrelationship between the cardiovascular system and certain endocrine disorders so that the appropriate therapeutic route can be followed.

THYROID DISEASE

It is well known that thyroxine has effects on the heart mediated not only by adrenergic stimulation but also by direct effects on the myocardium. The net cardiovascular impact of thyroid disease is multifaceted. The thyrotoxic patient may have electrocardiographic abnormalities related to myocardial ischemia, hypertrophy, or dilation. On the other hand, the hypothyroid patient may have electrocardiographic abnormalities related to myxedematous myocardial changes, electrolyte imbalances, deranged myocardial metabolism, pericardial effusion, anemia, or hypercholesterolemia.

Hyperthyroidism and Tachycardias

The recognition of the association of an enlarged thyroid gland and exophthalmos with tachycardia, palpitations, and cardiomegaly predates the description of hyperthyroidism by Graves about 150 years ago. Indeed, sinus tachycardia or atrial fibrillation may be present before other clinical symptoms of hyperthyroidism. Sinus tachycardia is more common than atrial fibrillation, occurring in about 40 percent of patients with hyperthyroidism. The incidence of atrial fibrillation in this condition, however, does increase with age. Hyperthyroid patients may present with paroxysms of atrial fibrillation, which may eventually give rise to chronic atrial fibrillation (see the chapter *Atrial Fibrillation*).

Atrial flutter is uncommon in hyperthyroidism, occurring in less than 2 percent of patients. Likewise, paroxysmal supraventricular tachycardia is infrequently associated with hyperthyroidism, in spite of increased automaticity and shortening of atrial refractoriness. This supports the theory that most paroxysmal supraventricular tachycardias are the result of reentrant phenomena and not of increased automaticity.

Supraventricular as well as ventricular premature complexes have been reported in hyperthyroid patients, although in many patients drug therapy (e.g., digoxin) may be the culprit, not the hyperthyroidism. Ventricular tachycardia is not associated with hyperthyroidism, although rare case reports of its occurrence in this setting do exist.

The approach to arrhythmias associated with hyperthyroidism should be directed toward correction of the underlying metabolic disorder. The optimal treatment of atrial fibrillation and other arrhythmias associated with hyperthyroidism is treatment of the primary endocrine disorder. Successful conversion to sinus rhythm after treatment with ^{131}I, surgical removal of thyroid tissue, or other antithyroid treatment is common.

Of particular note is the fact that arrhythmias in hyperthyroid patients are fairly resistant to conventional treatment with digitalis and its derivatives. The exact mechanism for this resistance is not clear. It may be the result of lowered serum glycoside levels secondary to increased volume of distribution. In addition, there is a reduction in the net prolongation of the atrioventricular node refractory period produced by digoxin in experimental studies. It is important to be aware of the decreased activity of cardiac glycosides, because toxicity may occur at doses that offer little therapeutic benefit. Moreover, direct current countershock is generally successful in establishing sinus rhythm only after the patient becomes euthyroid. While the hyperthyroidism is being treated, therapy is generally required to control the tachyarrhythmia.

Older studies found that centrally active agents such as reserpine or guanethidine were useful in controlling the tachycardia of hyperthyroidism. Since the introduction of beta-adrenergic blockers, these agents have been found to control many of the sympathetic effects of hyperthyroidism. Low doses, such as propranolol, 10 mg four times a day, may slow the rate of the tachycardias associated with hyperthyroidism in most patients; however, high doses may sometimes be required. Titration of the dosage of the beta-blocking agent to achieve an acceptable rate is required. As the hyperthyroid state resolves, downward titration is required.

Hyperthyroidism and Heart Block

Various degrees of heart block have been reported in hyperthyroidism. First-degree block is most common, occurring in 3 to 9 percent of hyperthyroid patients, even in the absence of any detectable heart disease. P-R interval prolongation, however, does not require any therapy in any setting. Once the patient becomes euthyroid, the P-R interval usually returns to normal.

Second- and third-degree heart block occur much less frequently. The mechanism of block is not understood. Treatment of type 2 second-degree or third-degree heart block in hyperthyroidism should be directed primarily at correction of the endocrine abnormality, as mentioned above. Temporary transvenous pacing is indicated until the patient becomes euthyroid, at which point the conduction should return to normal.

Hyperthyroidism and Preexcitation

There appears to be an increased frequency of preexcitation in patients with hyperthyroidism. The association is not clear, as several large series of patients with electrocardiographic evidence of preexcitation failed to reveal a large number of hyperthyroid patients. Reported cases of preexcitation in the presence of hyperthyroidism have shown cessation of the electrocardiographic changes when the euthyroid state was achieved. These cases may be caused by activation of a latent bypass tract by thyroid hormone. This finding is of particular importance because of the increased risk of atrial fibrillation in hyperthyroid patients. The combination of atrial fibrillation and preexcitation may result in rapid ventricular response.

Again, therapy should be based on correction of the underlying endocrine abnormality, which will resolve the rhythm disturbance. In this setting, digitalis is contraindicated. The effects of beta-adrenergic blockers, which are generally not recommended in patients with preexcitation and atrial fibrillation, may be beneficial in this unusual setting. Cautious use of short-acting beta blockers is appropriate.

Hypothyroidism

Sinus bradycardia with low-voltage T waves is a well-known finding in hypothyroidism. This is not usually of clinical significance and resolves with replacement of thyroid hormone.

Prolongation of the Q-T interval is almost always present. Although this does not appear to increase the risk of torsades de pointes or ventricular tachycardia, there are reports of ventricular tachycardia and fibrillation in patients with myxedema who do not have underlying cardiac disease. Whether this is directly related to hormone status or secondary to other alterations such as hypothermia is not clear.

As always in myxedema, thyroxine replacement should be slow and cautious. The ventricular arrhythmia should be approached in the same fashion as in euthyroid patients.

Myxedema is also associated with an increase in atrioventricular and intraventricular conduction disturbances. First-degree block is common. Complete atrioventricular heart block and syncope have been observed. Temporary pacing should be instituted until the patient is euthyroid.

PARATHYROID DISEASE

Hypoparathyroidism

Although parathyroid hormone has been found to have direct effects on isolated heart cells, causing increased beating and a positive inotropic action, it is not associated with abnormal heart rhythms.

Hypocalcemia caused by hypoparathyroidism results in prolongation of the Q-T interval. Although this abnormality may be associated with torsades de pointes, there are no data available to suggest an increased risk of this arrhythmia in hypoparathyroid patients. The Q-T interval in these patients returns to normal with calcium replacement.

Hyperparathyroidism

Hypercalcemia produced by hyperparathyroidism may produce arrhythmias; however, the incidence of rhythm disturbances in this syndrome is low. No relationship has been found between the elevated serum calcium concentration and heart rate. Atrial and ventricular premature complexes and atrial fibrillation have been reported but are rare.

Atrioventricular block rarely occurs in hyperparathyroidism. First-degree, type 1 second-degree atrioventricular block (Wenckebach phenomenon) and complete atrioventricular block have been reported. These generally resolve after surgical removal of the parathyroid adenoma.

Therapy in such cases should be evaluated on an individual basis. Lowering the serum calcium level is the primary treatment; however, the use of antiarrhythmic drugs or temporary pacing may occasionally be required.

DISEASES OF THE ADRENAL GLAND

Adrenal Cortex

Although Cushing's syndrome and hyperaldosteronism both have distinct cardiovascular manifestations, they are not associated with arrhythmias. Adrenal insufficiency (Addison's disease) may have associated sinus bradycardia or first-degree heart block, which responds to the administration of glucocorticoids. There are no data suggesting any predisposition to tachyarrhythmias in Addison's disease.

Adrenal Medulla

Pheochromocytoma, a catecholamine-producing tumor derived from chromaffin cells, is well known for its profound cardiovascular effects, in particular hypertension. Patients with pheochromocytoma may have sinus tachycardia, supraventricular premature complexes, and paroxysmal supraventricular tachycardia.

The tachyarrhythmias respond to beta-adrenergic blockage and should be treated with such an agent if they produce palpitations or are otherwise clinically significant. One must be careful not to treat patients who have pheochromocytoma with a beta blocker until after the blood pressure is controlled with an alpha-adrenoreceptor blocking agent, such as phenoxybenzamine or phentolamine. Beta blockade without adequate alpha blockade can produce hypertensive crisis in these patients. Surgical removal of the tumor should result in cessation of any arrhythmias. Persistent arrhythmias that require chronic treatment may occur if there has been permanent myocardial damage.

ACROMEGALY

Acromegaly (growth hormone excess) has well-documented cardiovascular sequelae. The most common of these are hypertension and cardiomegaly, which occur in up to 50 percent of cases. Other disorders such as congestive heart failure, intraventricular conduction abnormalities, and arrhythmias occur less frequently.

Ventricular premature complexes may occur and need be treated only if they produce symptoms. They can be treated with the usual antiarrhythmic drugs. Supraventricular tachyarrhythmias have been reported, but in most cases these were thought to be caused by concurrent hyperthyroidism. In fact, the presence of a supraventricular arrhythmia (e.g., sinus tachycardia, atrial fibrillation) in an acromegalic patient warrants an assessment of thyroid function.

Treatment of acromegaly is primarily accomplished by means of surgery or irradiation of the tumor. The secretion of growth hormone may be decreased in some patients with bromocriptine or somatostatin. One follow-up study, however, suggests that many cardiovascular effects, including arrhythmias, progress in spite of adequate control of growth hormone levels. The arrhythmias may require chronic treatment in these cases.

DIABETES MELLITUS

Diabetes mellitus is the most common endocrinopathy and certainly one of the leading health concerns in most nations. Most physicians are all too familiar with its profound cardiovascular effects: accelerated atherosclerosis, cardiomyopathy, congestive heart failure, and autonomic neuropathy. Cardiac arrhythmias in diabetic patients are secondary to the other cardiac manifestations of the disease as opposed to any direct effect on the heart by hyperglycemia. A discussion of the treatment of the broad cardiovascular effects of diabetes mellitus is beyond the scope of this chapter.

Of note is the fact that the autonomic neuropathy that frequently involves the heart is associated with sinus tachycardia and a fixed rapid heart rate.

This tends to be unresponsive to physiologic stimuli such as carotid sinus massage, Valsalva maneuver, tilting, or drugs such as beta-adrenergic blockers, atropine, or alpha-adrenergic agonists. Autonomic neuropathy, however, does not predispose one to other arrhythmias.

SUGGESTED READING

Surawicz B, Mangiardi ML. Electrocardiogram in endocrine and metabolic disorders. In: Rios JC, ed. Cardiovascular clinics: Clinical electrographic correlation. Philadelphia: FA Davis, 1977: 243.

Williams GH, Braunwald E. Endocrine and nutritional disorders of the heart. In: Braunwald E, ed. Heart disease. Philadelphia: WB Saunders, 1988: 1800.

CARDIAC ARRHYTHMIAS IN PULMONARY DISEASE

DAVID LEE SCHER, M.D.
LEONARD N. HOROWITZ, M.D.

Both supraventricular and ventricular arrhythmias occur with a high frequency in persons with chronic lung disease. Precipitating factors of arrhythmias in these subjects include acid-base disorders (respiratory, metabolic, or a combination), hemodynamic abnormalities (often seen in these patients who are hospitalized), electrolyte imbalance (notably hypokalemia and hypomagnesemia), and cardiac effects of bronchodilator drugs (theophylline preparations, beta-adrenergic agonists). Most commonly, more than one of the aforementioned conditions is present.

SUPRAVENTRICULAR ARRHYTHMIAS

Tachyarrhythmias predominate in these patients. The type of arrhythmia varies with the severity of illness. Although atrial premature complexes accompanying sinus rhythm are commonly noted in ambulatory patients, atrial fibrillation and multifocal atrial tachycardia (MAT) are observed in acutely ill hospitalized patients. The incidence of supraventricular arrhythmias is also variable, being much lower when standard 12-lead electrocardiograms are used (approximately 30 percent) and higher when ambulatory monitoring is utilized (80 to 90 percent).

APPROACH TO THE PULMONARY PATIENT WITH SUPRAVENTRICULAR ARRHYTHMIAS

In most instances, supraventricular arrhythmias in these patients are not life-threatening, and thus sufficient time is available to bring about correction of any of the underlying precipitating factors that are discussed further on. This is the most important therapeutic step, as in most cases it is sufficient to eradicate the rhythm disturbance. Specific antiarrhythmic therapy is then discussed.

Nonpharmacologic Treatment

Correcting Ventilation, Oxygenation, and Acid-Base Disorders

Correction of ventilation (as assessed by Pco_2 and pH via arterial blood gas monitoring) and oxygenation (assessed by arterial Po_2) should be the first step taken inasmuch as arrhythmias in these patients may be the first indication of respiratory decompensation and because these parameters may be readily correctable by pharmacologic (bronchodilators) or mechanical (intubation, ventilator parameter changes, endotracheal suctioning, physical therapy) means. It should be noted that alkalemic states may precipitate arrhythmias as well as acidemia.

Although beta-adrenergic agents and theophylline preparations may in themselves prompt supraventricular arrhythmias (MAT in particular), there should be no hesitation about the use of these agents if deterioration of pulmonary function is the precipitating arrhythmogenic factor.

Correction of Electrolyte Disturbances

It is not uncommon for these patients to exhibit electrolyte abnormalities, most commonly hypokalemia and hypomagnesemia. Depletion of magnesium usually accompanies that of potassium because the mechanism of electrolyte loss is similar (diuretic and theophylline use, edema with secondary hyperaldosteronism, and elevated circulating catecholamines). It should be noted that low intracellular stores of magnesium may not be adequately reflected in serum levels (which may even be normal).

Potassium may be given as solutions of the chloride salt in intravenous infusions of 20 to 40 mEq. Magnesium can be replaced by giving 10 to 15 mEq of magnesium (as a 2 percent solution of magnesium sulfate) per hour intravenously, for 5 to 7 hours. The kidneys retain magnesium until the deficit is replaced. Thus, measuring urine magnesium concentration may help to guide therapy. Serum potassium levels may fall further during magnesium infusion. Therefore, it may be advantageous to give simultaneous potassium supplementation.

Adjustment of Bronchodilator Therapy

The mechanism by which theophylline causes arrhythmias has not been fully elucidated. However, it does increase circulating catecholamines (probably by means of direct adrenal stimulation and decreased cellular re-uptake), and it can produce triggered activity (the presumed mechanism of MAT) in vitro. MAT is a common theophylline-induced toxic rhythm and can occur even in the patient with serum theophylline levels within the accepted "therapeutic" range. We therefore recommend discontinuing theophylline preparations in patients with MAT if this is clinically feasible. If not, serum levels should be kept in the "low normal" therapeutic range (10 to 12 mg per deciliter).

Although the inhaler or nebulized form of beta-adrenergic agonists is reported to produce fewer cardiac effects than other routes of administration, it may nonetheless precipitate tachyarrhythmias. It may be necessary to decrease the dose or increase the interval at which the drug is administered. When this is not possible (or the drug is ineffective in either abolishing the arrhythmia or treating the pulmonary disease), we substitute ipratropium bromide (Atrovent), an anticholinergic agent without significant cardiac effect.

Improvement of Hemodynamics

It is not unusual for patients with pulmonary disease who experience arrhythmias to be elderly and to have concomitant cardiac disease (cor pulmonale, coronary artery disease, or congestive heart failure). Assessing the relative contributions of cardiac and pulmonary pathologic processes to the arrhythmia may be clinically impossible, and because abolition of the arrhythmia is so dependent upon correction of precipitating factors, pulmonary artery catheterization may be a necessary adjunct to monitor and adjust therapy. It should be noted that these patients usually require higher right ventricular filling pressure because of chronic pulmonary hypertension.

Specific Antiarrhythmic Therapy

Atrial Fibrillation and Atrial Flutter

A rapid ventricular response accompanying atrial fibrillation or atrial flutter can precipitate congestive heart failure, myocardial ischemia, and a decrease in cardiac output. If this occurs, in addition to the nonpharmacologic measures discussed above, it is advisable to institute digitalis therapy. If atrial fibrillation or atrial flutter of new onset persists longer than 24 to 48 hours, the addition of a class IA antiarrhythmic agent (preferably procainamide, as quinidine increases digoxin levels) should be considered to convert the patient to sinus rhythm.

On physical examination and on a single channel rhythm strip, MAT may be misdiagnosed as atrial fibrillation. Because MAT is a rhythm that is unresponsive to digitalis and because patients with pulmonary disease are more sensitive to digitalis (rendering them more susceptible to digitalis toxicity), a 12-lead electrocardiogram should be performed to confirm the presence of atrial fibrillation.

Digitalis Use in Patients With Pulmonary Disease

It is generally accepted that patients with lung disease have an increased sensitivity to digitalis and that this hypersensitivity correlates with hypoxemia, hypercapnia, and clinical cor pulmonale. However, arrhythmias traditionally associated with digitalis toxicity are also seen in patients with severe lung disease who are not given digitalis. This may reflect hemodynamic and metabolic derangements associated with respiratory failure, which themselves increase susceptibility to digitalis toxicity. Therefore, when using digoxin in these patients, digitalis-induced toxic arrhythmias may occur at relatively low serum digoxin levels, and higher doses of digoxin should be avoided.

Multifocal Atrial Tachycardia

MAT is the most characteristic of all arrhythmias in patients with lung disease and the most common supraventricular rhythm disturbance encountered in patients with acute respiratory failure.

MAT is defined by the following electrocardiographic criteria: an atrial rate of more than 100 beats per minute, three or more diverse P-wave morphologies in the same electrocardiographic lead, varying P-P and P-R intervals, and an isoelectric baseline between P waves (Fig. 1). As mentioned previously, MAT may at first be mistaken for atrial fibrillation, and a 12-lead electrocardiogram will clarify this.

The mainstay of treatment for MAT is the correction of reversible precipitating factors, as discussed above. Digitalis, procainamide, phenytoin, quinidine, direct current cardioversion, and lidocaine have all uniformly failed in the treatment of MAT.

The presumed mechanism of MAT is triggered activity that may be produced by the various clinical situations discussed previously, and it manifests itself at the cellular level by an accumulation of intracellular calcium. It was the finding of this cellular phenomenon that led to the initial use of the calcium channel antagonist, verapamil, in MAT. Intravenous doses of 4 to 30 mg have been more successful in slowing MAT than in converting it to sinus rhythm. Successful therapy for chronic MAT with oral verapamil is anecdotal, but we have seen recurrent MAT in patients taking up to 120 mg every 8 hours.

Adverse reactions seen with verapamil in these patients have included a decline in systemic blood pressure (which has been shown to be attenuated by pretreatment with 1 g of intravenous calcium gluconate) and increasing ventilation-perfusion mismatching (by dilating pulmonary arterioles and thus increasing perfusion to poorly ventilated portions of the lung) evidenced by increased pulmonary shunt fractions and alveoloarterial oxygen gradients.

Because of the hyperadrenergic state of these patients and the role of catecholamines in the genesis of triggered activity, beta-adrenergic blocking agents would theoretically be useful for the treatment of MAT. Unfortunately and ironically, it is the pulmonary disease (specifically, chronic obstructive pulmonary disease) that theoretically interdicts the use of these agents. Because of its cardioselectivity at low doses (and the absence of clinically significant adverse pulmonary effects at intravenous doses up to 0.2 mg per kilogram), the beta-1 selective blocker metoprolol has been used in treating MAT in intravenous doses up to 10 mg and oral doses of 50 mg (although 25 mg orally has the same efficacy). At these doses, no deterioration of cardiac or pulmonary function has been seen. Our experience has been that metoprolol is more effective than verapa-mil in converting MAT to sinus rhythm. Chronic therapy with 25 mg orally twice daily has been used effectively and without side effects.

The successful treatment of MAT with verapamil and metoprolol must be tempered by the fact that most studies using these agents have employed strict patient selection criteria. Among exclusionary criteria were systolic blood pressure less than 100 mm Hg, congestive heart failure, bronchospasm, acidemia, anemia, hypoxemia, hypercarbia, electrolyte abnormalities, greater than first-degree heart block, and elevated serum theophylline levels.

The potential for both verapamil and metoprolol to cause deterioration of pulmonary function (metoprolol by bronchoconstriction and verapamil via increasing ventilation-perfusion mismatching) and hypotension cannot be overstated. However, in selected patients, they remain the drugs of choice for specific antiarrhythmic therapy of MAT.

Whether conversion to sinus rhythm is a better therapeutic end point than a controlled ventricular rate has not been established. Theoretically it seems to offer more stability, as MAT is often associated with paroxysmal atrial fibrillation that has associated loss of atrial contribution to cardiac output and increased risk of embolic events and may lead to overzealous use of digoxin.

Of most significance is that it is not known whether successful treatment of MAT alters the high mortality rate associated with it (40 to 50 percent of hospitalized patients). In fact, this is not likely to be the case, because the mortality is most certainly linked to the underlying predisposing and precipitating factors.

VENTRICULAR ARRHYTHMIAS

As is the case with supraventricular arrhythmias, the frequency of ventricular arrhythmias in these patients is dependent upon the stability of the lung disease and the method used for detecting these arrhythmias (electrocardiogram or Holter monitor).

The most common ventricular arrhythmia observed is ventricular premature complexes. Ventricular tachycardia (defined as three or more consecutive ventricular premature complexes) is seen in 10 to 20 percent of patients. The frequency of ventricular premature complexes has been linked to the degree of hypoxemia and the presence of edema in particular, but it is also a function of the same factors mentioned previously in reference to supraventricular arrhythmias.

The significance of ventricular arrhythmias in these patients has not yet been established. However, the frequency of ventricular ectopy in patients with pulmonary disease has been likened to that in post–myocardial infarction patients. Results of a trial currently underway to determine the efficacy of antiar-

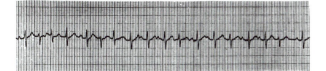

Figure 1 Electrocardiographic rhythm strip of multifocal atrial tachycardia.

rhythmic therapy in this latter group may influence the approach to the patient with pulmonary disease.

APPROACH TO THE PULMONARY PATIENT WITH VENTRICULAR ARRHYTHMIAS

Until prospective controlled studies are undertaken to determine the effect of antiarrhythmic agents on survival in these patients, we recommend the following approach. Underlying correctable precipitating conditions should be sought and rectified as described above for supraventricular arrhythmias. Life-threatening arrhythmias (sustained ventricular tachycardia and ventricular fibrillation) should be treated promptly with antiarrhythmic drugs and/or cardioversion. In other than life-threatening arrhythmias, drug therapy should be instituted only if the arrhythmia is symptomatic and persists after reversible precipitants have been corrected. The role of programmed electrical stimulation in guiding drug therapy in the patients just described (i.e., patients with multiple but not frequent episodes of unsustained ventricular tachycardia) is not clear at this time.

Lidocaine is a drug used frequently in these patients when they are hospitalized. Because these patients have clinical or subclinical hepatic dysfunction due to cor pulmonale, care should be taken in the lidocaine dosages used because the drug is cleared by the liver.

SUGGESTED READING

Arsura EL, Lefkin AS, Scher DL, et al. A randomized double-blind placebo controlled study of verapamil or metoprolol in multifocal atrial tachycardia. Am J Med 1988; 85:519–524.
Green LH, Smith TW. The use of digitalis in patients with pulmonary disease. Ann Intern Med 1988; 87:459–465.
Iseri LT, Fairshter RD, Hardemann JL, Brodsky MA. Magnesium and potassium therapy in multifocal atrial tachycardia. Am Heart J 1985; 110:789–794.
Levin JH, Michael JR, Guarnieri T. Treatment of multifocal atrial tachycardia with verapamil. N Engl J Med 1985; 312:21–24.
Scher DL, Arsura EL. Multifocal atrial tachycardia: Mechanism, clinical correlates, and treatment. Am Heart J 1989; 118:574–580.

INFECTIVE ENDOCARDITIS

T. JOHN MERCURO, M.D.
LEONARD N. HOROWITZ, M.D.

Infective endocarditis may be defined as an infective process involving the endocardium, including the heart valves, produced by microorganisms. The infection results in primary destruction of cardiac tissue with diverse manifestations. Infective endocarditis was initially characterized as acute or subacute. However, there is great variation in the rapidity with which the disease may develop, depending in part upon the nature of the infecting organism and also on the underlying cardiac substrate. The disease is a great masquerader, often presenting as a pulmonary, central nervous system, or orthopedic disorder, in association with constitutional symptoms such as fever, weight loss, and general malaise.

In the preantibiotic era, infective endocarditis was invariably fatal. Although today effective medical and surgical management exists, life-threatening complications of endocarditis continue to be a problem. The complications may be grouped broadly into two main categories, extracardiac and cardiac.

Extracardiac complications include embolic phenomena, metastatic infection, mycotic aneurysm, cutaneous and musculoskeletal involvement, central nervous system involvement, and renal abnormalities. Often the cardiac manifestation of endocarditis is a new heart murmur or a change in a previously diagnosed heart murmur. Other cardiac presentations include congestive heart failure, pericarditis, and conduction system abnormalities with varying degrees of heart block and arrhythmias.

The anatomy of the conduction system and its relationship to the surrounding cardiac structures, including the valves and septa, is fundamental to the pathophysiology of the conduction system abnormalities and certain arrhythmias seen in endocarditis.

The sinus node is located at the junction of the superior vena cava and the right atrial appendage. The anterior, middle, and posterior internodal bands extend across the atrium from the sinus node leading toward the AV node. The AV node is located just anterior to the orifice of the coronary sinus. It sits just under the endocardium on the right side of the atrial septum at the junction of the septal leaflet of the tricuspid valve with the central fibrous body.

The distal portion of the AV node and the bundle of His enter the right fibrous trigone and then course through the posteroinferior aspect of the membranous ventricular septum. Early in the course through the ventricular septum, the conductive fibers of the common bundle begin to form discrete fascicles of the left and right bundle branches. The left and right bundle branches pass to the left and right surfaces of the ventricular septum, respectively. Early in its course, the left bundle branch fans out and quickly divides into anterior and posterior fascicles. The right bundle branch continues just beneath the surface of the endocardium in the right side of the ventricular septum to the base of the anterior papillary muscle.

Localized pathology may develop in a small area, resulting in the block of a specific fascicle. The AV node and the bundle of His have a close proximity to the posteromedial aspect of the mitral valve apparatus and the medial tricuspid annulus. The distal bundle of His and the proximal bundle branches, specifically the proximal right and the left anterior branches, come into close proximity to the noncoronary and right cusps of the aortic valve while in the ventricular septum.

It is easily imagined how the extension of any myocardial infection interrupting the conduction system at a specific site will result in a particular form of conduction system disease. Because of the proximity of the heart valves to the conduction system, the infection of any of the heart valves may result in marked conduction system disease. The development of bundle branch block or heart block is most commonly associated with aortic valve ring abscess that has burrowed through the myocardium to involve the conduction system. This can be an early warning sign of risk of sudden death or abrupt hemodynamic compromise.

The extension of infection from the aortic valve to involve the surrounding conduction system is a common manifestation seen in endocarditis. No particular bacterial organism is more commonly responsible for aortic valve ring abscess. Ring abscess may develop from both virulent and nonvirulent bacterial species. It is clear, however, that ring abscess occurs more commonly in acute bacterial endocarditis involving the aortic valve rather than subacute forms. The presence of pericarditis and new aortic insufficiency adds further clinical evidence suggesting aortic valve ring infection.

The infection of a mitral valve that has undergone mitral annular calcification is not an uncommon substrate for mitral annular ring abscess. Typically, the posterior leaflet of the mitral valve is involved.

The incidence of infective endocarditis with resultant aortic or mitral valve ring abscess is rare with the exception of acute staphylococcal and streptococcal infections. In this setting, the incidence of ring abscess approaches 10 percent. In contrast, ring abscesses develop in a majority of patients with prosthetic valve endocarditis. The frequency of aortic valve ring involvement is slightly higher compared with that of the mitral valve apparatus.

Valve ring abscess, which may be inferred from conduction disturbances noted on the electrocardiogram and clinical findings of changing heart murmurs, provides strong evidence for surgical correction and treatment of the underlying disease process. It should be noted that although transient first-degree heart block may imply myocardial abscess and be a marker for increased mortality and further cardiac complications, other considerations should be taken into account before surgical treatment is recommended. Other causes unrelated to myocardial abscess must be excluded before the conduction abnormality may be attributed to valve ring disruption. Myocardial infarction should be excluded on the basis of serial creatinine kinase enzyme monitoring. Drug effects, especially those of digoxin, should be considered, and if possible, suspected drugs should be discontinued. Myocarditis resulting from ischemia induced by embolic phenomena of the coronary arteries, immunologic reactions, and toxin-related inflammatory reactions may contribute to the generation of transient first-degree heart block. Noninfectious heart block must be excluded before a recommendation for surgery can be made. The persistence of first-degree heart block over a period of days while the patient is on maximal antibiotic treatment lends strong support to surgical intervention. Careful observation seems reasonable when first-degree heart block appears transient. Close monitoring is necessary, however, because complete heart block may develop quite suddenly.

Abscess formation involving the interventricular septum can produce conduction disturbances, the nature of which varies with the anatomic location of the abscess. The lower aspect of the interventricular septum is usually infected by contiguous spread from disease in the mitral valve ring. In this setting, characteristic electrocardiographic findings are manifested by the gradual prolongation of the P-R interval. Prolongation of the Q-T interval is noted at times as well. With the progression of the septal abscess, left bundle branch block develops as a final consequence. Surgical treatment is essential. Abscess in the upper ventricular septum is usually associated with aortic valve disease. This diagnosis is more difficult to make, since the changes on serial electrocardiograms are usually vague. The arrhythmias noted are not specific and may vary. Various degrees of heart block may be found, including complete heart block and runs of ventricular tachycardia and high-grade ventricular ectopy.

Conduction system abnormalities, specifically those of high-grade heart block, may require the insertion of a transvenous pacemaker to avoid hemodynamic compromise. Indications for transvenous pacemaker insertion in the setting of endocarditis are consistent with the general indications

Table 1 Indications for Temporary Pacing in the Setting of Infective Endocarditis

---

Mobitz I atrioventricular block (symptomatic only)
Mobitz II atrioventricular block
Left bundle branch block (during right-sided heart
   catheterization)
Complete atrioventricular block
Acute myocardial infarction secondary to embolic phenomenon
   Bifascicular block
   New bundle branch block associated with transient complete
   heart block

---

for cardiac pacing (Table 1). In the settings of myocarditis and pericarditis, the right ventricle tends to be more irritable, and precautionary measures should be exercised to minimize ventricular arrhythmias. Prevention of subsequent line infection must also be a consideration. The incidence of embolic phenomenon is increased in right-sided endocarditis, as is septal perforation in the presence of interventricular septal abscess.

Pericardial involvement in the setting of subacute endocarditis is a rare complication in contrast to its acute counterpart. Pericarditis is usually seen following the perforation of a ring abscess. The organism most often isolated in this setting is *Staphylococcus aureus*. The inflammation of the pericardium and the myocardium increases overall cardiac irritability. Arrhythmias such as atrial fibrillation and increased ventricular and supraventricular ectopy are common in this setting. This complication usually requires surgical drainage. Addressing the underlying pathophysiology coupled with standard pharmacologic measures usually suffices in treating these complications.

Infective endocarditis is associated with an increased risk of sudden cardiac death. Although the risk is real, it is surprisingly relatively small. Most often the setting is that of acute hemodynamic compromise rather than that of an arrhythmogenic death. When death is related to arrhythmia, it is postulated that an embolic phenomenon to the coronary arteries resulting in acute ischemia and electrical instability is the primary event. High-grade heart block and various cardiac arrhythmias associated with infective endocarditis should be managed promptly by temporary transvenous pacemaker placement and appropriate drug therapy, such as lidocaine for ventricular arrhythmias and digitalization for atrial fibrillation. The primary goal of treatment, however, should be directed at the underlying pathophysiology, i.e., aortic valve ring abscess or suppurative pericarditis. Despite effective surgical and antibiotic treatments for infective endocarditis, morbidity and mortality remain high. It is hoped that prevention of infection by identification of high-risk patients and implementation of antibiotic prophylaxis will have a positive impact on the disease process.

SUGGESTED READING

Karckman AW, Eisenberg E, Frishman W. Infective endocarditis in the 1980s: Clinical features and management. Cardiol Series 1984; 7:13–13.

Mayo Clinic Proceedings—A symposium on infective endocarditis. Mayo Clin Proc 1982; 57:81–86, 155–170.

Robbins M, et al. Infective endocarditis: A pathophysiologic approach to therapy. Cardiol Clin 1987; 5:545–562.

CARDIAC SURGERY AND CARDIAC TRAUMA

MARIE-NOELLE S. LANGAN, M.D.
LEONARD N. HOROWITZ, M.D.

ARRHYTHMIAS AND OPEN HEART SURGERY

The perioperative period following open heart surgery is frequently associated with disturbances of cardiac rhythm. These are generally transient and managed by standard modes of therapy. There are, however, several characteristics unique to these patients that may change the management.

Bradyarrhythmias

Cardiac surgery causes numerous physiologic and biochemical perturbations which, not surprisingly, are frequently accompanied by either sinus tachycardia or bradycardia. Bradyarrhythmias are the most frequent arrhythmias seen in the surgical arena. A number of factors have been recognized as contributory causes, including hyperkalemia, inadequate cardioplegia, atrial ischemia, abnormal vagal tone, and damage to the central nervous system. Bradycardia is a frequent occurrence during intubation and anesthesia induction, precipitated by the agents currently in use. Preoperative medications may contribute to bradyarrhythmias; patients treated with both calcium channel blockers and beta blockers are at increased risk for intra- and postoperative bradycardia. Amiodarone given preoperatively has been associated with bradycardias that are particularly resistant to atropine.

During weaning from cardiopulmonary bypass and during the rewarming period immediately following the surgery, up to 20 percent of patients manifest a bradycardic rhythm. Since sinus bradycardia or significant atrioventricular (AV) block is frequently accompanied by a deleterious drop in cardiac output and may lead to the development of supraventricular tachycardias or ventricular arrhythmias, prompt recognition and treatment are important. Occasionally complete atrial quiescence occurs, with or without an AV junctional escape rhythm. During induction, atropine usually reverses bradycardia; however, in many cases esophageal pacing has been helpful. Postoperatively, use of the epicardial pacing leads placed during surgery allows restitution of a desirable rate by atrial pacing or, in cases of AV block, AV dual-chamber pacing. With atrial quiescence, in addition to lack of spontaneous electrical activity, the atrium is often refractory to pacing. The administration of intravenous isoproterenol may restore atrial excitability, thereby allowing effective pacing.

Sinus and AV Junctional Tachycardias

Sinus tachycardia is common in the first perioperative days and is most important as a hallmark of potentially reversible physiologic problems, including anemia, hypovolemia, fever, and tamponade. The first step in the management of this arrhythmia is therefore to search for the underlying cause (see the chapter *Sinus Tachycardia*).

The presence of epicardial electrodes may help to simplify the differentiation of sinus tachycardia from other supraventricular tachycardias. In the setting of sinus tachycardia, overdrive atrial pacing at a rate exceeding that of the tachycardia is usually associated with a temporary slowing of the rate when pacing is stopped and a gradual return to the original tachycardia with a warming-up period.

Although these temporary wires are frequently helpful in the diagnosis and treatment of the different tachycardias, their use in open heart surgery was once controversial. At present they have become routine, following several reports showing benefit and little risk, with no deaths attributed to their presence or removal and the rare complications of bleeding, pneumothorax, and pneumomediastinum.

AV junctional tachycardia is also common and usually transient, frequently caused by trauma to the AV junction during the surgery. It typically resolves in a few days. The treatment of this rhythm with antiarrhythmic medications (class IA drugs or calcium channel blockers) may be successful. Digitalis, however, is contraindicated because it may increase the automaticity of the AV junctional pacemaker. Even when the rate is controlled, overdrive pacing may be required for patients who rely on the atrial contribution to cardiac output. It is important to note that AV junctional tachycardia is frequently associated with significant antegrade block.

Atrial Fibrillation

Atrial fibrillation is a common postoperative rhythm, even in patients who were in normal sinus rhythm preoperatively (see the chapter *Atrial Fibrillation*). It has been reported to occur in up to 70 percent of patients in the first week after open heart surgery. Many factors have been proposed to account for its frequency, including the irritation of the atria by surgical cannulation, attachment of the pacemaker wires, high endogenous catecholamine secretion, left atrial hypertension and distention, and ischemic injury during the reperfusion phase. Although atrial fibrillation is prevalent, older patients and/or those with enlarged atria are particularly at risk.

In atrial fibrillation with a rapid ventricular response in which the diagnosis may be obscured, the pacemaker wires may once again be helpful in establishing a diagnosis. A recording of an atrial electrogram should show atrial complexes with myriad sizes, shapes, and polarities. There is great variability in the beat-to-beat intervals measured.

The use of antiarrhythmic drugs in this setting is common. The atrial epicardial electrodes are not helpful for treatment, as atrial fibrillation cannot be terminated by pacing. Cardioversion, despite the acuteness of the arrhythmia, is not recommended in the early postoperative period because the atrial fibrillation is most likely to recur. Of course, if atrial fibrillation causes marked hemodynamic compromise, immediate cardioversion is mandatory. Cardioversion may be considered later in the hospital course when the physiologic stimuli have stabilized.

Atrial Flutter

In the postoperative patient, the diagnosis of atrial flutter, a common rhythm postoperatively, is greatly enhanced by recording the atrial electrogram (see the chapter *Atrial Flutter*). The presence of atrial complexes of uniform morphology, polarity, and amplitude with regular beat-to-beat intervals is diagnostic. Atrial flutter is divided into two types: type 1 has an atrial rate of 230 to 340 beats per minute; type 2 has an atrial rate of 340 to 430 beats per minute. The distinction is important because of the difference in response to overdrive pacing.

Type 1 atrial flutter may be abolished by pacing the high right atrium at rapid rates. Pacing should start at just above the flutter rate and increase by increments of 10 beats per minute. While monitoring is performed with the surface electrocardiographic lead II, the atrial rate is gradually increased until the F waves become frankly positive. At this point pacing should be abruptly discontinued. This is usually followed by a termination of atrial flutter and return to sinus rhythm. Alternatively, the pacemaker may initially be set to 125 percent of the atrial flutter rate and maintained for 30 seconds, to be discontinued abruptly at that point. If this is unsuccessful, a 30-second overdrive pacing interval should be repeated at a rate 5 to 10 beats per minute higher.

Occasionally the rhythm that follows the cessation of the atrial pacing is atrial fibrillation. This is generally found only after pacing at a rate greater than 135 percent of the baseline rate. Most commonly, the atrial fibrillation is only temporary and reverts spontaneously to sinus rhythm. In the presence of atrial fibrillation, the rate of the ventricular response is usually lower than that seen during the preceding atrial flutter. If pacing attempts are not initially successful, digitalis and propranolol may ease conversion. Quinidine or procainamide should be added to suppress the atrial flutter.

Type 2 atrial flutter is usually unresponsive to overdrive pacing and should be treated pharmacologically in a manner similar to the treatment of atrial fibrillation with rapid ventricular response, as described earlier.

Paroxysmal Supraventricular Tachycardia

Paroxysmal supraventricular tachycardia is not common but may be distinguished from atrial flutter by recording of the atrial electrogram, which will reveal in the latter case 1:1 AV conduction with an atrial rate between 130 and 220. Differentiation of paroxysmal supraventricular tachycardia from sinus, AV junctional, sinus node reentrant, and ventricular tachycardia can be more difficult. The P-R versus R-P interval seen on the electrogram may be helpful, as the PR:RP ratio is usually less than one in atrial or sinus tachycardia and greater than one in junctional or ventricular tachycardia.

Paroxysmal supraventricular tachycardia, however, is one of the easiest to convert with overdrive pacing, frequently only requiring interruption by a single premature atrial depolarization. Because of this, one can start pacing at a low rate (of approximately 100 beats per minute) and await proper timing of an atrial premature complex. If this is not successful, the method described for type I atrial flutter may be attempted. If conversion is not possible and the patient is symptomatic because of the rapid rate, pacing the atrium at a rate of 180 to 230 beats per minute usually produces 2:1 AV block, with a resulting slower ventricular rate and less hemodynamic compromise. Even if successful conversion results, we suggest beginning therapy with digitalis, quinidine, or procainamide because recurrences are frequent.

Ectopic Atrial Tachycardia

Ectopic atrial tachycardia produces an atrial rate of 130 to 240 beats per minute. If the rate is above 160 beats per minute, it is frequently associated with second-degree AV block, which is helpful in distinguishing it from paroxysmal supraventricular tachycardia. An atrial electrogram shows remarkable beat-to-beat variability in the atrial cycle length, which distinguishes it from the reentrant supraventricular tachycardias. In the postoperative patient this rhythm is not uncommon and should not lead to suspicion of digitalis toxicity, as it might in the preoperative patient.

Because of the associated AV block, this rhythm frequently is not associated with rapid ventricular rates and may not require treatment. If this is not the case, drug therapy is usually not effective and indeed procainamide, if involved, should be stopped, as it seems to potentiate rather than alleviate the problem. Overdrive pacing, as for type I atrial flutter, occasionally converts the ectopic atrial tachycardia to normal sinus rhythm or one that is more readily treatable (atrial fibrillation or type I flutter).

Drug Therapy for Supraventricular Tachyarrhythmias

A number of studies have investigated the use of several different drugs in the patient who has undergone coronary artery bypass grafting both to treat and to prevent supraventricular tachycardias. The prevalence of these arrhythmias (11 to 100 percent) and the associated hemodynamic instability make this issue important. They tend to occur in the first postoperative days, two-thirds of them in the first 72 hours.

The problem of beta-blocker withdrawal has been addressed, and indeed patients previously treated with these drugs do have a greater incidence of supraventricular tachyarrhythmias. The patient who was not previously treated with beta blockers is nevertheless still prone to supraventricular tachyarrhythmias postoperatively, and it has been noted that the drug dosage required to suppress the arrhythmia is greater in these patients. The use of low-dose propranolol in all patients undergoing coronary artery bypass grafting has been shown to decrease the occurrence of postoperative supraventricular tachyarrhythmias to 5 to 20 percent.

The perioperative prophylactic use of digitalis has been slightly more controversial, as some studies have shown a significant decrease in the presence of supraventricular tachyarrhythmias but others have detected no difference. It has been postulated that the high sympathetic tone of the perioperative period tends to counteract most of the digitalis effect. In general, however, its use in the treatment of the supraventricular tachyarrhythmia is associated with a drop in the ventricular rate. It is important to recognize the potential for digitalis toxicity after coronary bypass, as the procedure causes digitalis to leave the tissues and produces an elevation in the serum concentration of the drug.

Because of the high sympathetic state, one might expect verapamil to be more helpful. Its use has resulted in slowing of the ventricular response, but no difference in conversion has been documented. There were significant side effects in these patients. Attempts at diminishing the side effects associated with longer-acting medications were made using esmolol. Although esmolol was successful in reducing ventricular response, there still were moderate problems with hypotension in association with its use. Various other combinations of drugs have been used to try to eliminate the occurrence of supraventricular tachyarrhythmia in the population, even lower than the 5 to 20 percent still seen with prophylactic beta blockade. These have included propafenone, disopyramide (with digoxin), sotalol, and flecainide. Overall they are all quite effective in the treatment of supraventricular tachyarrhythmia with rapid efficient conversion, but their use is limited by the associated side effects (Table 1).

Premature Complexes

Ventricular premature complexes are a common occurrence postoperatively, although their true relevance has not been defined. They may be suppressed by increasing the heart rate above the baseline rate by pacing or by use of antiarrhythmic drugs. Some have suggested that at the time of discharge these patients require ongoing therapy, but this has not been conclusively demonstrated.

Atrial premature complexes may be harbingers of atrial fibrillation, paroxysmal atrial tachycardia, or atrial flutter, and it may therefore be prudent to

Table 1 Drug Doses in the Acute Treatment of Supraventricular Tachyarrhythmias

Propranolol: 2 mg every 4 hours, then 10 mg every 6 hours
Atenolol: 50 mg/day
Sotalol: 1 mg/kg bolus intravenously, plus 0.2 mg/kg over 12 hours; then 160 mg b.i.d.
Digoxin: 0.75 mg intravenously; then 0.25 mg intravenously b.i.d.
Disopyramide: 2 mg/kg intravenously over 10 minutes; then 0.4 mg/kg per hour for 10 hours, followed by 150 mg q.i.d. (used if digitalis is unsuccessful)
Procainamide: 50 mg/min. intravenously to total dose of 15–25 mg/kg.
Propafenone: 2 mg/kg intravenously over 10 minutes
Flecainide: 2 mg/kg intravenously over 20 minutes, followed by 0.2 mg/kg per hour for 12 hours; then 100 mg b.i.d.
Esmolol: 500 µg/kg bolus over 1 minute followed by 4 min. infusion at 50 µg/kg/min. If inadequate response, repeat 500 µg/kg bolus and increase maintenance infusion to 100 µg/kg/min. Increase maintenance by 50 µg/kg/min after bolus to maximum of 200 µg/kg/min.

suppress them, especially in already compromised patients. Again, pacing may be the best way of abolishing the arrhythmia. The addition of procainamide or quinidine is then recommended.

Ventricular Tachycardia

Ventricular tachycardia is reported in 20 to 50 percent of postoperative patients. It is usually seen in the first 12 hours after surgery. Most commonly, only short runs of unsustained ventricular tachycardia are seen, in which case efforts to eliminate predisposing factors—hypokalemia, hypomagnesemia, ischemia, underlying bradycardia (if the underlying rate is less than 70 beats per minute, temporary pacing should be used)—will suffice. When unsustained runs of more than 6 to 10 beats of ventricular tachycardia occur, besides rectifying any of the above factors, intravenous lidocaine should be instituted in the routine manner (see the chapter *Lidocaine*). This therapy should be maintained for approximately 48 hours, following which the patient should be watched with electrocardiographic monitoring for the duration of the hospital stay. If unsustained ventricular tachycardia continues during convalescence, further evaluation, possibly including electrophysiologic studies, should be considered. Nonmalignant arrhythmias need not be treated chronically, as studies have shown that early postoperative ventricular tachycardia does not indicate a poor prognosis.

If the ventricular tachycardia is sustained and not tolerated hemodynamically, standard cardioversion should be used. The drug of first choice is usually lidocaine. This is frequently effective and has minimal negative inotropic effects (see the chapter *Lidocaine*). If lidocaine is ineffective, intravenous procainamide (see the chapter *Procainamide*) and then bretylium (see the chapter *Bretylium*) should be used. We prefer to use these agents singly initially and then to employ combinations if no single agent is effective.

Atrial pacing may be helpful occasionally. If the tachycardia is tolerated, atrial pacing can be tried, as the ventricular tachycardia may be suppressed by overdrive pacing at a rate slightly higher than that of the tachycardia. After stabilization and after the acute postoperative period has passed, further evaluation, including electrophysiologic studies, should be undertaken.

Conduction Disturbances

Conduction disturbances are extremely common but tend to be transient and without long-lasting clinical significance. Right bundle branch block is the most common (52 percent) and is often associated with left anterior hemiblock (13 percent). Left bundle branch block accounts for only 2 percent of the conduction disturbances documented postoperatively. The AV node may be vulnerable to early rewarming, which occurs because of the warmer noncoronary collateral flow in which it is bathed following the completion of the procedure. Hyperkalemia may also play a part. There has been some correlation between the type of cardioplegic solution used and the frequency of occurrence of conduction disturbances. These are less frequent when blood is used and most frequent with high-volume crystalloid solutions.

Occasionally high-grade or complete AV block occurs. Temporary pacing is required in these situations. If AV block is persistent, a permanent pacemaker should be considered.

VALVE SURGERY

Although many of the preceding comments apply to all open heart surgery, most studies and observations have been based on patients who have undergone coronary artery bypass grafting. There are certain particularities in patients who undergo valve surgery. Supraventricular tachyarrhythmia in these patients is frequent, perhaps more so than in the postbypass patients. This is particularly true in those with mitral regurgitation or high pulmonary capillary wedge pressure. Supraventricular tachyarrhythmia is often more serious in this group of patients because some prosthetic valves have worsening regurgitation and higher-grade stenosis in the face of elevated heart rates.

Factors predisposing to arrhythmias are not clearly established, but as with coronary bypass, older age groups are at higher risk, as are patients who undergo multiple valve replacements. It appears that preoperative arrhythmias are not predictive of increased risk. Conduction abnormalities are frequent in this group of patients, particularly after mitral valve repair. Complete heart block usually occurs in the first 48 hours and is transient in 85 percent, but some patients require a permanent pacemaker.

BLUNT CHEST TRAUMA

Cardiac arrhythmias are a common complication of cardiac trauma and have been implicated as one of the frequent causes of mortality in these patients. Both supraventricular and ventricular arrhythmias have been reported, with varying frequencies (Table 2).

Ventricular Arrhythmias

Ventricular arrhythmias are more often caused by injury to the left ventricle than to the right. Ventricular fibrillation generally occurs immediately at

Table 2 Arrhythmias Associated With Cardiac Trauma

Arrhythmia	Percentage of Patients
Any arrhythmia	73
Paroxysmal supraventricular tachycardia/atrial fibrillation	6
Ventricular premature complexes, uniform	54
Ventricular premature complexes, multiform	16
Bigeminy/trigeminy	11
Ventricular couplets/triplets	9
Ventricular tachycardia	3
Ventricular fibrillation	0
Right bundle branch block	9
Left bundle branch block	1
Atrioventricular block	2
Sinus bradycardia	2

the time of impact, and in the experimental setting it has been irreversible. However, it may be preceded by ventricular tachycardia or complete AV block. Ventricular tachycardia is mostly unsustained. It should be noted that there have been reports of ventricular tachycardia up to years after the injury, particularly in patients who suffered myocardial damage and later developed a ventricular aneurysm. Premature ventricular complexes have been documented in a large number of patients, but there is little evidence that they are significant.

Atrial Arrhythmias

Atrial arrhythmias are frequent and generally transient. The majority of patients have sinus tachycardia. However, a significant number have been reported with sinus bradycardia, particularly those who have suffered right-sided cardiac injury. Although this arrhythmia is usually well tolerated and transient, a rare patient may develop transient asystole.

The occurrence of AV block has been well documented. Specific criteria have been proposed for its diagnosis in this setting, including (1) youthful age, (2) absence of preexisting heart disease or conduction defects, (3) great magnitude of injury or force, (4) associated traumatic heart disease, and (5) absence of long latent period between time of injury and discovery of block. (These criteria might well be applied to the other arrhythmias in this setting.)

Electrocardiographic Changes

In addition to the ST-T segment abnormalities associated with true cardiac contusion, trauma patients may develop right bundle branch block, with or without associated left anterior hemiblock. These conduction abnormalities are most transient. Left bundle branch block is decidedly rare, most likely because the right ventricle is the more frequent site of impact.

Clinical studies have been unable to correlate the occurrence and severity of cardiac arrhythmias with more common indicators of thoracic injury. Experimental animal studies have shown that the higher the energy of impact, the more frequent the associated arrhythmias. However, even in these studies, minor trauma occasionally led to serious arrhythmias. High-energy impact is more likely to result in cardiac contusion, coronary artery trauma, and/or myocardial infarction, all of which provide electrical instability at a locus of unevenly perfused myocardium. Also of importance, it has been found that isolated blunt chest trauma is more often complicated by arrhythmias than is chest trauma associated with injury to other parts of the body, presumably because the chest alone absorbs all the kinetic energy of the impact.

The overall physiologic effect of the trauma on the victim is as important as the direct cardiac effect. Changes in vagal and sympathetic tone have been shown to precipitate arrhythmias and exacerbate their consequences. Acidosis, electrolyte abnormalities (particularly hyperkalemia secondary to myonecrosis), and hypovolemia are equally important factors. Apnea is a common consequence of chest trauma and results in low myocardial oxygenation and hypercapnia, both of which contribute to arrhythmogenesis.

Finally, the role of alcohol, a common culprit in trauma, must be remembered. Alcohol has been shown to decrease conduction in the myocardium and therefore may contribute to AV and bundle branch blocks. It has also been shown to enhance automaticity and therefore may participate in the genesis of arrhythmias.

Treatment

The management of trauma-induced arrhythmia is similar to the treatment of arrhythmia found in other settings. Specific recommendations may be summarized as follows:

1. The victim of significant thoracic trauma, with or without arrhythmia at presentation, requires 48 hours of close monitoring as well as serial electrocardiograms and cardiac enzyme determinations.
2. Antiarrhythmic drug therapy should be reserved for those patients with arrhythmias that have deleterious hemodynamic effects. This applies to both supraventricular and ventricular tachyarrhythmias.
3. Antiarrhythmic prophylaxis is generally not required.
4. When treatment of ventricular tachycardia is indicated, class IA drugs are useful because they affect both the ventricular and atrial myocardias and therefore may obviate associated supraventricular tachycardias. In su-

praventricular tachycardia alone, the ventricular rate is usually controlled by digitalis or a beta-blocking agent.
5. It is important to avoid positive inotropes (dobutamine and dopamine) if possible, because of their potential for precipitating arrhythmias.

In the case of AV block, more prolonged episodes require temporary pacing to prevent the progression to ventricular tachycardia or asystole. These blocks are often related to injury, bleeding, and edema in the region of the AV node, and this may require several weeks to resolve. If AV block persists after 2 to 3 weeks, placement of a permanent pacemaker should be considered.

Finally, in the face of ventricular arrhythmias in a patient with a more remote history of cardiac trauma, the possibility of the development of a ventricular aneurysm remains and should be investigated.

ELECTROCUTION

Cardiac arrhythmias and/or electrocardiographic changes have been reported in 10 to 20 percent of patients sustaining electrical injuries. All types of electrical current, including lightning and electroshock therapy, may affect the heart. Several factors determine the severity of cardiac injury sustained, including voltage, type of current site, pathway, and duration. These historical details are helpful in further assessing risk of the development of complications.

Several theories have been proposed to explain the effects of electricity on the heart, including coronary artery spasm, coronary artery endarteritis, and diffuse or patchy myocardial necrosis. The only pathologic correlation that has been found is the occasional presence of endocardial and pericardial petechial hemorrhages. In general, lightning acts as a massive direct current countershock, depolarizing the entire myocardium at once, after which the heart's normal rhythm may resume.

Ventricular fibrillation is the most common cause of death and can occur with even low-voltage electrocution. Significantly, respiratory arrest often lasts longer than asystole, and the victim may die from hypoxia if cardiopulmonary resuscitation is not started promptly. The cardiopulmonary resuscitation efforts should be prolonged, as the return of a rhythm may be prolonged despite minimal damage to the heart. Atrial fibrillation and sinus tachycardia have also been reported.

In general, these arrhythmias occur immediately after the electrical injury; however, there have been a few reports of delays of up to 12 hours after the injury. The right bundle branch block has also been documented, but little is documented regarding the natural history of this conduction defect in this setting.

Because of the potential delay in the onset of arrhythmias, patients should be monitored for 24 hours after injury in which current passes through the thorax. The treatment of these arrhythmias has not been adequately investigated. Digoxin has been successful in treatment of the atrial arrhythmias. Cardioversion and cardiopulmonary resuscitation are crucial in the acute situation.

SUGGESTED READING

Cheitlin MD, Abbott JA. The internist's role in the recognition and management of cardiovascular trauma. Med Clin North Am 1979; 63:201–221.

Liedtke AJ, DeMuth WE. Nonpenetrating cardiac injures: A collective review. Am Heart J 1973; 86:687–697.

Michelson EL, Morganroth J, MacVaugh H. Postoperative arrhythmias after coronary artery and cardiac valvular surgery detected by long-term electrocardiographic monitoring. Am Heart J 1979; 97:442–448.

Rubin DA, Niemenski KE, Monteferrante JC, et al. Ventricular arrhythmias after coronary artery bypass graft surgery: Incidence, risk factors and long-term prognosis. J Am Coll Cardiol 1985; 6:307–310.

Waldo AL, Henthorn RW, Epstein AE, Plumb VJ. Diagnosis and treatment of arrhythmias during and following open heart surgery. Med Clin North Am 1984; 68:1153–1159.

Waldo AL, MacLean WA, Karp RB, et al. Continuous rapid atrial pacing to control recurrent or sustained supraventricular tachycardias following open heart surgery. Circulation 1976; 54:245–250.

Zeldis SM, Morganroth J, Horowitz LN, et al. Fascicular conduction disturbances after coronary artery bypass surgery. Am J Cardiol 1978; 41:860–864.

DIGITALIS INTOXICATION

PHILLIP A. KOREN, M.D.
LEONARD N. HOROWITZ, M.D.

Digitalis preparations have been used for more than 200 years to treat cardiac disorders. Their basic structure is an aglycone coupled with one to four sugar molecules. The quantity of sugar molecules affects the pharmacokinetics and, to a lesser degree, the potency of the drug. The smaller the number of sugar molecules, the more water-soluble and the shorter the half-life of the digitalis preparation. Digitoxin is more lipid-soluble and is metabolized in the liver. On the other hand, digoxin, being more water-soluble, is excreted by the kidneys, primarily in its unchanged form. Digoxin is less bound to plasma proteins and has a half-life of 1.7 days, whereas digitoxin has a half-life of 7 days, since it is bound to a large extent to protein. The volume of distribution of digitoxin and digoxin is extensive and is most concentrated in certain tissues, with the highest concentration in the kidneys, followed by the heart.

The kinetics of digoxin is altered in various situations. In infants and children, the binding to tissues is more extensive and the half-life is shorter. The opposite situation occurs in the elderly. Obesity does not affect digoxin pharmacokinetics. Renal failure significantly prolongs digoxin half-life, and the volume of distribution is smaller. Hepatic failure and pregnancy do not seem to alter digoxin pharmacokinetics. It has been reported that thyroid abnormalities alter serum digoxin concentrations as well.

PHARMACOLOGIC EFFECTS

In 1785, Withering first demonstrated that digitalis glycoside had a diuretic effect on his patients. It is thought that the digoxin increases the utilizable calcium available during excitation and contraction coupling, thus enhancing contractility. In addition, it enhances parasympathetic activity and decreases sympathetic activity. Digoxin has been shown to be a direct vasoconstrictor in human arteries and veins. Its electrophysiologic effects have been widely studied, and primarily the sinoatrial node, atrium, atrioventricular node, and accessory pathways are affected.

Digitalis preparations have been used for two primary purposes: the treatment of congestive heart failure and the treatment of supraventricular arrhythmias. The latter include paroxysmal supraventricular tachycardia, atrial fibrillation or flutter, multifocal atrial tachycardia, and tachycardias caused by bypass tracts.

Drug interactions are extensive and clinically relevant. Several drugs are known to change the serum digoxin levels. Cholestyramine, metoclopramide, sulfasalazine, neomycin, and certain chemotherapeutic drugs are known to decrease serum digoxin levels. More important, quinidine, quinine, amiodarone, verapamil, erythromycin, tetracycline, and probanthine increase serum digoxin levels.

DIGITALIS TOXICITY

The incidence of digitalis toxicity during the 1960s and 1970s has been shown in several series to range between 6 and 23 percent of hospitalized patients receiving the drug. Mortality rates as high as

41 percent have been observed in these patients. Manifestations of digitalis toxicity are both cardiac and noncardiac. The noncardiac symptoms and signs are nonspecific and are primarily gastrointestinal and neurologic. In as many as one-third of patients with digitalis toxicity, extracardiac symptoms may be present for weeks before cardiac symptoms appear.

Gastrointestinal symptoms include anorexia, vomiting, nausea, diarrhea, bloating, and abdominal cramps. Neurologic manifestations can be diverse. They range from fatigue and weakness to visual disturbances, which include a yellow-green-red haziness around objects. Also, foxglove frenzy (known as digitalis delirium), psychosis, and restlessness have all been associated with digitalis toxicity. Myriad skin lesions have been described, and painful gynecomastia can occur.

Factors that predispose the patient to digitalis toxicity must be recognized when a clinician starts a patient on this drug or when a patient on digitalis has new symptoms or signs. The elderly are more likely to have a higher risk for development of digitalis toxicity. Patients with certain cardiac disorders, typically amyloidosis, have been known to be more likely to develop rhythm disturbances. Renal failure alters the volume of distribution of digitalis preparations, and in the case of digoxin, which is cleared by the kidneys, a much smaller daily requirement may be necessary. Hypoxia and electrolyte disturbances, specifically hypokalemia, hypomagnesemia, and alkalosis; must be avoided in these patients because they predispose to the development of digitalis toxicity.

The toxic cardiac effects seen are clearly the most dangerous (Table 1). Practically all arrhythmias have been described with digoxin use. Wellens has suggested that "digitalis toxicity should be suspected when there is the appearance of a slow heart rate in patients with fast or normal heart rate, the appearance of a fast heart rate in a patient with a normal heart rate, the appearance of regular rhythm in a patient with an irregular rhythm, and the appearance of a regularly irregular rhythm."

Certain rhythms are highly suggestive of digitalis toxicity, for example, junctional tachycardia, paroxysmal atrial tachycardia with 2:1 atrioventricular conduction, bidirectional tachycardia, nonconducted atrial premature complexes, regularization of the ventricular response in atrial fibrillation, and ventricular tachycardia with exit block. The clinician must be able to recognize when the situation suggests digitalis toxicity. Certain rhythms are not suggestive of toxicity, and these include sinus tachycardia, multifocal atrial tachycardia, paroxysmal atrioventricular junctional tachycardia without atrioventricular block, atrial flutter or atrial fibrillation with rapid conduction, and Mobitz type II second-degree atrioventricular block.

Management of Digitalis Toxicity (Table 2)

Initial assessment of the patient with possible digitalis toxicity must include the determination of the arrhythmias and evaluation of the noncardiac manifestations. In general, patients require hospitalization and cardiac monitoring. For minor toxicity, which may include slow response to atrial fibrillation in an asymptomatic patient with an otherwise normal laboratory profile, the patient may be carefully followed outside a hospital setting. Discontinuation of digoxin for 24 to 48 hours or of digitoxin for 4 to 5 days may be an adequate treatment in these patients.

The patient should be assessed, including evaluation of electrolytes, renal and hepatic function, acid-base and oxygen status, and hemodynamic monitoring, including telemetry. The use of serum digoxin levels can be helpful in diagnosing and following toxicity. Levels should be obtained in a steady state or several hours after the last dose. The therapeutic window for inotropy is quite narrow, and there are no beneficial inotropic effects at levels higher than 2 mg per milliliter. It has been shown that levels above 3.0 mg per milliliter are more than 12 times more likely to produce toxicity. On the other hand, therapeutic levels do not exclude digoxin toxicity. Approximately 10 percent of patients with "therapeutic" levels of digoxin manifest cardiac digoxin toxicity. There is considerable overlap in drug levels and noncardiac symptoms as well. When the clinical situation strongly suggests digoxin toxicity, the presence of "therapeutic" levels does not exclude toxicity, especially in the setting of hypokalemia, hypomagnesemia, and acid-base disturbances. When managing a patient conservatively, measurement of daily digoxin or digitoxin levels may be helpful, along with clinical correlation of patient improvement.

For acute overdose situations, oral activated charcoal every 6 hours for approximately 24 hours should be used. Cholestyramine and cholestipol rapidly decrease the serum concentration by shortening the half-life of the drug.

Table 1 Arrhythmias Associated With Digitalis Intoxication

Sinoatrial exit block or arrest
Type I second-degree atrioventricular block
Third-degree atrioventricular block
Atrial fibrillation with slow ventricular rate
Accelerated junctional rhythms (nonparoxysmal)
Frequent ventricular premature complexes
Ventricular bigeminy and trigeminy
Ventricular tachycardia
Atrial tachycardia with atrioventricular block

Table 2 Therapy of Digitalis Toxicity

	Indication	Comments
Discontinue drug	All suspected patients	Observe in monitored setting
Electrolyte correction	Hypo-/hyperkalemia	Hypokalemia: best if corrected intravenously slowly over 4–8 hours
		Hyperkalemia: immediate treatment necessary with glucose, insulin, bicarbonate, potassium-binding resins, and dialysis, if necessary; poor prognostic sign
Lidocaine	Hemodynamically significant ventricular arrhythmias	Central nervous system toxicity is common, and suppression of rhythm may lead to asystole
Phenytoin	Hemodynamically significant ventricular arrhythmias	Suppression of rhythm may lead to asystole
Other antiarrhythmics	Refractory ventricular arrhythmias	Judicious selection necessary
Atropine	Hemodynamically significant bradycardia and heart block	Effect is short-lasting
Temporary pacemaker	Severe bradycardia and advanced heart block	External or right ventricular transvenous pacemaker.
		Clinical decision necessary; must weigh benefit/risk ratio
Digitalis-specific antibodies	Severe life-threatening toxicity	Rapid onset of action may precipitate hypokalemia, ?congestive heart failure
Cardioversion	Ventricular tachycardia/ventricular fibrillation	May precipitate asystole
		Begin with low energy and increase if necessary
Activated charcoal	Massive acute overdose	Decreases absorption, may clear digitalis preparation via enterohepatic circulation

Electrolyte and acid-base disturbances should be corrected. Potassium replacement is particularly important in suppressing ventricular tachycardia and ectopy, and atrial and atrioventricular tachycardia with block. Potassium replacement enhances sodium pump activity, which decreases intracellular calcium and secondary afterdepolarizations. It should not be given when serum levels are unknown or normal. Hyperkalemia may be an additive to digoxin toxicity by increasing resting membrane potentials and may potentiate digoxin's effect on the atrioventricular node. In patients with digitalis intoxication, potassium replacement may raise the electrolyte level to a higher than expected value owing to inhibition of the sodium-potassium pump. Intravenous magnesium may suppress digitalis-induced ventricular arrhythmias but may cause atrioventricular block and hypotension. Its use should be reserved.

Marked bradycardia, atrioventricular block, and sinoatrial block often respond to atropine administered intravenously. Repeated symptomatic episodes of bradycardia requiring atropine or unresponsiveness to atropine may necessitate the use of temporary pacing. In situations in which atrioventricular conduction is preserved, atrial pacing is preferable, since it avoids the risk of worsening ventricular arrhythmias caused by the presence of a pacemaker catheter in the ventricle. Overdrive pacemaking the rhythm should be avoided, as it occasionally can accelerate the tachycardia and worsen the situation.

The use of antiarrhythmic medications to treat various toxic rhythms can often be lifesaving. Phenytoin may be particularly helpful in treating ventricular arrhythmias, atrial tachycardia with block, and nonparoxysmal junctional tachycardia. The pharmacologic effects of phenytoin include suppression of digitalis-induced automaticity and delayed afterdepolarizations. In addition, it may reverse depression of sinoatrial and atrioventricular conduction. Phenytoin should be administered intravenously via slow infusion up to 15 mg per kilogram of body weight. Close monitoring of blood pressure is required, since hypotension is common.

Lidocaine may be particularly helpful in digitalis-induced ventricular ectopy to control toxic ectopic rhythms. Care must be taken that lidocaine does not abolish the ectopic rhythm and precipitate asystole. In general, class IA agents (procainamide, quinidine, disopyramide) should be avoided, since they may precipitate asystole by depression of atrioventricular and His-Purkinje conduction. Quinidine may displace digoxin from protein-binding sites and elevate serum levels. The newer antiarrhythmic drugs, such as mexiletine, propafenone, flecainide, and encainide, have not been evaluated in the treatment of digitalis toxicity and therefore should be avoided.

In this setting, amiodarone has been reported to control ventricular arrhythmias but may increase atrioventricular nodal block. In addition, it may also raise serum digoxin levels. Therefore, one should avoid this medication in patients with digitalis toxicity. Similarly, verapamil may worsen atrioventricular block but may suppress delayed afterdepolarizations and triggered activity. Because serum digoxin levels are further elevated with verapamil use, verapamil should be avoided in these patients.

Beta blockers may decrease automaticity and shorten the refractory periods of atrial, ventricular, and Purkinje fibers. They may, however, cause depression of sinoatrial and junctional pacemakers and atrioventricular conduction. In the presence of atrioventricular conduction abnormalities, bradycardia, and congestive heart failure, beta blockers should not be used.

Bedside maneuvers such as carotid sinus massage and the Valsalva maneuver should be avoided because they may precipitate asystole, ventricular arrhythmias, and advanced atrioventricular block.

In patients in whom cardioversion is considered for life-threatening arrhythmias, the risk of inducing serious arrhythmias should be recognized. Digoxin lowers the threshold for cardioversion-induced arrhythmias and may precipitate both malignant refractory ventricular arrhythmias and asystole. The mechanism may involve release of catecholamines from nerve endings and a change in potassium gradients, thus causing membrane instability. Energy requirements for cardioversion are reduced, and therefore lower energy should be used. Cardioversion should be reserved for patients with life-threatening arrhythmias that do not respond to pharmacologic approaches.

Hemodialysis and peritoneal dialysis have both been ineffective in removing digoxin and have no useful role in digoxin toxicity.

The development of digoxin-specific antibodies over the last 20 years has enabled clinicians to treat patients with toxic levels safely and rapidly. Isolation and purification of Fab antibody fragment from sheep gamma G immunoglobulin have made digoxin antibodies commercially available. Such antibodies have been tested in many centers and shown to be both safe and efficacious.

The use of digoxin antibodies is somewhat controversial. Cost analysis has shown that rapid digoxin reversal is in fact cost effective, reducing both the length and the cost of the hospital stay. At present, indications for their use include severe life-threatening arrhythmias (both brady- and tachyarrhythmias), digoxin-induced hyperkalemia, and overdoses with severely elevated levels (>10 to 15 mg per milliliter).

Although digoxin antibodies are approved for digoxin toxicity, they are effective in treating digitoxin toxicity as well. The drug is administered intravenously over a 15- to 30-minute period. The dosage of digoxin antibodies with steady-state digoxin levels in milligrams is

$$\text{serum digoxin concentration} \times 5.6 \text{ L/kg} \times \text{weight (kg)} \times 60/1000$$

In patients with toxic digitoxin levels, the above formula is altered by substituting 0.56 as the mean volume of distribution. Each vial contains 40 mg of digoxin-specific Fab fragments, which will bind approximately 0.6 mg of digoxin. Dosages required are quite varied. Patients who have attempted suicide or accidentally taken overdoses may need larger amounts than patients in whom toxicity occurs while they are taking prescribed dosages of digitalis preparations.

In general, the onset of action of digoxin antibodies is rapid, and those patients who respond do so within 30 minutes. In severely toxic patients, serum potassium levels are varied. A low serum potassium level is associated with more frequent digitalis-induced arrhythmias. On the other hand, hyperkalemia often occurs as a result of severe intoxication. The mechanism involves severe inhibition of the sodium-potassium adenosine triphosphatase. After treatment with digoxin antibodies, potassium levels usually normalize and in some cases drop to below normal levels.

Side effects of digoxin antibodies are minimal. There may be a loss of inotropic support provided by the digitalis preparation, and as mentioned earlier, hypokalemia may occur. The elimination of the digoxin-Fab complex occurs slowly, with a half-life of 16 to 20 hours. Renal dysfunction may prolong the drug's half-life.

SUGGESTED READING

Braunwald E. Heart Disease: A textbook of cardiovascular medicine. Philadelphia: W.B. Saunders, 1984:504.

Wenger TL, Butler VP, Haber E. Treatment of 63 severely digitalis-toxic patients with digoxin specific antibody fragments. J Am Coll Cardiol 1985; 5(5):118A–123A.

PROARRHYTHMIA

HARRY A. KOPELMAN, M.D.

Although the phenomenon of proarrhythmia has been appreciated for well over 100 years; its full clinical impact has become apparent only recently. As physicians, our ability to uncover clinically relevant arrhythmias requiring antiarrhythmic drug therapy has never been greater. Therefore, it stands to reason that the likelihood of discovering proarrhythmic events has never been greater than at the present time. The recent proliferation of antiarrhythmic drugs and the development of methods by which therapy may be guided have only increased the complexity of this clinical dilemma.

By definition, proarrhythmia is either the aggravation or provocation of arrhythmias. In the broadest sense, this refers to bradyarrhythmias, supraventricular tachyarrhythmias, and ventricular tachyarrhythmias. It implies one of the following three events in the presence of antiarrhythmic drugs: (1) the occurrence of a new arrhythmia not previously observed, (2) a previously unsustained arrhythmia becomes sustained or incessant, and (3) a previously well-tolerated arrhythmia becomes associated with hemodynamic compromise. In summary, proarrhythmia refers to that aspect of antiarrhythmic drugs that can worsen native arrhythmias or induce arrhythmias not previously seen. This chapter deals specifically with the recognition and management of proarrhythmic responses to drug therapy.

APPROACH TO THE PATIENT WITH SUSPECTED PROARRHYTHMIA

The key to appropriate management of the patient with proarrhythmia is recognition that an antiarrhythmic drug is in fact playing a provocative role. *All* antiarrhythmic drugs have this potential. Fortunately, in most cases, there are characteristics of proarrhythmia that are diagnostic.

The various forms of proarrhythmia that may be observed are listed in Table 1. These are best classified according to arrhythmia rate and predominant site of origin within the myocardium.

Bradyarrhythmias

Antiarrhythmic drug-induced sinus bradycardia is fairly common and may be loosely classified as a proarrhythmic response. This may occur from overdose of antiarrhythmic drugs, such as beta blockers, in the absence of abnormalities of impulse generation (automaticity) and conduction (exit block).

Alternatively, it may occur in the setting of therapeutic plasma concentrations of class I antiarrhythmic drugs such as quinidine if underlying sinus node dysfunction exists. The tendency of class I antiarrhythmic drugs to cause an asystolic event or marked sinus bradycardia following conversion from atrial fibrillation is well known. Therefore, as a minimal precaution, it makes good clinical sense to initiate antiarrhythmic drug therapy for patients with known sinus node dysfunction (sick sinus syndrome) while they are being monitored.

Beta-adrenergic blocking drugs, calcium channel antagonists, and digitalis may cause prolongation of atrioventricular nodal refractoriness and conduction delay. Patients with a prolonged P-R interval and perhaps with second-degree atrioventricular block during sleep (or at other times when hypervagotonia occurs) may develop severe atrioventricular block during treatment. Of greater concern are patients with significant His-Purkinje system dysfunction in the setting of extensive underlying organic heart disease who require treatment with class I antiarrhythmic drugs. Class IA (disopyramide, procainamide, quinidine) and class IC (encainide, flecainide) antiarrhythmic drugs have the greatest propensity to cause aggravation of His-Purkinje system disease. These drugs significantly prolong the

Table 1 Nomenclature of Proarrhythmic Responses

Drug-Induced Bradyarrhythmias
  Sinus bradyarrhythmias (abnormal automaticity, exit block)
  Atrioventricular conduction disturbances
  Accelerated idioventricular rhythm
Drug-Induced Tachyarrhythmias
  Supraventricular
    Atrial tachycardia with block
    Nonparoxysmal atrioventricular junctional tachycardia
    Incessant supraventricular tachycardia
      Automatic
      Reentrant
  Ventricular
    Increased frequency of spontaneous ventricular ectopy
      Fourfold increase in frequency of premature ventricular complexes
      Tenfold increase in repetitive forms
    Bidirectional ventricular tachycardia
    Prolonged Q-T interval with torsades de pointes polymorphic ventricular tachycardia
    Spontaneous sustained monomorphic ventricular tachycardia
    Response at electrophysiologic study
      Conversion of unsustained to sustained ventricular tachycardia
      Hemodynamically unstable ventricular tachycardia as the result of faster rate and/or negative inotropic drug effect
      Induction of ventricular tachycardia with a less aggressive stimulation mode
      Spontaneous ventricular tachycardia following intraveous administration of antiarrhythmic drug
  Ventricular fibrillation
  Proarrhythmia associated with class IC antiarrhythmic drugs

HV interval; the class IC agents potentially cause the greatest degree of impairment. Prolongation of intra-ventricular conduction is routinely observed with the class I antiarrhythmic drugs, in with particular class IC agents, and does not constitute a proar-rhythmic drug effect.

For proarrhythmia of the bradycardic type, dis-continuation of the antiarrhythmic drug is the treat-ment of choice. Infrequently, temporary or even per-manent pacemaker back-up is required, in particular if the drug is necessary for control of a symptomatic tachyarrhythmia.

Supraventricular Tachyarrhythmias

The most commonly observed supraventricular tachyarrhythmias that occur as the result of antiar-rhythmic drug therapy are associated with digitalis. Paroxysmal atrial tachycardia with block and non-paroxysmal atrioventricular junctional tachycardia are so characteristic of digitalis toxicity that they are virtually diagnostic. The diagnosis is confirmed by the attendant clinical and chemical manifestations of digitalis toxicity.

The treatment of choice for these arrhythmias is discontinuation of digitalis and repletion of electro-lytes, including potassium and magnesium, which may be contributing to the arrhythmia. If these elec-trolyte disturbances coexist, plasma digitalis concen-tration may be found to be within the therapeutic range. The interaction between digitalis and other antiarrhythmic drugs (amiodarone, quinidine, vera-pamil) may also play a clinically relevant role. Rec-ognition of digitalis-toxic supraventricular arrhyth-mias and the contributing factors is key to their management, as further addition of digitalis or at-tempted cardioversion (which may be complicated by ventricular fibrillation) may exacerbate the prob-lem. Antiarrhythmic drugs that increase serum digi-talis concentration or augment its action should also be withheld.

The class I antiarrhythmic drugs are also asso-ciated with supraventricular proarrhythmia, particu-larly in the setting of arrhythmic substrates such as ectopic atrial tachycardia and atrioventricular reen-trant tachycardia. The mechanism in these cases probably relates to marked changes in automaticity or slowing of conduction within the reentrant circuit without a significant change in refractoriness. In the majority of these cases, the cycle length of the ar-rhythmia is significantly slower. However, the ar-rhythmia may be more frequent, even incessant, and unresponsive to pace termination or electrical car-dioversion. These findings in general are most char-acteristics of class IC antiarrhythmic drug-related proarrhythmias. Under these circumstances, the treatment of choice is removal of the inciting agent and close observation.

Ventricular Arrhythmias

The most clinically relevant and common form of proarrhythmia involves provocation or aggrava-tion of ventricular arrhythmias. Ventricular proar-rhythmias vary on the basis of antiarrhythmic drug, characteristics of the arrhythmia, and specific treat-ment.

Increased Frequency of Spontaneous Ventricular Ectopy

It has been proposed that a fourfold increase in the frequency of premature ventricular complexes and a tenfold increase in repetitive forms should be considered criteria for identifying proarrhythmia by ambulatory electrocardiographic monitoring. Using these criteria, proarrhythmic responses to antiar-rhythmic therapy have been estimated to occur in up to 5 to 15 percent of antiarrhythmic drug trials and in 20 to 35 percent of patients treated. The sensitiv-ity, specificity, and predictive value of these observa-tions require further study. Clearly, they do not carry the same clinical significance as the malignant ven-tricular arrhythmias to be discussed.

Digitalis-Related Ventricular Proarrhythmia

The classic occurrence of bidirectional ventricu-lar tachycardia is diagnostic of digitalis toxicity. It occurs infrequently. The characteristic arrhythmia is relatively slow, with rates between 150 and 200 beats per minute, with QRS complex polarity alternating on a beat-to-beat basis.

The specific treatment for this arrhythmia is the same as other supraventricular tachyarrhythmias as-sociated with digitalis. In addition, intravenous phe-nytoin administered slowly may be a specific and useful treatment for this arrhythmia. Electrical car-dioversion is contraindicated because of the risk of ventricular fibrillation complicating digitalis toxic-ity. Digitalis antibody therapy has clinical applicabil-ity only in rare cases and is typically reserved for massive digitalis overdose.

Proarrhythmia Related to the Acquired Long Q-T Interval Syndrome — Polymorphic Ventricular Tachycardia

Acquired torsades de pointes (polymorphic ven-tricular tachycardia) typically occurs in the setting of a long Q-T interval as the result of recent initiation of class IA antiarrhythmic drug therapy. It has been documented to be the cause of quinidine syncope. It has also been reported with class III antiarrhythmic drugs (amiodarone and bretylium). The arrhythmia has a characteristic initiation pattern and morphol-ogy (Fig. 1). Typically, a preinitiation sequence occurs, followed by a prolonged pause with subse-

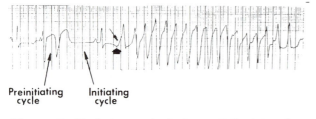

Preinitiating cycle   Initiating cycle

Figure 1 Typical acquired long Q-T interval—polymorphic ventricular tachycardia.

quent Q-T interval prolongation and an initiating premature ventricular complex that originates at the end of the T wave. The resultant polymorphic ventricular tachycardia occurs in an undulating pattern with the QRS complex "twisting" about the isoelectric baseline. The rate of tachycardia is typically between 200 and 250 beats per minute, significantly slower than ventricular fibrillation. A Q-T interval in excess of 600 msec and bizarre repolarization changes during sinus rhythm are part of the syndrome. This arrhythmia tends to occur in a bradycardia-dependent "triggered" fashion. Contributing factors are frequently present, including beta-adrenergic blocking drugs, digitalis, hypokalemia, and hypomagnesemia. Another frequent feature of this arrhythmia is self-termination, although on occasion it may culminate in ventricular fibrillation.

Pharmacogenetic factors may also contribute to this arrhythmia. A specific example of this is N-acetyl procainamide, the active metabolite of procainamide that primarily affects ventricular repolarization. In patients who are "rapid acetylators" of procainamide, N-acetyl procainamide may reach concentrations that are antiarrhythmic and in some cases proarrhythmic, especially in the presence of renal dysfunction. This usually occurs with plasma concentrations in excess of 30 μg per milliliter.

The treatment of choice for torsades de pointes is removal of the culprit antiarrhythmic drug. In addition, aggressive repletion of potassium clearly is of benefit. Recently, magnesium sulfate administered by slow intravenous infusion has been demonstrated to be remarkably effective.

The mainstay of therapy for antiarrhythmic drug-related long Q-T syndrome has been the administration of isoproterenol infusion and/or temporary atrial or ventricular pacing. The resultant increase in heart rate and regularization of the R-R interval decrease dispersion of ventricular refractoriness, which appears to be responsible for this arrhythmia. Maintenance of heart rates in excess of 70 beats per minute while washout of the antiarrhythmic drug occurs is usually effective in the prevention of recurrence. Intracardiac electrophysiologic studies have been found to be of little value in inducing torsades de pointes, whether it is acquired or congenital.

In the absence of significant organic heart disease, acquired long Q-T syndrome is associated with an excellent prognosis. However, many patients who have a proarrhythmic response of this sort also have significant preexisting underlying organic heart disease.

Whether or not cross-reactivity within the same class of antiarrhythmic drug occurs remains controversial. In general, other class I antiarrhythmic drugs may be safely initiated for the initial indication that resulted in torsades de pointes. However, it is recommended that these patients be closely monitored; if significant prolongation of the corrected Q-T interval occurs (in excess of 500 msec), the antiarrhythmic drug should be discontinued.

Sustained Monomorphic Ventricular Tachycardia

Proarrhythmia of this type may occur as new-onset sustained ventricular tachycardia, such as in the patient with unsustained ventricular tachycardia that becomes sustained, or it may present as hemodynamically unstable ventricular tachycardia attributable to shorter cycle length or worsening ventricular function. The incidence of this type of proarrhythmia is in the range of 5 to 15 percent. It has been reported with class IA, IB, IC, and III antiarrhythmic drugs. Patients at highest risk for this complication include those with depressed left ventricular function in the setting of significant coronary artery disease or cardiomyopathy and a history of malignant ventricular arrhythmias, sustained ventricular tachycardia, or ventricular fibrillation (Table 2).

Conventional wisdom suggests that sustained monomorphic ventricular tachycardia as a complication of antiarrhythmic drug therapy occurs soon after the initiation of the drug, typically within 5 days. However, with the availability of some of the newer antiarrhythmic drugs with longer elimination half-lives (amiodarone, encainide, flecainide), many of which have important active metabolites, this complication may occur weeks or even months after the initiation of therapy.

At times this type of proarrhythmia may be difficult to diagnose because of its somewhat capricious and unpredictable nature. Therefore, the most reasonable management approach is to remove the antiarrhythmic drug, which is clearly ineffective, cor-

Table 2 Risk Factors for the Development of Ventricular Proarrhythmia

Malignant ventricular arrhythmias on presentation
Organic heart disease (significant left ventricular dysfunction)
Clinical congestive heart failure (requiring digitalis and diuretics)
Concomitant electrolyte imbalance
High doses of class IC antiarrhythmic drugs

rect any potential contributing factors such as ischemia, congestive heart failure, or electrolyte imbalance, and identify an effective antiarrhythmic drug, surgical, or device therapy, as required. Intracardiac electrophysiologic studies are clearly indicated in circumstances in which a malignant ventricular arrhythmia is documented, even if it is uncertain whether or not a proarrhythmic event has occurred. Programmed ventricular stimulation better defines the pathophysiologic-anatomic substrate responsible, determines the risk of recurrent sustained ventricular tachyarrhythmias, and if necessary guides selection of appropriate antiarrhythmic therapy.

It has been suggested that the proarrhythmic effects of antiarrhythmic drugs in patients with malignant ventricular arrhythmias may be prospectively evaluated invasively with intracardiac electrophysiologic testing. Several endpoints have been used as criteria for proarrhythmia, as shown in Table 1. Of these, conversion of unsustained to sustained ventricular tachycardia and hemodynamically unstable ventricular tachycardia as the result of faster rate and/or negative inotropic drug effect appear to have the most clinical relevance, occurring in 5 to 20 percent of studies. Although induction of ventricular tachycardia with a less aggressive stimulation mode occurs more frequently, it is unclear whether or not this represents proarrhythmia or just variability of the test on a day-to-day basis. Spontaneous ventricular tachycardia following intravenous administration of antiarrhythmic drugs occurs infrequently, in less than 1 percent of studies, and reflects clear-cut proarrhythmic response to intravenous antiarrhythmic therapy administered during the intracardiac electrophysiologic study. Since any of these criteria are clearly unsatisfactory end points at serial electrophysiologic drug testing, it is appropriate to discontinue the drug. It remains unclear, at present, whether or not such testing will be predictive of clinical proarrhythmia.

Proarrhythmia Culminating in Cardiac Arrest

Fortunately, ventricular fibrillation as a result of antiarrhythmic drug therapy is an infrequent event, occurring in 4 to 5 percent of patients in whom antiarrhythmic drug therapy is initiated for malignant ventricular arrhythmias. Predictors of which patients are prone to this complication include the presence of depressed left ventricular function, congestive heart failure (requiring digitalis and diuretic therapy), and a history of sustained ventricular tachycardia or ventricular fibrillation (see Table 2). Drug-associated ventricular fibrillation tends to be an early event, and there may be an increased risk of its recurrence with subsequent antiarrhythmic drug trials.

As with sustained monomorphic ventricular tachycardia, intracardiac electrophysiologic studies are recommended in such patients. Noninducibility in the setting of a "remediable cause" such as a proarrhythmic drug response is associated with an acceptable 1-year survival from sudden cardiac death. Management then includes removal of the inciting medication and correction of the hemodynamic and metabolic parameters previously noted.

Proarrhythmia Associated with Class IC Antiarrhythmic Drugs

Proarrhythmia caused by class IC antiarrhythmic drugs (encainide and flecainide) is characteristically incessant. It usually occurs in patients with a history of spontaneous sustained ventricular tachycardia and depressed left ventricular function. In general, it tends to occur early after starting the medication or increasing the dose, particularly if it has been increased rapidly (see Table 2). This arrhythmia is characteristically slow and sinusoidal in morphology, with a wide QRS complex (Fig. 2). It recommences immediately after pace termination. In addition, it does not respond to electrical cardioversion and/or may resume immediately after delivery of the electrical shock or after a few sinus beats. In many cases, these patients develop associated congestive heart failure and/or cardiogenic shock.

Supportive care, including correction of electrolyte imbalance (specifically potassium repletion), administration of intravenous magnesium sulfate, protection of the airway (elective and/or emergent endotracheal intubation with ventilatory support), and hemodynamic support (cardioactive pressors, intraaortic balloon pump), may be necessary to reverse the toxic drug effects, allow for washout from the myocardium, and stabilize the patient. In general, administration of intravenous lidocaine is ineffective. Intravenous amiodarone may be effective under some circumstances but is not approved at present by the Food and Drug Administration for these indications. Preliminary experimental studies have suggested that the administration of hypertonic saline may reverse the effect of these antiarrhythmic drugs or isoproterenol, but clinical efficacy of such treatment remains controversial.

Although the proarrhythmic potential of class IC drugs in patients with malignant ventricular arrhythmias has long been appreciated, of great concern is the same potential they may have in patients with asymptomatic or mildly symptomatic ventricular arrhythmias after myocardial infarction. The Cardiac Arrhythmia Suppression Trial (CAST), a multicenter, placebo-controlled study, was designed to test whether or not suppression of asymptomatic or mildly symptomatic ventricular arrhythmias after myocardial infarction was associated with a reduced mortality rate. The study was discontinued prema-

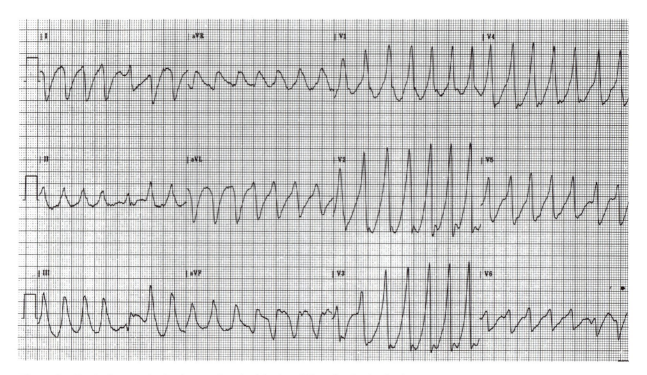

Figure 2 Typical proarrhythmia associated with class IC antiarrhythmic drugs.

turely for both encainide and flecainide once it was determined that treatment with these antiarrhythmic medications was associated with a substantial increase in sudden death rate and total mortality. These findings were remarkable in that they were observed across all patient subgroups and existed despite the effective suppression of spontaneous ventricular premature complexes by these agents. Although it is not entirely clear, the outcome is best explained as the result of provocation of malignant ventricular arrhythmias. Whereas previous uncontrolled studies suggested that patients like those entered in CAST without a history of sustained ventricular arrhythmias were at extremely low risk of ventricular arrhythmias caused by class IC drugs, this widely held view is no longer acceptable. In addition, the survival analysis in CAST demonstrated that an excess rate of sudden death persisted throughout the 10-month follow-up period among patients treated with encainide and flecainide. This observation challenges conventional wisdom, the long-held assumption that patients are susceptible to

drug-induced arrhythmias only in the early period of drug exposure. The mechanism by which these drugs increase the risk of sudden death and total mortality in this population remains unclear.

SUGGESTED READING

Minardo JD, Heger JJ, Miles WM, et al. Clinical characteristics of patients with ventricular fibrillation during antiarrhythmic drug therapy. N Engl J Med 1988; 319:257–262.

Nguyen PT, Scheinman MM, Seger J. Polymorphous ventricular tachycardia: Clinical characterization, therapy, and the QT interval. Circulation 1986; 74:340–349.

Podrid PJ, Lampert S, Graboys TB, et al. Aggravation of arrhythmia by antiarrhythmic drugs—incidence and predictors. Am J Cardiol 1989; 59:38E–44E.

Rae AP, Kay HR, Horowitz LN, et al. Proarrhythmic effects of antiarrhythmic drugs in patients with malignant ventricular arrhythmias evaluated by electrophysiologic testing. J Am Coll Cardiol 1988; 12:131–139.

Special Report: Effect of encainide and flecainide on mortality in a randomized trial of arrhythmia suppression after myocardial infarction. N Engl J Med 1989; 321:406–412.

VIII PHARMACOLOGIC MANAGEMENT

ADENOSINE TRIPHOSPHATE AND ADENOSINE

BERNARD BELHASSEN, M.D.

Adenosine triphosphate (ATP) and its related nucleoside adenosine play an important role in the physiologic regulation of cardiac function, particularly coronary blood flow and myocardial contractility. In addition, these agents have been known for many years for their potent cardiac electrophysiologic effects. These include a negative chronotropic action on the sinus node, junctional pacemaker, and ventricular escape rhythm as well as a negative dromotropic action on the atrioventricular (AV) node. The latter property has mainly led to the use of ATP and adenosine as antiarrhythmic agents for the acute management of paroxysmal supraventricular tachycardia (PSVT) caused by a reentrant mechanism involving the AV node. The AV nodal depressant effects of adenosine compounds have also been used for determining the actual mechanism of supraventricular tachyarrhythmias and for differentiating supraventricular tachyarrhythmias with aberrant conduction from ventricular tachycardia. More recently, adenosine compounds have been found to be effective in the treatment of a specific type of ventricular tachycardia. The clinical use of ATP and adenosine in the management of supraventricular and ventricular tachyarrhythmias is reviewed here.

ACUTE MANAGEMENT OF SUPRAVENTRICULAR TACHYCARDIA

Clinical Pharmacology of ATP and Adenosine

The effects of ATP and adenosine are dose-dependent, maximal after 10 to 30 seconds, and short-lasting; they disappear within 1 minute following drug administration. In humans, the effects of ATP are believed to depend mainly on its conversion to adenosine and to a lesser extent to a vagal reflex. The transient effects of adenosine and ATP are due to the very short half-life of adenosine (less than 10 seconds), which is quickly degraded to the electrophysiologically inactive inosine. When quickly administered intravenously, ATP and adenosine exert marked depressant effects on the AV node without affecting infranodal conduction. Conduction over accessory pathways is generally not affected by these drugs.

Despite the fact that ATP and adenosine are potent vasodilators, they do not usually decrease blood pressure at clinical doses effective for terminating PSVT. On the contrary, blood pressure typically increases upon termination of PSVT (Fig. 1). Should a decrease in blood pressure occur, it would be minimal, very brief, and thus not clinically significant. We have given ATP to many patients with hemodynamically poorly tolerated supraventricular tachycardia without any harmful effects.

Clinical Efficacy of ATP and Adenosine

The largest clinical experience with ATP has been acquired in Europe for the past 20 years, whereas that with adenosine has been acquired in both Europe and the United States for the last 7 years. Both agents have been found to terminate successfully 90 to 100 percent of episodes of AV junctional reentrant PSVT, both in adult and pediatric patients (see the chapter *Paroxysmal Reentrant Supraventricular Tachycardia Without Preexcitation: Pharmacologic Therapy*). In these patients, termination of PSVT with adenosine compounds is almost always related to conduction block in the antegrade slow pathway in patients with AV nodal reentrant tachycardia of the slow-fast type and to a block in the AV node in patients with orthodromic AV reentrant tachycardia involving an accessory pathway (Figs. 1 through 3). Termination of PSVT resulting from block in an accessory pathway has been observed in the rare cases of PSVT involving a retrogradely conducting accessory pathway with decremental AV nodal-like properties. Termination of PSVT is occasionally caused by premature atrial or

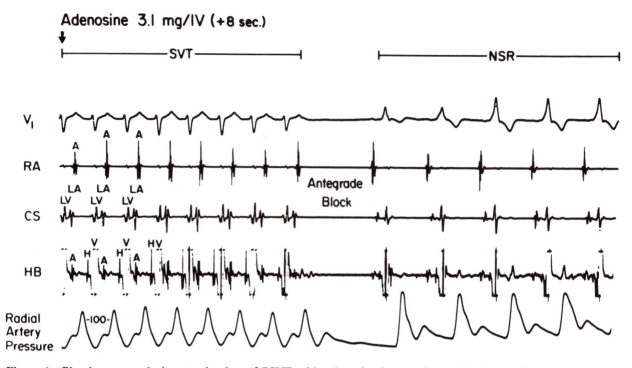

Figure 1 Blood pressure during termination of PSVT with adenosine in a patient with the Wolff-Parkinson-White syndrome. Shown are electrocardiographic lead V_1 and intracardiac recordings from the right atrium (RA), the coronary sinus (CS) showing a left atrial (LA) electrogram, and the region of the His bundle (HB). The radial artery pressure is shown in the bottom tracing. Adenosine, 75 μg per kilogram, produces antegrade block in the AV node that terminates the tachycardia and restores sinus rhythm with varying degrees of preexcitation. Radial artery pressure, which has been constant at 118/66 mm Hg during the tachycardia, increases to 140/82 mm Hg when sinus rhythm is restored. (Reprinted from DiMarco JP, Sellers TD, Berne RM, Adenosine: Electrophysiologic effects and therapeutic use for terminating paroxysmal supraventricular tachycardia. Circulation 1983; 68:1254–1263, with permission from the author and the American Heart Association.)

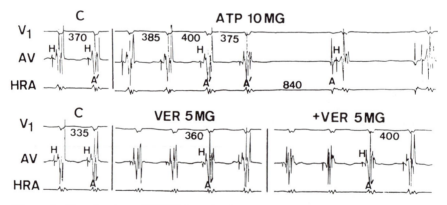

Figure 2 Termination of PSVT by ATP but not verapamil in a patient with AV nodal reentry. Shown are electrocardiographic lead V_1 and intracardiac electrograms from the atrioventricular junction (AV) and high right atrium (HRA). ATP (10 mg) terminates PSVT 25 seconds after administration owing to block in the slow antegrade AV nodal pathway following cycle length alternans (A'H alternans). In contrast, PSVT is slowed but not terminated by 5 mg of verapamil (VER) or an additional dose of 5 mg verapamil. C = control. (Reprinted from Belhassen B, Glick A, Laniado S. Comparative clinical and electrophysiologic effects of adenosine triphosphate and verapamil or paroxysmal reciprocating junctional tachycardia. Circulation 1988; 77:795–805; with permission from the American Heart Association.)

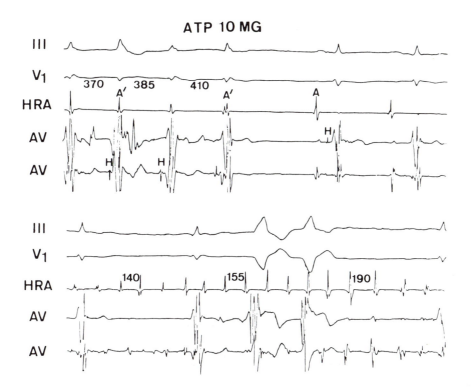

Figure 3 Termination of PSVT and occurrence of atrial fibrillation after administration of ATP in a patient with AV nodal reentry tachycardia. Shown are electrocardiographic leads III and V_1 and intracardiac electrograms from the high right atrium (HRA) and atrioventricular junction (AV). Tracings from upper and lower panels are continuous. Twenty-one seconds after administration of 10 mg ATP, PSVT terminates owing to block in the antegrade slow nodal pathway after progressive prolongation of the A′H interval. Two seconds after conversion to sinus rhythm, atrial fibrillation occurs. Normal sinus rhythm resumed 72 seconds later (not shown). Note two wide QRS complexes during atrial fibrillation that probably have a ventricular origin. (Reprinted from Belhassen B, Glick A, Laniado S. Comparative clinical and electrophysiologic effects of adenosine triphosphate and verapamil on paroxysmal reciprocating junctional tachycardia. Circulation 1988; 77:795–805; with permission from the American Heart Association.)

ventricular complexes, which are frequently triggered by these drugs (Fig. 4).

Termination of PSVT almost always occurs within 30 seconds following drug injection, depending on the rate and route of administration. A very rapid rate of injection (less than 2 sec) is mandatory for achieving a negative dromotropic effect on the AV node and termination of PSVT. Conversely, slower injection rates may paradoxically transiently increase the PSVT rate because of reflex response following systemic vasodilation caused by adenosine compounds that is unbalanced by their negative AV nodal dromotropic effects. In addition, an injection of the drugs through a central vein results in a more frequent and quicker termination of PSVT than after drug injection through a peripheral vein, probably because of the rapid intravascular degradation of adenosine.

Dosage and Administration of ATP and Adenosine

As pointed out above, the rate and route of drug administration are critical for achieving successful conversion of PSVT. The drugs should be injected

very quickly, in less than 1 to 2 sec through a large antecubital vein. Flushing with 5 to 10 ml of saline solution is recommended although not mandatory.

Because of the different molecular weights of ATP and adenosine (551 versus 267), the posology of the two drugs should be different. The following recommended posology applies to adults or adolescents. For ATP, I start with a dose of 5 mg; if patients fail to respond, I give increasing doses in 2.5- to 5-mg increments at 1-minute intervals until conversion of PSVT is obtained. Worldwide experience has shown that in the great majority of patients, tachycardias are terminated with doses of 10 mg or less. Only 10 to 20 percent of patients require doses higher than 10 mg. For adenosine, the starting dose is 2.5 mg; increasing doses of 2.5-mg increments are given if patients fail to respond. Most episodes of PSVT are terminated by doses of 5 to 10 mg of adenosine.

In pediatric patients, doses of ATP and adenosine should be adapted to the patient's body weight. The recommended starting and incremental doses are 80 μg per kilogram and 40 μg per kilogram for ATP and adenosine, respectively.

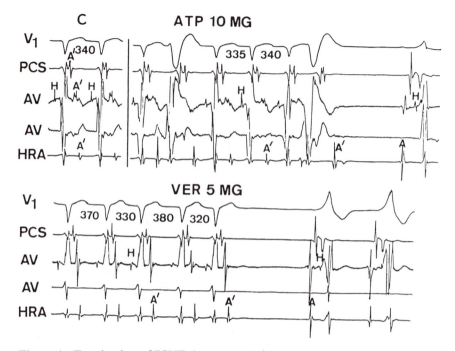

Figure 4 Termination of PSVT due to a ventricular premature complex triggered by ATP in a patient with the Wolff-Parkinson-White syndrome. Shown are electrocardiographic lead V_1 intracardiac recordings from the proximal coronary sinus (PCS), the atrioventricular junction (AV), and the high right atrium (HRA). Administration of 10 mg ATP results in termination of PSVT 24 seconds after drug administration owing to a ventricular premature complex followed by retrograde atrial activation over the accessory pathway. Another ventricular premature complex that occurs a few beats before but has a lesser degree of prematurity does not affect the tachycardia. Note that during a 5-minute control period of PSVT, no arrhythmias were observed. In the bottom panel, termination of tachycardia with 5 mg verapamil is shown in the same patient. Note that tachycardia terminates owing to AV nodal block following cycle length alternans, without any ventricular arrhythmias.

Administration of ATP and adenosine should always be performed under continuous electrocardiographic monitoring. Prior to drug injection, the patients should be informed about the possibility and nature of side effects (see further on) and their transient character.

Side Effects of ATP and Adenosine

The administration of ATP and adenosine has been associated with various cardiac and noncardiac side effects. As expected from the pharmacokinetics of the drugs, these side effects are always transient, reach a maximum within approximately 30 seconds, and completely disappear within 1 to 2 minutes. The side effects are dose-dependent and vary from patient to patient for a given drug dose.

The common cardiac side effects include sinus bradycardia, sinus arrest, and various degrees of AV nodal block. Because of their short-lasting character (less than a few seconds), the resulting bradycardias are usually well tolerated and do not require any intervention. Atrial and ventricular premature complexes are also frequently observed at the time or within the first minute following PSVT termination (see Fig. 4). These arrhythmias almost always have a benign course. Occasionally, however, they may be the source of atrial fibrillation (usually unsustained) (see Fig. 3), recurrent PSVT, or unsustained ventricular tachycardia (Fig. 5). Significantly, despite the potential ability of adenosine compounds to induce various types of brady- and tachyarrhythmias, I am not aware of a single case of death or severe permanent cardiac complication following administration of adenosine compounds in any clinical setting, even in critically ill patients with congestive heart failure, hypotension, or acute myocardial infarction.

Noncardiac side effects are frequent and mostly include flushing, malaise, headache, and hyperpnea. Cough, nausea, and chest pains are observed less commonly. Very rare cases of bronchospasm related to the bronchoconstrictive effects of the drugs have been reported in predisposed patients.

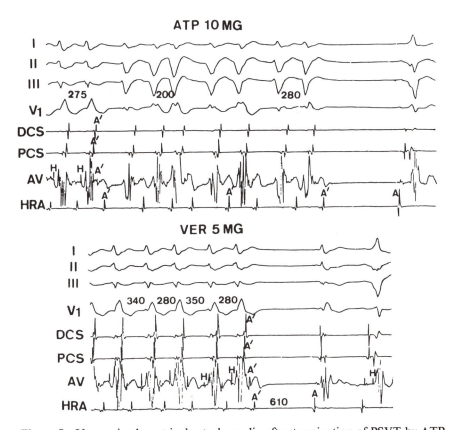

Figure 5 Unsustained ventricular tachycardia after termination of PSVT by ATP but not verapamil in a patient with the Wolff-Parkinson-White syndrome. Shown are electrocardiographic leads I, II, III, and V_1 and intracardiac electrograms from the distal coronary sinus (DCS), proximal coronary sinus (PCS), atrioventricular junction (AV), and high right atrium (HRA). PSVT terminates 18 seconds after administration of 10 mg ATP owing to AV nodal block. Immediately after conversion, unsustained irregular ventricular tachycardia (seven beats) with 1:1 retrograde conduction over the accessory pathway is observed. In contrast, 5 mg verapamil (VER) terminates PSVT 30 seconds after administration owing to AV nodal block following cycle length alternans but with no ventricular arrhythmia. (Reprinted from Belhassen B, Glick A, Laniado S. Comparative clinical and electrophysiologic effects of adenosine triphosphate and verapamil on paroxysmal reciprocating junctional tachycardia. Circulation 1988; 77:795–805; with permission from the American Heart Association.)

Contraindications and Precautions

Because of their very short half-lives, contraindications for the use of ATP or adenosine are rare. An absolute contraindication should be a previously documented history of bronchial asthma. Advanced age, hypertension, chronic obstructive lung disease, acute myocardial ischemia or infarction, a previous history of sick sinus syndrome, and atrial fibrillation or ventricular tachyarrhythmias are not contraindications to treatment, although special caution is justified in these instances. Patients with PSVT complicating the Wolff-Parkinson-White syndrome should also be closely observed, since adenosine compounds not infrequently induce atrial fibrillation, which could have potential severe consequences in case the accessory pathway has a very short refractory period. However, I am not aware of any

reported case of atrial fibrillation–triggered life-threatening tachyarrhythmias in patients with pre-excitation syndromes and PSVT treated with adenosine compounds. A possible explanation for this finding could be that atrial fibrillation induced by adenosine compounds is usually of short duration (see Fig. 3).

The following drugs that affect adenosine metabolism have been shown in experimental settings to potentiate the effects of ATP and adenosine: dipyridamole, cardiac glycosides, verapamil, and benzodiazepines. Therefore, I recommend reducing starting doses of ATP or adenosine in patients pretreated with these drugs, especially in those pretreated with dipyridamole, which is a potent inhibitor of adenosine metabolism. Aminophylline and other methylxanthines, on the other hand, antagonize the effects of adenosine, and therefore high doses of ATP or adenosine could be required for terminating PSVT in patients pretreated with these adenosine antagonists.

THE DRUG OF CHOICE FOR PSVT: ATP, ADENOSINE, VERAPAMIL?

Among the many other antiarrhythmic agents that have been shown to be effective in the management of acute AV junctional reentrant PSVT, the agent most utilized worldwide is verapamil (see the chapters *Paroxysmal Reentrant Supraventricular Tachycardia Without Preexcitation: Pharmacologic Therapy* and *Calcium Antagonists*). This drug effectively terminates about 90 percent of episodes of PSVT, in both adult and pediatric patients. Although verapamil is slightly less effective (see Fig. 2) and less rapid than ATP or adenosine for converting PSVT, it has several important advantages over ATP and adenosine: (1) its use is well known by both general physicians and cardiologists; (2) it is better tolerated; (3) it results in a lower incidence of conduction disturbances and cardiac arrhythmias; (4) because of its longer half-life, it would make reinitiation of PSVT more difficult in the event that premature complexes occur after drug administration. Therefore, in patients with hemodynamically well-tolerated PSVT who represent the vast majority of cases observed in clinical practice, I prefer to give verapamil as the first drug of choice for terminating PSVT.

I give ATP or adenosine only to the following groups of patients with PSVT: (1) those who do not respond to a cumulative dose of 10 to 15 mg of verapamil or those who develop hypotension after receiving a lower dose of verapamil that fails to convert PSVT, (2) those in whom verapamil is contraindicated (because of hypotension, left ventricular failure, or pretreatment with beta blockers), and (3) those in whom very rapid conversion in sinus rhythm is needed. For the latter group of patients, I recommend a starting dose of 10 mg of ATP or 5 mg of adenosine. As a result of our using such a protocol during the last decade, all cases of AV junctional reentrant PSVT observed in our institution have been successfully and safely terminated without resorting to additional antiarrhythmic agents, cardioversion, or cardiac pacing.

There are few data on the comparative effects of ATP and adenosine on PSVT. Despite the fact that ATP, but not adenosine, triggers a vagal reflex in humans, a recent preliminary study has not found substantial differences in the conversion rate of PSVT or in the incidence of side effects with these two drugs. The only significant difference was that the effective dose of ATP was greater than that of adenosine (8.5 versus 5 mg). This could be explained by the differences in molecular weight of the two drugs.

CLINICAL USE AS A DIAGNOSTIC TOOL

Diagnosis of the Mechanism of a Supraventricular Tachycardia

The identification of the mechanism underlying a supraventricular tachycardia can sometimes be difficult, even after direct (intracardiac) or indirect (esophageal) recording of the electrical atrial activity (Fig. 6). Adenosine compounds may be used for facilitating such diagnosis. Indeed, these agents usually do not have any effect on atrial tachyarrhythmias (atrial fibrillation or flutter, ectopic or reentrant atrial tachycardia), whereas they are highly effective in terminating AV junctional reentrant PSVT. In addition, in patients with atrial tachyarrhythmias, adenosine compounds produce a high-grade AV nodal block, thus allowing a clear demonstration of atrial activity (see Fig. 6).

Diagnosis of Mechanism of a Wide QRS Complex Tachycardia

Another interesting use of adenosine compounds is in the diagnosis of a wide QRS complex tachycardia (see the chapter *Wide QRS Complex Tachycardia*). Although in most instances, electrocardiographic criteria allow a clear differentiation between ventricular tachycardia and supraventricular tachycardia with aberrant intraventricular conduction, the diagnosis may sometimes be difficult. Except for rare exceptions (see below), adenosine compounds do not affect sustained ventricular tachycardia, especially that most frequently encountered in patients with coronary heart disease. In contrast, these agents either terminate or slow almost all types of supraventricular tachyarrhythmias. In addition, administration of adenosine compounds to patients with ventricular tachycardia does not have any deleterious effect. Verapamil has also been recommended for differentiating ventricular tachycardia from supraventricular tachycardia with aberration. However, I strongly recommend against using verapamil for this purpose for two reasons. First, verapamil may be highly effective for terminating certain types of ventricular tachycardia, especially those of idiopathic origin. Second, administration of verapamil to patients with sustained ventricular tachycardia (especially that related to coronary heart disease) may lead to hemodynamic catastrophes because of the negative inotropic effect and long half-life of the drug.

When adenosine compounds do not affect a wide regular QRS complex tachycardia, two very rare alternatives to ventricular tachycardia as a possible mechanism of the tachycardia should be considered: (1) atrial flutter or atrial tachycardia with antegrade conduction over an accessory pathway, and (2) reentrant tachycardia involving an accessory

A. Control

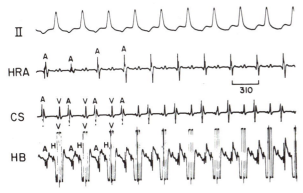

B. Adenosine – 7.2 mg IV (+ 9 sec.)

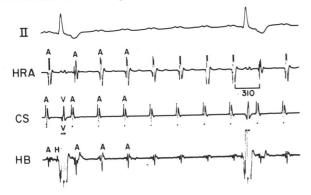

Figure 6 Diagnosis of mechanism of supraventricular tachycardia with adenosine. Shown are electrocardiographic leads II and intracardiac electrograms from the high right atrium (HRA), coronary sinus (CS), and the His bundle area (HB). *A*, A regular tachycardia is induced in which the earliest atrial activation is recorded by the coronary sinus electrode catheter. The atrial cycle length is 310 msec and there is a 1 : 1 AV conduction. *B*, Nine seconds after injection of adenosine, 112.5 μg per kilogram, high-grade AV nodal block occurs with no alteration in the atrial cycle length or activation sequence. The patient returned to 1 : 1 AV conduction 3.5 seconds after the end of this tracing (not shown). Thus, the mechanism of supraventricular tachycardia in this patient is atrial tachycardia originating close to the left atrium and not orthodromic AV reentrant PSVT involving a left accessory pathway. Actually, the tachycardia of this patient met the criteria for supraventricular tachycardia due to intraatrial reentry. (Reprinted from DiMarco JP, Sellers TD, Berne RM, et al. Electrophysiologic effects and therapeutic use for terminating paroxysmal supraventricular tachycardia. Circulation 1983; 68:1254–1263; with permission from the author and the American Heart Association.)

Adenosine 6 mg IV

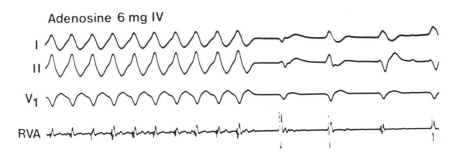

Figure 7 Adenosine-sensitive ventricular tachycardia in a young patient with no structural heart disease. Shown are electrocardiographic leads I, II, and V_1 and an intracardiac electrogram from the right ventricular apex (RVA). Administration of 6 mg of adenosine during sustained ventricular tachycardia induced at electrophysiologic study results in termination of the tachycardia 7.5 seconds after drug administration. At the termination of ventricular tachycardia, temporary sinus slowing and AV nodal block were observed associated with an idioventricular escape rhythm that lasted 6 seconds. (Reprinted from Lerman BB, Belardinelli L, West A, et al. Adenosine-sensitive ventricular tachycardia: Evidence suggesting cyclic AMP-mediated triggered activity. Circulation 1986; 74:270–280; with the permission of the author and the American Heart Association.)

pathway both in the antegrade and retrograde conduction.

MANAGEMENT OF A SPECIFIC TYPE OF VENTRICULAR TACHYCARDIA

As outlined above, ATP and adenosine do not affect most sustained ventricular tachycardias, especially those secondary to heart disease. Only one type of ventricular tachycardia has been convincingly demonstrated to be responsive to adenosine compounds. This type of tachycardia occurs in patients with morphologically normal hearts, is related to exertion, and is frequently induced by programmed ventricular stimulation or isoproterenol or both (Fig. 7). Although most of these reported cases exhibit a left bundle branch block morphology, I am aware of a few cases that show a right bundle branch block morphology. The mechanism of this type of ventricular tachycardia is assumed to be cyclic adenosine monophosphate–mediated triggered activity. Interestingly, this type of ventricular tachycardia also responds to verapamil, in agreement with its assumed mechanism.

SUGGESTED READING

Belhassen B, Pelleg A. Electrophysiologic effects of adenosine triphosphate and adenosine on the mammalian heart: Clinical and experimental aspects. J Am Coll Cardiol 1984; 4:414–424.

Belhassen B, Pelleg A, Shoshani D, et al. Electrophysiologic effects of adenosine-5-triphosphate on atrioventricular reentrant tachycardia. Circulation 1983; 68:827–833.

Belhassen B, Glick A, Laniado S. Comparative clinical and electrophysiologic effects of adenosine triphosphate and verapamil on paroxysmal reciprocating junctional tachycardia. Circulation 1988; 77:795–805.

DiMarco JP, Sellers TD, Lerman BB, et al. Diagnostic and therapeutic use of adenosine in patients with supraventricular tachyarrhythmias. J Am Coll Cardiol 1985; 6:417–425.

DiMarco JP, Sellers TD, Berne RM, et al. Adenosine: Electrophysiologic effects and therapeutic use for terminating paroxysmal supraventricular tachycardia. Circulation 1983; 68: 1254–1263.

Greco RF, Musto B, Arienzo V, et al. Treatment of paroxysmal supraventricular tachycardia in infancy with digitalis, adenosine-5-triphosphate, and verapamil: A comparative study. Circulation 1982; 66:504–508.

Griffith MJ, Linker NJ, Ward DE, Camm AJ. Adenosine in the diagnosis of broad complex tachycardia. Lancet 1988; i:672–675.

Lerman BB, Belardinelli L, West A, et al. Adenosine-sensitive ventricular tachycardia: Evidence suggesting cyclic AMP-mediated triggered activity. Circulation 1986; 74:270–280.

Overholt ED, Rheuban KS, Gutgesell HP, et al. Usefulness of adenosine for arrhythmias in infants and children. Am J Cardiol 1988; 61:336–340.

AMIODARONE

JAMES B. WATERS, M.D.
CHARLES I. HAFFAJEE, M.D.

Amiodarone was first synthesized by Labaz Laboratories in Belgium. It is a compound based on the benzofuran moiety of the khellin molecule and its congeners. It was initially developed as an antianginal agent because of its coronary vasodilatory effects, a property shared by this class of compounds. Because other derivatives in the benzofuran series showed serious side effects in early clinical trials, amiodarone came to the forefront of compounds in this series and has been the subject of intense study. Probably more papers have been devoted to this antiarrhythmic in the English literature than to any other comparable agent.

In the 1960s, Charlier and associates revealed some of the unique biologic properties of amiodarone, namely, slow onset and offset of action, with steady state effects noted at about 5 weeks following initiation of oral therapy and reversal of effects following discontinuation of drug still incomplete after 5 weeks. In 1967, Vastesaeger and coworkers published the first clinical study showing the antianginal effects of amiodarone.

In 1969, Charlier and coworkers documented the antiarrhythmic effect of amiodarone in animals. A proposed mechanism of action of amiodarone's antiarrhythmic properties was first suggested in 1970 by Singh and Vaughan-Williams. In the early 1970s clinical studies documenting amiodarone's antiarrhythmic properties appeared, first with the intravenous and later with the oral preparation. In 1974, Rosenbaum and colleagues published the earliest clinical study using oral amiodarone as an antiarrhythmic for control of a variety of tachyarrhythmias, including those associated with the Wolff-Parkinson-White syndrome.

Over the past two decades, scores of papers have been published documenting amiodarone's efficacy in treating atrial and ventricular tachyarrhythmias. During this time, amiodarone has become possibly the most effective antiarrhythmic drug for ventricular arrhythmias and symptomatic atrial tachyarrhythmias and is usually used when they are refractory to conventional agents.

PHARMACOKINETICS: CLINICAL PHARMACOLOGY; DOSING

Since the kinetics of amiodarone is unusual, somewhat unique, and not completely understood, the everyday use of this drug is less guided by the kinetics and is still empirical, based on reported clinical observations. High performance liquid chromatography provides a sensitive and specific means of detecting amiodarone and its major metabolite in serum, other body fluids, and body tissue. With this method it has been shown that single oral dose and intravenous bolus of amiodarone both result in high peak serum levels ($>5\mu g$ per milliliter) for a very short time (1 to 2 hours). Serum levels decline rapidly for the next 3 to 7 hours, during which time no measurable amiodarone is found in urine or feces. This observation, together with the progressive accumulation of amiodarone and its metabolite, desethylamiodarone, in almost all body tissues is consistent with tissue deposition. A three-compartment model helps best explain amiodarone's incompletely defined pharmacokinetics: first, the central component of distributional volume of amiodarone "fills" rapidly and "overflows" into other compartments; second, the peripheral compartment comprising most organs "fills" in about 5 days (discontinuance at this point "empties" this compartment rapidly); third, steady state is delayed until the deep compartment (fat) "fills," which takes 3 to 10 months.

Discontinuation empties this compartment very slowly. Therefore the volume of distribution is very large (300 to 500 liters); body fat contains the highest accumulation of amiodarone. The bioavailability of amiodarone is quite variable around 30 to 50 percent (range 22 to 85 percent), and excretion is minimal via the hepatic route and in the feces. Amiodarone is extensively metabolized in all tissues to desethylamiodarone (DEA), whose serum levels generally parallel those of parent amiodarone. Certain tissues have variable concentrations of DEA, with liver being the highest and fat the lowest, suggesting a difference in tissue metabolism of amiodarone. Amiodarone and DEA are excreted in small amounts in the biliary system during chronic therapy (Table 1).

The pharmacokinetic data are in keeping with the clinical observations that it takes several weeks of high daily dosing (1,200 to 1,600 mg) with amiodarone to achieve consistent arrhythmia suppression. During steady state (which takes 3 to 6 weeks to achieve), the daily dose can be reduced to around 400 mg per day. During steady state (or chronic therapy) serum amiodarone and DEA levels are similar, in the range of 1.5 to 2.5 μg per milliliter. Disparity is noted, however, in the levels of the parent amiodarone and DEA in various body tissues, with fat having the highest concentration of amiodarone and the lowest concentration of DEA. In those stud-

ies that have looked at distribution and tissue accumulation, high levels of amiodarone and DEA are consistently found in liver and lung tissue. In biopsy samples in patients with hepatic and pulmonary toxicity, high levels of both amiodarone and DEA were noted by Heger and coworkers and DEA levels were two- to three-fold higher than amiodarone levels, suggesting a possible relationship between DEA and toxicity and/or side effects. The tissue storage of amiodarone suggests a long elimination half-life.

The slow release of amiodarone from tissue binding sites seems to be the rate-limiting step and is responsible for the long elimination half-life. Wide variation exists among patients in this regard, with elimination half-life ranging from 13.7 to 129 days (Table 2).

Thus dosing of amiodarone involves a loading phase to steady state that is in the range of 1,200 to 1,600 mg daily in divided doses for 10 to 20 days, followed by a maintenance phase of 400 to 600 mg

Table 1 Pharmacokinetics

Absorption rate: 2–12 hours
Bioavailability: 30%–50%
Protein binding: >90%
Metabolism: All tissues: hepatic highest
Metabolite(s): Desethylamiodarone
Elimination: Minimal; ?biliary; non detectable in urine
Volume of distribution: Very large; >500 liters (7–50 liters per kilogram)
Elimination half-life: Several weeks to months
Total body clearance: 8–15 liters/hour (1.0–10.77 liters per minute)
Probable serum therapeutic range: 1.0–2.5 mg per milliliter

Table 2 Clinical Implications of Known Pharmacokinetics

Modest bioavailability:	Highest tolerable oral dosing initially given three times a day
Large volume of distribution	Long oral loading phase, 2–6 weeks
Minimal excretion	Low daily maintenance dosing 200 mg–400 mg/day
Long half-life	Once a day dosing
	Long and variable time period for drug elimination
Tissue accumulation	Facial discoloration, photosensitivity
	Asymptomatic corneal deposits
	Organ dysfunction and other side effects
Protein binding	Reduced clearance of other drugs and exaggeration of their effects, necessitating dosage reduction of most drugs used concomitantly with amiodarone (warfarin, quinidine, digoxin, flecainide, phenytoin, propafenone, and others)
Iodine content/ structural similarities	Iodine metabolism; increase in reverse thyroxine level
	Clinical hypo- and hyperthyroidism

daily, followed by a further reduction to 200 to 400 mg a day after 4 to 6 months of therapy.

MECHANISMS OF ACTION: ELECTROPHYSIOLOGIC EFFECTS

The exact mechanism of the antiarrhythmic action of amiodarone is not yet known. Its action as a coronary vasodilator may contribute minimally to its antiarrhythmic effect. Amiodarone appears to act as an adrenergic antagonist. It has been shown that amiodarone acts as a noncompetitive antagonist to beta receptors. It has also been documented to lower the number of beta receptors in ventricular muscle without altering receptor affinity. These actions can attenuate the positive chronotropic effects of catecholamines. Hypothyroidism also results in reduced beta-receptor density. An inference has been made that amiodarone might inhibit triiodothyronine (T3) action on heart muscle. Concomitant use of amiodarone and thyroid replacement hormone has been shown to prevent the prolongation of the repolarization phases of the action potential, implicating a possible mechanism of action, i.e., induced myocardial hypothyroid effect. One major electrophysiologic effect of amiodarone has consistently been shown to be the homogeneous prolongation of the action potential duration in atrial and ventricular tissue. The absolute and effective refractory periods are increased. These changes in repolarization are observed from 1 week into therapy until steady state is reached. These changes increase in stepwise fashion until a maintenance dose is reached. These effects have been noted in atria, ventricle, atrioventricular node, His-Purkinje system, and accessory pathways. The electrocardiogram usually shows an increase in the P-R and Q-T intervals and a sinus bradycardia. The sinus bradycardia may be the result of the decrease in the phase 4 depolarization of the sinoatrial nodal tissue. This finding is consistent with the possible blocking of the calcium-dependent slow channels.

Intravenous administration of amiodarone causes little or no change in refractoriness of ventricular muscle. Its main effect is to prolong antegrade and retrograde atrioventricular nodal refractoriness and intranodal conduction. Accessory pathway conduction in both orthodromic and antidromic directions is slowed.

In patients undergoing programmed electrical stimulation prior to and after receiving a loading dose of amiodarone, several investigators have noted significant prolongation of atrial and ventricular effective refractory periods and the lengthening of the paced cycle length at which atrioventricular nodal Wenckebach's block occurs. Haffajee and colleagues have shown that these effects were more pronounced than those caused by therapeutic quinidine and pro-

Table 3 Electrocardiographic and Electrophysiologic Effect of Amiodarone in Humans

Electrocardiographic Effect	Electrophysiologic Effect
Sinus bradycardia	Increase in sinoatrial conduction times and sinoatrial nodal recovery times
Increase in P-R interval	Prolongation of A-H interval
	Increase in cycle length to Wenckebach's block
Minimal QRS complex effects	Rarely increase in H-V interval
Prolongation of Q-Tc interval	Increase in ventricular effective refractory periods
Development of U waves	Prolongation of the action potential duration and increase in repolarization
Attenuation or disappearance of preexcitation in patients with Wolff-Parkinson-White syndrome	Increase in refractory period of accessory tract

cainamide administration in the same patients (Table 3).

EFFICACY PROFILE

Ventricular Tachycardia and Ventricular Fibrillation

Most studies reporting the use of amiodarone as treatment for serious ventricular arrhythmias (ventricular tachycardia and ventricular fibrillation— VT/VF) have numerous logistic shortcomings. There were no uniform treatment protocols; studies were not blinded or placebo-controlled; numbers of patients were small; disease populations were not uniform; and clinical or therapeutic end points were different. Most of the reported efficacy data for amiodarone do not include the outcome during the loading period (2 to 4 weeks) and instead begin reporting success or failure data after 4 to 6 weeks of loading therapy.

In the United States at present amiodarone is approved only for the treatment of documented life-threatening VT/VF, specifically recurrent VF and recurrent hemodynamically unstable VT when these arrhythmias have not responded to adequate doses of other available agents or when other agents cannot be tolerated. Generally this is how amiodarone has been used in the United States even prior to its full approval by the Federal Drug Administration. Its efficacy in these situations has been well documented. Amiodarone is the most widely prescribed drug for survivors of sudden cardiac death.

In several studies, amiodarone has been shown to suppress simple and complex ventricular premature complexes (VPCs) in over 85 percent of patients. It appears that the success of amiodarone can be predicted by long-term electrocardiographic monitoring once adequate high-dose oral loading and probable steady state (approximately 4 to 6 weeks) is reached. If suppression of VPCs and elimination of couplets and ventricular tachycardia are achieved by this method, then long-term success for amiodarone should be anticipated.

Amiodarone's effectiveness for suppression of VT is similar in patients given empirical amiodarone or in those in whom conventional antiarrhythmics failed during testing by programmed electrical stimulation. Furthermore, persistent inducibility of VT or VF during such testing while the patient is on chronic amiodarone does not preclude long-term clinical success of amiodarone as compared with conventional agents. If VT or VF remains inducible during programmed stimulation on Class I agent testing, several studies suggest a recurrence or sudden cardiac death rate of approximately 65 percent. In similar patients treated with amiodarone, the rate of VT recurrence or sudden cardiac death might be as low as 35 percent. Patients who relapse while on chronic amiodarone predominantly come from the group in which VT or VF remained inducible and is unchanged from baseline study as shown by Haffajee and coworkers and Horowitz and coworkers in 1983. Bauman and colleagues in 1987 showed that 73 percent of their patients with more easily induced VT and 60 percent of their patients whose VT during amiodarone administration was similar to baseline VT continued to experience VT recurrences or sudden cardiac death during follow-up. In 1987, Yazaki and coworkers examined the predictive value of programmed electrical stimulation testing after high-dose oral amiodarone loading (4 to 6 weeks) in 54 VT/VF survivors. Eleven percent of their patients had noninducible VT. In a mean follow-up period of 32 months, this non-inducible group of patients remained free of VT or sudden cardiac death. The other 89 percent continued to have inducible VT. This group of patients, however, could be subdivided into two groups: those with modified VT (slower and better tolerated VT 20 patients) and those with unchanged VT (28 patients). In the modified group there was a 15 percent recurrence rate of well-tolerated VT and no sudden deaths. In the unchanged VT group, 16 of 28 patients had recurrences of VT or VF, and sudden cardiac death occurred in six of these patients.

In 1989 Manolis and coworkers concluded that early programmed electrical stimulation testing may have prognostic value in patients receiving amiodarone for drug-refractory VT/VF. Patients with inducible sustained VT 10 to 14 days following high-dose oral loading had more arrhythmia recurrences and sudden death episodes than those patients who had nonsustained VT or no inducible VT. In the studies by Horowitz and coworkers, patients in whom VT or VF remained inducible after amiodarone loading had significantly shorter arrhythmia-free intervals than those patients in whom the arrhythmia was no longer inducible.

None of the many studies that evaluate amiodarone's efficacy can conclude that amiodarone improves survival. However, amiodarone's efficacy in treating VT, VF and sudden cardiac death has recently been summarized by Greene in an extensive review of the major studies. Success was defined when patients remained on amiodarone without recurrent sustained VT. In 13 major amiodarone studies, success rates varied from 39 to 78 percent, and arrhythmic deaths of 5 to 24 percent were reported in these studies, with a mean follow-up time varying between 8.5 and 24.4 months (Table 4).

In the largest reported VT study to date in which 427 patients received chronic oral amiodarone with follow-up to 98 months, Herre and coworkers have shown the incidence of both recurrent VT and sudden cardiac death in patients on chronic amiodarone to be 19 percent at 1 year, 33 percent at 2 years and 43 percent at 5 years as compared with recurrence rates for conventional therapy of approximately 67 percent at 6 months and 89 percent at 18 months. Herre also noted that the incidence of sudden cardiac death in patients on amiodarone therapy was 9 percent, 15 percent, and 21 percent at 1, 3, and 5 years respectively, which was half the incidence when compared with conventional drug therapy.

Most of the VT/VF reported experience has been with oral amiodarone. In a few studies intravenous amiodarone has been evaluated for efficacy of termination of sustained ventricular tachycardia,

Table 4 Reported Clinical Experience for Ventricular Tachycardia/Ventricular Fibrillation

Group	No. of Patients	Mean Follow-Up (Months)	Daily Dose (mg)	Success (%)
Wheeler	7	11	200–400	86
Kaski	23	21.5	200–1200	67
Podrid	96	27.3	200–600	78*
Waxman	51	8.6	400–800	50–78*
Nadamanee	96	15	200–600	78–83*
Haffajee	96	12.4	200–400	81
Fogoros	77	8.5		53
Smith	77	24.4	200–400	52
DiCarlo	104	15.7	600	48
Greene	66	11	200–600	52
Morady	154	14.2		69
Lavery	49	15		55
Horowitz	100	13.2		41
Peter	77	20.6	465	68
Heger	196	16.2	200–600	57
McGovern	42	9.8		52

*Twenty-two, nine, and six patients on additional antiarrhythmic drugs in these series.

suppression of frequent ventricular tachycardia episodes, and suppression of unsustained ventricular tachycardia and ventricular ectopic activity. Overall such studies show an acute efficacy of higher than 50 percent. Two studies (Morady and coworkers and Harriman and associates) examined VT inducibility on intravenous amiodarone by programmed electrical stimulation and found that 6 out of 15 patients had no inducible, sustained VT about 5 minutes after administration of intravenous (5 to 10 mg per kilogram) amiodarone. To date, there is no demonstrable concordance between the efficacy of oral and intravenous amiodarone based on the limited results of acute intravenous amiodarone therapy.

Supraventricular Tachyarrhythmias

Amiodarone is not as yet approved in the United States for treatment of supraventricular tachycardias, including atrial fibrillation. Thus the indications for treatment of patients with supraventricular tachyarrhythmias and/or atrial fibrillation are still considered investigational although an extensive experience both reported and clinical has been accumulated using amiodarone in this group.

In the treatment of atrial fibrillation, amiodarone has been used for conversion to normal sinus rhythm and its maintenance with or without the aid of cardioversion and for slowing of the ventricular response in patients with difficult to control atrial fibrillation.

The conversion rate from atrial fibrillation to normal sinus rhythm using amiodarone has been reported to be 50 to 96 percent. Santos and colleagues reported an 86 percent conversion rate in 83 patients with atrial fibrillation of long-standing duration. Most of their patients had underlying organic heart disease. However, enlarged left atrial size by chest x-ray study was highly predictive of failure of amiodarone to achieve cardioversion.

Oral amiodarone appears to be quite effective in maintaining normal sinus rhythm following cardioversion and in the prevention of recurrences in patients with paroxysmal atrial fibrillation. Several studies on patients whose atrial fibrillation was refractory to conventional agents show efficacy ranging from 53 to 96 percent. Most series have shown that prophylaxis can be accomplished chronically with relatively low daily doses (200 mg per day).

Left atrial size according to echocardiography has been shown by Naccarelli and coworkers to be predictive of clinical response to amiodarone. They reported an 88 percent response rate in patients with left atrial size less than or equal to 4.6 cm and a 33 percent response rate in patients with left atrial size greater than 5 cm. Horowitz and coworkers reported similar findings of reduced response rates in patients with left atrial size greater than 5.5 cm. Gold and

associates and Yee and colleagues, however, did not find a correlation of left atrial size with conversion of atrial fibrillation to normal sinus rhythm on administration of amiodarone. Gold and coworkers did report lower response rates in patients with atrial fibrillation of more than 1 year's duration. Haffajee and coworkers found a high conversion rate from atrial fibrillation to normal sinus rhythm in patients with corrected mitral valve disease with refractory, chronic atrial fibrillation when treated with amiodarone for 4 to 6 weeks followed by electrical cardioversion. The majority of their patients have remained in normal sinus rhythm during a longer than 12-month mean follow-up.

Intravenous amiodarone has also been used for acute conversion of atrial fibrillation to normal sinus rhythm, and most reports show success in the range of 80 percent when amiodarone is given as a bolus of 5 to 7 mg per kilogram, with or without a continuous infusion.

At the present time we suggest that amiodarone be used cautiously in patients with symptomatic or hemodynamically compromising atrial fibrillation that is unresponsive to more conventional and less toxic agents that are approved for this indication at this time.

In patients with drug-refractory supraventricular tachycardias, success rates of 55 to 100 percent have been reported. The long-term efficacy in this group is approximately 80 percent. The daily maintenance dose in this group generally is 200 mg to 400 mg. Several studies in patients with Wolff-Parkinson-White syndrome with recurrent supraventricular tachycardia have reported success rates between 70 and 80 percent when patients were subjected to electrophysiologic testing.

In addition to the electrophysiologic effects noted earlier, amiodarone in both oral and intravenous preparations has been shown to prolong significantly the antegrade and retrograde refractory periods of the accessory pathway in patients with the Wolff-Parkinson-White syndrome. Wellens and coworkers reported that circus-movement tachycardia could still be induced in 23 out of 30 patients during programmed electrical stimulation. However, during chronic amiodarone therapy in these patients with a mean follow-up of 40 months, only 13 percent had a recurrence of spontaneous tachycardia.

This may suggest, as others have, that amiodarone may also exert its effects by suppressing premature complexes that can initiate the tachycardia. Feld and coworkers, in a study of 10 patients, reported the prevention of induction of sustained supraventricular tachycardias in nine of ten patients during electrophysiologic study. In the majority of these patients, the antegrade refractory period of the accessory pathway was greater than 260 msec. Kappenberger and colleagues reported on 12 patients with Wolff-Parkinson-White syndrome who had programmed electrical stimulation testing before and after 3 months of amiodarone therapy. All patients had a baseline antegrade effective refractory period of the accessory pathway of less than or equal to 280 msec. In 58 percent of these patients, there was no change in the accessory pathway refractory periods after 3 months of therapy, and only 33 percent of patients had their arrhythmias rendered noninducible. Alboni and colleagues tested intravenous amiodarone in 27 patients by programmed electrical stimulation. Sustained reciprocating tachycardia was suppressed in 43 percent of the patients. In an additional 10 patients with concealed atrio-His tract, intravenous amiodarone had a 62 percent success rate. They concluded that suppression of reciprocating tachycardias by intravenous amiodarone may be used as a predictor of efficacy of oral amiodarone.

Wellens and colleagues, in a study of 76 patients with Wolff-Parkinson-White syndrome in a mean follow-up period of 67 months, showed that low-dose oral amiodarone was extremely effective in preventing circus movement tachycardia. The dose used in these patients ranged from 100 mg to 200 mg per day. In patients with Wolff-Parkinson-White syndrome and atrial fibrillation, they found that higher doses of amiodarone were generally required, in the range of 200 mg to 400 mg per day. Most of the studies in patients with Wolff-Parkinson-White syndrome suggest that amiodarone has its highest efficacy in those with antegrade refractory periods of the accessory pathway longer than 260 msec to 280 msec.

Amiodarone appears to be quite effective in controlling atrial tachyarrhythmias associated with sick sinus syndrome and a low incidence of marked sinus node depression requiring pacemaker intervention.

POTENTIAL SUDDEN CARDIAC DEATH PROTECTION

Cardiomyopathies

Ventricular arrhythmias are common in patients with hypertrophic cardiomyopathy. McKenna and coworkers reported that 29 percent of their patients with hypertrophic cardiomyopathy had ventricular tachycardia on at least one occasion. They also have shown a significant difference in the cumulative survival rate in patients with ventricular tachycardia treated with conventional drugs compared with those without ventricular tachycardia. Supraventricular tachycardias are also quite common in patients with hypertrophic cardiomyopathy. McKenna and coworkers reported that 41 percent of their patients either had established atrial fibrillation or episodes of supraventricular tachyarrhythmias, especially atrial fibrillation. They have reported no deaths in 21 consecutive patients with hypertrophic cardiomyopathy with a history of ventricular tachycardia treated with amiodarone and followed over a 3-year period. The same authors reported a 7 percent annual mortality in these patients when previously treated with disopyramide, quinidine, or mexiletine. They concluded that amiodarone improves survival in these high-risk patients, in whom they used a mean amiodarone dose of 300 mg daily.

Amiodarone has been shown to be effective in restoring sinus rhythm in hypertrophic cardiomyopathy patients with refractory and long-standing atrial fibrillation and in patients with paroxysmal supraventricular tachyarrhythmias. Amiodarone has also been reported to improve symptoms and exercise tolerance in these patients with refractory chest pain and dyspnea who did not respond well to beta-blocker therapy, calcium-blocker therapy, or surgical therapy.

Whether or not amiodarone improves survival in patients with dilated congestive cardiomyopathy and ventricular and supraventricular tachyarrhythmias remains to be confirmed. It has been shown to be efficacious in treating both ventricular and supraventricular tachyarrhythmias in this condition and does not seem to exacerbate ventricular dysfunction. Amiodarone probably should be considered the agent of choice in patients with dilated cardiomyopathy who are in the extreme stages of the disease, when their arrhythmias lead to serious hemodynamic compromise.

Postmyocardial Infarction Patients

Two controlled/randomized trials (Canadian and European) are currently being conducted in postmyocardial infarction asymptomatic patients with low-dose (200 mg per day) amiodarone compared with placebo to determine if there is a reduction in sudden cardiac death in long-term follow-up. Preliminary observations suggest that in the short term (up to 2 years), amiodarone is relatively safe and well tolerated, and there is a trend toward decrease in sudden cardiac death and arrhythmic events in the amiodarone-treated group.

With respect to survivors of sudden arrhythmic death, there is, as yet, no trial addressing the potentially protective effects of empiric amiodarone. Not uncommonly, patients surviving arrhythmic death in whom inducible ventricular tachyarrhythmias are not suppressible by conventional antiarrhythmic agents are given empiric amiodarone, especially when they are not candidates for arrhythmia surgery or the automatic implantable cardioverter defibrillator. The results and rationale of this approach produce more questions than answers at this time.

DRUG INTERACTIONS

Amiodarone's interaction with other commonly used cardiac and noncardiac drugs is a major concern. Several of the drug interactions are attributable to pharmacodynamic interactions (increasing effect of other drugs), and others are pharmacokinetic (alteration in the metabolism, excretion, and serum level of the other drug) (Table 5).

In patients using warfarin, the prothrombin time may increase significantly during the early loading phase, and this effect may persist if amiodarone therapy is continued. Prothrombin times in patients taking concomitant amiodarone have to be carefully monitored during amiodarone therapy, and invariably warfarin dosage needs to be decreased by 50 percent.

Amiodarone and digoxin interact by several mechanisms. The net effect is decreased digoxin elimination and elevated serum digoxin levels. The dose of digoxin should be reduced by about one-third to one-half when amiodarone is started. The dose of class 1 antiarrhythmic agents (quinidine, procainamide) should also be decreased by 30 to 50 percent because their serum levels increase during amiodarone therapy, which can result in a proarrhythmic effect and intraventricular conduction delays. Torsade de pointes has been rarely reported in patients on amiodarone alone but has been seen more often when patients are taking concomitant class IA antiarrhythmic agents. Neurologic toxicity is associated with aprinidine; hypotension and bradycardia with propafenone; and exacerbation of ventricular tachycardia, polymorphic ventricular tachycardia, increased side effects, widening of the QRS complex, and atrioventricular block with flecainide and encainide.

When beta blockers are used concomitantly with amiodarone, an exaggerated negative inotropic and chronotropic response may occur that includes sinus arrest and sinus bradycardia. Sinus arrest and marked atrioventricular nodal blockage have been noted with concomitant use of calcium antagonists. Use of anesthetic drugs during amiodarone therapy may cause mild cardiac depression, bradycardias, hypotension, and pulmonary complications, especially in patients undergoing prolonged cardiopulmonary bypass procedures. Adult respiratory distress syndrome has been reported in two patients who had pulmonary angiography using standard intravenous contrast agents.

SIDE EFFECTS AND TOXICITY

Early studies mainly from Argentina and France suggested that side effects necessitating termination of amiodarone therapy rarely occurred. This lower incidence of side effects was thought to reflect the lower maintenance doses used by these investigators as opposed to the experience in the United States. Around 12 percent of patients required discontinuation of the drug because of adverse effects in short-term therapy. In the American experience, a high incidence of clinical and potential side effects has been encountered; however, the majority are not serious and do not limit short-term treatment to any great extent (Table 6).

Pulmonary toxicity (interstitial pneumonitis, alveolitis) is the most serious side effect and is potentially fatal. In studies in which low daily doses were used, the incidence may be as low as 2 to 7 percent, but in patients treated with higher doses and for

Table 5 Drug Interactions

Concomitant Drug	Effect
Warfarin	Increased prothrombin time and bleeding
Digoxin	Sinoatrial and atrioventricular nodal depression
Quinidine/procainamide	Torsades de pointes and increased side effects
Flecainide	VT exacerbation—polymorphic VT Bradycardia and atrioventricular block
Beta blockers	Sinus arrest, sinus bradycardia, heart failure
Calcium antagonists	Sinus arrest, atrioventricular nodal depression
Anesthetic drugs	Hypotension and bradycardia
Phenytoin	Increased central nervous system side effects

Table 6 Side Effects of Amiodarone

System	Side Effects
Cardiac	Exacerbation of arrhythmia (2%–5%) Bradycardia, sinus arrest, and suppression of escape focus (2%–4%)
Pulmonary	Alveolitis, interstitial fibrosis (2%–15%)
Neurologic	Ataxia, tremor, sleep disturbance, myopathy, peripheral neuropathy (25%)
Thyroid	Hypothyroidism/hyperthyroidism (5%–10%)
Gastrointestinal	Nausea and vomiting, constipation, anorexia, elevated liver function test (>25%)
Skin	Photosensitivity and blue-gray skin discoloration (>10%)

Amiodarone and Thyroid Function

Thyroxine	Increased
Triiodothyronine	Decreased
Reverse triiodothyronine	Increased
Thyroid-stimulating hormone	Increased
Hyperthyroid	Triiodothyronine >200 ng/dl
Hypothyroid	Thyroxine <5 ng/dl; thyroid-stimulating hormone ≥ 15 ng/dl; reverse triiodothyronine

longer periods of time, the incidence may be closer to 15 percent. Pulmonary function studies reveal decreased diffusing capacity (DL_{co}) and reduced lung volumes. Hypoxemia is the rule. Fever is rare, and results of gallium scanning are often positive. Therapy includes reduction of dose and careful monitoring for mild early signs with or without the use of steroid therapy. In more advanced cases of pulmonary toxicity, discontinuation of amiodarone is recommended and use of steroids should be considered, although their exact role in the recovery process remains unclear. Pulmonary fibrosis often resolves slowly, although in a significant number of patients it can be fatal or irreversible.

Neurologic side effects are probably the commonest and include tremors, ataxic gait, and sleep disturbance, which are generally more noticeable in the loading phases of therapy and are often tolerable with dose reduction. Gastrointestinal side effects of nausea, vomiting and constipation are reported in 10 to 33 percent of patients. Liver enzyme levels are frequently elevated (more than 20 percent of patients), but asymptomatic in the majority of patients. Amiodarone rarely can cause hepatitis, cirrhosis, and even fatal hepatic failure.

Amiodarone may cause hypothyroidism or hyperthyroidism, the former being more common. Thyroid profiles typically reflect changes in the various parameters of thyroid function, but patients usually remain clinically euthyroid, even with modest elevation of serum thyroxine levels. If any new signs of arrhythmia appear, hyperthyroidism should be ruled out as a possible etiology. A low serum thyroxine level nearly always reflects clinical hypothyroidism.

In about 10 percent of patients, photosensitivity may result and can cause sunburn in exposed body areas. Over long-term therapy a small percentage of patients develop an asymptomatic blue-gray discoloration of sun-exposed skin. Corneal microdeposits are universally seen in patients on amiodarone. They are composed of intracytoplasmic lipid inclusions that cause a whorl-shaped epithelial keratopathy. This brownish-white lesion only rarely causes visual disturbances. The lesions are reversible on reduction or discontinuation of amiodarone.

SUGGESTED READING

Haffajee CI. Clinical pharmacokinetics of amiodarone. Clin Cardiol 1987; 10(Suppl):I-6–19.

Herre JM, Sauve MJ, Malone P, et al. Long term results of amiodarone therapy in patients with recurrent sustained ventricular tachycardia or ventricular fibrillations. J Am Coll Cardiol 1989; 13:442–449.

Kehoe RF, Zheutlin T eds. Amiodarone I, II, III. Prog Cardiovasc Dis 1989; 31:249–294, 319–366, 393–453.

Yazaki Y, Haffajee CI, Gold RL, et al. Electrophysiologic predictors of long-term clinical outcome with amiodarone for refractory ventricular tachycardia secondary to coronary artery disease. Am J Cardiol 1987; 60:293–297.

BETA-ADRENERGIC BLOCKING AGENTS

WILLIAM H. FRISHMAN M.D.

The introduction of beta-adrenoceptor blocking drugs in clinical medicine has provided one of the major pharmacotherapeutic advances in this century. Beta blockers initially were conceived for the treatment of patients with angina pectoris and arrhythmias; it soon became clear, however, that they had much to offer in the management of a diversity of clinical disorders, including systemic hypertension, hypertrophic cardiomyopathy, mitral valve prolapse, migraine, glaucoma, and thyrotoxicosis. Recent clinical trials encompassing 1 to 6 years of active treatment with these agents have demonstrated that some beta blockers are effective in reducing the risk of cardiovascular death and reinfarction in patients who are recovering from an acute

myocardial infarction. Beta blockers also have been suggested as a treatment modality for reducing the extent of myocardial injury and mortality during the acute phase of myocardial infarction, but their role in this situation is unclear.

In this chapter the clinical pharmacology of beta-adrenergic blockers is reviewed and their use in treatment of arrhythmias is discussed.

BASIC PHARMACOLOGIC DIFFERENCES

As a class of drugs, the beta-adrenoceptor blockers have been so successful that many of them have been synthesized, and more than 15 are available on the world market. The application of these agents has been accelerated by the development of drugs possessing a degree of selectivity for two beta-adrenoceptor subgroups: beta-1 receptors in the heart and beta-2 receptors in the peripheral circulation and bronchi. More controversial has been the introduction of beta-blocking drugs with alpha-adrenergic blocking actions, varying amounts of intrinsic sympathomimetic activity (partial agonist activity), and nonspecific membrane-stabilizing effects. There also are pharmacokinetic differences among beta-blocking drugs that may be of clinical importance.

As of 1989, with the introduction of betaxolol, carteolol, and penbutolol, 12 beta blockers are marketed for approved uses in the United States. These are propranolol for angina pectoris, arrhythmia, systemic hypertension, essential tremor, prevention of migraine headache, and reducing the risk of mortality of survivors of acute myocardial infarction; nadolol for angina pectoris and hypertension; timolol for hypertension, open angle glaucoma, and reducing the risk of mortality and reinfarction in survivors of acute myocardial infarction; atenolol and metoprolol for hypertension, angina pectoris, and reducing the risk of mortality in survivors of acute myocardial infarction; acebutolol for hypertension and ventricular arrhythmias; betaxolol, carteolol, penbutolol, and pindolol for hypertension; intravenous esmolol for supraventricular tachycardias; and labetalol for hypertension and hypertensive emergencies. Five beta blockers (bisoprolol, bevantolol, carvedilol, celiprolol, dilevalol) are now under consideration by the Food and Drug Administration for marketing approval or are being studied actively in clinical trials. Oxprenolol has been approved for use in hypertension but has not yet been marketed.

Despite the extensive experience with beta blockers in clinical practice, there are no studies suggesting that any one of these agents has major advantages or disadvantages over any other for treatment of cardiovascular diseases. When any available beta blocker is titrated properly, it can be effective in patients with arrhythmias, hypertension, or angina pectoris. However, one agent may be more effective in reducing adverse reactions in some patients and clinical situations.

Potency

Beta-adrenoceptor blocking drugs are competitive inhibitors of catecholamine binding at beta-adrenoceptor sites. In the presence of a beta blocker, the dose-response curve of the catecholamine is shifted to the right; that is, a higher concentration of the catecholamine is required to provoke the response. The potency of a beta blocker tells us how much of the drug must be administered in order to inhibit the effects of an adrenergic agonist. Potency can be assessed by noting the dose of the drug that is needed to inhibit tachycardia produced by an agonist or by exercise. Potency differs from drug to drug, pindolol being the most potent and esmolol the least potent. Although differences in potency explain the different dosages needed to achieve effective beta-adrenergic blockade, they have no therapeutic relevance, except when switching patients from one drug to another.

Structure-Activity Relationships

The chemical structures of most beta-adrenergic blockers have several features in common with the agonist isoproterenol, which consists of an aromatic ring with a substituted ethanolamine side chain linked to it by an $-OCH_2$ group. Among the beta blockers, timolol is unique in that it has a catecholamine-mimicking side chain; this is attached to a five-membered heterocyclic ring containing nitrogen and sulfur (a thiadiazole), which is, in turn, attached to another heterocyclic ring containing nitrogen and oxygen (a morpholino compound). It remains to be determined whether or not this thiadiazole-morpholino structure gives timolol properties not found in the other beta blockers.

Most beta blockers exist as pairs of optical isomers and are marketed as racemic mixtures. Almost all of the beta-blocking activity is found in the negative (−) levorotatory stereoisomer, which can be up to 100 times more active than the positive (+) dextrorotatory isomer. The two stereoisomers of beta-adrenergic blockers are useful to investigators seeking to differentiate between the pharmacologic effects of the beta blockade and other unrelated effects. If the effect is produced when only a d-isomer is present, it can be assumed to be unrelated to catecholamine inhibitory actions. D-isomers of beta-blocking drugs have, of themselves, no clinical value except for d-sotalol, which has class III antiarrhythmic properties.

Membrane-Stabilizing Activity

At very high concentrations, certain beta blockers have a quinidine or local anesthetic effect on the cardiac action potential. There is no evidence that membrane-stabilizing activity is responsible for any direct negative inotropic effect of the beta blockers, because drugs with and without this property depress left ventricular function equally. In therapeutic situations, the concentration of the beta blocker is probably too low to produce the membrane-stabilizing activity. Only during massive beta blocker intoxication is the activity manifested.

Selectivity

The beta-adrenoceptor blockers can be classified as selective or nonselective, according to their relative abilities to antagonize the actions of sympathomimetic amines in some tissues at lower doses than those required in other tissues. Drugs have been developed with a degree of selectivity for two subgroups of the beta-adrenoceptor population: beta-1 receptors, such as those in the heart, and beta-2 receptors, such as those in the peripheral circulation and bronchi. It has been known for some time that selective beta-1 blockers, such as acebutolol, atenolol, and metoprolol, inhibit cardiac beta-1 receptors but have less influence on bronchial and vascular beta-2 adrenoceptors.

Because selective beta-1 blockers have less of an inhibitory effect on beta-2 receptors, they offer theoretical advantages. In patients with asthma or obstructive pulmonary disease, in which beta-2 receptors must remain available to mediate adrenergic bronchodilation, relatively low doses of beta-1 selective drugs have been shown to cause a lower incidence of side effects than similar doses of a nonselective drug, such as propranolol. It should be noted that even selective beta-1 blockers may aggravate bronchospasm in some patients; therefore, these drugs are not generally recommended for patients with asthma and other bronchospastic disease.

Selective beta-1 blockers also have less of an inhibitory effect on the beta-2 receptors that mediate dilation of arterioles and are thus less likely to impair peripheral blood flow. In the presence of epinephrine, nonselective beta blockers can cause a pressor response by blocking beta-2-receptor–mediated vasodilation (since alpha-adrenergic vasoconstriction receptors remain operative). Selective beta-1 blockers may not induce this effect.

The theoretical advantages associated with the use of selective beta-1 blockers may translate into clinical advantages. For example, because selective beta-1 blockers in low doses do not block the beta-1 receptors that mediate dilation of arterioles, these drugs may offer advantages in treatment of hypertension (a possibility that has yet to be clearly demonstrated). In general, leaving beta-2 receptors unblocked and responsive to epinephrine may be important in treating patients who have asthma, hypoglycemia, hypertension, or peripheral vascular disease.

Intrinsic Sympathomimetic Activity (Partial Agonist Activity)

Certain beta-adrenoceptor blockers (acebutolol, dilevalol, pindolol, and possibly labetalol) possess partial agonist activity. These drugs cause a slight to moderate activation of the beta receptor, even as they prevent the access of natural and synthetic catecholamines to the receptor sites. The result is stimulation of the receptor, which is, of course, much weaker than the receptors of the agonists epinephrine and isoproterenol.

Quantitative assessment of the partial agonist activity of a beta blocker is made by observing the actions of the drug in animals whose resting sympathetic tone has been abolished by adrenalectomy and pretreatment with reserpine or syringoserpine. If the beta blocker increases the heart rate or force of myocardial contraction, the drug has partial agonist activity. The effects are known to be mediated through

beta-adrenergic stimulation because they can be antagonized by propranolol. The pharmacologic effects of beta-adrenoceptor blocking drugs are, of course, much weaker than those of the agonists epinephrine and isoproterenol. In laboratory animals, pindolol, for example, may have as much as 50 percent of the agonist activity of isoproterenol; the activity is probably lower in humans, however.

Whether partial agonist activity in a beta blocker offers an overall advantage in cardiac therapy remains a matter of controversy. Some investigators suggest that drugs with this property may reduce peripheral vascular resistance and may depress atrioventricular conduction less than other beta blockers. Other investigators claim that partial agonist activity in a beta blocker protects against myocardial depression, bronchial asthma, and peripheral vascular complications in patients receiving therapy. However, these claims have not yet been substantiated by definitive clinical trials.

Pharmacokinetic Properties

Although the beta-adrenergic blocking drugs have similar therapeutic effects, their pharmacokinetic properties differ significantly in ways that may influence their clinical usefulness in some patients. Among individual drugs, there are differences in completeness of gastrointestinal absorption, amount of first-pass hepatic metabolism, lipid solubility, protein binding, extent of distribution in the body, penetration into the brain, concentration in the heart, rate of hepatic biotransformation, pharmacologic activity of metabolites, and renal clearance of the drug and its metabolites.

On the basis of their pharmacokinetic properties, the beta blockers can be classified into two broad categories: those eliminated by the hepatic metabolism, and those eliminated unchanged by the kidney. Drugs in the first group, for example propranolol and metoprolol, are lipid-soluble, are almost completely absorbed by the small intestine, and are largely metabolized by the liver. They tend to have highly variable bioavailability and relatively short plasma half-lives. In contrast, drugs in the second category are more water-soluble, are incompletely absorbed through the gut, and are eliminated unchanged by the kidney. They show less variable bioavailability and have longer half-lives.

Many of the beta blockers, including those with short plasma half-lives, can be administered as infrequently as once or twice daily. Of course, the longer the half-life, the more useful the drug is likely to be for patients who experience difficulty in complying with beta blocker therapy. A recent addition to the list of available beta blockers is a long-acting, sustained-release preparation of propranolol that provides beta blockade for 24 hours. Studies have shown that this compound provides a much smoother curve of daily plasma levels than comparable divided doses of conventional propranolol and that it has fewer side effects.

Ultra–short-acting beta blockers, with half-lives of no more than 10 minutes, also offer advantages to the clinician, for example in patients with questionable congestive heart failure in whom beta blockers may be harmful. Such drugs are now being tested, and one, esmolol, has already been approved for clinical use in patients with supraventricular tachycardias. The short half-life of esmolol relates to the rapid metabolism of the drug by blood tissue and hepatic esterases.

In medical practice, the pharmacokinetic properties of the different beta-adrenergic blockers become important. The dose of the drug, for example, depends on its first-pass metabolism; if the first-pass effect is extensive, not much of an orally administered drug will reach the systemic circulation, and so the oral dosage will have to be higher than the intravenous dose would be. Knowing if the drug is transformed into active metabolites as opposed to inactive metabolites is important in gauging the total pharmacologic effect. Finally, for some beta blockers, lipid solubility has been associated with the entry of these drugs into the brain, resulting in side effects that are probably unrelated to beta blockade, such as lethargy, mental depression, and even hallucinations. Whether drugs that are less lipid-soluble cause fewer of these adverse reactions remains to be determined.

ELECTROPHYSIOLOGIC EFFECTS

Beta-adrenoceptor blocking drugs have two main effects on the electrophysiologic properties of specialized cardiac tissue (Table 1). The first results from the specific blockade of adrenergic stimulation of cardiac pacemaker potentials. This undoubtedly is important in the control of arrhythmias caused by enhanced automaticity. In concentrations causing significant inhibition of adrenergic receptors, the beta blockers produce little change in the transmembrane potentials of cardiac muscle. By competitively inhibiting adrenergic stimulation, however, beta blockers decrease the slope of phase 4 depolarization and the spontaneous firing rate of sinus or ectopic pacemakers, thereby decreasing automaticity. Arrhythmias occurring in the setting of enhanced automaticity, as seen in myocardial infarction, digitalis toxicity, hyperthyroidism, and pheochromocytoma, would therefore be expected to respond well to beta blockade.

The second electrophysiologic effect of beta blockers involves membrane-stabilizing activity, also known as "quinidine-like" or "local anesthetic" action. Characteristic of this effect is a reduction in the rate of rise of the intracardial action potential without an effect on the spike duration of the resting potential. This effect and its attendant changes have been explained by inhibition of the depolarizing inward sodium current.

Sotalol is unique among the beta blockers in that it possesses class III antiarrhythmic properties, causing prolongation of the action potential period and thus delaying repolarization. Clinical studies have verified the efficacy of sotalol in the control of arrhythmias, but additional investigation is required to determine whether its class III antiarrhythmic properties contribute significantly to its efficacy as an antiarrhythmic agent.

The most important mechanism underlying the antiarrhythmic effect of beta blockers, with the possible exclusion of sotalol, is thought to be beta blockade with resultant inhibition of pacemaker potentials. If this view is accurate, all beta blockers would be expected to be similarly effective at a comparable level of beta blockade. In fact, this appears to be the case. No superiority of one beta-blocking agent over another in the therapy of arrhythmias has been convincingly demonstrated. Differences in overall clinical usefulness are related to their other associated pharmacologic properties.

THERAPEUTIC USES IN CARDIAC ARRHYTHMIAS

Beta-adrenergic blocking drugs have become an important treatment modality for various cardiac arrhythmias (Table 2). It has long been thought that beta blockers are more effective in treating supraventricular than ventricular arrhythmias, and only recently has it been appreciated that this may not be the case. These agents can be quite useful in the treatment of ventricular tachyarrhythmias. Intravenous and oral propranolol and intravenous esmolol are approved formally for the treatment of supraventricular tachyarrhythmias and oral acebutolol and propranolol for the treatment of ventricular arrhythmias.

Table 1 Antiarrhythmic Mechanisms of Beta-Blockers

Beta-Blockade:
  Electrophysiology; depress excitability; depress conduction
  Prevention of ischemia; decrease automaticity; inhibit reentrant mechanisms
Membrane-Stabilizing Effects:
  Local anesthetic "quinidine-like" properties; depress excitability; prolong refractory period; delay conduction
  Clinically: probably not significant
Special Pharmacologic Properties:
  Beta-1 selectivity and intrinsic sympathomimetic activity do not appear to contribute to antiarrhythmic effectiveness

From Frishman WH. Clinical pharmacology of the β-adrenoceptor blocking drugs. 2nd ed. Norwalk, CT: Appleton-Century-Crofts, 1984: 34; with permission.

Table 2 Effects of Beta-Blockers on
Various Arrhythmias

Supraventricular

Sinus Tachycardia: Treat underlying disorder; excellect
response to beta-blocker if need to control rate (e.g., ischemia).

Atrial Fibrillation: Beta-blockers reduce rate, rarely restore
sinus rhythm, and may be useful in combination with digoxin.

Atrial Flutter: Beta-blockers reduce rate, sometimes restore
sinus rhythm.

Atrial Tachycardia: Beta blockers are effective in slowing
ventrficular rate and may restore sinus rhythm; useful in
prophylaxis.

Ventricular

Premature Ventricular Complexes: Good response to beta
blockers, especially complexes that are digitalis-induced,
exercise (ischemia)-induced, or caused by mitral valve
prolapse or hypertrophic cardiomyopathy.

Ventricular Tachycardia: Beta blockers are effective as
quinidine, most effective in digitalis toxicity or exercise
(ischemia)-induced tachycardias.

Ventricular Fibrillation: Electrical defibrillation is treatment of
choice. Beta blockers can be used to prevent recurrence in
cases of excess digitalis or sympathomimetic amines; appear
to be effective in reducing the incidence of ventricular
fibrillation and sudden death after myocardial infarction.

From Frishman WH. Clinical pharmacology of the β-adrenoceptor
blocking drugs. 2nd ed. Norwalk, CT: Appleton-Century-Crofts, 1984: 100;
with permission.

Supraventricular Arrhythmias

These arrhythmias have a variable response to
beta blockage. Beta blockers are not only therapeutically useful but also diagnostically important in
managing these arrhythmias; by slowing a very rapid
heart rate, the drug may permit an accurate electrocardiographic diagnosis of an otherwise puzzling
arrhythmia.

Sinus Tachycardia. This arrhythmia usually
has an obvious cause (e.g., fever, hyperthyroidism,
congestive heart failure) and therapy should be directed at correcting the underlying condition. However, if the rapid heart rate itself is compromising the
patient, for example causing recurrent angina in a
patient with coronary artery disease, direct intervention with a beta blocker may be an effective and
indicated therapy. Patients with heart failure, however, should not be treated with beta blockers unless
they have been placed on diuretic therapy and cardiac glycosides, and even then only with extreme
caution. Some patients with primary cardiomyopathy with congestive heart failure appear to benefit
from prolonged very low dose beta-blocker therapy;
the mechanisms for such beneficial effect, however,
remain unclear.

Premature Supraventricular Complexes. As
with sinus tachycardia, specific treatment of these
premature complexes seldom is required, and therapy should be directed at the underlying cause. Although premature supraventricular complexes often

are the precursors of atrial fibrillation, there is no
evidence that prophylactic administration of beta
blockers can prevent the development of atrial fibrillation. Premature supraventricular complexes
caused by digitalis toxicity generally respond well to
beta blockade.

Paroxysmal Supraventricular Tachycardia. By
delaying atrioventricular conduction (e.g., increased
A-H interval in His bundle electrocardiograms) and
prolonging the refractory period of the reentrant
pathways, beta blockers are effective in terminating
many cases of paroxysmal supraventricular tachycardia. Vagal maneuvers that were previously unsuccessful may effectively terminate an arrhythmia
after beta blockade. Even when beta blockers do not
convert an arrhythmia to sinus rhythm, by increasing atrioventricular nodal refractoriness, they often
slow the ventricular rate. The use of beta blocking
drugs also still allows the option of direct current
countershock cardioversion.

Atrial Flutter. Beta blockade can be used to
slow the ventricular rate (by increasing atrioventricular block) and may restore sinus rhythm in a large
percentage of patients. This is a situation in which
beta blockade may be of diagnostic value; given intravenously, beta blockers slow the ventricular response and permit the differentiation of flutter
waves, ectopic P waves, or sinus mechanism.

Atrial Fibrillation. The major action of beta
blockers in rapid atrial fibrillation is the reduction in
the ventricular response caused by increasing the
refractory period of the atrioventricular node. Although beta-blocking drugs have been effective in
slowing ventricular rates in patients with atrial fibrillation, they are less effective than quinidine or direct
current cardioversion in converting atrial fibrillation
to sinus rhythm.

Beta blockers must be used cautiously when
atrial fibrillation occurs in the setting of a patient
with a severely diseased heart that depends on high
levels of adrenergic tone to avoid myocardial failure.
These drugs may be particularly useful in controlling
the ventricular rate in situations where this is difficult to achieve with maximally tolerated doses of
digitalis (e.g., thyrotoxicosis, hypertrophic cardiomyopathy, mitral stenosis, and postcardiac surgery).

Many patients with paroxysmal atrial fibrillation or flutter may have sick sinus or tachybrady
syndrome, and administration of beta blockers may
precipitate severe bradycardic episodes. These patients often require both antiarrhythmic therapy and
a pacemaker.

Ventricular Arrhythmias

Beta-adrenoceptor blocking drugs can decrease
the frequency of or abolish ventricular premature
complexes in various conditions. Beta blockers are
particularly useful if these arrhythmias are related to

excessive catecholamines (e.g., exercise, halothane anesthesia, pheochromocytoma, exogenous catecholamines), myocardial ischemia, or digitalis.

Ventricular Premature Complexes. The response of these arrhythmias to beta blockers such as acebutolol and propranolol is similar to responses to quinidine. The best response can be expected in patients with ischemic heart disease, particularly when the arrhythmia is secondary to an ischemic event. Because beta blockers are effective in preventing ischemic episodes, malignant arrhythmias generated by these episodes may be prevented. Beta blockers are also quite effective in controlling the frequency of ventricular premature complexes in hypertrophic cardiomyopathy and in mitral valve prolapse. In these situations, a beta blocker generally is the antiarrhythmic drug of first choice.

Ventricular Tachycardia. Beta-blocking drugs should not be considered agents of choice in the treatment of acute ventricular tachycardia. Cardioversion or other antiarrhythmic drugs should be the initial mode of therapy. Beta blockers recently have been shown to be of benefit for prophylaxis against recurrent ventricular tachycardia, particularly if sympathetic stimulation and/or myocardial ischemia appears to be a precipitating cause. Several studies have been reported showing the prevention of exercise-induced ventricular tachycardia by beta blockers; in many previous cases, these patients had shown a poor response to digitalis or quinidine.

Prevention of Ventricular Fibrillation. Beta-blockade agents can attenuate cardiac stimulation by the sympathetic nervous system and perhaps attenuate the potential for reentrant ventricular arrhythmias and sudden death. Experimental studies have shown that beta blockers raise the ventricular fibrillation threshold in the ischemic myocardium. Placebo-controlled clinical trials have shown that beta-blockers reduce the number of episodes of ventricular fibrillation and cardiac arrest during the acute phase of myocardial infarction. The long-term beta blocker post–myocardial infarction trials and other clinical studies with beta blockers have demonstrated that they produce a significant reduction of complex ventricular arrhythmias.

Use in Survivors of Acute Myocardial Infarction

The results of placebo-controlled long-term treatment trials with some beta-adrenergic blocking drugs in survivors of acute myocardial infarction have demonstrated a favorable effect on total mortality, cardiovascular mortality (including sudden and nonsudden cardiac deaths), and the incidence of nonfatal reinfarction. These beneficial results with beta-blocker therapy can be explained by both the antiarrhythmic and the anti-ischemic effects of these drugs. Two nonselective beta blockers, propranolol and timolol, have been approved by the Food and Drug Administration for reducing the risk of mortality in infarct survivors when started 5 to 28 days after an infarction. Metoprolol and atenolol, two beta selective blockers, are approved for the same indication and can be used in both intravenous and oral forms. Beta blockers have also been suggested as a treatment for reducing the extent of myocardial injury and mortality during the hyperacute phase of myocardial infarction, but their exact role in this situation remains unclear.

OTHER CARDIOVASCULAR APPLICATIONS

Mitral Valve Prolapse

This auscultatory complex, characterized by a nonejection systolic click, a late systolic murmur, or a midsystolic click followed by a late systolic murmur, has been studied extensively over the last 15 years. Atypical chest pain, malignant arrhythmias, and nonspecific S-T and T-wave abnormalities have been observed with this condition. By decreasing sympathetic tone, beta-adrenergic blockers have been shown to be useful for relieving the chest pains and palpitations that many of these patients experience and for reducing the incidence of life-threatening arrhythmias and other electrocardiographic abnormalities.

Q-T Interval Prolongation Syndrome

The syndrome of Q-T interval prolongation is usually a congenital condition associated with deafness, syncope, and sudden death. Abnormalities in sympathetic nervous system functioning in the heart have been proposed as explanations for the electrophysiologic aberrations seen in these patients. Propranolol appears to be the most effective drug for treatment of this syndrome. It reduces the frequency of syncopal episodes in most patients and may prevent sudden death. This drug may reduce the duration of the Q-T interval.

NONCARDIOVASCULAR APPLICATIONS

Thyrotoxicosis

Many of the symptomatic and physical manifestations of thyrotoxicosis resemble those produced by the sympathetic nervous system or by the administration of catecholamines. The physiologic basis for these sympathomimetic features of thyroid hormone excess is obscure. Possible mechanisms include (1) an enhanced tissue sensitivity to catecholamines caused by increased numbers of beta receptors, to more efficient coupling of catecholamine binding, and to activation of adenylate cyclase or inhibition of tissue phosphodiesterase activity; (2) increased delivery of circulating catecholamines caused by increased tissue perfusion; and (3) the occurrence of similar but separate and additive effects of thyroid hormones and catecholamines.

Despite the inability to define precisely the relationship between catecholamines and hyperthyroidism, certain antiadrenergic agents (e.g., reserpine, guanethidine, and beta blockers) are capable of alleviating many of the sympathomimetic manifestations of the thyrotoxic state. Because of their relative freedom from side effects, ease of administration, and rapid onset of action, beta blockers are the agents of choice. The exact mechanism of beta blocker benefit in hyperthyroidism is not fully defined. It is not resolved whether the effects of beta blockage are mediated by adrenergic blockade or by blocking the peripheral conversion of triiodothyronine to thyroxine.

Particular benefit has been obtained with beta-blocking drugs in the management of thyrotoxic excess (thyrotoxic storm). In this situation, beta blockade produces a rapid reduction in fever, heart rate, and adverse central nervous system effects, such as restlessness and disorientation. Most of the experience with beta blockers in "thyroid storm" to date has been with propranolol, although other beta blockers also be effective. Beta blockers also have been used preoperatively in thyrotoxic patients undergoing partial thyroidectomy and other surgical procedures.

As part of routine medical management for hyperthyroidism, beta-blocking drugs are of less certain value. All are capable of reducing the heart rate, although drugs with partial agonist activity probably are less effective. Other manifestations of thyrotoxicosis—tremor, hyperreflexia, agitation, hemodynamic changes, hyperkinesia, and those eye signs attributable to sympathetically innervated smooth muscle—may be reduced by beta-1 selective and nonselective beta blockers.

When employed chronically as the sole therapeutic agent, beta blockers alleviate but do not eliminate the symptomatic and physiologic manifestations of thyrotoxicosis. The drugs have no effect on thyroid hormone secretion, the peripheral disposal of the hormone, or the thyrotropic or prolactin responses to thyrotropin-releasing hormone. Patients fail to gain weight satisfactorily, and evidence of an increased metabolic rate persists. Beta blockers therefore cannot be considered a substitute for specific antithyroid therapies.

ADVERSE EFFECTS OF BETA BLOCKERS

Comparing and tabulating adverse effects from different studies of beta-adrenergic blockers is diffi-

cult because of the definition of side effects, the kinds of patients studied, and study design features. Methods of ascertaining and reporting adverse side effects also differ significantly from study to study. When these differences are taken into account and results are analyzed, it appears that the types and frequencies of side effects attributed to various beta-blocker compounds are similar. The profile of side effects of beta blockers also is remarkably close to that seen with concurrent placebo treatments, attesting to the remarkable safety margin of the beta blockers as a group.

The adverse effects of beta-adrenoceptor blockers can be divided into two categories: those that result from known pharmacologic consequences of beta-adrenoceptor blockade, and those that do not appear to result from beta-adrenoceptor blockade.

Side effects of the first type are widespread because of the ubiquitous nature of the sympathetic nervous system in the control of physiologic and metabolic functions. They include asthma, heart failure, hypoglycemia, bradycardia, and heart block, intermittent claudication, and Raynaud's phenomenon. The incidence of these adverse effects varies with the type of beta blocker used.

HOW TO CHOOSE A BETA BLOCKER

The various beta-blocking compounds given in adequate dosages appear to have comparable antihypertensive, antiarrhythmic, and antianginal effects. The beta-blocking drug of choice in an individual therefore is determined by the pharmacodynamic and pharmacokinetic differences among the drugs, in conjunction with the patient's other medical conditions.

SUGGESTED READING

Cruickshank JM, Prichard BNC. Beta blockers in clinical practice. Edinburgh: Churchill-Livingstone, 1987.

Frishman WH: β-Adrenergic blockers. Med Clin North Am 1988; 72:37–81.

Frishman WH. Clinical pharmacology of the β-adrenoceptor blocking drugs. 2nd ed. Norwalk, CT: Appleton-Century-Crofts, 1984.

Frishman WH, Laifer LI, Furberg CD. β-Adrenergic blockers in the prevention of sudden cardiac death. In: Josephson M, ed. Cardiovascular clinics. Philadelphia: FA Davis, 1985:249.

Frishman WH, Skolnick AE, Lazar EJ, Fein S. β-Adrenergic blockade and calcium channel blockade in myocardial infarction. Med Clin North Am 1989; 73:409–436.

Frishman WH, Sonnenblick EH. Beta-adrenergic blocking drugs. In: Hurst JW, ed. The heart. 7th ed. New York:McGraw-Hill, 1989:1712–1731.

BRETYLIUM

WALTER REYES, M.D.
SIMON MILSTEIN, M.D.
MARY ANN GOLDSTEIN, M.D.
DAVID G. BENDITT, M.D.

Bretylium is a bromobenzyl quaternary ammonium compound originally developed in the mid-1950s during a search for antihypertensive compounds having selective adrenergic neuronal blocking properties (Fig. 1). However, because of its variable and incomplete gastrointestinal absorption and frequent undesirable side effects, bretylium did not became widely used for the treatment of hypertension.

About 10 years after its initial discovery, bretylium's antiarrhythmic actions became recognized. Today, bretylium is typically characterized among the class III antiarrhythmic agents, along with amiodarone and sotalol. Most important, owing to its potent antifibrillatory and defibrillatory actions in the ventricle, bretylium occupies a unique place in the acute pharmacologic management of life-threatening ventricular tachyarrhythmias.

MECHANISMS OF ACTION

Bretylium exerts both antiadrenergic and direct electrophysiologic actions on the heart; both influences probably contribute to its antiarrhythmic effects.

Antiadrenergic Action

After parenteral administration, bretylium is selectively concentrated in the peripheral adrenergic nerve terminal. Initially, bretylium induces abrupt norepinephrine release with a consequent transient sympathomimetic response lasting from 30 minutes to several hours. Depletion of peripheral norepinephrine stores by reserpine pretreatment prevents this effect. Subsequently, bretylium prevents norepinephrine release and also blocks its reuptake by the nerve terminal, resulting in both an antiadrenergic effect and an increasing sensitivity to circulating catecholamines. The magnitude of the net antiadrenergic effect depends not only on the bretylium dose but also on the preexisting levels of both sympathetic discharge and circulating catecholamines; therefore, it is usually impossible to anticipate the magnitude of this action in a particular patient.

The importance of the antiadrenergic action of bretylium for its antiarrhythmic efficacy is unclear. However, canine studies suggest that the sympathetic nervous system plays a role in bretylium's antifibrillatory actions. For example, in dogs pretreated with nortriptyline (an antidepressant tricyclic that antagonizes the adrenergic neuron blocking effect of bretylium), the acute antifibrillatory effect of bretylium has been shown to be attenuated.

Direct Electrophysiologic Effects

Bretylium exerts direct electrophysiologic effects that are unaffected by reserpine pretreatment, adrenoreceptor blockade, or surgical denervation. In isolated normal ventricular muscle and Purkinje fibers, bretylium typically increases action potential duration and ventricular refractoriness, without altering (unlike most other membrane-active antiarrhythmic drugs) the transmembrane action potential upstroke, conduction velocity, or membrane responsiveness. Prolongation of action potential duration is caused by lengthening in phase 2 depolarization (presumably by diminishing potassium conductance at this level of membrane potential and thereby slowing outward movement of potassium ions from the cell).

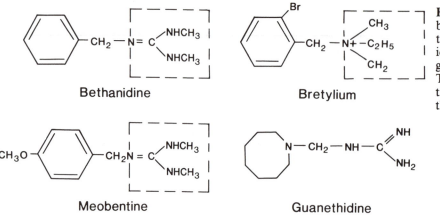

Figure 1 Structural formulas of bretylium, bethanidine, meobentine, and guanethidine. Guanethidine is the prototype of postganglionic adrenergic blocking drugs. The principal side-chain substitution differences are highlighted by the dashed lines.

In ischemic myocardium, it is widely believed that surviving subendocardial Purkinje fibers play a role in the genesis of ventricular arrhythmias. In cellular electrophysiologic studies of tissues removed from regions of left ventricular infarction, Cardinal and Sasyniuk pointed out that bretylium produced greater increases in action potential duration and refractoriness in normal cells within the infarct zone. Potentially bretylium's antiarrhythmic action may be attributable in part to a reduction in dispersion of excitable states within and around diseased myocardium.

Increased prostaglandin levels (probably prostaglandin I_2) after bretylium administration may contribute to bretylium's antifibrillatory action. Prostaglandin I_2 prevented ventricular fibrillation in dogs after induced myocardial infarction. Conversely, bretylium's ability to increase the ventricular fibrillation threshold was prevented by previous administration of cyclo-oxygenase inhibitors such as indomethacin.

Hemodynamic Effects

At high doses, bretylium has been shown experimentally to exert a positive inotropic effect; it is still unclear whether this is a direct effect or an indirect result of catecholamine release. In humans, the hemodynamic response after a single parenteral bretylium dose has two phases: initially there is a transient (about 15-minutes' duration) increase in heart rate and systemic arterial pressure caused by catecholamine release. Subsequently, heart rate, systemic arterial pressure, and systemic vascular resistance fall with a maximal effect at around 2 hours. Therefore, by decreasing afterload without negative inotropic effects (and possibly with a positive inotropic effect), bretylium can improve overall left ventricular performance. On the other hand, the diminished peripheral resistance can be responsible for aggravation of preexisting hypotension, particularly if the patient is not maintained in a recumbent position. Overall, keeping in mind the fact that the clinical setting in which the agent is used is often complex, with severe cardiac dysfunction accompanying life-threatening arrhythmias, bretylium's hemodynamic track record appears to be relatively good.

PHARMACOKINETICS AND ROUTES OF ADMINISTRATION

Bretylium exhibits a complex pharmacokinetic profile that is not yet fully understood. The drug is poorly absorbed after oral administration (absolute oral bioavailability 18 to 23 percent). Consequently, dosages of 5 to 10 g per day are necessary to achieve therapeutic response in patients receiving long-term oral therapy. Unfortunately, these doses are often not tolerated because of resulting hypotension. Although bretylium can be administered by the intramuscular route, the drug is most often employed for emergency control of life-threatening ventricular arrhythmias, and in this setting the intravenous route is more reliable.

Bretylium is negligibly bound to plasma proteins but appears to exhibit extensive tissue binding. In animals, bretylium uptake by adrenergic nerves and myocardium has been demonstrated; 12 hours after infusion, myocardial concentration is 6- to 12-fold that of plasma concentration. There is no apparent relation between plasma concentration and myocardial concentration, antiarrhythmic effect, symptoms of catecholamine release, or hypotension.

Bretylium is cleared by the kidneys. Its clearance is independent of dose or route of administration and correlates with creatinine clearance. Approximately 70 to 80 percent of the administered dose is recovered in urine within 24 hours. Elimination half-life after oral or intravenous administration is similar (10 and 9 hours, respectively). Because of its extensive tissue binding, hemodialysis has a negligible impact on bretylium clearance.

Tricyclic antidepressant drugs are inhibitors of neuronal and myocardial bretylium uptake. Consequently pretreatment with these drugs can reduce bretylium-related hypotensive effects, although they do not seem to impair antiarrhythmic efficacy. On the other hand, one should be aware that acute reversal of adrenergic blocking action may aggravate underlying arrhythmia susceptibility and increase myocardial catecholamine sensitivity.

ANTIARRHYTHMIC ACTIONS

Bretylium and Ventricular Fibrillation

Classic antiarrhythmic (antiectopic) drugs provoke, in variable degrees, slowing of conduction and increased refractoriness in normal and ischemic tissue and also tend to suppress abnormal automaticity. The impact of drugs on conduction and refractoriness affects the stability of reentry circuits, whereas the latter impedes spontaneous firing of cells, which under normal conditions remains quiescent. As a result, these agents are often effective in preventing premature complexes, which are presumed to be potential trigger events of ventricular tachycardia or fibrillation. On the other hand, these same actions may be proarrhythmic in some patients. Indeed, whether or not this antiectopic treatment prevents sudden death has been called into even greater question given the demonstrated increase in mortality associated with typical class IC drugs during the recent Cardiac Arrhythmia Suppression Trial sponsored by the National Institutes of Health.

Bretylium is considered primarily an antifibrillatory agent with only modest antiectopic activity (Fig. 2). Antifibrillatory agents, such as bretylium, are believed to act by decreasing the capability for multiple micro-reentrant circuits to exist and thereby diminishing vulnerability to ventricular fibrillation. Bacaner has shown that the reduction of fibrillation threshold associated with acute ischemia can be dramatically reversed by bretylium. In fact, fibrillation threshold was elevated beyond control levels. This effect appeared approximately 2 minutes after high intravenous doses and lasted more than 12 hours. Presumably bretylium decreases the degree of ischemia-induced dispersion of electrical excitability among myocardial fibers and thereby diminishes susceptibility to ventricular fibrillation (lidocaine in higher doses than are commonly employed also shares this effect).

In canine models, the antifibrillatory effects of bretylium have been shown to be superior to those of lidocaine, quinidine, procainamide, phenytoin, and propranolol. In the same model, bretylium reduced energy requirements to defibrillate the heart, a finding not yet conclusively demonstrated in humans. However, the success rate of electrical countershock improves with bretylium, particularly if it is used early during resuscitative maneuvers. Bretylium is the only available drug that has been effective both in treating countershock refractory ventricular fibrillation and in inducing chemical defibrillation in animals and humans.

The electrophysiologic and antifibrillatory effects of bretylium are dependent on myocardial drug concentration. With low doses, myocardial concentration increases slowly, and consequently effects on ventricular refractory period and fibrillation threshold are delayed. With high initial doses, myocardial concentration rises promptly, and therapeutic effects are more immediately evident.

Bretylium and Ventricular Tachycardia

Bretylium has not generally been included as a candidate antiarrhythmic drug during provocative electropharmacologic testing in humans with ventricular tachyarrhythmias. The principal reason for this is the lack of an effective oral form for chronic therapy. Further, difficulty differentiating between bretylium's direct effects and its indirect effects resulting from transient early catecholamine-releasing

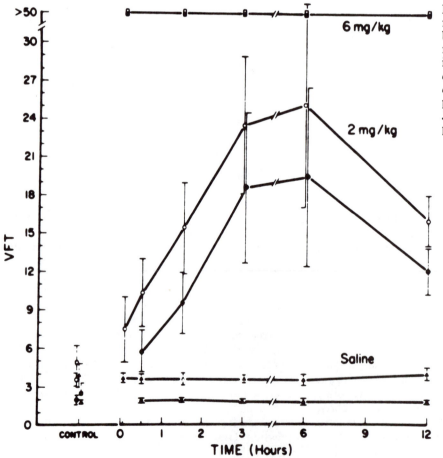

Figure 2 Graphs illustrating the marked increase in ventricular fibrillation thresholds (VFT, ordinate) following bretylium administration in ischemic (*filled circles*) and nonischemic (*unfilled circles*) canine myocardium. (Reprinted from Anderson JL. Am J Cardiol 1980; 46:588; with permission.)

action complicates interpretation of electropharmacologic studies. Several studies suggest that bretylium's direct electrophysiologic actions are largely masked by sympathomimetic effects due to early neural norepinephrine release. It appears that in chronic stable heart disease, bretylium does not modify the electrophysiologic substrate of sustained reentrant ventricular tachycardia, at least in the doses and conditions usually tested. Whether its antiarrhythmic actions may be more readily demonstrable in the presence of an acute ischemic episode remains to be explored.

Bretylium and Acute Myocardial Infarction

An antifibrillatory agent without clinically significant negative inotropic effects seems ideal for prophylactic use in acute coronary events. For example, in a study lasting 10 years and including 1,255 patients with acute myocardial infarction, 843 patients treated prophylactically with bretylium (10 mg per kilogram per day by continuous intravenous infusion for 5 to 7 days) and the remainder with a conventional antiarrhythmic approach, Torresani and coworkers reported primary ventricular fibrillation in only 1.3 percent of bretylium-treated patients compared with 5.9 percent in the no bretylium group. On the other hand, others have found no difference when comparing bretylium with placebo or lidocaine.

Bretylium has also been effective for control of refractory ventricular fibrillation after open heart surgery, not only in patients who cannot be defibrillated while coming off the pump but also for patients with recurrent ventricular arrhythmias in the immediate postoperative period. It appears that bretylium can be used effectively in a prophylactic antifibrillatory role for patients with acute ischemic events.

The predilection of bretylium to induce hypotension is a concern but can be minimized by careful attention to dosing, especially since these patients tend to be kept in bed during the early postinfarction phase. At present, bretylium's role in the treatment of ventricular tachyarrhythmias complicating acute myocardial infarction is as a back-up when conventional class I agents (e.g., lidocaine, procainamide) have failed. Under these circumstances, bretylium has shown remarkable effectiveness against resistant arrhythmias, particularly given the severe left ventricular dysfunction or shock often present in these patients.

Although no controversy exists about the use of bretylium in this desperate clinical situation, it is useful to remember that the efficacy of the drug has been said to be enhanced when it is administered in the absence of other conventional antiarrhythmic agents. Consequently, it may prove most effective when used as initial therapy.

Bretylium and Torsades de Pointes

Bretylium does not typically prolong the Q-T interval and is not known to induce torsades de pointes. On the other hand, bretylium is not useful in the treatment of torsades de pointes. In the presence of acute myocardial infarction, bretylium appears to help normalize and stabilize prolonged Q-T intervals and in this sense may be helpful in the prevention of ischemia-related polymorphic ventricular tachyarrhythmias or ventricular fibrillation.

Bretylium and Arrhythmias Due to Digitalis Toxicity

Bretylium is usually considered contraindicated for use in digitalis-induced arrhythmias because of experimental findings suggesting the potential for worsening of ventricular arrhythmias after bretylium administration. In this setting, the arrhythmogenic action of bretylium has been attributed to transient bretylium-induced norepinephrine release. Pretreatment with propranolol prevents this deleterious effect. On the other hand, in the single report documenting use of bretylium in severe ventricular arrhythmias associated with digitalis intoxication in humans, the drug was effective in the two cases discussed.

DOSES AND ROUTES OF ADMINISTRATION

The initial bretylium dose is usually an intravenous bolus of 5 to 10 mg per kilogram, repeated 15 to 30 minutes later if necessary. Therapeutic levels can be maintained with a continuous infusion of 1 to 2 mg per minute or intramuscular administration of 5 to 10 mg per kilogram every 6 or 8 hours. Considering a daily turnover in the tissues of 15 percent, the amount of drug necessary to maintain constant tissue levels (after loading doses) could be supplied by oral administration of 1 to 2 g daily (absorption 10 to 15 percent).

SIDE EFFECTS

Hypotension is the most common side effect of bretylium and is usually orthostatic in nature. Reduction in blood pressure is typically less than 20 mm Hg when the patient is supine; in some patients a greater fall in blood pressure may occur, warranting fluid or vasopressor therapy. The use of concomitant tricyclic antidepressant administration (e.g., protriptyline) has been helpful in ameliorating the hypotension without compromising antiarrhythmic efficacy.

Nausea and vomiting can occur after rapid intravenous injection of the drug. Similarly, injection may result in adrenergic side effects owing to catecholamine release (e.g., tachycardia, hypertension, flushing, or premature ventricular complexes). Minor adverse effects include parotid gland pain and swelling, headache, and nasal congestion.

RELATED DRUGS

Bretylium's clinical usefulness has been limited primarily because of poor oral absorption. In the search for an orally active drug with similar antifibrillatory actions, many experimental and a few clinical studies have been performed with bethanidine sulfate and meobentine sulfate.

Bethanidine

The substitution of bretylium quaternary ammonium by a dimethylguanidine side chain characterizes bethanidine sulfate (see Fig. 1). This chemical modification increases lipid solubility and facilitates transport across intestinal mucosa (60 to 70 percent absorption after oral administration). Bethanidine has essentially the same antifibrillatory and inotropic actions as bretylium. Although antiadrenergic effects are identical, the direct electrophysiologic effects of bethanidine may differ: action potential duration shortens and, at high concentrations, action potential phase 0 upstroke velocity is depressed. As with bretylium, it is difficult clinically to separate bethanidine's direct effects from those caused by the initial transient catecholamine release. Experimentally, bethanidine has been associated with a marked increase in ventricular fibrillation threshold in either normal or infarcted myocardium and also with spontaneous termination of induced ventricular fibrillation. In humans, bethanidine has been useful in the control of unstable ventricular tachyarrhythmias in patients resuscitated after out-of-hospital cardiac arrest, a result that could be acceptably predicted by electropharmacologic testing.

As with bretylium, bethanidine failure during laboratory testing may not preclude clinical effectiveness in suppressing spontaneous tachyarrhythmias. Long-standing worldwide experience with bethanidine as an antihypertensive agent supports its safety, although the antiarrhythmic dose is higher (typically 400 to 600 mg four times daily). Like bretylium, bethanidine induces marked orthostatic hypotension but differs in that tolerance to this effect rarely develops. Concomitant administration of protriptyline (at lower doses than those used for antidepressant therapy) has been effective in antagonizing bethanidine-induced hypotension without interfering with antiarrhythmic and antifibrillatory actions.

Meobentine

Meobentine sulfate was synthesized in the search for an absorbable bretylium-like antiarrhythmic agent without adrenergic blocking properties in order to avoid orthostatic hypotensive side effects (see Fig. 1). Experimentally meobentine exhibits neither significant adrenergic neuron blocking action nor sympathomimetic activity. Meobentine sulfate has been shown to decrease sinus rate and depress the rate of rise of the transmembrane action potential upstroke. Also, it shortens action potential duration at 50 percent repolarization and lengthens it at 100 percent repolarization, with an overall prolongation of the effective refractory period. This effect on the action potential is similar to the effect produced by high doses of bethanidine. Meobentine prolongs ventricular refractoriness in ischemic and nonischemic myocardial areas, with a greater effect in the former. This difference from bretylium suggests that the common antifibrillatory property of both drugs is not related solely to differential effects on refractoriness of normal and ischemic cardiac tissues. Also experimentally, meobentine showed antifibrillatory actions, increasing the threshold of induced ventricular fibrillation and preventing reinitiation of ventricular tachyarrhythmias.

Dr. Milstein was supported in part by a grant from the American Heart Association—Minnesota Affiliate. Dr. Reyes was supported by a grant from the Minnesota Medical Foundation–Electrophysiology Research Fund. Dr. Goldstein is a recipient of the Kenneth N. Rosen Fellowship of the North American Society of Pacing and Electrophysiology (NASPE). The authors would like to thank Wendy Markuson and Barry L.S. Detloff for assistance in preparation of the manuscript.

SUGGESTED READING

Anderson JL. Bretylium tosylate: Profile of the only available class III antiarrhythmic agent. Clin Ther 1985; 7:205.

Anderson JL, Brodine WN, Patterson E, et al. Serial electrophysiologic effects of bretylium in man and their correlation with plasma concentrations. J Cardiovasc Pharmacol 1982; 4:871.

Bacaner MB. Quantitative comparison of bretylium with other antifibrillatory drugs. Am J Cardiol 1968; 21:504.

Bacaner MB, Benditt DG. Antiarrhythmic, antifibrillatory and hemodynamic actions of bethanidine sulfate: An orally effective analog of bretylium for suppression of ventricular tachyarrhythmias. Am J Cardiol 1982; 50:728.

Benditt DG, Tobler HG, Benson DW, et al. Antiarrhythmic actions of bretylium, bethanidine and related compounds. Clin Prog Pacing Electrophys 1983; 1:349.

Bexton RS, Camm AJ. Drugs with class III antiarrhythmic action. Pharmacol Ther 1982; 17:315.

Cardinal R, Sasyniuk BI. Electrophysiological effects of bretylium tosylate on subendocardial Purkinje fibers from infarcted canine hearts. J Pharmacol Exp Ther 1978; 204:159.

Heissenbuttel RH, Bigger JT. Bretylium tosylate: A newly available antiarrhythmic drug for ventricular arrhythmias. Ann Intern Med 1979; 91:229.

Kopia GA, Lucchesi BR. Antifibrillatory action of bretylium: Role of sympathetic nerve system. Pharmacology 1987; 34:37.

Puddu PE, Jouve R, Saadjian A, Torresani J. Experimental and clinical pharmacology of bretylium tosylate in acute myocardial infarction: A 15 years journey. J Pharmacol 1986; 17:223.

Rapeport WG. Clinical pharmacokinetics of bretylium. Clin Pharmacol 1985; 10:248.

Symposium on the Management of Ventricular Dysrhythmias. Bretylium Tosylate Symposium. Am J Cardiol 1984; 54: 14A–33A.

CALCIUM ANTAGONISTS

HARVEY L. WAXMAN, M.D.
LOU-ANNE M. BEAUREGARD, M.D.
KENT J. VOLOSIN, M.D.

ELECTROPHYSIOLOGY

There are currently four calcium antagonists available for clinical use, including verapamil, diltiazem, nifedipine, and most recently, nicardipine. Nifedipine and nicardipine both have in vitro but no significant in vivo electrophysiologic activity. This probably relates to a complicated interaction between reflex responses to vasodilation and additional pharmacologic properties. Verapamil has the most potent in vivo electrophysiologic effects and is currently the only calcium antagonist approved for treatment of supraventricular tachyarrhythmias. Diltiazem also has significant in vivo electrophysiologic effects, and there is considerable evidence for the use of intravenous and oral diltiazem for the management of supraventricular tachyarrhythmias. Bepridil is a new antiarrhythmic medication currently undergoing investigation that has both calcium channel and sodium channel blocking properties. Although of considerable electrophysiologic interest, it is unlikely that this medication will ever be marketed for this use because of significant proarrhythmic effects.

At the cellular level, calcium antagonists block the slow calcium channel that is responsible for action potential generation in the regions of the sinus and atrioventricular (AV) nodes. In other regions of the heart, the sodium channel, which has a lower threshold potential, more rapid upstroke, and higher maximal potential, overshadows the calcium channel. It has been shown that in damaged His-Purkinje and ventricular muscle fibers, which are usually dependent upon the sodium-dependent fast channel, the slow channel may predominate. In these circumstances, at least theoretically, calcium channel blockers might be expected to have antiarrhythmic effects.

The above cellular electrophysiologic effects of the calcium antagonists translate into significant clinical electrophysiologic effects of these agents on both the sinus and AV nodes (Table 1). Specifically, verapamil and diltiazem depress automaticity and prolong conduction and refractoriness in the sinus and atrioventricular nodes. Nifedipine and nicardipine have little or no electrophysiologic effects and are not useful as antiarrhythmic agents (Table 1).

DOSAGE AND ADMINISTRATION

The usual dosage of intravenous verapamil is 0.075 to 0.15 mg per kilogram, infused over 1 to 3 minutes. This translates into 5 to 10 mg for the average 70-kg adult. This dosage can be repeated in 10 to 20 minutes if the initial amount is ineffective and significant hypotension does not develop. In young patients with no evidence of organic heart disease and rapid supraventricular tachycardia, the intravenous dose can be given more rapidly with better effect. In elderly people with underlying heart disease and depressed left ventricular function, the dosage should be given more slowly and cautiously in order to avoid hypotension and congestive heart failure.

The oral dosage of verapamil is 40 up to 200 mg every 8 hours. The new, slower-release form can be given every 12 hours; however, there is little information in the literature concerning the use of the long-acting form for treatment of arrhythmias.

Table 1 Electrophysiologic Effects of Calcium Antagonists

	Verapamil		Diltiazem	Nifedipine	Bepridil
	(IV)	(Oral)	(Oral)	(Oral and IV)	(Oral and IV)
SNRT	−	↑	↑	−	↑
Atrial ERP	−	−	−	−	↑
Atrioventricular node ERP	↑↑↑	↑↑↑	↑↑	−	↑↑
HPS ERP	−	−	−	−	↑↑
Ventricular ERP	−	−	−	−	↑↑
Accessory pathway ERP	−↓	?	?	−	↑

SNRT = sinus node recovery time; ERP = effective refractory period; HPS = His-Purkinje system.

The major nuisance side effects of verapamil include constipation and peripheral edema. There is little organ toxicity, and the initial reports of findings of cataracts produced in beagle dogs do not seem to have been borne out in humans. The major cardiac side effects include bradycardia, AV block, hypotension, and suppression of left ventricular function.

The dosage of intravenous diltiazem is 0.25 mg per kilogram, administered over 1 minute. This dosage can be repeated in approximately 15 minutes if the initial amount is not effective. It can be increased to 0.35 mg per kilogram of body weight. Oral diltiazem can be administered in dosages of 30 to 120 mg every 6 hours.

In a small number of studies, the overall incidence of adverse effects using intravenous diltiazem has been low, although they have been of a nature similar to those seen with verapamil. There are no studies comparing intravenous verapamil and diltiazem in the same patients.

There has been more experience with the use of intravenous and oral verapamil in the management of arrhythmias; however, the drugs probably have similar efficacy. In the discussions that follow, most references to verapamil can probably also be applied to diltiazem.

SUPRAVENTRICULAR TACHYARRHYTHMIAS

Supraventricular tachyarrhythmias in humans are most often caused by a reentrant mechanism and less commonly by enhanced automaticity. It is hypothesized that rarely, some types of supraventricular tachyarrhythmias are due to triggered automaticity related to delayed afterpotentials, although this has never been documented. The calcium channel antagonists are most useful for treatment of reentrant supraventricular tachyarrhythmias when the reentrant circuit incorporates the AV node. In addition, calcium antagonists are useful for control of the ventricular rate during atrial tachycardias or atrial fibrillation by slowing conduction through the AV node. Theoretically, calcium antagonists might also be useful for automatic rhythms attributable to delayed afterdepolarizations, such as might occur with digitalis toxicity.

Atrial Fibrillation

Atrial fibrillation is the most common atrial arrhythmia. For acute management of atrial fibrillation, intravenous verapamil is extremely effective in slowing the ventricular rate. The dosage of intravenous verapamil, particularly in the therapy of atrial fibrillation, should be individualized. Atrial fibrillation often occurs in the setting of significant underlying heart disease, and verapamil is a potent negative inotropic agent that can precipitate severe congestive heart failure, cardiogenic shock, and death in patients with poor ventricular function. Accordingly, intravenous verapamil should not be used in patients with overt heart failure and should be used with extreme caution in patients with depressed left ventricular function. In patients with mildly to moderately depressed left ventricular function and no overt heart failure, the drug should be given in a lower dosage and over longer periods of time. In order to produce a more prolonged control of the ventricular rate, other medications such as digoxin should be started concomitantly.

Although intravenous verapamil is an extremely effective agent for rate control during atrial fibrillation, it is not very effective for conversion of atrial fibrillation to sinus rhythm. From numerous studies, it appears that intravenous verapamil results in conversion to sinus rhythm in, at most, 10 to 15 percent of patients. Conversion rates are higher for patients with more recent onset atrial fibrillation and essentially nil for those with chronic atrial fibrillation. Thus, after the acute control of ventricular rate with intravenous verapamil, in combination with either oral verapamil or digoxin, it is usually necessary to employ an additional medication to effect conversion to sinus rhythm. Beta blockers are relatively contraindicated in combination with verapamil for control of the ventricular rate. Occasionally in patients with good left ventricular function and ventricular rates that are extremely difficult to control, beta blockers may be added cautiously to verapamil. An ultrafast-acting beta blocker, e.g., esmolol, may be useful in this regard because its very short half-life allows rapid discontinuance of the medication if side effects such as hypotension, bradycardia, or heart failure occur.

Beta blockers are probably more effective for conversion of atrial fibrillation to sinus rhythm than the calcium channel blockers, particularly in patients with recent-onset atrial fibrillation. However, in most cases, to convert from atrial fibrillation to sinus rhythm, a class IA agent is needed in combination with either verapamil or a beta blocker after the ventricular rate is controlled. If rapid conversion is desirable, an intravenous agent, most often procainamide, can be employed. Procainamide can be infused at a rate of up to 50 mg per minute and a total dose of 10 to 15 mg per kilogram as a bolus dose. If conversion to sinus rhythm is achieved, the class IA agent should be continued as an infusion or started orally to maintain sinus rhythm. The need for long-term therapy depends on the clinical setting, e.g., early postoperative surgery patients may require only short-term therapy, whereas patients with left atrial enlargement and valvular disease may require chronic therapy. For patients with paroxysmal atrial fibrillation, verapamil is not very useful to prevent recurrences and, in fact, has been reported to prolong the episodes even though the ventricular rate may be better controlled. Occasionally, if paroxysmal atrial fibrillation cannot be prevented, verapamil either alone or in combination with digoxin may be useful to provide rate control during the episodes. However, approximately 50 percent of patients with paroxysmal atrial fibrillation remain symptomatic during episodes, even with a well-controlled ventricular rate.

Multifocal Atrial Tachycardia

Multifocal atrial tachycardia most often occurs in the setting of other illnesses, such as chronic obstructive pulmonary disease or multisystem disease often associated with hypoxia and sepsis. Verapamil has been reported to be of use in this arrhythmia for both control of the ventricular rate and conversion of the tachycardia to sinus rhythm. Verapamil appears to produce an actual reduction in the number of premature P waves rather than to increase the number of nonconducted P waves during multifocal atrial tachycardia. Thus, it has a primary antiarrhythmic effect. This response may be attributable to verapamil's effect on a triggered automatic rhythm or suppression of damaged atrial fibers that may be calcium channel–dependent. Verapamil is preferable to beta blockers because it does not precipitate bronchospasm. Nevertheless, verapamil should be used cautiously in this situation because of the frequently concomitant left-sided and/or right-sided heart failure. The mainstay of treatment for long-term control of this arrhythmia remains with the correction of underlying metabolic derangements such as hypoxia, sepsis, ischemia, and electrolyte abnormalities.

Automatic Atrial Tachycardia

Automatic atrial tachycardia is the least common of the atrial arrhythmias. There are few data concerning the efficacy of verapamil for automatic atrial tachycardia, since it is so rare and there are no large series. Nevertheless, it appears that verapamil is most useful in slowing the ventricular rate and not very effective in terminating or suppressing automatic atrial tachycardia. Accordingly, either intravenous or oral verapamil may be used for acute and chronic control of the ventricular rate with little expectation that it will result in either conversion or long-term maintenance of normal sinus rhythm.

Intraatrial Reentrant Tachycardia

Intraatrial reentrant tachycardia is the most common cause of uniform atrial tachycardia. This arrhythmia most often occurs in the setting of organic heart disease. As is the case with automatic atrial tachycardia, there are no large series evaluating

verapamil when used to manage this entity; however, it has been reported to be effective for both control of the ventricular rate and conversion to sinus rhythm. One form of intraatrial reentrant tachycardia is sinus node reentrant tachycardia. In this instance, the P waves are very similar in morphology to sinus rhythm and the reentrant circuit occurs in the perinodal fibers. Verapamil is quite effective for termination and suppression of this arrhythmia.

AV Nodal Reentrant Tachycardia

The most common cause of supraventricular tachycardia, in patients with a normal electrocardiogram, is AV nodal reentrant tachycardia. This accounts for approximately two-thirds of the episodes of supraventricular tachycardia in humans when the resting electrocardiogram does not show evidence of preexcitation. This arrhythmia has been well demonstrated to be caused by functional dissociation of the AV node into two distinct pathways, each of which has different electrophysiologic properties. The slow pathway has a shorter refractory period but conducts more slowly, whereas the fast pathway has a longer refractory period but conducts impulses more rapidly. Verapamil suppresses conduction and prolongs refractoriness in both the slow and fast pathways in both the antegrade and retrograde directions.

Intravenous verapamil is an extremely effective agent for termination of AV nodal reentrant supraventricular tachycardia and is effective in over 90 percent of cases. Oral verapamil is also effective for maintenance therapy to suppress recurrence of AV nodal reentrant tachycardia; however, it is less effective than the intravenous medication. This difference is probably due to at least three reasons: (1) The levels achieved with oral verapamil are not as high as those achieved with intravenous verapamil. (2) One isomer of verapamil, the *l*-isomer, is more potent than the *d*-isomer in depressing AV conduction. Higher levels of the *l*-isomer are achieved after intravenous compared with oral administration. (3) AV nodal tissue is significantly influenced by the autonomic nervous system, and the effects of oral verapamil can sometimes be overcome by circulating catecholamines or other autonomic influences. Nevertheless, oral verapamil is sometimes effective alone and is often useful in combination with digoxin or other AV nodal blocking drugs to prevent recurrences of AV nodal reentrant supraventricular tachycardia.

In refractory cases of AV nodal reentrant supraventricular tachycardia, electrophysiologic testing is often utilized to select pharmacologic therapy. The intravenous form of verapamil has been used with some success to predict the efficacy of oral verapamil. Nevertheless, it seems prudent to test the oral medication for efficacy with electrophysiologic testing for the above-mentioned reasons.

In the usual form of AV nodal reentrant supraventricular tachycardia, antegrade conduction occurs across the fast pathway and retrograde conduction occurs across the slow pathway. In the unusual form of AV nodal reentrant supraventricular tachycardia, antegrade conduction occurs down the fast pathway and retrograde conduction occurs up the slow pathway. The unusual form of tachycardia is rare and even somewhat difficult to diagnose electrophysiologically, since some forms of the so-called unusual AV nodal reentry may, in fact, be due to a slowly conducting retrograde accessory pathway. Nevertheless, intravenous and oral verapamil are sometimes effective for termination of suppression of the unusual form of AV nodal reentry. In fact, intravenous verapamil may be helpful in defining the mechanism of this unusual tachycardia in the electrophysiology laboratory by implicating AV nodal tissue in the circuit if verapamil can be demonstrated to have an electrophysiologic effect on the retrograde limb.

Accessory Pathway Tachycardias

Three general types of tachycardia occur in the Wolff-Parkinson-White syndrome (see Section IV, *Preexcitation Syndromes*): orthodromic circus movement tachycardia with antegrade conduction over the AV node and retrograde conduction over the accessory pathway; antidromic circus movement tachycardia with antegrade conduction over the accessory pathway and retrograde conduction over the AV node; and atrial fibrillation or flutter with antegrade conduction over the AV node, accessory pathway, or both.

Since intravenous verapamil is an excellent AV nodal blocker, it is usually quite effective for termination of orthodromic AV reciprocating tachycardia by interruption of the circuit at the AV nodal level. However, care must be exercised when using intravenous verapamil in patients with known manifest Wolff-Parkinson-White syndrome, i.e., patients in whom there is antegrade conduction over the accessory pathway during sinus rhythm. It has been well demonstrated that intravenous verapamil can accelerate conduction over the accessory pathway during atrial fibrillation or flutter, resulting in ventricular fibrillation. The ability of verapamil to accelerate conduction over the accessory pathway is most likely caused by hypotension produced by the intravenous medication, resulting in reflex catecholamine discharge. This results in a shortening of the effective refractory period of the accessory pathway. In addition, verapamil blocks the AV node, resulting in decreased retrograde concealment into the accessory pathway, which can lead to a more rapid ventricular response during atrial fibrillation over the accessory

pathway. Finally, verapamil may have a direct effect, resulting in shortening of the accessory pathway's effective refractory period. Usually, verapamil can be safely used during orthodromic supraventricular tachycardia, but it must be realized that occasionally supraventricular tachycardia may spontaneously convert to atrial fibrillation or atrial flutter, with the risk of intravenous verapamil accelerating conduction over the accessory pathway. Thus, if intravenous verapamil is to be used in suspected orthodromic supraventricular tachycardia in a patient with manifest Wolff-Parkinson-White syndrome, it should be done in a controlled setting with the ability to perform cardioversion promptly if the need arises.

Antidromic circus movement tachycardia is unusual, and there is little evidence for the clinical use of verapamil in this setting, although it is quite possible that verapamil will result in termination of the tachycardia by interruption of retrograde conduction through the AV node. However, it is often extremely difficult using electrocardiography to differentiate antidromic circus movement tachycardia from atrial flutter with 2:1 conduction over the accessory pathway; moreover, in the latter case, intravenous verapamil is contraindicated, since it can result in acceleration from 2:1 to 1:1 conduction over the accessory pathway and potentially precipitate cardiac arrest.

As mentioned above, atrial fibrillation in the setting of Wolff-Parkinson-White syndrome, with either total or intermittent conduction over the accessory pathway, is a contraindication to the use of intravenous verapamil because it may accelerate conduction over the accessory pathway. Whether oral verapamil has similar effects is not well defined. If oral verapamil is to be used in patients with manifest Wolff-Parkinson-White syndrome, its effects on conduction over the accessory pathway should be fully evaluated with electrophysiologic testing before the patient is discharged on oral verapamil.

VENTRICULAR ARRHYTHMIAS

Calcium antagonists play a minor role in the management of most ventricular arrhythmias. However, some experimental data suggest that verapamil may be useful in the management of ischemic ventricular arrhythmias, although there is little substantiating clinical information. It has been hypothesized that calcium antagonists may be effective by suppressing calcium-dependent action potentials that may be present in damaged His-Purkinje or ventricular muscle fibers or by improving conduction through ischemic areas by reduction of ischemia. In this regard, calcium antagonists may occasionally be useful in patients with ventricular arrhythmias that are mediated by acute ischemia, particularly in the first 48 hours after acute myocardial infarction. Certainly calcium antagonists should be used cautiously and probably avoided in the treatment of sustained ventricular arrhythmias even in this setting, because it has been well documented that they may result in profound hypotension and cardiac arrest.

Verapamil has been demonstrated to be useful in selected patients with ventricular tachycardia who usually have no evidence of organic heart disease. One group of patients has been described with exercise-induced ventricular tachycardia that has a left bundle branch block morphology and right axis deviation. Another group of patients with syncope and torsades de pointes, with a normal Q-T interval and an exceptionally short coupling interval of the complex initiating the tachycardia, has been reported to respond to intravenous and oral verapamil. Finally, a third group of patients with ventricular tachycardia of right bundle branch block and left axis deviation morphology that respond to verapamil has been described. These patients, once again, have no demonstrable organic heart disease. In patients with ventricular tachycardia and no organic heart disease, it has been hypothesized that the ventricular tachycardia may be caused by triggered activity and the calcium antagonists are effective by means of suppression of calcium-dependent delayed afterdepolarizations.

WIDE COMPLEX TACHYCARDIA

Special mention should be made of the use of intravenous verapamil in the setting of wide complex tachycardia. There have been a number of reports of cardiac arrest precipitated by the use of intravenous verapamil in patients with ventricular tachycardia. Unless the patient has a well-known history of documented supraventricular tachycardia with aberration or the patient has preexisting bundle branch block with an identical match during supraventricular tachycardia, intravenous verapamil should not be used in patients with wide complex tachycardia. In patients with either a history of underlying heart disease or previous myocardial infarc-

tion who present with wide complex tachycardia, the diagnosis is most often ventricular tachycardia, and intravenous verapamil *should not be administered.*

DRUG INTERACTIONS

The most important drug interactions are those between the calcium antagonists and digoxin, and calcium antagonists and beta blockers. Verapamil and nifedipine have been reported to increase the serum digoxin level during concomitant administration. The clinical significance of this finding is unclear; however, the digoxin dose should probably be decreased and the level and clinical effects monitored carefully during the concomitant administration of digoxin and a calcium channel blocker. When verapamil or diltiazem are given together with beta blockers, signs and symptoms of congestive heart failure should be carefully watched for, particularly in people with abnormal ventricular function. In addition, this combination can result in significant bradyarrhythmias. Nifedipine, in combination with quinidine, can usually result in lowered quinidine levels during concomitant administration and, more important, elevated quinidine levels approximately 24 hours after discontinuation of the nifedipine.

SUGGESTED READING

Buxton AE, Marchlinski FE, Doherty JU, et al. Hazards of intravenous verapamil for sustained ventricular tachycardia. Am J Cardiol 1987; 59:1107–1110.

Huycke EC, Sung RJ, Dias VC, et al. Intravenous diltiazem for termination of reentrant supraventricular tachycardia: A placebo-controlled, randomized, double-blind, multicenter study. J Am Coll Cardiol 1989; 13:538–544.

Russell RP. Side effects of calcium channel blockers. Hypertension Suppl II 1988; 11:42–44.

Singh BN, Nademanee I. Use of calcium antagonists for cardiac arrhythmias. Am J Cardiol 1987; 59:153B–162B.

Waxman HL, Myerburg RJ, Appel R, Sung RJ. Verapamil for control of ventricular rate in paroxysmal supraventricular tachycardia and atrial fibrillation or flutter. Ann Intern Med 1981; 94:1–6.

DISOPYRAMIDE

MAURICE PYE, M.B.
ALAN P. RAE, B.Sc., M.D.

The antiarrhythmic activity of disopyramide was first described in 1962 by Motsler and Van Arman. It is a pyridinacetamide-type agent, chemically unrelated but electrophysiologically similar to the class IA antiarrhythmic agents procainamide and quinidine. The drug was first marketed in France in 1969 and approved in the United States in 1977. Its initial use was limited by side effects, but with increasing experience it has become a valuable part of antiarrhythmic therapy.

ELECTROPHYSIOLOGIC EFFECTS

Disopyramide is a class IA antiarrhythmic drug (Vaughan Williams classification) but also has some class III effects, which are often masked by its anticholinergic actions. In vitro it causes a rate-dependent depression of V_{max} of phase 0 (fast sodium channel blockade). The repolarization phase is lengthened, but it prolongs the effective refractory period more than it prolongs action potential duration. It reduces the difference in action potential duration between normal and infarcted tissues by lengthening the action potential of cells from the infarcted regions of the heart, resulting in a more homogeneous repolarization and reduced disparity of refractoriness, which may favor suppression of ventricular arrhythmias relying on a reentrant mechanism. It produces a concentration-dependent decrease in the slope of phase 4 diastolic depolarization in Purkinje fibers. This effect may account for its efficacy in control of arrhythmias caused by abnormal automaticity. In vitro it lengthens conduction time in normal and depolarized Purkinje fibers but does not affect slow response action potentials, except at high concentrations. These effects on conduction and repolarization can lead to a widening of the QRS complex and lengthening of the Q-T interval on the surface electrocardiogram.

Disopyramide and its major metabolite, N-mono dealkylated disopyramide, have potent anticholinergic activity and increase the sinus node discharge rate and shorten atrioventricular nodal conduction time and refractoriness when the nodes are restrained by cholinergic influences. This can lead to a dramatic acceleration in the ventricular response rate to atrial flutter or fibrillation. In higher doses it can have a direct effect on slowing the sinus node discharge rate. Although this is not important in patients with normal sinoatrial activity, it can significantly depress sinus nodal activity at therapeutic concentrations in patients with sinus node dysfunction (sick sinus syndrome).

CLINICAL EFFICACY AND INDICATIONS

Disopyramide with its class IA profile has a wide spectrum of antiarrhythmic activity. Much of the published data on its clinical efficacy have been obtained from open studies using variable dosages and imprecise methods of evaluation (Tables 1 and 2).

Supraventricular Arrhythmias

Junctional Reentrant Tachycardias

In junctional reentrant tachycardias (atrioventricular nodal and atrioventricular reentrant or reciprocating tachycardia), disopyramide can be used for arrhythmia termination and as prophylaxis. Its usual site of action is either on the retrograde fast pathway in atrioventricular nodal reentrant tachycardia or on the retrograde accessory pathway in orthodromic atrioventricular reentrant tachycardia

Table 1 Indications for Disopyramide

	Termination	Prophylaxis	Choice
Supraventricular arrhythmias			
Atrioventricular nodal reentry	+	+	3rd/4th
Atrioventricular reentry	+	+	3rd/4th
Atrial flutter	+ (after direct current conversion or pacing)	+ only with atrioventricular blocking drugs	3rd
Atrial fibrillation	+ (direct current conversion	+ only with atrioventricular blocking drugs	3rd
Wolff-Parkinson-White syndrome	+	+	2nd
Ventricular arrhythmias	+	+	?

Table 2 Contraindications to Disopyramide

Relative	Absolute
Compensated congestive heart failure	Untreated uncompensated congestive heart failure, hypertension
Prostatism	Untreated urinary retention, glaucoma
Treated glaucoma or family history of glaucoma	Long Q-T interval syndrome or history of torsades de pointes
Sinus node dysfunction	Myasthenia gravis
Hypokalemia	

(see the chapter *Paroxysmal Reentrant Supraventricular Tachycardia Without Preexcitation: Pharmacologic Therapy*). With both a direct depressant effect on atrioventricular conduction and a more potent indirect anticholinergic effect, its action on the antegrade limb may be very variable. Intravenously it has a 30 to 60 percent success rate in acute termination of these arrhythmias, which is less than intravenous verapamil, beta-adrenoceptor blocking agents, or more recently the adenyl compounds, e.g., adenosine triphosphate.

Used as prophylaxis, disopyramide is successful in up to 70 percent of cases when administered in the higher dosage range of 800 to 1,600 mg per day, although frequently lower dosages may be effective.

Although there have been few comparative studies with other antiarrhythmic agents, disopyramide is probably as effective as quinidine and procainamide. Electrophysiologic studies have shown that suppression of induction of the tachycardia by disopyramide equates well with its long-term efficacy.

In the Wolff-Parkinson-White syndrome, disopyramide slows conduction and prolongs both antegrade and retrograde refractoriness in the accessory pathway. It is effective prophylactically, but for this type of use it should be combined with an atrioventricular nodal blocking agent to offset its effect on atrioventricular nodal conduction.

Atrial Tachycardia

Disopyramide can terminate paroxysmal atrial tachycardias in up to 70 percent of cases, although its long-term efficacy in preventing recurrences in this group is only about 60 percent.

Atrial Flutter and Fibrillation

When disopyramide is given intravenously in patients with atrial flutter, chemical cardioversion occurs in only 30 percent of patients, but if it is used together with overdrive atrial pacing, it improves the pacing success rate to about 75 percent. In atrial fibrillation chemical cardioversion to sinus rhythm occurs in about 50 percent of cases, perhaps more often with higher intravenous doses, and it prevents a return to fibrillation after direct current conversion in about 60 percent of cases. In established atrial fibrillation or flutter, higher intravenous doses are often necessary to convert to sinus rhythm, e.g., 2 mg per kilogram. In paroxysmal atrial fibrillation, its ability to maintain sinus rhythm has been compared with that of quinidine (40 to 50 percent), although it is probably less effective than amiodarone.

It should be emphasized that disopyramide (and similar class IA drugs) should not be used unless the ventricular rate during atrial flutter or fibrillation has first been slowed with either digoxin, a beta blocker, or verapamil, and it should not be used prophylactically without these agents. Disopyramide has a vagolytic action that may increase conduction through the atrioventricular node temporarily, together with a direct action to slow the atrial rate; therefore, atrioventricular conduction may be facilitated to cause a rapid increase in the ventricular response or result in a 1:1 ventricular response in atrial flutter.

Ventricular Arrhythmias

Many early studies compared disopyramide to other class I agents in suppressing ventricular premature complexes (VPCs). It can significantly reduce the frequency of VPCs in Lown's grades II to IV in 70 to 80 percent of patients. An intravenous bolus injection of disopyramide followed by an infusion can terminate ventricular tachycardia in 70 to 80 percent of cases, but more often overdrive pacing, direct current conversion, or other agents are used in this situation because of disopyramide's negative inotropic effects.

More important, oral disopyramide, 400 to 1,600 mg per day, can prevent induction of ventricular tachyarrhythmias by programmed stimulation in approximately 35 percent of patients, and this includes patients whose disease is refractory to other class I drugs. It has been successful in preventing spontaneous recurrences of sustained ventricular tachycardia during long-term (2 years) follow-up in 60 percent of cases. Disopyramide is comparable in efficacy to mexiletine, tocainide, procainide, quinidine, propafenone, atenolol, propranolol, and prajmalium in suppression of VPCs or induction of ventricular tachycardia. Only a few studies including small numbers of patients have compared disopyramide with flecainide, encainide, or amiodarone, each of which has been found to be more effective than disopyramide in preventing recurrence of sustained ventricular tachycardia and suppression of VPCs. Further studies are needed to determine the relative efficacy of disopyramide in comparison with these newer agents.

Patients whose ventricular arrhythmias are controlled and noninducible with intravenous disopyramide can be successfully maintained during long-term oral administration of the drug, i.e., electrical programmed stimulation studies have a high positive predictive accuracy (approximately 90 percent).

Although disopyramide is electrophysiologically similar to procainamide and quinidine, in studies employing programmed stimulation the concordance rate is low (failure of suppression of inducibility with procainamide or quinidine does not predict the response with disopyramide).

In acute myocardial infarction, disopyramide can be used for "lidocaine failures," but its profound negative inotropic effect can lead to problems in this situation. No trial has shown that disopyramide reduces the incidence of ventricular tachycardia or fibrillation in the post–myocardial infarction period if given prophylactically (UK Rhythmodan Multicentre Group, 1984).

DOSAGE AND PHARMACOKINETICS

The phosphate salt and free base of disopyramide both have similar bioavailability and pharmacokinetics. The majority (80 to 90 percent) of the oral drug is absorbed, and peak blood levels occur at 2 to 3 hours. Bioavailability exceeds 80 percent with a first pass metabolism of 15 percent. The drug has a mean elimination half-life of 8 to 9 hours in healthy volunteers but is prolonged to about 10 hours in cardiac failure and up to 18 hours in renal failure. About 60 percent is excreted unchanged in the urine and 40 percent is metabolized first by N-alkylation. The metabolites exert less antiarrhythmic effects than the parent compound, but its major metabolite, a mono d-alkylate, has very potent anticholinergic properties.

The extent of plasma protein binding of disopyramide is concentration-dependent, and the higher the blood level the lower the percentage bound to plasma protein, so that potential toxicity is greatly enhanced at higher drug levels; however, over clinically relevant concentrations of 2 to 16 μg per milliliter, the free fraction varies little. The usual dose is 100 to 200 mg every 6 hours, with a maximum recommended dose of 800 mg daily, although this may be increased to as much as 1,600 mg daily if tolerated in patients with good left ventricular function. Therapeutic blood levels are between 2 and 5 μg per milliliter, with toxicity often reported at levels higher than 7 μg per milliliter.

If a rapid onset of action is required, an initial loading dose of 300 mg is given, but this should be omitted in the elderly (because of their reduced renal excretion) or in patients with cardiac and renal failure. Therapy should be carefully titrated beginning with lower doses of 100 mg every 6 hours and allowing ample time for steady state equilibrium to be achieved. Disopyramide kinetics cannot be pre-

dicted accurately from the creatinine clearance. The recommended dose regimen is 100 mg every 8, 12, or 24 hours for creatinine clearances of 40 to 30, 30 to 15, or less than 15 ml per minute, respectively. Less than 2 percent of a dose of disopyramide is removed during hemodialysis, and therefore the same dosing criteria apply to this group of patients.

Several controlled release long-acting preparations require dosing only every 12 hours. These preparations may improve compliance and reduce side effects, as they smooth out fluctuations in free drug levels.

Disopyramide can be given intravenously at a dose of 0.5 mg per kilogram over 10 to 15 minutes, repeated after 15 minutes to a maximum of 2 mg per kilogram. This can be followed by an infusion of 1 mg per kilogram per hour for the next 3 hours, reducing to 0.5 mg per kilogram per hour for the next 3 to 28 hours in patients who are unable to take oral preparations (Table 3).

Many aspects of the pharmacokinetics of disopyramide remain unclear, and all kinetic features show substantial interpatient variability.

Dose increments should be small, as the active free component increases proportionately more than the total concentration.

The antiarrhythmic efficacy and left ventricular function and anticholinergic effects correlate best with the free disopyramide concentration.

Phenytoin, rifampin, phenobarbital and other inducers of hepatic metabolism may lower disopyramide concentrations by increasing its metabolism. There is no significant interaction with warfarin, digoxin, or cimetidine.

SIDE EFFECTS

When disopyramide was first marketed, the incidence of side effects was very high because the dosage recommendations were based on the pharmacokinetics of normal volunteers, and loading doses now known to depress myocardial contractility significantly were used. Also the nonlinear plasma protein binding properties of disopyramide were not considered (Table 4).

Myocardial Depression

Disopyramide has a dose-related negative inotropic effect. It can cause profound cardiovascular collapse and death in patients with uncompensated

Table 3 Dosage of Disopyramide

Oral	100–200 mg q6h, loading dose 200–300 mg, maximum 800 mg daily
Intravenous bolus	0.5–2 mg/kg maximum over 15 minutes Infusion: 1 mg/kg/hour for 3 hours 0.5 mg/kg/hour for 3–28 hours

Table 4 Side Effects of Disopyramide

Negative inotropic
Anticholinergic:
    Dry mouth, eyes, nose, throat (prevented by anticholinesterase inhibitors)
    Constipation
    Urinary hesitancy, retention
    Blurred vision
Proarrhythmic ($<5\%$) + torsades de pointes (1%)
Nausea
Dizziness
Intrahepatic cholestasis (very rare)
Skin rashes, photosensitivity ($<1\%$)
Fasting hypoglycemia (in the elderly)
Acute psychosis (very rare)

heart failure and is contraindicated in such patients. The drug can precipitate a worsening of heart failure in approximately 50 percent of patients with preexisting but well-compensated heart failure, although this figure is likely to be lower if the dosage is carefully titrated and loading doses are avoided. The left ventricular effects of disopyramide occur early, usually in the first few days of treatment, and hence patients should be observed closely during this period. In patients with normal or mildly impaired left ventricular function, the decrease in cardiac performance is not clinically significant, and heart failure is a rare complication. Disopyramide, along with flecainide, probably exerts a larger negative inotropic effect than other available antiarrhythmic agents.

Anticholinergic Effects

Disopyramide has potent anticholinergic effects, which include dry mouth, nose, throat, and eyes (40 percent), blurred vision (10 percent), difficulty with micturition (20 percent), urinary retention (5 percent), and constipation (10 percent). There is a risk of precipitating closed-angle glaucoma, and use of the drug is contraindicated in patients with this problem or a family history of glaucoma. These side effects can be prevented by the concomitant use of acetylcholinesterase inhibitors such as neostigmine or pyridostigmine, and these do not reduce antiarrhythmic efficacy.

Sinus Node Dysfunction and Atrioventricular Conduction Abnormalities

Disopyramide is a membrane depressant and can potentially depress sinus node function, but this is often offset by its anticholinergic effects. Studies have shown that disopyramide can significantly depress sinus node function in a sizable proportion of patients with the sick sinus syndrome, especially in the subgroup that demonstrates spontaneous sinus pauses or sinoatrial block, and the drug is contraindicated in this group. Patients who have only sinus bradycardia without sinus pauses tolerate disopyramide; however, serial ambulatory electrocardiographic recordings should be obtained after therapy is started in this subgroup.

The drug mildly prolongs infranodal conduction times (increase in H-Q interval of 15 to 20 percent) in both normal subjects and patients with bundle branch block. The drug does not precipitate atrioventricular block in such patients. It should not be used in patients with second- or third-degree atrioventricular block.

Proarrhythmia and Torsades de Pointes

By its effect on the ventricular refractory period, disopyramide can prolong the Q-T interval. This is probably the mechanism of induction of torsades de pointes, which can occur at both therapeutic and toxic blood levels of the drug. However, the ventricular proarrhythmic effect of the drug is low (1 to 3 percent) in comparison with that of other antiarrhythmic agents. Some patients have cross-sensitivity to both quinidine and disopyramide and develop torsades de pointes while receiving either drug. It is recommended that Q-T interval prolongation of more than 25 percent of the corrected interval or significant widening of the QRS complex (more than 25 percent) requires discontinuation of the drug.

PLACE IN THERAPY

The marked negative inotropic effect of disopyramide makes it unsuitable for a large proportion of the patients at whom it is aimed, i.e., patients with life-threatening ventricular arrhythmias and with moderate to severe left ventricular impairment caused by ischemic or congestive cardiomyopathy. Early reports on the incidence of the drug's inducing heart failure were probably excessive as a result of ignorance concerning proper dosage and pharmacokinetics. The avoidance of loading doses, adequate reductions of maintenance doses in the setting of renal insufficiency, gradual dose titration for additional drug action, and omission of patients with decompensated heart failure or significant left ventricular dysfunction should improve the safety of this agent. Even allowing for these considerations, a significant number of patients cannot tolerate this drug on the basis of its hemodynamic impact. One advantage is that the hemodynamic effects of disopyramide occur early (usually in the first few days of use) and late side effects on ventricular function are rare. It remains difficult to delineate precisely the role of disopyramide in the treatment of ventricular arrhythmias, since its efficacy is similar to that of other class IA and IB drugs. The choice of drug depends primarily on its toleration by the individual patient.

Disopyramide has an efficacy comparable to that of quinidine and procainamide in supraventricular arrhythmias and is frequently better tolerated. Its major noncardiac side effects relate to its anticholinergic activity, which is predictable and tends to be of little importance if patients are selected appropriately. It should certainly be used with caution in the elderly, who may have occult prostatism.

Although less effective than flecainide and amiodarone, disopyramide does not possess the potential long-term toxicity of the latter and more particularly does not exhibit the potential for proarrhythmia manifested by the former. Indeed with the major concerns with class IC compounds, especially flecainide, in light of the recent observations in the Cardiac Arrhythmia Suppression Trial, the use of disopyramide may increase dramatically.

SUGGESTED READING

DiBianco R, Gottdiener JS, Singh SN, Fletcher RD. A review of the effects of disopyramide phosphate on left ventricular function and the peripheral circulation. Angiology 1987; 38:174–182.

Brogden LM and Todd PA. Focus on disopyramide. Drugs 1987; 34:151–187.

Morady F, Scheinman MM, Desai J. Disopyramide. Ann Intern Med 1982; 96:337–343.

Ribeiro C, Longo A. Procainamide and disopyramide. Eur Heart J 1987; 8(Suppl A):11–19.

Willis PW. The clinical scope of disopyramide seven years after introduction—an overview. Angiology 1987; 38:165–173.

ELECTROLYTE SOLUTIONS

BORYS SURAWICZ, M.D.

The chief use of parenterally administered electrolyte solutions in clinical practice is to correct appropriate electrolyte deficiencies and to treat arrhythmias resulting from such deficiencies. However, both potassium and magnesium ions have nonspecific antiarrhythmic properties that encompass a wide range of cardiac arrhythmias unrelated to electrolyte deficiencies. This discussion focuses on treatment with potassium and magnesium salts, followed by treatment of hyperkalemia, hypocalcemia, and hypercalcemia.

TREATMENT WITH POTASSIUM SALTS

The human body contains approximately 50 mEq of potassium per kilogram. The normal diet of an adult man contains about 100 mEq of potassium per day, of which about 90 percent is excreted in the urine and 10 percent in the feces. Potassium depletion may be attributable to an inadequate intake, excessive loss, or both. When the intake of potassium is low, the kidneys usually continue to excrete about 40 to 60 mEq of potassium daily for several days. Afterwards, the kidneys begin to conserve potassium more efficiently, and the urinary potassium excretion decreases. Thus, from the history, a rough estimate of urinary potassium losses in patients with inadequate potassium intake can be made. It may be more difficult to estimate potassium losses in gastric secretions and in the stools of patients with a history of vomiting and diarrhea.

Hypokalemia may be caused by potassium depletion, hemodilution, or shift of potassium from the extracellular fluid into the cells. The causes of potassium shift into the cells include alkalosis, administration of glucose and insulin, and unknown factors, e.g., attacks of familial periodic paralysis. Loss of about 200 mEq or 5 to 10 percent of total body potassium in an adult person results in a decrease of plasma potassium concentration by 0.75 to 1.5 mEq per liter. Loss of 20 to 30 percent of body potassium results in a moderately severe hypokalemia with electrocardiographic abnormalities. Several investigators have stressed poor correlation between total body potassium and plasma potassium concentration.

An important factor that determines plasma potassium concentration is plasma pH. For each 0.1 unit change of plasma pH, there is an inverse change in approximately 0.4 to 1.2 mEq per liter in plasma potassium concentration. Therefore, the relation between the plasma potassium concentration and total body potassium depends on plasma pH. In patients with severe alkalosis, plasma potassium concentration must fall below 2.5 mEq per liter to reflect significant intracellular potassium depletion. However, in patients with severe acidosis, even a slight lowering of plasma potassium concentration reflects a significant intracellular potassium depletion.

The amount of potassium required to correct potassium deficiency is usually determined by the magnitude of the depletion, the patient's weight, and the excretory function of the kidneys. Severely depleted patients may have deficits up to 15 or 17 mEq per kilogram. The maximum amount of potassium that can be efficiently utilized is about 3 mEq per kilogram of body weight per day. Although some adult patients may retain about 300 mEq daily, the commonly recommended therapeutic doses in patients with potassium depletion range from 65 to 130 mEq daily. The rate of potassium administration necessary for the correction of potassium depletion is usually slower than that used for the treatment of arrhythmias. However, in severely depleted patients without renal insufficiency, potassium has been administered intravenously at a rate of from 0.4 to 1.0 mEq per minute.

In patients with congestive heart failure who are unable to take potassium supplements by mouth, potassium must be administered intravenously using small amounts of fluids. For moderate hypokalemia, e.g., potassium concentrations of 3.3 to 3.7 mEq per liter, the recommended initial dose is 30 mEq of potassium chloride in 50 ml of saline administered intravenously over a period of 2 hours. In patients with more severe hypokalemia, the recommended initial dose is 50 mEq of potassium chloride in 100 ml of saline over a period of 3 hours. Plasma potassium concentration should be rechecked 1 hour after the end of infusion, and the therapy may be repeated if hypokalemia persists and the patient is unable to tolerate oral potassium therapy.

Potassium salts have been used in the treatment of cardiac arrhythmias since 1930. The effectiveness of therapy with potassium is determined largely by the rate of administration. When the rate is too slow, the treatment may not be effective; when the rate is too rapid, potassium may produce toxic effects. The margin between the therapeutic and toxic doses of potassium is rather narrow. Plasma potassium concentration must usually increase by 0.5 to 1.5 mEq per liter in order to suppress ectopic complexes, but an absolute increase to above 6.5 mEq per liter is not desirable.

The effect of potassium on arrhythmias is nonspecific. Potassium is equally effective in abolishing ectopic complexes in patients with low and normal plasma potassium concentrations and in patients both receiving and not receiving digitalis. However, potassium is most frequently used for the treatment of ectopic rhythms and atrioventricular conduction disturbances precipitated by hypokalemia and for the treatment of ectopic supraventricular tachycardias with 1:1 or 2:1 conduction and ventricular tachycardias induced by digitalis. When the ectopic rhythms are not caused by hypokalemia or digitalis toxicity, the duration of the nonspecific antiarrhythmic potassium effect may be short, and the arrhythmias may recur as soon as the treatment is discontinued and potassium concentration returns to the control value. Even in patients without hypokalemia or digitalis toxicity, the use of potassium may sometimes be desirable because it has no hypotensive effect. Potassium is very effective in the treatment of ectopic complexes and rapid ectopic rhythms after open heart operations. Even when these patients are not hypokalemic before surgery, their total body potassium concentration is frequently low. After the operation, hypokalemia may appear because of he-

modilution, use of glucose, and large potassium losses in the urine. The effectiveness of oral therapy with potassium on arrhythmias is difficult to evaluate because the treatment is usually combined with other agents and extended over a longer period of time, and the electrocardiogram is seldom monitored.

To suppress ectopic complexes and ectopic rhythms, potassium can be administered intravenously either continuously or intermittently under electrocardiographic monitoring. The therapeutic dose is not readily predictable. Frequently only a few milliequivalents of potassium are required to suppress the ectopic complexes. Should the undesirable arrhythmia reappear, potassium is again administered until the arrhythmia is suppressed. The intermittent method is particularly advantageous in patients with digitalis-induced ectopic tachycardia when potassium excretion is impaired by low cardiac output or hypotension. In these patients, small amounts of potassium salts administered rapidly may suppress the arrhythmia. However, as long as excessive amounts of digitalis remain in the body, arrhythmias are likely to recur, even when plasma potassium concentration is higher than normal. If potassium administration is continued during the arrhythmia-free intervals, even at a slow rate, hyperkalemia may be produced. This precludes further use of potassium if the arrhythmia recurs. Therefore, potassium should be discontinued during intervals free from arrhythmia in patients with an inadequate urinary output.

The rate of potassium administration is governed by the following factors:

1. *Plasma potassium concentration or the electrocardiographic pattern at the onset of therapy.* In patients with hypokalemia and potassium depletion, a more rapid rate of administration is recommended because the cellular uptake or excretion of potassium may be so rapid that plasma potassium concentration fails to rise, even during administration of 0.65 mEq per minute. This applies particularly to the administration of potassium with glucose, probably because the latter facilitates the cellular potassium uptake.

2. *Renal function as related to the ability to excrete potassium in the urine.* In patients with renal insufficiency, administration of potassium is usually considered dangerous, although with careful electrocardiographic monitoring, early manifestations of potassium toxicity can be readily recognized and a safe rate of administration can be maintained.

3. *The patient's tolerance of pain caused by intravenous administration of potassium salts.* The pain threshold varies. Some patients

may object even to a rate of 0.5 mEq per minute or less, but most experience pain at 1 mEq per minute. Local application of hot packs or administration through a catheter threaded into a vein is frequently effective in combating the pain.

4. *The observed effects on the electrocardiogram during therapy.* In monitoring the electrocardiogram during intravenous potassium administration, attention must be paid not only to the configuration of the atrial and ventricular complex but also to atrioventricular conduction.

The amount and the composition of the diluent depend to some extent on clinical considerations. A solution containing 80 mEq (6 g) of potassium chloride in a liter of "one-half strength saline" (4.25 g sodium chloride) is nearly isotonic and is frequently employed. If sodium is contraindicated, a 2.5 percent glucose solution can be used. When the intake of fluid must be restricted, a concentration of 160 mEq of potassium (12 g potassium chloride) per liter can be employed.

TREATMENT WITH MAGNESIUM SALTS

The increased availability of serum magnesium concentration determinations has established hypomagnesemia as a common electrolyte disturbance in patients with nutritional deficiencies, starvation, alcoholism, gastrointestinal disorders, certain types of renal disease, and a variety of other clinical conditions. In patients with heart disease, the occurrence of hypomagnesemia is facilitated by treatment with diuretics. An increased incidence of magnesium deficiency, independent of treatment with diuretics, has been reported in patients with ischemic heart disease, myocardial infarction, and mitral valve prolapse.

The cardiac effects of magnesium deficiency have largely escaped precise definition, but numerous investigators share the view that hypomagnesemia provokes and aggravates cardiac arrhythmias. The clinical evidence of the association between hypomagnesemia and arrhythmias is frequently based on the suppression of arrhythmias by administration of magnesium salts. However, the latter effect is nonspecific and does not prove that the arrhythmia suppressed by magnesium results from the deficiency of this cation.

Prolonged hypomagnesemia may be associated with hypocalcemia but has no effect on the levels of serum sodium, chloride, potassium, or cholesterol. However, magnesium deficiency causes depletion of muscle potassium. This depletion persists in spite of a large intake of potassium. This suggests that magnesium deficiency may have an influence on the ability of cells to maintain an appropriate potassium gradient. This particular finding, believed to be present in magnesium-depleted patients, is the basis of the hypothesis that intracellular potassium depletion predisposes to cardiac arrhythmias, which would defy correction in the absence of magnesium.

The evidence that hypomagnesemia is responsible for cardiac arrhythmias is limited to case reports. In some of these, other associated causes could be suspected because of either Q-T interval prolongation or the presence of hypokalemia on hospital admission. Most of the indirect evidence linking hypomagnesemia with cardiac arrhythmias stems from the effectiveness of magnesium salts in the treatment of cardiac arrhythmias. Magnesium sulfate solution administered intravenously has been used empirically to suppress a variety of supraventricular and ventricular arrhythmias in the absence and in the presence of digitalis therapy. Recently, magnesium sulfate has been used in the treatment of torsades de pointes. The precise mechanism of antiarrhythmic action of acute magnesium administration has not been elucidated. In humans, infusion of magnesium salts lengthens sinus node recovery time, atrioventricular conduction time, and QRS complex duration during ventricular pacing.

The lack of answers to the question of whether hypomagnesemia causes arrhythmias makes it difficult to assess the clinical importance of magnesium deficiency and to define the therapeutic goals of magnesium administration. In most cases, the correction of hypomagnesemia and magnesium deficiency is probably desirable, but an overzealous treatment may not be innocuous, particularly in patients with impaired renal function.

The suggested mode of intravenous magnesium sulfate administration is a bolus of 25 percent solution containing 1 to 3 g injected within 1 to 2 minutes, followed by a continuous infusion of 3 to 20 mg per minute. A second bolus can be given from 5 to 15 minutes after the first one. The total amount of magnesium used for suppression of arrhythmias ranges from 2 to 12 g over 5 hours. To avoid flushing and hypotension, some authors have suggested a slower rate of magnesium sulfate administration, 50 mg per minute for 20 to 30 minutes followed by a prophylactic infusion at a rate of 30 mg per minute twice a day.

TREATMENT OF HYPERKALEMIA

Hyperkalemia is frequently associated with serious life-threatening disturbances of rhythm and conduction requiring emergency treatment with electrolyte solutions. The most common cause of hyperkalemia is renal insufficiency. Potassium homeostasis during renal failure is not adequately maintained when the glomerular filtration rate falls to less than 20 ml per minute. Another cause of hyperkalemia frequently associated with renal failure is severe acidosis, which displaces potassium from intracellular to extracellular space. Less common causes of hyperkalemia include treatment with potassium-sparing diuretic drugs, tissue necrosis (e.g., crush injury), excessive administration of potassium (e.g., treatment with potassium penicillin), use of salt substitutes, and hyperthermia.

Treatment of life-threatening hyperkalemia should be guided by monitoring the electrocardiogram, which is a sensitive indicator of changes in the transmembrane potential resulting from an increased extracellular potassium concentration. Peaking of the T wave is the earliest electrocardiographic manifestation of hyperkalemia, which occurs when the plasma potassium concentration exceeds 5.5 mEq per liter, usually before the electrocardiogram shows any measurable alteration of the QRS complex. The diagnosis of hyperkalemia cannot be made with certainty on the basis of T-wave changes alone. When the plasma potassium concentration exceeds 6.5 mEq per liter, QRS complex changes are usually present. A correct electrocardiographic diagnosis of hyperkalemia can usually be made in all cases in which the plasma potassium concentration exceeds 6.7 mEq per liter.

When the plasma potassium concentration exceeds 7.0 mEq per liter, the P wave amplitude usually decreases and the duration of the P wave increases because of the slower conduction in the atria. The P-R interval is frequently prolonged as a result of slower atrioventricular transmission. When the plasma potassium concentration exceeds 8.8 mEq per liter, the P wave is frequently invisible. When the QRS complex is wide, a low amplitude or absence of the P wave helps to differentiate the pattern of hyperkalemia from intraventricular conduction disturbances of other origin.

The pattern of advanced hyperkalemia is almost identical to that recorded in hearts of dying patients. Sometimes in advanced hyperkalemia the S-T segment deviates significantly from the baseline and simulates the pattern of acute injury, which may result in an incorrect diagnosis of infarction or pericarditis. An increase in plasma potassium concentration above 12 to 14 mEq per liter causes ventricular asystole or ventricular fibrillation. The latter may or may not be preceded by acceleration of the ventricular rate.

The most rapid improvement of intraventricular and atrioventricular conduction can be accomplished by administration of calcium, e.g., 10 ml of 10 percent calcium chloride or calcium gluconate solution within 1 to 2 minutes. A similar effect can be achieved using either a 5 percent sodium chloride infusion administered intravenously at a rate of about 50 to 100 ml per hour or 100 mEq of sodium bicarbonate administered within 5 minutes. In cases of lesser emergency, glucose and insulin are the preferred therapeutic agents. Treatment should be started with a 30 percent dextrose solution in 500 ml of water, with 30 U of insulin and 100 mEq of sodium bicarbonate at a rate of 100 ml during the first hour, followed by 20 to 30 ml per hour. In less urgent situations, sodium polystyrene sulfonate (Kayexelate) is administered either orally or as an enema, and the control of potassium homeostasis is achieved by means of dialysis.

TREATMENT OF HYPOCALCEMIA

Severe hypocalcemia causing tetany or marked depression of cardiac contractility may constitute a medical emergency requiring intravenous administration of 1 to 2 ampules of 10 percent calcium gluconate (100 to 200 mg of elemental calcium) over a period of 10 minutes. Similar treatment may be required for severe verapamil toxicity associated with depressed myocardial contractility and hypotension.

TREATMENT OF HYPERCALCEMIA

Hypercalcemia rarely requires parenteral treatment. In emergency situations, plasma calcium concentration can be effectively lowered by administration of disodium ethylendiaminetetraacetic acid (EDTA) (50 mg per kilogram in 500 mg of saline over a period of 4 hours). However, the procedure may result in renal damage. Monitoring the duration of the S-T segment on the electrocardiogram during Na_2 EDTA therapy is helpful in assessing the changes in plasma calcium concentration.

Supported in part by the Herman C. Krannert Fund; by Grants HL-06308 and HL-07182 from the National Heart, Lung and Blood Institute of the National Institutes of Health, U.S. Public Health Service; and the American Heart Association, Indiana Affiliate, Inc.

SUGGESTED READING

Bettinger JC, Surawicz B, Bryfogle JW, et al. Effect of intravenous administration of potassium chloride on ectopic beats and A-V conduction disturbances. Am J Med 1956; 21:521.

Garcia-Palmieri MR. Reversal of hyperkalemic cardiotoxicity with hypertonic saline. Am Heart J 1962; 64:483.

Kunin AS, Surawicz B, Sims EAH. Decrease in serum potassium concentrations and appearance of cardiac arrhythmias during infusion of potassium with glucose in potassium-depleted patients. N Engl J Med 1962; 266:228.

Lown B, Weller JM, Wyatt N, et al. Effects of alterations of body potassium on digitalis toxicity. J Clin Invest 1952; 31:648.

Surawicz B. Relationship between electrocardiogram and electrolytes. Am Heart J 1967; 73:814.

Tzivoni D, Banai S, Schuger C, et al. Treatment of torsade de pointes with magnesium sulfate. Circulation 1988; 77:392.

ENCAINIDE

MAGDI SAMI, M.D.

Encainide hydrochloride is one of a new generation of powerful antiarrhythmic drugs that has had a high rate of success in suppressing ventricular premature complexes and has been well tolerated by the majority of patients receiving it chronically.

Recently, however, preliminary results from the Cardiac Arrhythmia Suppression Trial (CAST) have raised concerns about the safety of the long-term use of encainide in patients who have sustained a myocardial infarction. They have also raised doubts about the conventional wisdom that the suppression of ventricular premature complexes is beneficial in preventing sudden cardiac death. With this in mind, several aspects of the clinical use of encainide are still in question. This report attempts to summarize the current knowledge about this drug and put it in a clinical context based on the experience of the author.

ELECTROPHYSIOLOGY

Encainide has been classified as a class IC antiarrhythmic agent according to the modified Vaughan Williams classification. Class IC drugs are so designated because they markedly slow conduction in the His-Purkinje system without significantly affecting the action potential duration or ventricular muscle refractoriness.

The electrophysiologic effects of encainide are similar in both ischemic and healthy myocardial tissue; however, they are more marked in ischemic tissue. This differential activity may contribute to the antiarrhythmic action of encainide and perhaps to its proarrhythmic effects.

The antiarrhythmic and electrophysiologic effects of encainide result from the unchanged drug and its two major metabolites, O-demethylencainide (ODE) and 3-methoxy-O-demethylencainide (MODE). The relative proportions of encainide and its metabolites in plasma vary considerably, depending on the patient's genetically determined ability to metabolize the drug (oxidizer phenotype) and on the route and the length of administration of the drug. In patients with the extensive oxidizer phenotype, the electrophysiologic effects appear to be correlated principally with levels of ODE and to a lesser extent with levels of MODE. In patients with the poor oxidizer phenotype, these effects are correlated with the levels of the unmodified drug.

Encainide and its metabolites produce a dose-related decrease in intracardiac conduction throughout the heart, with a most marked effect on conduction within the His-Purkinje system. The effects of the drug on intraatrial and atrioventricular conduction are less pronounced than its effects on intraventricular conduction, particularly following acute administration. Following chronic oral administration, refractoriness in most parts of the heart may also increase; however, the effect on refractoriness is less pronounced than the effect on intracardiac conduction ODE, and to a lesser degree MODE, appear to decrease intracardiac conduction and to increase refractoriness to a greater extent than encainide.

The effect of encainide and its metabolites on the surface electrocardiogram is dose-related and consists of an increase in the P-R interval and QRS complex. Q-T intervals remain unchanged in most patients. Although there is prolongation in some cases, the P-R and QRS intervals increase in a linear manner at encainide dosages ranging from 30 to 225 mg per day. With chronic oral administration of therapeutic dosages of the drug, increases in P-R and QRS intervals generally range from about 10 to 30 percent and 24 to 40 percent, respectively. During chronic oral administration, the Q-T interval may increase by about 10 percent; however, this increase is almost entirely due to the increase in QRS duration and not to the J-T interval (Q-T-QRS). Only MODE appears to prolong the corrected J-T interval (J-Tc). Based on changes in the J-T interval observed during chronic oral administration, some data suggest that encainide may have a lesser effect on ventricular repolarization than flecainide, another class IC agent; however, direct comparative studies are not available.

PHARMACOKINETICS

Encainide is rapidly and almost completely absorbed from the gastrointestinal tract following oral administration. In most patients (those with the extensive oxidizer phenotype) it is modified extensively and undergoes first-pass metabolism in the liver, producing the two major active metabolites ODE and MODE. In patients with poor oxidizer phenotype, encainide is very poorly metabolized and remains unchanged in the plasma. The rate of absorption of encainide hydrochloride may be slightly decreased by the presence of food, but the extent of absorption is not affected. Following oral administration, plasma encainide concentration usually occurs within 0.5 to 1.5 hours; however, peak plasma concentrations of ODE and MODE occur after substantially longer periods, ranging from 2 to 10 hours. The kinetics of encainide do not appear to be affected by age or sex. There is considerable interpatient variability in plasma concentration of the drug and its metabolites after a given oral dosage. There is also a poor correlation between adverse effects of the drug and the plasma concentration of encainide or its metabolites. It is therefore not clinically useful to measure the plasma concentration of encainide or its metabolites on a routine basis.

Following repeated oral administration of encainide, steady-state plasma concentrations of the drug and its metabolites are obtained within 3 to 5 days in most patients with normal hepatic and renal function.

Although encainide has not been studied during pregnancy, our own unpublished data suggest that it does cross the placental barrier and is excreted in milk. The animal data available and the isolated case reports of women who have received the drug during their pregnancy have shown no teratogenic effects.

Following oral or intravenous administration of encainide, the drug and its metabolites are excreted in feces and urine in approximately equal amounts. The elimination half-life of encainide averages about 1 to 3 hours in patients with extensive oxidizer phenotypes and normal renal or hepatic function, but the half-life of encainide is prolonged to about 13 hours in adults with poor oxidizer phenotypes. The elimination half-life of ODE and MODE in adults with normal renal and hepatic function average about 3 to 11 hours and 12 hours, respectively.

In patients with cirrhosis of the liver, plasma clearance of encainide is markedly reduced; however, the elimination half-life remains within the normal range, apparently because of an associated decreased protein binding and an increased volume of distribution. Therefore, it is probably not necessary to alter the dosage of encainide for patients with liver disease. Elimination of ODE and MODE is reduced substantially in patients with renal impairment; therefore, comparatively lower doses of encainide should be used in those patients, and dose increments should not take place at intervals of less than 1 week. It is not known whether encainide and its metabolites are removed by hemodialysis or peritoneal dialysis.

CLINICAL USES

It is well known that patients who most need antiarrhythmic drugs, those with malignant ventricular arrhythmias and poor left ventricular function, are also those who are the least likely to tolerate them. This is true for any antiarrhythmic drug and is no less so for encainide.

Encainide has been shown to be very effective in the suppression of ventricular premature complexes, whether single or repetitive. In this respect, it surpasses in efficacy most other class I agents. However, it is less successful against more malignant arrhythmias, such as ventricular tachycardia or recurrent ventricular fibrillation. In such cases, encainide's efficacy is comparable to that of other class I agents

and is probably somewhat less than that of amiodarone. In the absence of studies directly comparing the efficacy of encainide in malignant arrhythmias with that of other antiarrhythmic agents, one must rely on the overall literature, results showing most class I agents to be effective in some 30 to 40 percent of such patients.

Who, then, should receive encainide? In view of the recent results from CAST, I would not recommend the use of encainide in any patient with benign or asymptomatic ventricular arrhythmias. In patients with symptomatic or malignant ventricular arrhythmias, the potential benefit of using encainide must be carefully weighed against the possible risks of proarrhythmia, which may range from a mere increase in the frequency of ventricular premature complexes to the development of sustained ventricular tachycardia or sudden death. The risk of proarrhythmia appears to be increased in patients with a previous myocardial infarction, a history of sustained ventricular tachycardia or ventricular fibrillation, the presence of congestive heart failure, or conduction disease. The reported incidence of proarrhythmia varies considerably from one center to another and depends largely on the population studied and the method of titration of the antiarrhythmic drugs.

In my view, all patients with a history of sustained ventricular tachycardia/ventricular fibrillation, congestive heart failure, or a left ventricular ejection fraction of 35 percent or less should be admitted to a monitored cardiac bed during the titration phase of antiarrhythmic drug therapy. This is especially true if the drug chosen for these patients is a class IC agent such as encainide. The initial dose of encainide should not exceed 25 mg every 8 hours, and the dose should not be increased except after 3 to 5 days, provided there is no evidence of proarrhythmia. Further increases in the dosage should take place gradually from 25 mg three times a day to 35 mg three times a day, then to 50 mg three times a day, then to 50 mg four times a day, and in very rare cases up to 75 mg three times a day. During the titration phase, QRS complex duration should not be allowed to increase beyond 0.16 to 0.18 second and P-R interval to increase beyond 0.24 second.

Should the patient develop a proarrhythmic sustained ventricular tachycardia, this is usually a wide complex, slow monomorphic ventricular tachycardia that is best treated by stopping encainide. The use of other antiarrhythmic agents or cardioversion should be avoided if possible. If the patient becomes hypotensive from the ventricular tachycardia, the use of a vasopressor such as norepinephrine for blood pressure support has been advocated as an alternative to cardioversion, which may prove to be risky in such a context.

As a general rule, when treating patients with ventricular arrhythmias, encainide should be reserved for those with symptomatic ventricular tachycardia, sustained or nonsustained, who have not responded to at least one other antiarrhythmic agent or those in whom the risk from using other agents appears to be greater.

Encainide in Supraventricular Arrhythmias

Because of the effect of the metabolites of encainide, ODE and MODE, on atrial and atrioventricular node refractoriness and on the conduction and refractoriness of accessory pathways, encainide may be suited for a variety of supraventricular arrhythmias, particularly those associated with an accessory pathway. Several preliminary studies in the literature show encainide to be useful in the conversion and prevention of paroxysmal supraventricular tachycardias, especially those associated with the Wolff-Parkinson-White syndrome. Encainide may also be extremely useful either in controlling the ventricular rate in cases of atrial fibrillation with the Wolff-Parkinson-White syndrome or in converting atrial fibrillation to sinus rhythm. However, these are only preliminary reports supporting this contention, and large controlled trials are needed to define further the role of encainide in supraventricular arrhythmia.

ADVERSE REACTIONS

Adverse reactions of any antiarrhythmic drug may be classified into cardiac and noncardiac. Cardiac adverse effects can be further subclassified into electrophysiologic and hemodynamic.

Cardiac Adverse Reactions

Electrophysiologic Adverse Effects

Encainide can occasionally cause sinus arrest of sinoatrial block in patients with preexisting sick sinus disease. However, in the experience of the author, these sinus pauses have never been symptomatic; many patients have been able to tolerate them while continuing to receive encainide.

A more significant, potential adverse effect is the effect on conduction. Patients with preexisting bundle branch block or bifascicular block or first- or second-degree atrioventricular block are at risk of further aggravation of the block. The effect of encainide and its metabolites on His-Purkinje conduction without concomitant increase in refractoriness may also in some cases be responsible for the development of proarrhythmic ventricular tachycardia.

Much has been said and written about the potential for class IC agents to worsen preexisting ventricular arrhythmia or to provoke new ones. The reported incidence of proarrhythmia with the use of encainide has varied widely, depending on the population studied, and ranges from 4 or 5 percent to 20 percent or more. Proarrhythmia is hard to define, since sometimes modest increases in frequency of ventricular premature complexes or ventricular tachycardic events per day have been considered proarrhythmia by some investigators but considered "spontaneous variability" by others. It is important for the clinician to realize that all antiarrhythmic drugs have the potential for proarrhythmic effects.

Although it is not always possible to predict who will have a proarrhythmic response to a given antiarrhythmic agent, it is fair to assume that the more severe the preexisting ventricular arrhythmia, the more severe the underlying heart disease; and the more severe the underlying conduction disease, the higher the risk for development of proarrhythmia. According to a recent report, 1,245 patients entered in various clinical studies using encainide for the control of ventricular arrhythmias were followed for a period ranging from 30 to 780 days. Of this total number, 84 percent had cardiac disease, and the incidence of proarrhythmia was 9.2 percent. The majority of these cases were identified within the first 20 days of therapy. Among 455 patients with previously documented sustained ventricular tachycardia, 12 percent developed proarrhythmia, and in 384 patients who had congestive heart failure, 11.7 percent developed proarrhythmia. In 187 patients with cardiomyopathy, 16 percent had proarrhythmia. Conversely, patients with no ventricular tachycardia with or without heart disease had a very low incidence of proarrhythmia, ranging from 3 to 6 percent. This represents the incidence of all forms of proarrhythmia, including those cases in which there was merely an increase in total frequency of ventricular premature complexes without sustained ventricular tachycardia. The overall incidence of new-onset sustained ventricular tachycardia believed to be caused by encainide was 2.7 percent. Although the risk of proarrhythmia is real, careful selection of the patient and careful titration of encainide might considerably reduce this risk.

Congestive Heart Failure

Like most antiarrhythmic drugs, encainide has the potential for worsening congestive heart failure in some patients with severe left ventricular dysfunction. However unlike many class I antiarrhythmics, encainide appears to be well tolerated by the majority of patients with left ventricular dysfunction. We had treated 25 patients with a mean ejection fraction of 23 percent, ranging from 6 to 45 percent at baseline. The New York Heart Association functional class was II in 24 percent, III in 36 percent, and IV in 40 percent. One to six weeks after initiation of therapy at a dose that controlled the ectopic activity (75 to 300 mg per day), the ejection fraction was unchanged and none of the patients had developed worsening of congestive heart failure. Twelve patients had a repeat study after 1 year and the ejection fraction remained unchanged. DiBianco and coworkers measured left ventricular function in 16 patients first on placebo and then on the dosage of encainide that suppressed ventricular premature complexes by 80 percent. Exercise duration while taking encainide (8.8 ± 3.8 minutes) was not significantly different from the 9.3 ± 3.8 minutes achieved at baseline. The average ejection fraction, heart rate, blood pressure, and rate-pressure product at rest or with exercise did not differ significantly from pre-drug values. Similar results were obtained by Tordjman and colleagues. In the safety report on encainide, one patient of 859 (0.1 percent) probably had new congestive heart failure related to the use of encainide and three of 386 patients (0.8 percent) had a worsening of congestive heart failure.

Noncardiac Adverse Reactions

The most common noncardiac adverse reactions encountered with encainide are dizziness and abnormal blurred vision. These may occur in up to 25 percent of patients. However, they are usually mild effects that frequently subside by reducing the total daily dose or by further dividing the drug into smaller doses. Other adverse reactions are rare, and the drug is particularly well tolerated by people with sensitive stomachs.

DRUG INTERACTIONS

Encainide has no significant effect on digoxin blood levels. It is of potential clinical relevance that cimetidine increases plasma levels of encainide and its metabolites by more than 30 percent. The mechanism of this effect is unknown. Although there are no systematic studies evaluating interactions between encainide and other drugs commonly used in cardiac patients, examination of the clinical course of the patients receiving concurrent medications suggests that digoxin, nifedipine, lidocaine, mexiletine, propranolol, tolbutamide, chlorpropamide, insulin, chlorpromazine, diazepam, warfarin, acenoumarol, and diuretics may be successfully used concurrently with encainide therapy. Concomitant administration of encainide and verapamil increases the incidence of heart block in dogs; however, retrospective data in humans do not seem to indicate serious drug interactions between these two drugs.

Other antiarrhythmic drugs may be dangerous to combine with encainide. For example, quinidine and amiodarone may be expected to interfere with encainide metabolism in patients with extensive oxidizer phenotype, and hence caution should be ob-

served if either of these drugs is administered concurrently with encainide. Drugs that are potentially useful in combination with encainide include lidocaine, which has resulted in additive suppression of arrhythmias in a small number of patients without pharmacokinetic interactions; mexiletine, because its electrophysiologic effects are similar to those of lidocaine; and sotalol, because its major electrophysiologic effect is on refractoriness (class III action), which may have synergistic antiarrhythmic action with encainide and at the same time reduce its potential for proarrhythmia. In the experience of the author, several patients with resistant ventricular arrhythmias have received combinations of sotalol and encainide successfully.

SUGGESTED READING

Abdollah H, Brugada P, Green M, et al. Clinical efficacy and electrophysiologic effects of intravenous and oral encainide in patients with accessory atrioventricular pathways and supraventricular arrhythmias. Am J Cardiol 1984; 54:544–549.

Barbey JT, Thompson KA, Echt DS, et al. Antiarrhythmic activity, electrocardiographic effects and pharmacokinetics of the encainide metabolites O-desmethyl encainide and 3-methoxy-O-desmethyl encainide in man. Circulation 1988; 77:380–391.

Bergstrand RH, Wang T, Roden DM, et al. Encainide disposition in patients with chronic cirrhosis. Clin Pharmacol Ther 1986; 40:148–154.

Bergstrand RH, Wang T, Roden DM, et al. Encainide disposition in patients with renal impairment. Clin Pharmacol Ther 1986; 40:64–70.

Brugada P, Abdollah H, Wellens HJJ. Suppression of incessant supraventricular tachycardia by intravenous and oral encainide. J Am Coll Cardiol 1984; 4:1255–1260.

Campbell RWF, Nicholson MR, Julian DG. Ventricular tachycardia—management with encainide (abstract). Eur Heart J 1981; 2 (Suppl A):185.

Capos NJ Jr, Kates RE, Harrison DC. Increased incidence of heartblock induced by combined encainide, encainide metabolites, and verapamil in dogs (abstract). Circulation 1983; 68(Suppl III):III–270.

The Cardiac Arrhythmia Pilot Study (CAPS) Investigators. Effects of encainide, flecainide, imipramine and moricizine on ventricular arrhythmias during the year after myocardial infarction: The CAPS. Am J Cardiol 1988; 61:501–509.

The Cardiac Arrhythmia Suppression Trial (CAST). Preliminary report: Effect of encainide and flecainide on mortality in a randomized trial of arrhythmia suppression after myocardial infarction. N Engl J Med 1989; 321:406–412.

Carey EL Jr, Duff HJ, Roden DM, et al. Encainide and its metabolites; comparative effects in man on ventricular arrhythmia and electrocardiographic intervals. J Clin Invest 1984; 73:539–547.

Caron JF, Libersa CC, Kher AR, et al. Comparative study of encainide and disopyramide in chronic ventricular arrhythmias: A double-blind placebo-controlled crossover study. J Am Coll Cardiol 1985; 5:1457–1463.

Chesnie B, Podrid P, Lown B, Raeder E. Encainide for refractory ventricular tachyarrhythmia. Am J Cardiol 1983; 52:495–500.

Davy J-M, Dorian P, Kantelip J-P, et al. Qualitative and quantitative comparison of the cardiac effects of encainide and its three major metabolites in the dog. J Pharmacol Exp Ther 1986; 237:907–1911.

DiBianco R, Fletcher RD, Cohen AI, et al. Treatment of frequent ventricular arrhythmia with encainide: Assessment using serial ambulatory electrocardiograms, intracardiac electrophysiologic studies, treadmill exercise tests and radionuclide cineangiographic studies. Circulation 1982; 85:1134–1147.

Guengerich FP, Umbenhauer DR, Churchill PF, et al. Polymorphism of human cytochrome P-450. Xenobiotica 1987; 17:311–316.

Horowitz LN. Encainide in lethal ventricular arrhythmias evaluated by electrophysiologic testing and decrease in symptoms. Am J Cardiol 1986; 58:83C–86C.

Jackman WM, Zipes DP, Naccarelli GV, et al. Electrophysiology of oral encainide. Am J Cardiol 1982; 49:1270–1278.

Kates RE, Harrison DC, Winkle RA. Metabolite cumulation during long-term oral encainide administration. Clin Pharmacol Ther 1982; 31:427–432.

Larrey D, Tinel M, Letteron P, et al. Formation of an inactive cytochrome P-450Fe(II)-metabolite complex after administration of amiodarone in rats, mice and hamsters. Biochem Pharmacol 1986; 35:2213–2220.

Lineberry MD, Davies RF, Chaffin PL, et al. Safety and efficacy of combining encainide and lidocaine. Circulation 1987; 76 (Suppl IV):IV–511. Abstract.

Markel ML, Prystowsky EN, Heger JJ, et al. Encainide for treatment of supraventricular tachycardias associated with the Wolff-Parkinson-White syndrome. Am J Cardiol 1986; 58:41C–48C.

Mason JW, Peters FA. Antiarrhythmic efficacy of encainide in patients with refractory recurrent ventricular tachycardia. Circulation 1981; 63:670–675.

McAllister CB, Wolfenden HT, Aslanian WS, et al. Oxidative metabolism of encainide: Polymorphism, pharmacokinetics and clinical considerations. Xenobiotica 1986; 5:483.

Morganroth J, Horowitz LN. Flecainide: Its proarrhythmic effect and expected changes on the surface electrocardiogram. Am J Cardiol 1984; 53:89B–94B.

Morganroth J, Pool P, Miller R, et al. Dose-response range of encainide for benign and potentially lethal ventricular arrhythmias. Am J Cardiol 1986; 57:769–774.

Nicholson MR, Campbell RWF, Julian DG. Encainide in management of ventricular tachycardia (abstract). Aust NZ J Med 1982; 12:313.

Quart BD, Gallo DG, Sami M, et al. Drug interaction studies and encainide use in renal and hepatic impairment. Am J Cardiol 1986; 58:104C–113C.

Rinkenberger RL, Prystowsky EN, Jackman WM, et al. Drug conversion of nonsustained ventricular tachycardia to sustained ventricular tachycardia during serial electrophysiologic studies: Identification of drugs that exacerbate tachycardia and potential mechanisms. Am Heart J 1982; 103:177–184.

Roden DM, Reele SB, Higgins SB, et al. Total suppression of ventricular arrhythmias by encainide: Pharmacokinetic and electrocardiographic characteristics. N Engl J Med 1980; 302:877–882.

Sami M, Derbekyan VA, Lisbona R. Hemodynamic effects of encainide in patients with ventricular arrhythmia and poor ventricular function. Am J Cardiol 1983; 52:507–511.

Sami M, Harrison DC, Kraemer H, et al. Antiarrhythmic efficacy of encainide and quinidine: Validation of a model for drug assessment. Am J Cardiol 1981; 48:147–156.

Sami M, Mason, JW, Oh G, Harrison DC. Canine electrophysiology of encainide, a new antiarrhythmic drug. Am J Cardiol 1979; 43:1149–1154.

Sami M, Mason JW, Peters F, Harrison DC. Clinical electrophysiologic effects of encainide, a newly developed antiarrhythmic agent. Am J Cardiol 1979; 44:526–532.

Sokya LF. Safety of encainide for the treatment of ventricular arrhythmias. Am J Cardiol 1986; 58:96C–103C.

Tordjman T, Podrid PJ, Raeder E, Lown B. Encainide for malignant ventricular arrhythmias. Am J Cardiol 1986; 58:87C–95C.

Velebit V, Podrid PJ, Lown B, et al. Aggravation and provocation of ventricular arrhythmias by antiarrhythmic drugs. Circulation 1982; 65:886–894.

Wang T, Roden DM, Wolfenden HT, et al. Influence of genetic polymorphism on the metabolism and disposition of encainide in man. J Pharmacol Exp Ther 1984; 228:605–611.

Winkle RA, Mason JW, Griffin JC, Ross D. Malignant ventricular tachyarrhythmias associated with the use of encainide. Am Heart J 1981; 102:857–864.

Winkle RA, Peters F, Kates RE, Harrison DC. Possible contribution of encainide metabolites to the long-term antiarrhythmic efficacy of encainide. Am J Cardiol 1983; 51:1182–1188.

Wong SS, Myerburg RJ, Ezrin AM, et al. Electrophysiologic effects of encainide on acutely ischemic rabbit myocardial cells. Eur J Pharmacol 1982; 80:323–329.

FLECAINIDE

JEFFREY L. ANDERSON, M.D.

Flecainide acetate (Tambocor) represents a prototype of a new class of antiarrhythmic agents (class IC). The development of new antiarrhythmic drugs over the past decade has been motivated by the recognition that traditional antiarrhythmic therapy is often problematic because of inadequate antiarrhythmic activity, intolerable side effects, or compliance problems as a result of unfavorable pharmacokinetics. In this setting, flecainide is of importance because of the improved tolerance and effectiveness

for certain ventricular and supraventricular arrhythmias that it demonstrates. Flecainide was synthesized in 1972, first tested in human trials in 1978, and approved for marketing in the United States in December, 1984. Flecainide shows antiarrhythmic activity for many ventricular and supraventricular arrhythmias. However, because of concern for its proarrhythmic effects and the results of the recently reported Cardiac Arrhythmia Suppression Trial (CAST), its only current officially approved indication is for life-threatening ventricular arrhythmias such as ventricular tachycardia or fibrillation. As the implications of CAST for flecainide and other class IC agents (such as encainide) and class I antiarrhythmic agents in general are clarified, the future application of this and similar drugs will be better defined.

GENERAL DESCRIPTION OF PHARMACOLOGY

Pharmacokinetics

Flecainide is a long-acting antiarrhythmic drug possessing a favorable pharmacologic profile that allows relatively precise correlations of dose, plasma concentration, electrocardiographic effects, and antiarrhythmic action (Table 1). Its half-life averages 14 hours after a single dose in normal subjects but about 20 hours (range 12 to 30) in patients with arrhythmias who are receiving multiple-dose therapy. Because of the drug's prolonged half-life, a steady state is not reached for 3 to 5 days during continued oral dosing. Twice daily dosing is adequate to establish therapeutic plasma concentrations and to maintain continuous arrhythmia control, and it allows for easy patient compliance. Flecainide is well absorbed after oral dosing. Bioavailability generally exceeds 90 percent and is relatively unaffected by food or antacid. Increases in dose lead to approximately proportionate increases in plasma concentrations. Flecainide excretion is accounted for almost entirely by urinary excretion of unchanged drug and metabolites. Alkalinization of urine increases renal drug clearance. Flecainide is only partially protein-bound (about 40 percent).

Clinical effects of flecainide are attributable almost entirely to parent drug that can be measured in plasma by a clinically available assay. The two major metabolites of flecainide (dealkylation products) possess little or no antiarrhythmic activity.

Minor drug interactions have been described with digoxin, propranolol, and cimetidine, resulting in 10 to 30 percent increases in plasma drug concentrations during coadministration.

Effects on Electrophysiology and Electrocardiography

Flecainide, like other class I antiarrhythmic agents, displays membrane-stabilizing activity because of its interaction with sodium channels. However, its electrophysiologic profile is relatively unique compared with that of traditional agents.

The result is a substantial depression of conduction velocity associated with only modest effects on refractoriness. Flecainide's potent antiarrhythmic effects are related to the intensity and duration of sodium channel blockade. Class IC agents have the longest associated time constant for membrane recovery from sodium channel blockade (flecainide = 30 seconds), class IA agents have intermediate effects (quinidine = 5.0 seconds), and class IB agents have the most transient actions (lidocaine = 0.3 seconds).

During oral therapy, flecainide has distinct effects on the electrocardiogram, including dose-dependent prolongation of P-R and QRS intervals and only modest increases in Q-T interval that are explained by QRS rather than J-T segment changes. Flecainide depresses conduction in all parts of the heart, with greatest effects on the His-Purkinje system. Modest effects on refractoriness are observed in the ventricle and atrium and few effects in atrioventricular nodal and His-Purkinje tissue. Accessory pathway refractory periods are often more dramatically changed (increased). Sinus node recovery times are usually little affected unless underlying conduction system disease (e.g., sick sinus syndrome) is present, in which case substantial prolongation may occur. In clinical practice, therapeutic doses of flecainide (200 to 400 mg every day) may be expected to increase P-R and QRS intervals by 10 to 30 percent and Q-T intervals by 5 to 10 percent.

Flecainide therapy may alter acute and chronic pacing thresholds to a clinically significant degree in patients receiving pacemakers.

Effects on Hemodynamics

Flecainide is generally well tolerated hemodynamically but does possess mild to moderate negative inotropic potential. Experience in clinical trials with flecainide showed an overall rate of heart failure of 5 percent during therapy, including a 1 percent incidence in patients with no prior history and a 10 to 20 percent rate in those with a prior history of heart failure. These figures suggest that flecainide is better tolerated hemodynamically than disopyramide. In the Cardiac Arrhythmia Pilot Study (CAPS), the incidence of heart failure during the first year after myocardial infarction was only modestly increased during flecainide therapy compared with placebo therapy (difference not significant) and also appeared to be greater than with encainide.

In patients receiving flecainide for serious ventricular arrhythmias, hemodynamic deterioration has been observed, primarily in those with advanced left ventricular dysfunction (ejection fraction less than 30 percent) and with advanced clinical heart failure class (New York Heart Association class III or IV).

Table 1 Pharmacokinetics Summary of Flecainide

Antiarrhythmic drug class: Vaughan Williams class IC
Route of administration: oral (also intravenous outside US)
Usual daily dose: 100–400 mg/day
Therapeutic plasma concentration: 0.2–1.0 μg/ml
Oral bioavailability: 90%
Plasma half-life: 12–30 hours (mean, 20 hours)
Plasma drug clearance: 8–10 ml/min/kg
Apparent volume of distribution: 10 liters/kg
Plasma protein binding: 40%
Urinary excretion of unchanged drug: 30%

ANTIARRHYTHMIC ACTIONS OF FLECAINIDE: EXPECTATIONS BASED ON A REVIEW OF CLINICAL STUDIES

Response of Ventricular Arrhythmias

Studies in patients with chronic, stable ventricular premature complexes (VPCs) of varying etiology demonstrated the ability of flecainide to suppress VPCs effectively (more than 80 percent) in about 85 percent of patients treated. Average suppression of total VPCs has averaged about 95 percent, and of repetitive VPCs, about 98 percent. Long-term effectiveness without adverse effects has been achieved in about 70 percent of patients. Flecainide has also been shown to suppress VPCs in the post–myocardial infarction population to a similar degree, but because of an increased risk of mortality associated with therapy (CAST study), treatment is not indicated in this group.

Flecainide has been compared with several traditional and newer antiarrhythmic agents given in clinically recommended doses. In several comparative trials, direct comparisons with quinidine have suggested that flecainide shows greater suppression of isolated and repetitive VPCs, increases P-R and QRS intervals more and Q-T interval less on electrocardiography than quinidine, and is better tolerated, with neurologic rather than gastrointestinal effects being more common. Similarly, comparison with disopyramide has suggested a superior suppression and tolerance for treatment of frequent VPCs with flecainide. Flecainide was more effective than propafenone, and both were more effective than mexiletine in another comparative study of VPC therapy. VPC suppression with flecainide has also been favorably compared with amiodarone in other studies. Flecainide and encainide were highly effective for therapy of post–myocardial infarction VPCs and more effective than the other agents tested (moricizine and imipramine) in the Cardiac Arrhythmia Pilot Study (CAPS), but they were later shown to increase the risk of cardiac arrest in this setting (CAST study).

Flecainide may be effective in about 60 percent of patients with a history of sustained ventricular tachycardia when ambulatory monitoring is used as an end point, but it is effective in a lower percentage (20 to 35 percent) when electrophysiologic testing, which is often preferred in these patients, is used as the therapeutic end point. Among patients with sustained ventricular tachycardia who undergo electrophysiologic testing, a lower complete response rate may be expected in those with coronary artery disease and left ventricular dysfunction (akinetic or dyskinetic segments, ejection fraction less than 30 to 40 percent) than in those without these characteristics. In patients in whom the ventricular tachycardia is not completely suppressed, flecainide typically slows the rate of induced ventricular tachycardia and may cause improved hemodynamic tolerance in some of these. More ready induction or more frequent spontaneous occurrences of ventricular tachycardia, and poor hemodynamic tolerance, whatever the ventricular tachycardia rate, are reasons to pursue alternative therapies.

Response of Supraventricular Tachyarrhythmia

Although it is still investigational for therapy of supraventricular tachyarrhythmia in the United States, flecainide has been used in several trials both intravenously (abroad) and orally (United States and abroad) for spontaneously occurring or electrophysiologically induced supraventricular tachyarrhythmia with promising results. In an overview of these studies, flecainide was judged to be effective in about 70 percent (73 percent of acute, intravenous trials and 66 percent of oral trials). Intravenous flecainide may be expected to terminate atrioventricular nodal reentrant tachycardia in 80 percent of patients and to be effective and well tolerated for oral prophylaxis in 70 to 80 percent. A similar experience may be observed with atrioventricular reentrant tachycardia using a concealed bypass tract.

Paroxysmal atrial fibrillation, a more difficult rhythm to treat, may be eliminated in about 35 percent of patients and substantially reduced in frequency overall. The average interval between attacks with therapy has been shown to be lengthened by four- to fivefold. Flecainide also has been effective for termination of atrial fibrillation of recent onset in about 60 percent of patients given intravenous and/or oral therapy. Atrial flutter and chronic atrial fibrillation, as expected, are much less responsive to therapy.

The Wolff-Parkinson-White syndrome is associated with ortho- and antidromically conducting atrioventricular reentrant tachycardias and paroxysmal atrial fibrillation that may be highly symptomatic and refractory to therapy. Flecainide has shown promise in these patients, being judged successful in about 75 percent of acute intravenous trials and in about 60 percent of patients tested after oral therapy. Approximately half of these patients show long-term benefit with maintained tolerance and effectiveness.

Recent experience suggests that flecainide may also be exceptionally effective and well tolerated in children with symptomatic supraventricular arrhythmias requiring therapy.

SAFETY AND ADVERSE POTENTIAL

Noncardiac Adverse Effects

Relative to other antiarrhythmic drugs, flecainide is unusually well tolerated, although minor adverse effects may be seen. Discontinuation of therapy because of noncardiac adverse effects may be required in only 5 to 10 percent of treated patients. Reports of biochemical or organ toxicity have not been characteristic of flecainide therapy and have rarely been reported.

Adverse effects most commonly take the form of visual symptoms, including blurred vision and difficulty in accommodation, particularly on lateral gaze. Lightheadedness or dizziness is frequently an accompanying or alternate symptom. About 30 percent of patients receiving an average daily dose of 400 mg may notice these effects, usually occurring transiently after a drug dose. Often they are minor and resolve with continued therapy, but in others they require downward adjustment of the dose. Complaints of nausea, headache, anxiety, ataxia, or chest pain associated with therapy may be reported in 5 percent or less of patients.

Cardiac Adverse Effects

Adverse rhythm effects and heart failure form two categories of important adverse cardiac potential. Their understanding is of great importance to the appropriate use of flecainide. Ventricular proarrhythmia may take the form of increased frequency of VPCs, increased salvos of repetitive complexes (either spontaneously or at electrophysiologic study), and, occasionally, induction of new arrhythmia or of clinical arrhythmia that is more frequent, incessant, and/or more difficult to convert.

The risk of ventricular proarrhythmia is dependent on the clinical substrate as well as the drug dosing regimen. In overall experience, proarrhythmic effects have been reported to occur in 7 percent of patients treated with flecainide; these were considered serious in 3 percent. Proarrhythmia risk is substantially higher and more serious in those with organic (especially ischemic) heart disease and a history of sustained ventricular tachycardia than in those without these factors. In one large data base, *serious* proarrhythmia occurred in 7 percent of patients with a history of sustained ventricular tachycardia, 1 percent with unsustained ventricular tachycardia, and none with isolated VPCs alone. Similarly, proarrhythmia occurred in 3 percent of those with structural heart disease (most commonly ischemic) versus 0.4 percent of those without organic disease. Death attributed to proarrhythmia was reported in 1.2 percent versus 0 percent of these two groups, respectively.

Of further interest is the differential effect on serious or fatal proarrhythmia of the dosing regimen. In initial experience, when high or rapidly incrementing doses of flecainide were used in seriously ill patients with ventricular tachycardia refractory to other agents, 10 percent (10 of 100 patients) suffered proarrhythmic death versus 0.5 percent (1 of 198 patients) in the subsequent low initial dose, slow incrementation regimen that is currently recommended. The vast majority of proarrhythmic events have been observed to occur within a few days to 2 weeks after dose initiation or incrementation.

Sudden arrhythmic death or cardiac arrest is a further proarrhythmic risk of flecainide, recently defined by the CAST study. In this study, prognostically important but asymptomatic ventricular arrhythmias in patients with recent myocardial infarction were treated with active antiarrhythmic therapy or matching placebo. Among 1,455 patients treated with the class IC agents encainide or flecainide, mortality over a follow-up period of 10 months was increased from 3.0 to 7.7 percent (22 versus 56 deaths), and sudden death or cardiac arrest was increased from nine (1.2 percent) to 33 (4.5 percent) events. The majority of the excess events occurred in patients with a history of *multiple* myocardial infarctions, low ejection fraction, recent myocardial infarction (within 90 days), and high-frequency initial ventricular ectopic activity. The mechanism of this excess cardiac arrest is unknown. It may have involved (1) the usual pattern of proarrhythmic events (however, all patients entering blinded therapy showed more than 80 percent VPC *suppression* on initial monitoring without proarrhythmia, and events occurred throughout the follow-up period), or (2) increased propensity to ventricular fibrillation in the setting of advanced ischemic heart disease with potentially recurrent ischemic events (e.g., reduced ischemic ventricular fibrillation threshold). In either case, it is apparent that the survival outcome with flecainide (or encainide) therapy in patients with high-risk characteristics in the post–myocardial infarction setting cannot be predicted by the response on Holter monitor recordings. There are other tests of risk and response, such as exercise treadmill, electrophysiologic study, and possibly signal averaged electrocardiography, that may perhaps be more accurate in predicting adverse as well as successful outcomes. Meanwhile, most myocardial infarction patients with prognostically important but asymptomatic VPCs should not be treated with flecainide (or encainide and possibly other class I drugs) as guided by Holter monitor recordings.

Proarrhythmia in patients with supraventricular tachyarrhythmia (such as atrial flutter or atrioventricular reentry) may also take the form of more readily occurring or readily induced or more incessant (although often slower) supraventricular tachyarrhythmia. Occasionally, patients with atrial flutter may present with a rapid (175 to 250 beats per minute), unstable rhythm ascribed to slowing of an atrial rate sufficient to allow 1:1 atrioventricular conduction. Treatment of paroxysmal atrial fibrillation may occasionally be associated with increased frequency or duration of attacks or the appearance of incessant atrial flutter. Unexpected episodes of ventricular tachycardia or ventricular fibrillation, often during extreme exercise, have been rarely reported in patients with chronic atrial fibrillation who received flecainide for control of ventricular rate.

Significant conduction disturbances have been reported in about 2 percent of patients receiving flecainide but have generally not proved fatal. These occurrences have related more to preexisting conduction system disease than to underlying ventricular dysfunction. These effects have taken the form of sick sinus syndrome, advanced atrioventricular block (second or third degree), or new bundle branch block. Significant preexisting disease of sinus or atrioventricular nodes or bi- or trifascicular His-Purkinje block should raise particular concern when considering flecainide therapy.

Flecainide has been observed to increase the threshold for pacemaker capture to a variable but occasionally dramatic degree. Thus flecainide may be best avoided or given cautiously in patients who are pacemaker-dependent.

Congestive Heart Failure

Flecainide is well tolerated hemodynamically in patients without preexisting ventricular dysfunction but shows moderate negative inotropic potential in those with a history of heart failure. Overall, heart failure has developed in about 1 percent of patients without a prior history compared with 10 to 20 percent of those with a prior history. In the CAPS, the actuarial 1-year incidence of heart failure was 27 percent during placebo and 35 percent during flecainide therapy (trend not significant). Treatment of these patients varied. In some, flecainide was continued with adjustment of medical therapy, and in others it was discontinued. In other experiences, the risk of adverse hemodynamic outcome was shown to reside in patients with functional class III or IV heart failure and/or an ejection fraction of less than 30 percent. Based on this experience, the author tends to avoid the use of flecainide in most patients with functional class III or IV failure and an ejection fraction of less than 25 to 30 percent.

ANTIARRHYTHMIC INDICATIONS FOR FLECAINIDE

Currently, flecainide is officially indicated only for life-threatening arrhythmias, such as ventricular tachycardia or fibrillation. However, the author believes that experimental trials and clinical experience suggest the beneficial application of flecainide for indications shown in Table 2. Such therapy must be balanced against the risk of flecainide, particularly in groups suggested in Table 3. A careful assessment of the benefit-risk ratio is important to all antiarrhythmic therapy and particularly so for class IC agents.

Table 2 Arrhythmias That May Benefit from Therapy with Flecainide

1. *Prevention†* of symptomatic paroxysmal supraventricular tachyarrhythmias, such as
   a. Paroxysmal supraventricular tachycardias (e.g., atrioventricular nodal reentrant tachycardias, atrioventricular [bypass tract–mediated] reentrant tachycardias, intraatrial reentrant or automatic or unspecified mechanisms)
   b. Paroxysmal atrial fibrillation or fibrillation/flutter
   c. Paroxysmal supraventricular tachycardia/paroxysmal atrial fibrillation associated with the Wolff-Parkinson-White syndrome

2. *Prevention of life-threatening ventricular arrhythmias,* such as
   a. Sustained ventricular tachycardia
   b. Ventricular fibrillation
   c. Symptomatic, hemodynamically significant unsustained ventricular tachycardia

3. Treatment of non–life-threatening‡ ventricular arrhythmias such as frequent premature ventricular complexes and/or unsustained ventricular tachycardia associated with *debilitating symptoms*

---

*In the author's view.
†When intravenous flecainide is available, it may also be used for acute termination of supraventricular tachycardias.
‡See also contraindications and precautions, Table 3.

PRACTICAL ASPECTS OF FLECAINIDE THERAPY: DOSING RECOMMENDATIONS

For most indications, the appropriate starting dose of flecainide is 100 mg every 12 hours. Initiation of therapy with 50 mg, two or three times a day, may be appropriate for patients with paroxysmal supraventricular tachycardia, a more responsive ar-

Table 3 Contraindications and Cautions for the Use of Flecainide

Contraindications
Ventricular arrhythmias (ventricular premature complexes and/or unsustained ventricular tachycardia) that are asymptomatic or mildly symptomatic non–life-threatening in patients with a history of myocardial infarction
Cardiogenic shock
Known flecainide hypersensitivity
Second- or third-degree atrioventricular block
Bifascicular, trifascicular bundle branch block (in the absence of a pacemaker)

Cautions (Relative Contraindications)
Heart failure (FC III or IV; ejection fraction <25–30%)
Permanent pacemaker with pacemaker-dependent rhythm
History of sustained ventricular tachycardia or ventricular fibrillation (and other potentially responsive rhythms) in association with advanced coronary artery disease, previous multiple myocardial infarctions, and/or severe left ventricular dysfunction
Need for concomitant use of other medications that depress conduction or contraction (especially verapamil, disopyramide)

rhythmia, and in small or elderly patients or those with disposition problems (see below). Dosage may be increased, as needed, in increments of 50 mg twice a day every 3 to 7 days or until efficacy has been achieved or a total dose of 200 mg every 12 hours (200 mg per day) has been reached. Increases in dosage beyond this level rarely improve the benefit-risk outcome, although it has been stated that in patients whose arrhythmias remain symptomatic and whose plasma levels remain suboptimal (below about 0.6 μg per milliliter), dosage may be cautiously further increased to a maximum of 600 mg per day. (I have not exceeded the 400 mg per day limit of flecainide in my personal practice over several years.) Use of higher initial doses and more rapid dosing adjustments than these have resulted in an increased incidence of adverse effects, including proarrhythmia and heart failure, particularly during the first days after dose initiation or dose change. For this reason as well, a loading dose is not recommended.

Flecainide therapy should generally be initiated on an inpatient basis for those being treated for a history of sustained ventricular tachycardia or ventricular fibrillation, those with significant left ventricular dysfunction and complex although unsustained arrhythmias, and those with the potential for developing sinus node dysfunction or other conduction disturbances. For patients with stable rhythm substrate without life-threatening arrhythmias (such as cases of supraventricular tachyarrhythmia) and highly symptomatic but prognostically nonlethal ventricular arrhythmias requiring treatment, outpatient initiation has often been used.

Conditions of Altered Dosing

In patients with severe renal failure, initial dosage should be 100 mg per day or less, given in one or two doses. Careful monitoring of response over an extended period of time (more than 1 to 2 weeks) and measurement of plasma drug concentrations are performed to guide therapy further. With less severe renal failure, a dose of 100 mg every 12 hours may be given but with more cautious dose incrementation. Other patients who should receive conservative dosing regimens include the elderly, those of low body weight (less than 50 kg), and those with hepatic dysfunction. Children are most effectively dosed on a milligram per kilogram or, preferably, a milligram per square meter of body surface area basis. When flecainide is given concurrently with amiodarone (rarely indicated), the usual dosage should be reduced by 50 percent and the patient monitored for adverse reactions. Concurrent therapy with digoxin, cimetidine, and propranolol has also been shown to cause modest increases in flecainide drug levels that may or may not require dose adjustment.

MANAGEMENT OF OVERDOSE OR ADVERSE RHYTHM EFFECTS OF STANDARD DOSING

Supportive care and continuous monitoring form the initial approach to the management of flecainide overdose or adverse dosing. After recent ingestion, the usual therapy (e.g., charcoal, magnesium citrate) may be used. Hypotension may be managed with expansion of intravascular volume with intravenous fluids and, if necessary, vasoconstrictors to support blood pressure. For associated proarrhythmic effects, there have been a few reports of successful use of sodium lactate or sodium bicarbonate. The mechanism of action of these agents is uncertain but may involve reversal of sodium channel blockade and treatment of acidosis. An attempt to convert sustained ventricular or atrial tachycardia with the usual measures (pacing, cardioversion) may be tried initially. If arrhythmias are incessant and refractory to conversion but the patient is hemodynamically stable, a period of supportive care is usually effective until flecainide is eliminated. Lidocaine has been used along with flecainide in some series without adverse effect and occasionally with benefit. Intravenous procainamide has occasionally been used in order to maintain slowing of ventricular tachycardia rate during gradual elimination of flecainide in patients with a proarrhythmic response and marginal, rate-dependent hemodynamic compensation.

Intravenous flecainide, often given in a dose of 2 mg per kilogram per 10 minutes, is available in many countries and has been used primarily for acute termination of supraventricular tachycardias. Hypotension or acute heart block or bradyarrhythmia is a potential complication of this form of therapy. The usual measures of blood pressure support for the former and temporary pacing for the latter two complications are appropriate.

ASSESSMENT OF THE RESULTS OF THERAPY

Table 4 outlines potential methods of assessing antiarrhythmic efficacy. These include noninvasive and invasive electrocardiographic and associated

Table 4 Methods of Arrhythmia Assessment and Therapy

Symptom history
Noninvasive: Electrocardiography
    Ambulatory (Holter) monitoring (24–48 hour)
    Exercise (treadmill) testing
    Transtelephonic event monitoring
    Signal-averaged electrocardiography*
Invasive: Electrophysiology
    Programmed electrical stimulation

*No role yet shown for assessing results of therapy.

symptom assessment and plasma drug concentration monitoring. In patients in whom therapy is primarily used to relieve symptoms, reduction in arrhythmia-related symptoms forms an important end point. However, because of the potential for proarrhythmic effects, I also prefer to make an objective (monitored) assessment of rhythm response during therapy and at baseline for comparisons. Ambulatory (Holter) monitoring has formed a standard approach to arrhythmia assessment for most of these patients and electrophysiologic study for those patients with malignant or life-threatening ventricular and occasionally supraventricular (e.g., Wolff-Parkinson-White syndrome–related) arrhythmias. Continuous telemetric or ambulatory (Holter) monitoring is first useful to exclude worrisome increases (sometimes asymptomatic) in rhythm in occasional patients.

Because proarrhythmia (wide complex tachycardia) may be manifested only during exercise testing even in patients with suppression of ambient arrhythmia during resting conditions, it has been suggested that exercise testing be used as an additional method of assessing outcome, complementary to Holter monitoring. Although such an approach has not been extensively tested and/or universally applied, it does appear inherently reasonable and is readily available. Its use may be particularly helpful in patients requiring therapy with flecainide who have special risk factors for proarrhythmia (e.g., coronary artery disease with angina or myocardial infarction, left ventricular dysfunction, chronic atrial fibrillation).

Plasma levels of flecainide may be measured by commercially available assays, and a therapeutic range has been broadly defined as 0.2 to 1.0 μg per milliliter. As noted, a general correlation between drug dose, plasma flecainide level, and drug efficacy and adverse effects exists. However, as with other drugs, assessment of an individual's specific response to a specific drug dose or plasma concentration is more important than comparisons to a group standard. Thus, use of plasma level monitoring is not routinely required but may be helpful in the following circumstances: (1) to ensure patient compliance when doubt exists, (2) to assist in monitoring potential drug toxicity in patients with potentially altered metabolism (see above), (3) to assess potential drug overdose, and (4) to help evaluate potentially drug-related adverse cardiac and noncardiac effects. For plasma concentrations of less than 1.0 μg per milliliter, up to 90 percent of patients achieve over 80 percent suppression of ventricular arrhythmias, whereas for levels over 0.8 to 1.0 μg per milliliter, an increasing incidence of cardiac and noncardiac adverse effects is noted, progressively narrowing the benefit-risk ratio.

SUGGESTED READING

Anastasiou-Nana MI, Anderson JL, Stewart JR, et al. Occurrence of exercise-induced wide-complex tachycardia during therapy with flecainide for complex ventricular arrhythmias: A probable proarrhythmic effect. Am Heart J 1987; 113:1071–1077.

Anderson JL, Stewart JR, Perry BA, et al. Oral flecainide acetate for the treatment of ventricular arrhythmias. N Engl J Med 1981; 305:473–477.

Anderson JL, Lutz JR, Allison SB. Electrophysiologic and antiarrhythmic effects of oral flecainide in patients with inducible ventricular tachycardia. J Am Coll Cardiol 1983; 2:105–114.

Flecainide Ventricular Tachycardia Study Group. Treatment of resistant ventricular tachycardia with flecainide acetate. Am J Cardiol 1986; 57:1299–1304.

Morganroth J, Anderson JL, Gentzkow GD. Classification by type of ventricular arrhythmia predicts frequency of adverse cardiac events from flecainide. J Am Coll Cardiol 1986; 8:607–615.

Pritchett ELC, Anderson JL, eds. International symposium on supraventricular arrhythmias: Focus on flecainide. Am J Cardiol 1988; 65:1D–67D.

Roden DM, Woosley RL. Flecainide. N Engl J Med 1986; 315:36–41.

Symposium on flecainide therapy for ventricular arrhythmias. Am J Cardiol 1984; 53:Suppl B.

The Cardiac Arrhythmia Suppression Trial (CAST) Investigators. Preliminary report: Effect of encainide and flecainide on mortality in a randomized trial of arrhythmic suppression after myocardial infarction. N Engl J Med 1989; 321:406–412.

LIDOCAINE

DANIEL S. CONTRAFATTO, M.D.

HISTORY

Lidocaine was introduced to clinical medicine in 1943 as a local anesthetic agent. It was first used as a treatment for ventricular arrhythmias in 1950 by Southworth and coworkers when it successfully terminated an episode of ventricular tachycardia during cardiac catheterization. Used primarily by anesthesiologists during the 1950s for intraoperative ventricular arrhythmias, it was not until 1959 that lidocaine began to be used for the treatment of ventricular arrhythmias during cardiac surgery. Lidocaine enjoyed immediate popularity as a first-line parenteral agent for ventricular arrhythmias, which continues to this day. This is because of its ease of administration, rapid therapeutic effect, short half-life, and lack of detrimental hemodynamic effects.

PHARMACOLOGY

Lidocaine is a class IB antiarrhythmic agent in the modified Vaughan Williams classification. It is a local anesthetic agent with no effect on the autonomic nervous system.

This agent demonstrates variable effects on phase 0 of the cardiac action potential, ranging from minimal depression of depolarization in normal tissue to moderate depression in ischemic or partially depolarized tissue. The effects are most exaggerated in the presence of elevated extracellular potassium levels and reduced pH or reduced membrane potential, all conditions common during ischemia. Lidocaine generally shortens action potential duration and repolarization. Therefore it does not prolong ventricular refractoriness. The electrophysiologic effects are less marked in atrial myocardium, which may explain this agent's limited effectiveness in the treatment of supraventricular arrhythmias.

Lidocaine has a variable but usually minimal effect on atrioventricular and intraventricular conduction. However, heart block may rarely be precipitated in the presence of bifascicular or trifascicular block in the setting of acute myocardial infarction. Effects on the surface electrocardiogram are minimal. The P-R, QRS, and Q-T (as well as J-T) intervals in general are not significantly affected. Lidocaine does not affect slow channel–dependent action potentials and therefore has little effect on sinus nodal automaticity.

In therapeutic doses, lidocaine has negligible hemodynamic effects. Although it can reduce arterial blood pressure, the effect is modest. It is essentially free from any significant negative inotropic effect and can be administered safely even in the setting of compromised left ventricular function.

Although it is readily absorbed from the gastrointestinal tract, oral administration of lidocaine is precluded by extensive first-pass hepatic metabolism. Although the drug is usually administered intravenously, intramuscular injections can also provide therapeutic blood levels. Significant liver dysfunction or conditions that decrease hepatic blood flow (cardiac failure, hypotension, cardiogenic shock) decrease lidocaine metabolism and clearance and increase the plasma concentration. Consequently a 50 percent reduction in the maintenance dose of lidocaine should be contemplated in patients with these disorders in order to avoid toxicity. Likewise, drugs that decrease hepatic blood flow, such as cimetidine, propranolol, or norepinephrine, can also decrease lidocaine clearance. In contrast, phenobarbital (by induction of the microsomal enzyme system) and isoproterenol (by increasing hepatic blood flow) can facilitate lidocaine clearance. These factors may all alter the therapeutic and toxic effects of the drug.

After intravenous administration of lidocaine, only 10 percent of the drug is excreted unchanged in the urine. Thus, abnormal renal function has no significant effect on lidocaine pharmacokinetics. Approximately 90 percent of the administered drug is rapidly metabolized in the liver into two major active metabolites—monoethylglycinexylidide (MEGX) and glycinexylidide (GX). In experimental preparations, MEGX was found to be 80 percent as potent as lidocaine and GX was found to be 10 percent as potent. Since MEGX can achieve significant concentrations in the body, it may contribute to the antiarrhythmic effect of lidocaine. Unlike lidocaine, these metabolites are excreted in the urine. Although GX can accumulate in patients with renal failure, MEGX generally does not because it is further de-ethylated to GX. Both compounds can contribute to central nervous system toxicity by causing or potentiating seizure activity.

The disposition of lidocaine injected intravenously follows a three-phase pattern described as peaking, distribution, and elimination. Phase 1 (peaking) involves the rapid distribution of the administered drug to the highly perfused organs. The rapidity with which lidocaine enters the heart probably accounts for the rapid therapeutic effect observed. Phase 2 (distribution) lasts approximately 20 minutes and involves the movement (i.e., diffusion) of drug from highly perfused organs to other tissues until equilibrium is achieved. This phase accounts for the short duration of therapeutic effect following bolus administration. Phase 3 (elimination) is the decline in blood level, primarily as a result of metabolic elimination of the drug. The elimination half-life of lidocaine is 1.5 hours in normal subjects, a mean of 3.2 hours in subjects with uncomplicated myocardial infarction when measured after discontinuing an infusion lasting longer than 24 hours, and longer than 10 hours in patients with myocardial infarction complicated by cardiac failure.

Seventy percent of lidocaine is bound to plasma proteins. The primary binding protein is alpha-1-acid glycoprotein. This is an acute phase reactant that increases in the setting of myocardial infarction. This accounts for increasing plasma concentrations of lidocaine during treatment of patients with myocardial infarction with constant infusion. As the level of alpha-1-acid glycoprotein increases, the total drug level also increases. Since enhanced binding reduces drug clearance, this explains the increased elimination half-life during uncomplicated myocardial infarction and the apparent effect of lidocaine's impairment of its own elimination after prolonged administration in this setting.

The therapeutic plasma level for lidocaine ranges from 1.6 to 5.0 μg per milliliter. Below 1.6 μg per milliliter, the antiarrhythmic effects of the drug are minimal. Above 5.0 μg per milliliter, toxic effects, particularly central nervous system depression, may predominate. In patients with normal hepatic blood flow and function, the plasma clearance of lidocaine is 10 ml per kilogram per minute. In patients with heart failure, the clearance is reduced by 50 percent. With this knowledge one can determine optimal infusion rates, since at steady state the infusion rate (micrograms per kilogram per minute) is equal to the desired steady-state plasma concentration (micrograms per milliliter) multiplied by the clearance (milliliters per kilogram per minute).

Although lidocaine can be administered intramuscularly, the intravenous route is most commonly used. Intramuscular administration of 4 to 5 mg per kilogram can produce effective serum levels in 15 minutes that last for 90 minutes. Several administration protocols have been devised for intravenous administration. The continuous infusion of 150 to 250 mg of lidocaine over 10 to 20 minutes or the administration of sequential 50-mg boluses every 5 minutes to a total dose of 200 to 250 mg will provide therapeutic plasma levels with minimal toxicity. These loading methods are followed by a continuous infusion of 1 to 5 mg per minute.

Another method involves the administration of a loading dose of 1 to 2 mg per kilogram at 50 mg per minute immediately followed by a maintenance infusion of 1 to 4 mg per minute. For this method, a second bolus needs to be administered 20 to 30 minutes after the initial bolus. Because the plasma concentration falls rapidly during phase 2 of the lidocaine disposition, it can become subtherapeutic. The maintenance infusion does not reach steady state for four half-lives (6 hours), providing a "first-hour gap" when the patient may not be protected from arrhythmias. The second bolus often maintains the plasma concentration within the therapeutic range. All doses should generally be reduced by 50 percent for patients in cardiac failure. If arrhythmia recurs after the patient is at steady state, he or she should be given another small bolus, and the maintenance infusion rate should be increased.

When lidocaine infusion therapy is discontinued at steady state, the rate of elimination is governed by the elimination half-life. This provides a natural taper, with the drug concentration being 50 percent of steady-state concentration at 90 minutes, 25 percent after 180 minutes, and 12.25 percent after 270 minutes. Completely discontinuing an infusion does not produce an abrupt change in plasma drug concentration. Therefore lidocaine needs no formal tapering.

The most commonly reported adverse effects of lidocaine involve the central nervous system and are dose-related. These include paresthesias, drowsiness, agitation, slurred speech, confusion, and in its most severe form, seizures and coma. These side effects are most commonly seen in the elderly and in patients with cardiac dysfunction. Although lidocaine has minimal effect on the cardiac conduction system, it may precipitate high-grade atrioventricular block in patients with His-Purkinje system dysfunction. In patients with complete heart block secondary to block in the His-Purkinje system, lidocaine can cause a marked decrease in the rate of the ventricular escape rhythm. Administration of lidocaine to patients with atrial tachyarrhythmias and rapid ventricular response has resulted in life-threatening increases in ventricular rate. Lidocaine does not cause torsades de pointes and rarely aggravates preexisting arrhythmias. As a rule, serious proarrhythmic effects are less common with class IB antiarrhythmic agents when compared with other classes.

INDICATIONS AND EFFICACY

Lidocaine is effective for the treatment of ventricular arrhythmias in various clinical settings (e.g., surgery, ischemia, digitalis toxicity). It is the drug of choice for emergency therapy because of the rapidity with which therapeutic plasma concentrations can be reached, a wide toxic-therapeutic ratio, and a low incidence of significant hemodynamic complications. The efficacy of lidocaine in the treatment of premature ventricular complexes and ventricular tachycardia has been reported to be 50 to 75 percent in various studies. However, lidocaine appears to be more effective in ischemia-related ventricular arrhythmias and less effective for chronic ventricular arrhythmias. Lidocaine is not effective and should not be used for the treatment of atrial arrhythmias. Lidocaine is most frequently used for prophylaxis against primary ventricular fibrillation (VF) in the setting of acute myocardial infarction, as the prototypical class IB agent during electrophysiologic testing to try to predict the response to tocainide or mexiletine for treating chronic ventricular arrhythmias, for the treatment of ventricular arrhythmias during acute myocardial infarction, and for control of the ventricular response in atrial arrhythmias in the presence of an accessory pathway.

The prophylactic use of lidocaine in the setting of acute myocardial infarction remains somewhat controversial; however, it is important to consider the prehospital and hospital phases of acute infarction separately. Obviously, the risk to life of primary VF is greater at home than in a fully staffed and equipped cardiac care unit. Early prophylactic administration of lidocaine may decrease mortality during the prehospital phase of acute myocardial infarction, especially when administered within 60 minutes of the onset of symptoms, and since intramuscular administration can achieve effective plasma levels "in the field," it is recommended that in the setting of acute myocardial infarction lidocaine be administered prior to the patient's arrival at the hospital.

Routine prophylaxis for the in-hospital patient

is less clearcut. Since warning arrhythmias lack sensitivity and specificity in predicting VF, monitoring patients in a cardiac care unit often does not help identify patients with the potential for developing VF. Lie and coworkers have demonstrated that in this group prophylactic lidocaine was highly effective in preventing primary VF. However, there was a 15 percent incidence of side effects and no difference in the in-hospital mortality compared with that of untreated patients, because in all instances prompt defibrillation terminated the VF. In fact, it has never been unequivocally demonstrated that the benefits of prophylactic lidocaine outweigh the risks in hospitalized patients, since other studies have shown no protective effect of lidocaine in preventing ventricular arrhythmias caused by infarction. In light of this, prophylaxis is not indicated for all patients because of the low risk of death from primary VF in a coronary care unit and the risk of adverse effects secondary to lidocaine administration. This is especially true because unlike secondary VF (associated with hypotension, cardiac failure, or shock), which has a 75 to 80 percent in-hospital mortality, primary VF as a primary electrical disturbance does not affect prognosis. Routine lidocaine prophylaxis can only be recommended in patients with acute myocardial infarction at high risk of developing VF. This includes younger patients (less than 60 years old) with extensive acute myocardial infarction seen within 6 hours of onset of infarction. Older patients (more than 70 years old) seen more than 6 hours after the onset of myocardial infarction are less likely to develop primary VF and more likely to demonstrate toxicity and should not routinely receive prophylaxis.

Lidocaine, the only class IB antiarrhythmic agent released in an intravenous form at present, is often used in the electrophysiology laboratory to help predict clinical response to the oral agents in this class, tocainide and mexiletine. Several investigators have demonstrated that a clinical response to lidocaine will predict a clinical response to oral tocainide only in approximately 50 percent of patients. Nonresponsiveness to lidocaine was associated with infrequent response to oral tocainide. Similarly, the efficacy of intravenous lidocaine when compared with oral mexiletine has a positive predictive value of only 50 percent, whereas the negative predictive value approaches 100 percent. A response to lidocaine may help to predict a favorable response to oral tocainide and oral mexiletine. However, when lidocaine fails to suppress ventricular arrhythmias, these agents should not be considered for long-term therapy because of the high likelihood of ineffectiveness.

Lidocaine's role in the treatment of an irregular wide complex tachycardia is uncertain. A wide complex tachycardia with gross irregularity (R-R interval variation greater than 120 msec) generally is indic-

tive of atrial fibrillation in the presence of an antegradely conducting accessory pathway. Ventricular rates greater than 200 beats per minute correlate with an accessory pathway antegrade refractory period of 280 msec or less. Lidocaine does not prolong refractoriness of the accessory pathway in patients whose antegrade refractory period is 300 msec or less. In fact, it has been shown that a number of patients actually demonstrate acceleration of the ventricular rate under these circumstances. Therefore, patients with irregular wide complex tachycardia with ventricular rates greater than 200 beats per minute or with a wide complex tachycardia and known Wolff-Parkinson-White syndrome should be treated, if hemodynamically stable, with intravenous procainamide rather than lidocaine.

Ventricular arrhythmias in the setting of acute myocardial infarction generally can be divided into three phases. Phase 1 begins at the onset of infarction and lasts for 6 hours. The arrhythmias range from ventricular premature complexes to primary VF. The incidence of VF peaks at 2 hours. The mechanism is reentry. Prophylactic therapy for primary VF was discussed earlier.

Ventricular tachycardia, either sustained or unsustained, is most frequently seen with transmural or extensive myocardial infarction. These rhythms should be treated with lidocaine if the patient is hemodynamically stable. If the arrhythmia fails to respond to lidocaine, procainamide should be administered.

Phase 2 starts at 6 hours and extends to 72 hours after infarction. Most commonly, one sees accelerated idioventricular rhythm or ventricular tachycardia. The mechanism is abnormal automaticity and is generally suppressible with pharmacologic therapy. Accelerated idioventricular rhythm is generally not treated unless it is associated with hypotension or decreased cardiac output from loss of atrioventricular synchrony. Under these circumstances, intravenous atropine in low doses should be used. Phase 2 ventricular tachycardia is usually controlled and suppressed by lidocaine.

Phase 3 begins 72 hours after infarction. The characteristic arrhythmia is primarily ventricular tachycardia secondary to reentry. Unlike arrhythmias in phase 1 or 2, these arrhythmias are secondary to a permanent structural abnormality and tend to be chronic, with a high rate of recurrence. Lidocaine is not generally useful. Chronic therapy is often required and is predicted on the results of invasive electrophysiologic testing.

SUGGESTED READING

Akhtar M, Gilbert CJ, Shanasa M. Effect of lidocaine on atrioventricular response via the accessory pathway in patients with Wolff-Parkinson-White syndrome. Circulation 1981; 63: 435–441.

Campbell RWF. Prophylactic antiarrhythmic therapy in acute myocardial infarction. Am J Cardiol 1984; 54:8E–13E.

Collingsworth KA, Kalman SM, Harrison DC. The clinical pharmacology of lidocaine as an antiarrhythmic drug. Circulation 1974; 50:1217–1230.

Danahy D, Aronow WS. Lidocaine-induced cardiac rate changes in atrial fibrillation and atrial flutter. Am Heart 1978; 95:474–482.

Lee KI, Wellens HJ, Van Capelle FJ, Durrer D. Lidocaine in the prevention of primary ventricular fibrillation. N Engl J Med 1974; 291:1324–1326.

LeLorier J, Grenon D, Latour Y, et al. Pharmacokinetics of lidocaine after prolonged intravenous infusions in uncomplicated MI. Ann Intern Med 1977; 87:700–702.

Valentine PA, Frew JL, Mashford ML, Sloman JC. Lidocaine in the prevention of sudden death in the pre-hospital phase of acute infarction. N Engl J Med 1974; 291:1327–1331.

Wyse DG, Kellen J, Rademaker AW. Prophylactic versus selective lidocaine for early ventricular arrhythmias of myocardial infarction. J Am Coll Cardiol 1988; 12:507–513.

Zehender M, Geibel A, Treese N, et al. Prediction of efficacy and tolerance of oral mexiletine by intravenous lidocaine application. Clin Pharmacol Ther 1988; 44:389–395.

MEXILETINE

RAYMOND L. WOOSLEY, M.D., Ph.D.

Mexiletine is an analogue of lidocaine and shares many of lidocaine's pharmacologic characteristics. These characteristics make it an effective agent for the treatment of experimental arrhythmias due to ischemia and may also make it of value in a postinfarction population with continuing ischemia. However, mexiletine is not a widely effective (broad-spectrum) antiarrhythmic agent; its efficacy is largely dependent on the type of arrhythmia being treated. It has been found not to reduce mortality when used as a single agent in a post–myocardial infarction population (IMPACT study). Mexiletine is not very effective in altering conduction velocity, which may explain its low degree of efficacy for the treatment of chronic arrhythmias such as sustained ventricular tachycardia, which presumably result from conduction over reentrant pathways. When mexiletine is used alone, arrhythmia control is achieved in only about 10 percent of patients with chronic arrhythmias as evaluated by programmed electrical stimulation. Although the rate of response to mexiletine is low when it is used alone, it has been combined successfully with other antiarrhythmic agents in the treatment of ventricular arrhythmias.

The intravenous formulation of mexiletine has not been developed in the United States. Oral mexiletine therapy is neither safe nor practical in situations requiring acute intervention.

MECHANISM OF ACTION

Mexiletine is an orally effective lidocaine congener, classified according to Vaughan Williams as having class IB action. It blocks fast sodium channels, thereby decreasing the maximal rate of depolarization ($\dot{V}$max) and shortening the repolarization phase of ventricular myocardium. Like lidocaine, the effects of mexiletine appear to be rate-dependent and are more prominent in hypoxic tissue. In usual doses, mexiletine has little effect on the surface electrocardiogram. It does not prolong the Q-T interval and may, in some cases, shorten it. It produces no apparent effects on calcium channels, nor have anticholinergic actions been seen.

DOSAGE AND DRUG ADMINISTRATION

Mexiletine is well absorbed and has little first-pass hepatic clearance. Since it is cleared mainly by hepatic metabolism, its disposition demonstrates considerable interindividual variability and is susceptible to induction or inhibition by other drugs. Induction of metabolism by agents such as phenytoin and barbiturates has been described, but the expected inhibition by cimetidine was not observed. Because of the variability of mexiletine clearance from patient to patient, dosage intervals can vary from 6 to 8 and in some cases 12 hours. In most patients for whom mexiletine is effective, arrhythmia control can be achieved with administration every 8 hours. The usual range for intrinsic clearance is 400 to 700 ml per minute and for half-life, from 8 to 20 hours (6 to 12 hours for healthy subjects); consequently, steady-state equilibrium should be reached after 2 to 3 days of dosing in most patients. Mexiletine has a large volume of distribution that reflects extensive tissue uptake of the drug. About 1 percent of total body content of mexiletine is in the plasma compartment, with approximately 70 percent of this bound to serum proteins.

The range of plasma concentrations usually associated with antiarrhythmic efficacy is from 1 to 2 μg per milliliter. However, routine monitoring of mexiletine plasma concentrations is of little value at present and is unnecessary for several reasons. There is poor correlation between drug action and mexiletine plasma concentration, and there is tremendous overlap between concentrations that prove effective and those causing toxicity. Recent studies, which recognize that mexiletine is actually a racemate, may explain these observations. The assays used in earlier studies failed to distinguish between the two isomers, which differ in their antiarrhythmic potency (in animal studies). Pharmacokinetic studies in humans have shown that the clearance of the two isomers is stereospecific, and there are differences in their ratio over time in the same individual. These ratios also appear to be different among individuals once steady state has been achieved.

As mentioned above, mexiletine is only moderately potent as an antiarrhythmic drug. In patients with acute myocardial infarction, it has been found to produce a statistically significant reduction in the frequency of premature ventricular complexes, but no effect on mortality or serious arrhythmias was found. In the IMPACT trial, similar results were found in a post-myocardial infarction population; however, the many weaknesses in this study make any conclusions tenuous. For example, patients were not required to have arrhythmias to be in the trial, and measurable levels of mexiletine were found in the plasma samples from some subjects receiving placebo.

During the development of mexiletine, it was tested extensively in patients with stable high-frequency ventricular ectopy (ventricular premature complexes) and found to have efficacy and tolerance similar to those of quinidine. Uncontrolled studies using programmed electrical stimulation in patients with life-threatening arrhythmias such as sustained ventricular tachycardia or in survivors of sudden death have found only a 5 to 15 percent response rate compared with 20 to 35 percent with other more potent agents. Considering the fact that programmed electrical stimulation testing has 85 to 90 percent reproducibility, a 10 to 15 percent response rate would not be distinguishable from placebo. In this population, mexiletine has proved useful when combined with other agents such as quinidine or disopyramide. When used in combination, mexiletine and the other agent can be given in lower (and better tolerated) doses with a higher response rate than seen with either agent alone. Patients whose arrhythmias are extremely sensitive to lidocaine can usually be successfully treated with mexiletine. However, the predictability is not perfect; there is about 20 percent discordance. Furthermore, even though some patients' arrhythmias seem to respond to lidocaine or mexiletine early in therapy, intolerable side effects prevent long-term use.

Individualization of Dosage

Because of large variability in clearance of mexiletine and overlap between dosages required for efficacy and those causing side effects, each patient's dosage must be titrated to an optimal response. Patients with normal renal and hepatic function should initially be given 150 mg every 8 hours. If no response is seen after 3 to 7 days, the dosage may be increased to 200 mg every 8 hours. Titration to 250 mg every 8 hours or 300 mg every 8 or 6 hours is necessary for some patients, but side effects usually limit the use of doses over 750 mg per day. The dosage for patients with hepatic disease or severe heart failure should be started at 150 mg every 12 hours. Patients with kidney disease usually require the same dosages as those with normal renal function. As mentioned above, combination of mexiletine with quinidine or disopyramide allows the use of lower doses of both agents.

COMPLICATIONS OF TREATMENT

One of mexiletine's attributes is its safety profile. Unlike the more potent agents, encainide and flecainide, it only rarely causes severe early worsening of arrhythmias. Unlike disopyramide and flecainide, it produces little depression of myocardial function when the usually effective dosages are used. Unlike its congener tocainide, mexiletine produces little organ toxicity or allergenicity. Rare instances of hepatitis have been described, but no cases of pulmonary fibrosis or agranulocytosis have been attributed to mexiletine therapy.

Although serious problems with mexiletine are rare, unpleasant side effects such as dizziness, lightheadedness, paresthesias, burning skin, nervousness, tremor, nausea, or dyspepsia are common. These are often dose-related or caused by rapid absorption of the drug, and administration with meals or with aluminum hydroxide gels can often reduce side effects without reducing bioavailability. For many patients, giving lower doses more frequently (every 6 hours) is necessary to prevent the occurrence of side effects or arrhythmia recurrence. However, some patients can be treated with doses every 12 hours without loss of efficacy.

ASSESSMENT OF THERAPEUTIC RESPONSE

Therapeutic response to mexiletine is usually determined using continuous 24-hour Holter monitoring or the treadmill exercise test to assess arrhythmia suppression. For patients receiving combination therapy (mexiletine plus quinidine or disopyramide), measurement of electrocardiographic intervals may be useful to prevent toxicity. Routine monitoring of mexiletine plasma concentration is of no value at present, except for detection of noncompliance. However, information about the activity of mexiletine's stereoisomers and eventual development of stereospecific assays may alter this situation. Invasive programmed electrical stimulation has been used to assess mexiletine efficacy, and as with all antiarrhythmic agents, some patients whose arrhythmias appeared to be suppressed when evaluated by Holter monitoring demonstrated continued arrhythmia induction by programmed electrical stimulation. The risks and costs associated with invasive techniques usually limit their use to only highly symptomatic and life-threatening arrhythmias.

PROS AND CONS OF TREATMENT

Although there are some patients for whom antiarrhythmic therapy is indicated without question, the tremendous gap in our knowledge of the risk:benefit ratio for use of antiarrhythmic drugs in many patients with arrhythmias is a major concern. For example, patients with recent myocardial infarction and evidence of left ventricular dysfunction have been found to be at higher risk for sudden death if ventricular arrhythmias are detected, but there is no data indicating that suppression of arrhythmias reduces the incidence of sudden cardiac death. On the contrary, the Cardiac Arrhythmia Suppression Trial (CAST) has found that two agents, encainide and flecainide, increase the incidence of sudden death and overall mortality. At this time, antiarrhythmic drug therapy is indicated for life-threatening arrhythmias only. Until further studies have been performed, we cannot assume that arrhythmia suppression per se is of benefit to asymptomatic patients or that the discomfort and risks associated with such therapy are justified.

SUGGESTED READING

Campbell RWF. Mexiletine. N Engl J Med 1987; 316:29–34.
CAST Investigators. Preliminary report: Effect of encainide and flecainide on mortality in a randomized trial of arrhythmia suppression after myocardial infarction. N Engl J Med 1989; 321:406–412.
Duff HJ, Kolodgie FD, Roden DM, Woosley RL. Electropharmacologic synergism with mexiletine and quinidine. J Cardiovasc Pharmacol 1986; 8:840–846.
Impact Research Group. International mexiletine and placebo antiarrhythmic coronary trial. I: Report on arrhythmia and other findings. J Am Coll Cardiol 1984; 4:1148–1163.
Woosley RL. Mexiletine and tocainide: A profile of two lidocaine analogs. Ration Drug Ther 1987; 21:1–7.
Woosley RL. Indications for antiarrhythmic therapy—a wealth of controversy, a dearth of data. Ann Intern Med 1988; 108:450–453.

MORICIZINE

CRAIG M. PRATT, M.D.

It has been established that the presence of ventricular premature complexes (VPCs) after acute myocardial infarction increases the risk of sudden death. The recent publication of the surprising results of the Cardiac Arrhythmia Suppression Trial (CAST) showing that both encainide and flecainide increased arrhythmic mortality rates more than threefold compared with placebo (despite suppression of VPCs in patients surviving acute myocardial infarction) mandates a rethinking of decisions regarding drug selection of antiarrhythmic therapy for ventricular arrhythmias. Moricizine is an investigational antiarrhythmic drug in the final stages of the review process by the Food and Drug Administration and is the only active antiarrhythmic drug still being tested in CAST. It is not yet marketed in the United States, but as of June, 1990, it is in the final stages of the approval process by the Food and Drug Administration.*

---

*FDA approved.

INITIAL DEVELOPMENT, ELECTROPHYSIOLOGIC EFFECTS, AND PHARMACOKINETICS

Moricizine is an unusual antiarrhythmic drug in many ways. First, it is a phenothiazine derivative and is unique among the antiarrhythmics used and investigated at present in this respect. Second, it is a drug that was initially developed by Soviet physicians. Podrid and Lown of the Harvard School of Public Health were instrumental in conducting clinical investigations of this drug in the Soviet Union and were responsible for bringing the drug to the United States for investigation.

During invasive electrophysiologic testing, moricizine significantly prolongs P-R and QRS intervals as well as A-H and H-V intervals. Additionally, moricizine increases the cycle length at which atrioventricular nodal block occurs but has minimal or no effect on repolarization or cardiac refractory periods. Thus, although moricizine is an electrophysiologic class I antiarrhythmic agent, it does not clearly fit into a IA, B, or C category. In patients in whom inducible sustained ventricular tachycardia (VT) is produced in the drug-free state and on moricizine therapy, the cycle length of the induced VT is significantly prolonged during moricizine therapy.

The pharmacokinetics of moricizine is complex and not well understood. In normal individuals, moricizine is almost completely absorbed by the gastrointestinal tract, with peak plasma levels being attained within 1 to 2 hours after an oral dose. The plasma half-life ranges from 3 to 12 hours but may be longer in patients with a low left ventricular ejection fraction. In most studies, moricizine has been administered every 8 hours, although its activity may extend to allow a longer interdosing interval (every 12 hours) in selected patients. The pharmacokinetics of moricizine is somewhat complicated by the presence of a number of active metabolites in the plasma that appear to be present for more extended periods than the native compound. In most studies, moricizine plasma levels have not accurately predicted the extent of arrhythmia suppression.

The normal therapeutic dose range for moricizine is somewhere between 8 and 14 mg per kilogram per day. Thus, standard oral doses are usually in the 600 to 900 mg per kilogram range, divided into three doses. Moricizine does not alter digoxin levels in patients with normal renal function, but this may not be true in patients taking concomitant cimetidine, which reduces the clearance of many drugs. The pharmacokinetics of moricizine is presented in Table 1.

Experience in patients with supraventricular arrhythmias is minimal, with uncontrolled observations made both in adults and children. Our review of moricizine for efficacy is limited to its use in treatment of ventricular arrhythmias.

EFFICACY OF MORICIZINE

Benign Ventricular Arrhythmia

At the time of this writing, the antiarrhythmic drug suppression of asymptomatic spontaneous ventricular arrhythmias is without proven patient benefit. Thus, much of the data regarding moricizine is similar to the data for most antiarrhythmics in that many studies focus on arrhythmia suppression in this population, which is a measure of antiarrhythmic drug activity and not of efficacy.

In moricizine studies, more than 1 day of baseline ambulatory electrocardiographic recording was done to ensure that the observed arrhythmia changes were not caused by variability. The percentage of suppression of VPCs, ventricular pairs, and unsustained ventricular tachycardia required to document a "drug effect" is contained in Table 2. Notice that the variability for VPCs and unsustained ventricular tachycardia is such that observed reductions of greater than or equal to 80 percent are necessary if only 1 day of monitoring is used, before and after treatment, to rule out arrhythmia variability with a high degree of confidence.

The first study to evaluate the ability of moricizine to suppress VPCs utilizing both 24-hour ambulatory electrocardiographic recordings and exercise testing was reported in 1977 by Podrid and coworkers. Effective suppression of VPCs was achieved when doses of at least 600 mg per day were used. In most trials, 600 mg per day (three times a day dosing) appears to be a minimal effective dose.

In our initial report of 39 patients enrolled in three placebo-controlled protocols, we demonstrated the efficacy of moricizine in daily doses of 8.5 to 11.5 mg per kilogram (mean 830 mg per day in three divided doses). We found an overall 80 percent reduction of VPCs, a 95 percent reduction in ventricular pairs, and a 99 percent reduction in the runs of unsustained ventricular tachycardia in the 19 out of 39 patients who had unsustained ventricular tachycardia during the placebo period. Arrhythmia suppression appeared to be as effective in patients with ischemic heart disease as in those with other types of organic heart disease. The side effect profile of moricizine in these early studies was promising, reveal-

Table 1 Moricizine Pharmacokinetic Variables After Administration of a 150 mg Intravenous Bolus

	Mean	Range
Distribution half-life	8.3 minutes	3.5–22.2
Elimination half-life	1.86 hours	0.82–4.2
Central volume of distribution	52 liters	19.8–98.7
Total volume of distribution	210 liters	102–447
Clearance	1.31 liters/minute	0.83–2.96

From Woosley et al. Am J Cardiol 1987;60:35F, with permission.

Table 2 Minimal Percent Hourly Arrhythmia Reduction Necessary to Document "Drug Effect" Versus Spontaneous Variability*

Length of Ambulatory ECG Recording (Days)		% Reduction Required		
C	T	VPCs/hour	Pairs/hour	VT/hour
1	1	78	83	77
2	2	66	72	64
3	3	58	65	57
4	4	53	59	52
5	5	49	55	48
6	6	46	52	45
7	7	44	49	42

*Based on a 95 percent confidence interval in 110 patients with ventricular tachycardia enrolled in investigational antiarrhythmic trials.

C = control; T = treatment; VPC = ventricular premature complexes; VT = ventricular tachycardia.

Adapted from Pratt CM, et al. Am J Cardiol 1985;56:67, with permission.

ing no serious toxicity or proarrhythmia of any magnitude.

One special population worth mentioning is composed of patients with symptomatic VPCs and/or unsustained ventricular tachycardia with mitral valve prolapse as their only evidence of organic heart disease. In 17 such patients whose disease was resistant to numerous other antiarrhythmic agents (mean of 3.3 antiarrhythmic drugs per patient), we found moricizine to be very helpful, without serious side effects and able to suppress both symptomatic VPCs and unsustained ventricular tachycardia long term. This is an important patient population to keep in mind because the labeled indications for antiarrhythmic drugs have vastly changed as a result of the CAST. Antiarrhythmic drug suppression of asymptomatic spontaneous ventricular arrhythmia is not indicated at present. In patients with significantly bothersome symptoms, such as severe palpitations and lightheadedness, antiarrhythmic therapy is also not targeted as a label indication, although clinicians realize the necessity of treating some of those individuals. In patients with mitral valve prolapse, moricizine is not only very safe but also appears to be very effective in suppressing both arrhythmia and symptoms.

Potentially Lethal Ventricular Arrhythmias

Moricizine was evaluated in patients with frequent VPCs who survived a recent (6 to 60 days) myocardial infarction in the Cardiac Arrhythmia Pilot Study (CAPS). Compared with baseline arrhythmia frequency, moricizine suppressed more than or equal to 70 percent of the VPCs in 66 percent of the patients tested. Moricizine appeared to have similar antiarrhythmic efficacy in patients with depressed as well as preserved left ventricular function. Compared with the other three study drugs, moricizine was most effective in the patients with the lowest left ventricular ejection fractions (21 to 29 percent).

We previously reported a placebo-controlled prospective long-term clinical trial of moricizine in 50 patients selected with frequent unsustained ventricular tachycardia at baseline. This group had depressed left ventricular function (mean left ventricular ejection fraction 36 percent), and nearly two-thirds had a calculated left ventricular ejection fraction of less than 40 percent and coronary artery disease. Initially, approximately three-fourths of the patients achieved a greater than or equal to 75 percent reduction in runs of unsustained ventricular tachycardia on moricizine. At the time of hospital discharge, 21 of the 33 patients still taking moricizine had total abolition of unsustained ventricular tachycardia. We observed that patients with an initial left ventricular ejection fraction of less than 30 percent were much less likely to have suppression of ventricular tachycardia than patients with more preserved left ventricular function, an observation that is typical for most antiarrhythmic drugs (Table 3).

Lethal Ventricular Arrhythmias

The largest single-center experience in this patient population was reported by Hession and associates on 102 patients, including 46 with documented sustained ventricular tachycardia, 31 with ventricular fibrillation, and an additional 25 with unsustained ventricular tachycardia. These investigators used a combination of ambulatory electrocardiographic recordings and electrophysiologic testing to evaluate patients taking moricizine in doses ranging from 600 to 1200 mg daily. Of the 75 patients evaluated by ambulatory electrocardiograms and exercise testing, 40 percent were considered responders to moricizine in that they had a greater than 90 percent reduction in ventricular pairs and runs of unsustained ventricular tachycardia as well as a greater than 50 percent reduction of VPCs. In those patients undergoing electrophysiologic testing, moricizine was successful in suppressing inducible sustained ventricular tachycardia in only 5 percent of the patients.

Table 3 Patient Outcome in Moricizine Ventricular Tachycardia Trial: Relationship to Left Ventricular Ejection Fraction at Entry (Mean ± SD)

Outcome	Left-Ventricular Ejection Fraction at Selected Intervals in Trial (%)		
	At Discharge	At 1 Month	At 3 Months
Successful therapy	38 ± 17 (N = 33)	40 ± 16 (N = 30)	42 ± 16 (N = 22)
Dropouts	31 ± 15 (N = 15)	29 ± 14 (N = 18)*	32 ± 16 (N = 26)†

*p < 0.01 versus successful group.
†p = <0.04 versus successful therapy.
From Pratt CM, Wierman A, Scals AA, et al. Circulation 1986;73:718, with permission.

The combined experience of moricizine during electrophysiologic study was presented in a symposium on the drug reporting on 60 patients. Despite a number of different electrophysiologic protocols and definitions of efficacy, moricizine was effective in suppressing inducible sustained ventricular tachycardia in 19 percent (7 of 38) of the patients. In the 22 patients with unsustained ventricular tachycardia, during their control electrophysiologic study, 27 percent had total abolition of their presenting arrhythmia during a repeat electrophysiologic study while on moricizine. To determine the value of the electrophysiologic study during moricizine therapy in this high-risk population, 37 of the initial 60 patients had follow-up data available while receiving moricizine for up to 10 months. It was concluded that the electrophysiologic study was useful in predicting which of these patients would or would not have a recurrence of the lethal tachyarrhythmia (sensitivity 82 percent, specificity 65 percent). In summary, moricizine appears to have only modest potency in suppressing inducible sustained ventricular tachycardia, probably effective in only 20 percent of the cases. It shares this limitation with other electrophysiologic class I agents. In selected patients in whom moricizine can suppress inducible sustained ventricular tachycardia, its advantages lie in its low proarrhythmia rate and its tolerance in patients with left ventricular dysfunction. Formal comparisons of efficacy in this population with other antiarrhythmic drugs have not been reported.

COMPARISON WITH OTHER ANTIARRHYTHMIC AGENTS

Published studies have compared moricizine to both propranolol and disopyramide. In our trial, which was a placebo-controlled, double-blind, crossover trial of 33 patients with non–life-threatening frequent VPCs, moricizine and disopyramide were compared. Moricizine was superior to disopyramide in mean VPC suppression (71 versus 53 percent, respectively), but both were comparable in suppressing runs of unsustained ventricular tachycardia. Although moricizine administration resulted in total VPC suppression in 30 percent of the patients, this was never seen during disopyramide therapy.

In a placebo-controlled, cross-over trial comparing moricizine to propranolol, Butman demonstrated potential additive efficacy of moricizine to propranolol in addition to showing that moricizine was superior to propranolol in suppressing VPCs. The dose of propranolol used in that trial was 120 mg daily. In addition to this small study, there has now been a great deal of experience accumulated with the safety of using moricizine in combination with beta blockers from both the CAPS and the ongoing CAST trial. Since beta blockers have been

shown to be effective in reducing mortality in patients surviving acute myocardial infarction, it is important to note that moricizine can be used with a high degree of safety in combination with the currently available beta-blocking drugs.

Left Ventricular Function

Since it is clear that many of the antiarrhythmic drugs have negative inotropic activity, the effect of moricizine on left ventricular function has been evaluated by multiple techniques. This includes our report of 81 patients enrolled in three placebo-controlled antiarrhythmic protocols that used two-dimensional echocardiographic assessment of left ventricular ejection fraction before and after moricizine therapy. The mean placebo left ventricular ejection fraction of 47 percent was unchanged during moricizine therapy (46 percent). In the 31 patients with left ventricular ejection fraction of less than 45 percent, moricizine therapy resulted in no change in the mean left ventricular ejection fraction. The only two patients we encountered who developed symptoms of congestive heart failure on moricizine had a prior history of congestive heart failure and baseline left ventricular ejection fractions of 19 percent and 26 percent, respectively.

The results of radionuclide ventriculographic assessment of left ventricular function in 24 patients who had severe lethal ventricular arrhythmias showed no change in the mean global left ventricular ejection fraction during moricizine therapy (38 percent) compared with the baseline measurement (40 percent). Moricizine was well tolerated, with no development of clinical congestive heart failure. Right ventricular ejection fraction measurements were unchanged during moricizine therapy. A separate analysis of the 15 patients with left ventricular ejection fraction of less than 45 percent and a history of clinical congestive heart failure likewise revealed no deterioration in left or right ejection fraction during moricizine therapy. In addition, exercise testing revealed no change in exercise performance during moricizine administration.

We have also performed right-sided heart catheterization for hemodynamic assessment of left ventricular function before and during 3 days of moricizine therapy in 19 patients who had frequent runs of unsustained ventricular tachycardia. In these patients with a mean left ventricular ejection fraction of 39 percent during the control phase, hemodynamics were unchanged after 3 days of moricizine administration at rest and during supine bicycle exercise.

Recently, Podrid and this author reported on the evaluation of the entire moricizine database forming the basis for approval by the Federal Drug Administration. As a result of the analysis of these 908 patients, it was found that new onset congestive heart failure during moricizine therapy occurred in only one patient. Of the 374 patients in the moricizine database with a history of congestive heart failure, 13 percent developed a repeat episode of congestive heart failure on moricizine, approximately half of whom had to discontinue therapy (Fig. 1). Moricizine was effective in suppressing spontaneous ventricular arrhythmias in approximately one-half of the patients with left ventricular dysfunction. As seen in Table 4, in the accepted dosing range of 600 to 900 mg per day, moricizine was nearly as effective in achieving VPC suppression in patients with depressed as in patients with preserved left ventricular ejection fractions. In the CAPS population, moricizine did not increase the incidence of congestive heart failure.

SIDE EFFECTS

Development of Proarrhythmia During Moricizine Therapy

Every antiarrhythmic drug has the potential to produce proarrhythmia, and moricizine is no exception. In general, the risk of proarrhythmia is related to the extent of the underlying heart disease and the severity of the presenting ventricular arrhythmia. For instance, patients with sustained ventricular tachycardia are much more likely to have a proarrhythmic effect from an antiarrhythmic drug than those with a benign arrhythmia. Proarrhythmic effects can be potentially lethal even in patients with potentially lethal arrhythmias, such as those patients who received encainide and flecainide in the CAST trial. Estimating the proarrhythmic potential of antiarrhythmic drugs is fraught with hazard. The encainide (N = more than 1,700) and flecainide (N = more than 1,300) databases used as the basis of Federal Drug Administration approval failed to indicate the lethal proarrhythmic potential of these drugs. Therefore the analysis that Morganroth and this author reported with the moricizine database has to be looked at with hope and yet with skepticism, since the proarrhythmic rates are estimated without the benefit of a parallel placebo group such as was present in CAST. Furthermore, the moricizine database contains few patients with a recent myocardial infarction, with the only published experience limited to the 100 patients receiving moricizine in the CAPS.

With those reservations, I still feel that moricizine has a low proarrhythmic potential compared with other electrophysiologic class I antiarrhythmic drugs. This may be related to the fact that it is well tolerated in patients with congestive heart failure. In our review of the 908 patients with ventricular arrhythmias in the moricizine database, the proarrhythmic event rate during moricizine therapy was quite low. Deaths that were felt to be attributable to the proarrhythmic effects of moricizine did not occur in any patients with benign ventricular arrhythmia, and occurred in less than 0.1 percent of patients with potentially lethal arrhythmia and in 0.4 percent of the patients treated whose initial arrhythmia was in the lethal category (Table 5). Torsades de pointes ventricular tachycardia can occur

Table 4 Relationship of Maximal Daily Moricizine Dose Administered, Left Ventricular Ejection Fraction at Baseline, and Resultant VPC Suppression

Total Daily Moricizine Dose	Baseline Left Ventricular Ejection Fraction		
	<30% (N = 46)	30–45% (N = 57)	>45% (N = 117)
	Percent of Patients Achieving >75% VPC Suppression		
<600 mg	0	0/1 (0%)	0/5 (0%)
600 mg	4/9 (44%)	4/7 (57%)	14/22 (64%)
750 mg	7/14 (50%)	8/18 (44%)	17/35 (48%)
900 mg	11/20 (54%)	13/20 (65%)	26/38 (68%)
>900 mg	1/3 (33%)	4/11 (36%)	12/17 (71%)

From Pratt CM, Podrvid P, Greatrix B, et al. Am Heart J 1990;119:1, with permission.

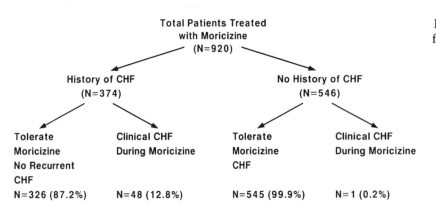

Figure 1 CHF = congestive heart failure

Table 5 Number of Patients by Ventricular Arrhythmia Classification and Proarrhythmic Categories

Classification of Ventricular Arrhythmias	Patients (N = 908)	Proarrhythmic Category		
		Death (N = 4)	Serious (N = 15)	Nonserious (N = 10)
Benign	89	0	0	0
Potentially lethal	509	1 (0.1%)	14 (1.5%)	4 (0.4%)
Lethal	310	3 (0.4%)	1 (0.1%)	6 (0.7%)

From Morganroth J, Pratt CM. Am J Cardiol 1989;63:172, with permission.

during moricizine therapy but appears to be very uncommon. Nonserious proarrhythmic events, for instance an increase in VPCs, occur more frequently but are of no known clinical consequence. Therefore, to the extent that the review of a non–placebo-controlled database can be reassuring, I feel that moricizine has a low proarrhythmic potential and has a small detrimental effect on left ventricular function.

Other Side Effects

In our experience, moricizine is well tolerated. Patients complained of occasional dizziness and minor gastrointestinal symptoms. The best way to assess the true side effect profile of any antiarrhythmic drug is to have a parallel placebo group. The best database published for the analysis of moricizine is the CAPS, in which approximately 100 patients were treated with moricizine and were compared with a parallel, 100 patient, placebo group. In that trial, the side effects of moricizine were similar to those of placebo (Table 6). In the CAPS, the incidence of proarrhythmia or congestive heart failure during moricizine therapy did not differ from

the incidence of either during placebo. It is possible and even likely that side effects may be more commonly seen in patients taking moricizine in the CAST trial, now limited to patients with ejection fractions of less than 40 percent. My experience is that most antiarrhythmic agents produce more side effects in sicker patients, often as a result of altered pharmacokinetics and drug accumulation.

RISK-BENEFIT CONSIDERATIONS OF MORICIZINE

Moricizine seems well tolerated and has a low incidence of side effects in most patient populations. It suppresses spontaneous ventricular arrhythmias to an extent comparable to that of other class IA and 1B agents, although it is not as potent in this area as class IC agents. Moricizine is well tolerated in patients with congestive heart failure. Many patients with low left ventricular ejection fractions still have arrhythmia suppression on moricizine, although in our experience, patients who have a left ventricular ejection fraction of less than 25 percent and unsustained ventricular tachycardia usually have no suppression. Experience in patients with life-threatening ventricular arrhythmias, such as sustained ventricular tachycardia, is somewhat limited, and no multi-center prospective electrophysiologic protocol has been completed. Based on limited data, moricizine appears to be of only modest efficacy in this area, preventing inducible sustained ventricular tachycardia in approximately 20 percent of patients. Moricizine appears to have a relatively low proarrhythmia potential, and its overall efficacy and safety profile appear favorable, indicating why it is currently being tested in the CAST in patients surviving acute myocardial infarction with ventricular arrhythmia and left ventricular ejection fractions of below 40 percent.

SUGGESTED READING

Cardiac Arrhythmia Pilot Study (CAPS) Investigators. Effects of encainide, flecainide, imipramine, and moricizine on ventricular arrhythmias during the year after acute myocardial infarction: The CAPS. Am J Cardiol 1988; 61:501–509.

Cardiac Arrhythmia Suppression Trial Investigators. Preliminary report: Effect of encainide and flecainide on mortality in a randomized trial of arrhythmia suppression after myocardial infarction. N Engl J Med 1989; 321:406–412.

Morganroth J, Pratt CM. Prevalence and characteristics of proarrhythmia from moricizine (Ethmozine). Am J Cardiol 1989; 63:172–176.

Podrid PJ, Lyakishev A, Lown B, Mazur N. Ethmozin, a new antiarrhythmic drug for suppressing ventricular premature complexes. Circulation 1980; 61:450–457.

Pratt CM, Brater C, Harrell FE, et al. Clinical and regulatory implications of the Cardiac Arrhythmia Suppression Trial. Am J Cardiol 1990; 65:103–105.

Pratt CM, Butman SM, Young JB, et al. Antiarrhythmic efficacy of Ethmozine. (moricizine HC1) compared with disopyramide and propranolol. Am J Cardiol 1987; 60:52F–58F.

Table 6 Comparison of Noncardiac Adverse Events Between Moricizine and Placebo Reported During the Cardiac Arrhythmia Pilot Study

Adverse Effect Category	CAPS Drug	
	Moricizine (N = 77)	Placebo (N = 87)
Cardiovascular	23%	21%
Skin reactions	6%	3%
Gastrointestinal	26%	21%
Genitourinary	18%	11%
Neurologic	34%	38%
Other	44%	43%
Any symptom	64%	60%

From Cardiac Arrhythmia Pilot Study (CAPS) Investigators. Am J Cardiol 1988;61:501, with permission.

Pratt CM, Podrid P, Greatrix B, et al. Efficacy and safety of moricizine in patients with congestive heart failure: A summary of the experience in the United States. Am Heart J 1990; 119:1–7.

Pratt CM, Podrid PJ, Seals AA, et al. Effects of Ethmozine. (moricizine HC1) on ventricular function using echocardiographic, hemodynamic and radionuclide assessments. Am J Cardiol 1987; 60:73F–78F.

Pratt CM, Wierman A, Seals AA, et al. Efficacy and safety of moricizine in patients with ventricular tachycardia: Results of a placebo-controlled prospective long-term clinical trial. Circulation 1986; 73:718–726.

Pratt CM, Yepsen SC, Taylor AA, et al. Ethmozine suppression of single and repetitive ventricular premature depolarizations

during therapy: Documentation of efficacy and long-term safety. Am Heart J 1983; 106:85–91.

Pratt CM, Young JB, Francis MJ, et al. Comparative effect of disopyramide and Ethmozine in suppressing complex ventricular arrhythmias by use of a double-blind, placebo-controlled, longitudinal crossover design. Circulation 1984; 69:288–297.

Pratt CM, Young JB, Wierman AM, et al. Complex ventricular arrhythmias associated with the mitral valve prolapse syndrome: Effectiveness of moricizine (Ethmozine) in patients resistant to conventional antiarrhythmics. Am J Med 1986; 80:626–632.

Wyndham CRC, Pratt CM, Mann DE, et al. Electrophysiology of Ethmozine (moricizine HC1) for ventricular tachycardia. Am J Cardiol 1987; 60:67F–72F.

PHENYTOIN

RICHARD N. FOGOROS, M.D.

HISTORY OF PHENYTOIN AS AN ANTIARRHYTHMIC AGENT

Once phenytoin was recognized as an effective anticonvulsant in 1938 (30 years after it was first synthesized), the drug soon came into widespread clinical use. By the early 1950s, some were suggesting that phenytoin might also be useful for the treatment of cardiac arrhythmias (based on the premise that seizures of the heart might be similar to seizures of the brain). The first clinical use of phenytoin as an antiarrhythmic agent was documented in 1958, with the published report of a patient whose ventricular tachycardia responded to phenytoin after failing to respond to quinidine and procainamide. During the 1960s, interest in phenytoin as an antiarrhythmic agent was relatively high. Numerous studies were published supporting the drug's efficacy in the treatment of several varieties of cardiac arrhythmias and proposing mechanisms for its antiarrhythmic effects. In the early 1970s, however, the Food and Drug Administration decided that the available data were insufficient (because of a lack of well-controlled studies) to warrant adding the treatment of cardiac arrhythmias to the list of approved indications for phenytoin. For this reason and because the more "convenient" drug lidocaine was by then in widespread use for most of the arrhythmias that were effectively treated by phenytoin, phenytoin largely fell out of favor.

Through the 1980s, the appropriate place of phenytoin in the treatment of cardiac arrhythmias has remained ambiguous. Although some cardiologists (including, apparently, most of those who have published lists of antiarrhythmic drugs) administer

the drug infrequently or not at all, others (including the author) prescribe the drug often and consider it very useful in managing some types of life-threatening arrhythmias.

ANTIARRHYTHMIC PROPERTIES OF PHENYTOIN

Experimental studies have shown phenytoin to possess properties similar to those of many other antiarrhythmic drugs.

Class I Antiarrhythmic Effects. Phenytoin has been demonstrated to have a lidocaine-like effect on ion transport across the cardiac cell membrane. Thus, phenytoin decreases the action potential duration and the refractoriness of cardiac cells. Those who consider phenytoin an antiarrhythmic agent, therefore, classify it as a class IB drug. Both animal and human studies have shown that phenytoin, by virtue of its class I effects, is capable of altering reentrant pathways and thus ameliorating reentrant arrhythmias.

Suppression of Automaticity. In animal models, phenytoin has been shown to suppress automaticity by depressing spontaneous diastolic (phase 4) membrane activity. Uncontrolled clinical studies have suggested that phenytoin may be of benefit in the treatment of arrhythmias that are caused by enhanced automaticity.

Suppression of Triggered Activity. Studies in animal models have shown that phenytoin can suppress the triggered afterdepolarizations seen with digitalis toxicity. This triggered activity is thought by many to be responsible for digitalis-toxic arrhythmias. The clinical efficacy of phenytoin in digitalis-toxic arrhythmias has been well recognized for many years.

Suppression of Sympathetic Tone. Phenytoin has a depressant effect on the sympathetic centers of the central nervous system and therefore decreases sympathetic activity in the cardiac nerves. Since several cardiac arrhythmias are mediated by increased sympathetic tone, the depressant influence of phenytoin on efferent sympathetic fibers may be an important component of the drug's antiarrhythmic effects.

INDICATIONS FOR PHENYTOIN IN THE TREATMENT OF CARDIAC ARRHYTHMIAS

Digitalis Toxicity. The most widely accepted indication for using phenytoin as an antiarrhythmic agent is in the treatment of arrhythmias caused by digitalis toxicity. Since the early 1960s, it has been recognized that phenytoin is effective at suppressing both the atrial and the ventricular tachyarrhythmias associated with toxic levels of digitalis. Digitalis toxicity is the only clinical setting in which phenytoin reliably treats atrial tachycardias. Among many experts, phenytoin remains the antiarrhythmic drug of choice in digitalis toxicity.

In treating digitalis-toxic arrhythmias, phenytoin is loaded intravenously, and the clinical response is usually rapid. The salutary effect of phenytoin in this setting may be attributable to the drug's suppression of digitalis-related triggered activity, as previously noted. In addition, intrathecal phenytoin has been shown to be effective in treating digoxin-induced arrhythmias in dogs, suggesting that a significant part of the drug's effect may be centrally mediated.

Ventricular Arrhythmias in Medically Unstable Patients. During the 1960s, phenytoin was often reported to be effective against ventricular arrhythmias associated with acute myocardial infarction and administration of general anesthesia, as well as against those arrhythmias observed in the early postoperative period and in the intensive care setting in general. Lidocaine, however, has almost entirely replaced phenytoin for the treatment of such arrhythmias, since lidocaine is relatively easy to use and since phenytoin has not been labeled or marketed for this purpose. Nonetheless, in our center, we have often found phenytoin to be effective in treating ventricular arrhythmias that occur in the intensive care setting, even in patients in whom lidocaine or procainamide has not been effective. Since the arrhythmias that occur in this setting are generally thought not to be reentrant in nature, it is likely that the success of phenytoin is related to its suppression of automaticity and/or suppression of triggered afterdepolarizations. Further, the centrally mediated effects of phenytoin may be important, since virtually all the arrhythmias occurring in such circumstances are accompanied by high adrenergic tone.

Late Ventricular Arrhythmias Following Surgery for Congenital Heart Disease. Several reports during the past decade have suggested that phenytoin may be especially efficacious in the treatment of chronic complex ventricular ectopy occurring after surgical repair of congenital heart disease. Such ectopy has been clearly associated with an increased risk of sudden death (especially in patients with persistently abnormal right ventricular hemodynamics) and has been generally regarded as difficult to suppress. Why phenytoin may be more effective than other antiarrhythmic agents in this clinical setting is unknown. Phenytoin, however, has been used as chronic therapy for epilepsy in young patients for decades and is a relatively attractive choice for long-term antiarrhythmic therapy in young patients.

Reentrant Ventricular Tachyarrhythmias. Phenytoin has usually been regarded as effective in treatment of ventricular tachyarrhythmias only when they are associated with digitalis toxicity or acute illness. The ventricular tachycardias associated with chronic underlying heart disease, however, are a much greater public health problem, since they cause the sudden deaths of hundreds of thousands of people each year. These arrhythmias are generally held to be reentrant in nature, largely because of their inducibility with programmed stimulation. Serial drug testing for these arrhythmias in the electrophysiology laboratory is predicated on the ability of drugs to alter reentrant circuits in order to render a previously inducible arrhythmia noninducible.

Although phenytoin is properly classified as a class I antiarrhythmic drug and should therefore have some activity against reentrant arrhythmias, few electrophysiologists have used it for serial drug testing. Recently, we and one other group (Epstein and associates) reported our respective experiences with the use of phenytoin in serial electrophysiologic testing in patients with inducible ventricular tachyarrhythmias. Both reports gave similar results, but the conclusions were disparate. We found that phenytoin suppressed inducible arrhythmias in 13 percent of the trials with that drug, compared with 11 percent in Epstein's study. However, whereas Epstein and coworkers concluded that phenytoin is effective only infrequently and implied that routine testing with phenytoin was not worthwhile, we concluded that the drug is sufficiently effective to warrant routine testing. Obviously, whether a 10 to 15 percent rate of efficacy is considered frequent or infrequent is largely based on one's expectations and on the rate of efficacy seen with other agents. In our laboratory, phenytoin's efficacy was comparable to that of other, commonly used antiarrhythmic agents (an updated list of the relative efficacy of phenytoin and other antiarrhythmic agents in our laboratory is presented in Table 1). Since long-term therapy with phenytoin is usually well tolerated (compared with some of the newer antiarrhythmic agents), we find the drug to be an attractive option for patients with inducible ventricular tachyarrhythmias, and we continue to test it routinely.

Table 1 Results of Electrophysiologic Drug Trials for Commonly Used Antiarrhythmic Drugs*

Drug	No. of Trials	No. of Success	% Success
Phenytoin	221	35	16
Procainamide	198	41	21
Quinidine	155	32	21
Lidocaine	55	4	7
Combination†	51	8	16
Disopyramide	44	6	14
Mexiletine	41	1	2
Class IC‡	25	3	12
Tocainide	24	2	8
Total	814	132	16

*Results of 814 consecutive trials using the antiarrhythmic drugs listed in patients with inducible ventricular tachyarrhythmias.
†Usually class IA + class IB drugs.
‡Encainide, flecainide, and lorcainide.

PHARMACOLOGY OF PHENYTOIN

Pharmacokinetics

After oral ingestion, absorption of phenytoin is relatively slow and can be erratic, especially when different preparations of the drug are used. Peak serum concentrations may occur anywhere from 3 to 12 hours after ingestion. When given intramuscularly, the drug precipitates and is absorbed only slowly. With intravenous injection, the drug can be delivered rapidly to target tissues. The pH of the injectable form is 12, however, and phlebitis can easily occur. Thus, intravenous phenytoin is given by intermittent injection (and not by infusion) and into a central vein if possible. Once absorbed, phenytoin is rapidly distributed to all tissues and is extensively protein-bound.

Phenytoin is metabolized by the liver to inactive compounds; less than 5 percent of the original drug is excreted in the urine. At lower plasma levels (less than 10 μg per milliliter), elimination of phenytoin is exponential (half-life is 6 to 12 hours). At higher plasma levels, elimination is dose-dependent (most likely because hepatic microsomal enzymes have been saturated), and plasma levels increase disproportionately as dosage is increased. The therapeutic plasma concentration of phenytoin for treating arrhythmias is similar to the therapeutic concentration for treating seizures, i.e., 10 to 20 μg per milliliter.

Administration of Phenytoin

Oral administration of phenytoin is used for long-term therapy and frequently for loading of the drug for testing in the electrophysiology laboratory. Because of phenytoin's slow absorption and relatively long and dose-dependent half-life, a "drug-

loading" regimen is usually recommended, especially if therapeutic levels are desired within 24 hours. A typical loading regimen would consist of giving 15 mg per kilogram on day one and 7.5 mg per kilogram on day two, followed by a maintenance dose of approximately 5 mg per kilogram (typically 300 to 500 mg per day). Daily doses are most often given as two or three divided doses. Because with higher (i.e., therapeutic) plasma levels the elimination of phenytoin is dose-dependent, chronic doses should be changed no more often than at 10- to 14-day intervals.

Intravenous administration is commonly used for the treatment of digitalis-toxic arrhythmias, for ventricular arrhythmias associated with acute medical conditions, and for the acute testing of inducible arrhythmias in the electrophysiology laboratory. As noted, intermittent injections should be used, preferably via a central vein. No more than 50 mg per minute should be given. In the electrophysiology laboratory, we attempt to load with a total of 7.5 to 10 mg per kilogram. We commonly give 50 mg every 2 minutes, monitoring blood pressure carefully (cuff pressures every minute have been adequate). If the blood pressure drops, the injection rate is slowed. We have found that sustained lateral gaze nystagmus is an early sign of achieving adequate drug levels (i.e., 10 μg per milliliter), and we check for lateral gaze nystagmus prior to each injection during acute intravenous loading.

ADVERSE EFFECTS

Compared with many other antiarrhythmic drugs, phenytoin is relatively well tolerated when given on both an acute and a chronic basis. When loading phenytoin to treat an acute condition, most adverse effects are related to the central nervous system. Patients typically develop drowsiness or vertigo when there is rapid loading to the therapeutic range. Ataxia and overt nystagmus (i.e., nystagmus while gazing straight ahead) are usually seen with plasma levels near or above 20 μg per milliliter. Since 90 percent of arrhythmias that respond to phenytoin respond at levels less than 18 μg per milliliter, if ataxia and overt nystagmus occur before an arrhythmia has responded, further administration of phenytoin is unlikely to be effective.

Gastrointestinal side effects can be seen with either acute or chronic use of phenytoin. The most common are nausea and vomiting, heartburn, and anorexia. These symptoms are sometimes related to toxic drug levels but can usually be ameliorated by dividing the daily dosage of phenytoin.

Gingival hyperplasia is seen in up to 20 percent of children and young adults who take phenytoin chronically and is probably related to poor oral hygiene. This side effect appears to be uncommon in older adults.

Relatively rare complications of phenytoin include osteomalacia (from interference with vitamin D metabolism), megaloblastic anemia (from interference with folate metabolism), and hypersensitivity reactions. Very rare complications have included systemic lupus erythematosus, hepatic necrosis, hematologic reactions, and pseudolymphoma.

Arrhythmia exacerbation (proarrhythmia), which can be seen with any antiarrhythmic drug, is relatively rare with phenytoin in our experience.

Several drug interactions have been documented with phenytoin. Increases in plasma phenytoin levels have been seen with cimetidine, isoniazid, sulfonamides, and amiodarone. Plasma levels of phenytoin can be reduced with concomitant administration of theophylline (and theophylline levels are reduced by phenytoin).

SUGGESTED READING

Epstein AE, Plumb VJ, Henthorn RW, Waldo AL. Phenytoin in the treatment of inducible ventricular tachycardia: Results of electrophysiologic testing and long-term follow-up. PACE 1987; 10:1049–1057.

Fogoros RN, Fiedler SB, Elson JJ. Efficacy of phenytoin in suppressing inducible ventricular tachyarrhythmias. Cardiovasc Drugs Ther 1988; 2:171–176.

Garson A, Kugler JD, Gillette PC, et al. Control of late postoperative ventricular arrhythmias with phenytoin in young patients. Am J Cardiol 1980; 46:290–294.

Wit AL, Rosen MR, Hoffman, BF. Electrophysiology and pharmacology of cardiac arrhythmias. VII. Cardiac effects of diphenylhydantoin. A. Am Heart J 1975; 90:265–272.

Wit AL, Rosen MR, Hoffman, BF. Electrophysiology and pharmacology of cardiac arrhythmias. VII. Cardiac effects of diphenylhydantoin. B. Am Heart J 1975; 90:379–404.

PROCAINAMIDE

JAMIE D. PARANICAS, M.D.
ALLAN M. GREENSPAN, M.D.

Procainamide is a class IA antiarrhythmic drug that was first introduced in 1951. Because of its availability in several oral forms and an intravenous form, it can be employed in the treatment of acute as well as chronic rhythm disturbances. Initially, procainamide was used almost exclusively for ventricular tachyarrhythmias, but during the last 25 years its success in suppressing a variety of supraventricular tachyarrhythmias has made it a mainstay of drug therapy for both types of rhythm abnormalities.

PHARMACOLOGY OF PROCAINAMIDE

Structure

Procainamide is a congener of procaine and differs from procaine only in that the ester linkage has been replaced by an amide bond.

Metabolism

After oral ingestion, the drug's effects can be observed in 1 hour, whereas the onset of action is almost immediate after intravenous administration. Seventy-five to ninety-five percent of the drug is absorbed after oral administration; however, absorption may be slow and incomplete following acute myocardial infarction. Approximately 15 percent of procainamide is protein-bound. The half-life of the drug is 2 to 3 hours. Fifty percent of the drug is excreted into the urine unchanged, and approximately 50 percent of the drug is metabolized by the liver to N-acetyl procainamide. The total amount of N-acetyl procainamide found in the plasma at any time depends on liver function and acetylator phenotype. The efficiency of the hepatic transferase enzyme system for the metabolism of procainamide is transmitted to offspring as an autosomal recessive trait. Slow acetylators, who constitute approximately 50 percent of the population, may be more prone to systemic lupus erythematosus–like side effects when given procainamide.

It is commonly recommended that the loading dose of procainamide be reduced in patients with congestive heart failure. It is theorized that because of reduced cardiac output, the absorption, hepatic metabolism, and urinary excretion of the drug and its active metabolite N-acetyl procainamide could be altered. Extreme caution in prescribing maintenance dosages of procainamide should be employed in the patient with renal insufficiency, since both procainamide and N-acetyl procainamide accumulate in this situation and may cause toxic side effects.

DRUG INTERACTIONS

Frequently, patients taking procainamide are also on several other medications for cardiac and noncardiac conditions. Careful attention should be given to the possibility of unfavorable drug interactions, e.g., that with potassium-wasting diuretics that can cause hypokalemia and acquired long Q-T syndromes. When procainamide is used with other antiarrhythmic agents, there may be additive toxicities. Procainamide enhances the effect of anticholinergic drugs and antagonizes the effects of anticholinesterases. When used in combination with antihypertensive drugs and thiazide diuretics, procainamide potentiates the hypotensive effects of these drugs because of its ganglionic blocking effect. Histamine (H_2) antagonists, specifically cimetidine and ranitidine, reduce the renal clearance of both N-acetyl procainamide and procainamide. Procainamide has been shown to enhance the effect of neuromuscular blocking agents that are commonly used during general anesthesia.

MECHANISM OF ACTION

Procainamide is classified as a class IA antiarrhythmic drug because it alters the action potential in ischemic and normal cardiac tissue, much like quinidine. It acts mainly by decreasing the influx of sodium into the cell via the rapid conducting sodium channel. This results in a reduction of upstroke velocity (phase 0) of the action potential, which in turn causes a slowing of conduction and a depression of excitability.

Procainamide and other class I antiarrhythmics also decrease the slope of phase 4 diastolic depolarization that causes a reduction in the automaticity of ectopic pacemakers. This reduction in automaticity does not affect the sinoatrial node function, since its impulses are generated by slow response (calcium dependent) action potentials.

Procainamide decreases impulse conduction in the atria, atrioventricular (AV) node, bundle of His, and the ventricles. Electrocardiographically, this is reflected as a prolonged P-R interval, widened QRS complex, and prolonged Q-T interval. Procainamide possesses anticholinergic properties (especially at low drug concentrations) that may antagonize its direct effects of AV conduction slowing and may produce a net acceleration of AV conduction in some circumstances.

Procainamide's ganglionic blocking effect and its direct vasodilatory effect on arteriolar tissue are responsible for its side effect of hypotension, which is encountered more commonly with intravenous administration.

What differentiates the class IA from other class I drugs is their prolongation of the effective refractory periods of most cardiac tissue. Procainamide increases the effective refractory periods of AV nodal, His-Purkinje, and ventricular muscle fibers.

SIDE EFFECTS

The side effects of procainamide can be categorized as acute and chronic. Hypotension, severe bradycardia, AV block, asystole, and ventricular tachycardia are acute side effects that may be encountered, especially with rapid intravenous administration. Gastrointestinal side effects including nausea, vomiting, and diarrhea can also occur acutely. Among the chronic side effects, agranulocytosis is the most serious one but fortunately is rare. Most cases of agranulocytosis are seen within the first 3 months of procainamide therapy. Fifty to eighty percent of patients who take procainamide long term convert to a positive antinuclear antibody (ANA) titer. Approximately 20 percent of patients develop a systemic lupus erythematosus type condition manifested clinically by fever, rash, arthralgias, pleuritis, or pericarditis. Slow acetylators more commonly develop this syndrome. When the drug is discontinued, symptoms should resolve in approximately 2 weeks.

Absolute contraindications to procainamide use are few but include prior procainamide-induced systemic lupus erythematosus, Mobitz type II second-degree or third-degree AV block, new onset of bifascicular block, long Q-T syndrome, severe sinus node dysfunction, or torsades de pointes related to type IA drug, tricyclic antidepressant administration, hypokalemia, or hypomagnesemia.

MONITORING PLASMA LEVELS

At this time, plasma procainamide and N-acetyl procainamide levels are readily available for both inpatient and outpatient monitoring. The therapeutic range for procainamide is 8 to 15 μg per milliliter, with toxicity more likely when the level is higher than 20 μg per milliliter. However, it should be noted that for life-threatening arrhythmias, plasma drug levels can be pushed as far as is necessary to achieve a therapeutic effect or until toxicity is encountered.

Although initially thought to have significant antiarrhythmic efficacy, N-acetyl procainamide is now monitored primarily to assess levels that can be associated with proarrhythmic and left ventricular depressant effects. These effects become a problem with plasma levels in excess of 30 μg per milliliter. Accumulation of N-acetyl procainamide is most commonly seen in fast acetylators, in patients with impaired renal or cardiac function, and in patients receiving the long-acting formulations of procainamide.

Once a therapeutic level is achieved with a specific dose, the timing of further determinations of drug levels should be based on the specific clinical needs. In the case of arrhythmia recurrence, procainamide and N-acetyl procainamide levels should be checked immediately to ensure that subtherapeutic levels were not the cause of drug failure. Drug levels should be checked when a new drug known to interact with procainamide metabolism is added to the medical regimen. When there is a significant change in renal or hepatic function or a significant reduction in left ventricular function, procainamide and N-acetyl procainamide levels should be checked to avoid dosage-related toxicities.

With long-term use of oral procainamide, ANA titers should be checked routinely. When conversion to a positive titer occurs, the decision to terminate the drug should be based on the risk-benefit ratio for the specific clinical situation. Generally for serious arrhythmias a (+) ANA titer alone does not necessitate termination of procainamide therapy. Only 25 to 40 percent of patients who develop (+) ANA titers go on to develop drug-induced lupus. When using procainamide on a long-term basis, periodic ANAs and white blood cell counts should be obtained.

In both short- and long-term therapy with procainamide, levels should be determined immediately if significant P-R, QRS, or Q-T interval prolongation is noted on an electrocardiogram. Prolongation of the QRS complex or Q-T interval by more than 25 to 35 percent of the baseline value is an indication to terminate therapy.

One of the reasons procainamide has gained great popularity in treating a variety of supraventricular and ventricular arrhythmias is its versatility of administration. Procainamide can be administered orally in a short-acting or slow-release form and intravenously as a bolus and maintenance infusion. In most patients, procainamide is well tolerated orally and intravenously. Significant side effects can frequently be avoided by careful monitoring of the blood pressure, electrocardiogram, and heart rate during acute intravenous administration and by monitoring plasma drug levels, white blood cell count, and patient symptoms during chronic oral administration. Hypotension occurring with intravenous bolus administration is attributable to the ganglionic blocking effect of the drug and frequently responds to volume replacement.

PROCAINAMIDE USE IN ATRIAL FIBRILLATION AND ATRIAL FLUTTER

Procainamide is a drug that can be effectively used in the conversion of atrial fibrillation or atrial flutter to sinus rhythm and the maintenance of normal sinus rhythm. Atrial fibrillation and atrial flutter are thought to be perpetuated by multiple reentrant wavelets and by an intraatrial reentry mechanism, respectively. Procainamide is effective in terminating these arrhythmias because it prolongs intraatrial conduction times and atrial refractoriness. Even without terminating the arrhythmia, procainamide may still improve hemodynamic tolerance of the arrhythmia by slowing the atrial mechanisms, thereby decreasing the ventricular response. However, before initiating procainamide therapy, AV nodal conduction should be adequately slowed with AV nodal blocking agents (e.g., digoxin or a beta or

calcium channel blocker) to prevent the paroxysmal acceleration of the ventricular response caused by procainamide's anticholinergic effect on AV conduction. Typically, we use digoxin, 0.5 mg intravenously, propranolol, 3 to 5 mg intravenously over 5 minutes, or verapamil, 10 mg intravenous push, before administering intravenous procainamide. Oral digoxin, 0.25 mg daily, or propranolol, 10 to 40 mg every 8 hours, or verapamil, 80 to 120 mg every 8 hours, can then be used along with procainamide on a chronic basis.

PROCAINAMIDE ADMINISTRATION IN ACUTE CONVERSION OF ATRIAL FIBRILLATION OR ATRIAL FLUTTER

In the emergency or hospital setting, atrial fibrillation or flutter with a rapid ventricular response is a frequently encountered arrhythmia. Despite variability in precipitating causes for the arrhythmia (e.g. "holiday heart," metabolic or ischemic derangements, exacerbation of pulmonary disease, or post-cardiac surgery), procainamide is an effective drug to convert the arrhythmia or slow the ventricular response. Intravenous procainamide should be infused at the rate of 50 mg per minute to a maximum loading dose of 20 mg per kilogram. The loading infusion can be terminated if the arrhythmia converts to normal sinus rhythm, if the patient becomes significantly hypotensive, if significant QRS or Q-T interval prolongation occurs, if second or third AV block develops, or if new ventricular dysrhythmias are seen. Once again, special attention must be given to appropriately blocking the AV node with a suitable agent. Once conversion of the atrial fibrillation or atrial flutter has been accomplished, a maintenance intravenous infusion or oral procainamide should be instituted. The maintenance infusion rate can vary from 2 to 6 mg per minute. For oral maintenance, slow-release procainamide hydrochloride 50–70 mg per kilogram in divided doses every 6 to 8 hours can be started immediately after termination of the loading infusion.

To use oral preparations for initial conversion of atrial fibrillation or atrial flutter, an initial dose of 1,250 mg of procainamide hydrochloride can be given, followed by 750 mg in 1 hour if the arrhythmia persists. An additional 500 mg to 1,000 mg of procainamide hydrochloride can be given every 2 hours until conversion has occurred or significant electrocardiographic changes or hypotension is observed. Once conversion is accomplished, slow-release procainamide hydrochloride 50 to 70 mg per kilogram, given every 6 to 8 hours in divided doses, can be started 2 hours after the last procainamide hydrochloride dose.

It is recommended that both procainamide and N-acetyl procainamide levels be measured when conversion of the atrial fibrillation or atrial flutter occurs. The procainamide level achieved at conversion can be used as a guide to levels required for adequate maintenance therapy.

PROCAINAMIDE USE IN ACUTE ATRIAL FIBRILLATION OR ATRIAL FLUTTER IN CONJUNCTION WITH CARDIOVERSION

Unfortunately, in many circumstances despite aggressive medical therapy, conversion of atrial fibrillation or atrial flutter to normal sinus rhythm is not accomplished. In this situation electrical cardioversion in combination with procainamide therapy can be employed. Prior to attempts at cardioversion, therapeutic levels of procainamide should be achieved, since this increases the probability of successful cardioversion and assists in the maintenance of normal sinus rhythm. Not infrequently, the combination of cardioversion and procainamide is used in emergency situations when the acute onset of atrial fibrillation or flutter is associated with hemodynamic compromise and is precipitated by an ongoing toxic or metabolic derangement that cannot be rapidly corrected. The occurrence of atrial fibrillation or flutter under these circumstances increases the probability that the arrhythmia will recur despite successful electrical cardioversion. The rapid intravenous infusion of 20 mg per kilogram of procainamide at 50 mg per minute followed by cardioversion is often effective in reestablishing and then maintaining sinus rhythm. Although worsening hypotension might be expected as a common side effect under these conditions, it is surprisingly rare, perhaps related to the afterload-reducing effect of the drug's ganglionic blockade action. The decision to maintain procainamide therapy after successful cardioversion depends on the clinical situation.

Special situations may arise when a temporary pacemaker should be inserted prophylactically for cardioversion of atrial arrhythmias. These would include a history of intermittent high-degree AV block, especially if associated with a slow ventricular response, and digoxin toxicity. In these instances, significant bradycardia or asystole can occur following cardioversion, and therefore temporary pacing capabilities should be available.

PROCAINAMIDE USE IN CHRONIC ATRIAL FLUTTER

In many patients, usually those with dilated left atria, atrial flutter remains a chronic condition. In most of these patients the atrial arrhythmia is well tolerated as long as cardiac output is maintained in an acceptable range. Depending on the situation, it may be elected to allow the atrial flutter to persist, especially when past attempts at conversion or maintenance of sinus rhythm have proved unsuccessful. In this case, slow-release oral procainamide hydrochloride can be used on a long-term basis to help control the ventricular response. The appropriate dosage would be 50 to 70 mg per kilogram in divided doses, given every 6 to 8 hours. Propranolol, digoxin, or another agent that slows AV nodal conduction should also be used in combination with the slow-release procainamide hydrochloride.

With the long-term use of any class IA agent, periodic electrocardiographic recordings should be obtained to monitor the P-R, QRS, and Q-T intervals. A life-threatening complication of procainamide use frequently seen in the elderly with chronic atrial arrhythmias is the development of torsades de pointes. Unexplained syncope or palpitations in this setting should alert the physician to that possibility, and procainamide therapy should be stopped and the patient monitored.

PROCAINAMIDE USE IN SUPRAVENTRICULAR TACHYCARDIAS

Supraventricular tachycardias are common and can be seen in a variety of clinical settings. Most paroxysmal supraventricular tachycardia (SVT) is due to reentry but can also be the result of increased automaticity. When SVT is caused by enhanced automaticity, it can be transient or chronic and is frequently related to specific underlying clinical circumstances. When SVT is the result of a reentrant mechanism, four different sites of reentry can be involved: the AV node, the sinoatrial node, the atrium, or the AV conduction system. Procainamide is effective both in termination and prophylaxis of SVT caused by both mechanisms.

PROCAINAMIDE USE IN AUTOMATIC ATRIAL TACHYCARDIA

Automatic atrial tachycardia (see the chapter *Automatic Atrial Tachycardia and Nonparoxysmal Atrioventricular Junctional Tachycardia*) can present in different settings, including acute myocardial infarction, exacerbation of chronic pulmonary disorders, pneumonia, hypokalemia, and excess alcohol ingestion. Automatic atrial tachycardia can also be provoked by catecholamine release, atrial stress, inflammation, drugs, and hypoxia. Automatic atrial tachycardia is caused by accelerated spontaneous depolarization of atrial cells that results from an increased slope of phase 4 of the cardiac action potential. Procainamide can be effective in terminating automatic atrial tachycardias primarily because of its ability to depress diastolic depolarization.

In the setting of symptomatic automatic atrial tachycardia, procainamide can be infused intravenously at the rate of 50 mg per minute to a maximal dose of 20 mg per kilogram until the tachycardia is terminated or signs of toxicity occur. Chronic oral therapy should be instituted if it is likely that the arrhythmia will recur, e.g., in the setting of pericardial infiltration with tumor. In this case, slow-release procainamide hydrochloride, 50 to 70 mg per kilogram, divided into every 6 to 8 hour doses, can be used. In most instances, further episodes of automatic atrial tachycardia can be prevented by correcting the metabolic derangement or avoiding the precipitating agent, which might obviate the need for long-term drug therapy.

PROCAINAMIDE USE IN REENTRANT SUPRAVENTRICULAR TACHYCARDIA

As many as 90 percent of all supraventricular tachycardias (SVTs) are caused by a reentrant mechanism (see the chapters *Paroxysmal Reentrant Supraventricular Tachycardia Without Preexcitation: Pharmacologic Therapy* and *Paroxysmal Atrioventricular Reentrant Tachycardia: Pharmacologic Therapy*). Reentrant SVT can be precipitated by any stress that alters automatic tone and in particular causes excess catecholamine release, e.g., exercise or emotional stress. Alcohol, nicotine, and caffeine have also been implicated in its occurrence.

Procainamide is effective in terminating reentrant SVT and preventing its recurrence. Acute administration of procainamide and long-term therapy are the same as described previously for automatic atrial tachycardia.

PROCAINAMIDE USE IN THE WOLFF-PARKINSON-WHITE SYNDROME

The Wolff-Parkinson-White (WPW) syndrome (see the section *Preexcitation Syndromes*) is a condition resulting from the presence of one or more accessory pathways that allow preexcitation of the ventricle. Patients with the WPW syndrome are sometimes plagued with frequent symptomatic episodes of SVT. They can also suffer bouts of paroxysmal atrial fibrillation or atrial flutter with rapid antegrade conduction over the bypass tract, resulting in a very rapid ventricular response. In this population of patients, prophylactic antiarrhythmic therapy is often necessary.

Reentrant Supraventricular Tachycardia in the Wolff-Parkinson-White Syndrome

Most of the tachyarrhythmias seen in the setting of the WPW syndrome are caused by reentry employing an accessory pathway retrogradely and the normal AV conduction system antegradely. An effective method to terminate such a reentrant SVT would be to slow accessory pathway conduction, and procainamide is effective in doing so.

When reentrant SVT is suspected as the mechanism for a tachycardia in a patient with the WPW syndrome, intravenous procainamide is an excellent agent for rapid termination of the arrhythmia. The infusion rate should be 50 mg per minute to a maximal dose of 20 mg per kilogram until termination of the arrhythmia or signs of toxicity occur. After successful termination, oral therapy with slow-release procainamide hydrochloride can be initiated at 10 to 20 mg per kilogram every 6 to 8 hours.

Atrial Fibrillation and Atrial Flutter in the Wolff-Parkinson-White Syndrome

Although they are less common than SVT, atrial fibrillation and atrial flutter can be devastating in patients with the WPW syndrome because of rapid antegrade conduction over the bypass tract, yielding very rapid ventricular rates (see the chapter *Atrial Fibrillation in the Wolff-Parkinson-White Syndrome*). When rapid atrial fibrillation or flutter occurs in a patient with the WPW syndrome, many clinicians consider parenteral procainamide to be the therapeutic modality of choice. Administration of procainamide can be carried out as described previously for SVT. In the event of hemodynamic compromise, cardioversion should be performed.

Wide Complex Tachycardia in the Wolff-Parkinson-White Syndrome

A potentially life-threatening situation often occurs when a patient with the WPW syndrome comes to the emergency room with a very rapid wide complex tachycardia. Sometimes the most experienced cardiologist has difficulty in determining whether the tachycardia is supraventricular or ventricular in origin. At best, even when it has been decided that the rhythm is supraventricular in origin, identification of the specific type of SVT may remain undetermined. In these situations, the use of parenteral procainamide or a class IB agent such as lidocaine is the most appropriate therapy in contrast to the use of intravenous verapamil. Although verapamil can terminate AV reentrant SVT utilizing a bypass tract, it accelerates the ventricular response in atrial fibrillation or atrial flutter with antegrade conduction over a bypass tract. The patient should be given a total loading dose of 20 mg per kilogram infused at a rate of 50 mg per kilogram and then maintained on an intravenous infusion of 3 to 6 mg per minute. Oral therapy can be instituted thereafter with slow-release procainamide hydrochloride 10 to 20 mg per kilogram given every 6 to 8 hours. Again, if hemodynamic compromise ensues, cardioversion should be performed.

PROCAINAMIDE USE IN ACUTE INCESSANT VENTRICULAR TACHYCARDIA

Regardless of the etiology, incessant ventricular tachycardia is a medical emergency that frequently deteriorates into ventricular fibrillation if untreated. A common cause of ventricular tachycardia, both unsustained (less than 30 seconds) or sustained (more than 30 seconds or causing acute hemodynamic compromise), is acute myocardial infarction. In this clinical situation, intravenous lidocaine is commonly used. However, if lidocaine fails to terminate the ventricular tachycardia, intravenous procainamide can be substituted for or added to lidocaine. In the case in which there is a contraindication to lidocaine therapy, intravenous procainamide may be used as the first line of therapy.

In treating ventricular tachycardia, the procainamide loading dose should be administered at the rate of 50 mg per minute. Ideally, even if the ventricular tachycardia has terminated, a total of 20 mg per kilogram should be given. Heart rate, blood pressure, and electrocardiographic recordings should be monitored frequently and loading slowed or terminated if intractable hypotension (unresponsive to intravenous fluids or dopamine) or heart block occurs. Procainamide should also be stopped if marked Q-T interval prolongation occurs. When loading is completed, a maintenance infusion of procainamide at 2 to 6 mg per minute should be continued. Plasma levels of procainamide and N-acetyl procainamide should be checked to ensure appropriate dosing. In some cases, procainamide levels higher than the accepted therapeutic levels may be necessary to suppress the arrhythmia, in which case the procainamide infusion should be maintained unless clinical toxicity occurs. Occasionally procainamide will not completely suppress ventricular tachycardia, even at high levels. Since procainamide substantially increases the cycle length of ventricular tachycardia (slows the rate), it might render the arrhythmia better tolerated hemodynamically and can be used as a temporizing measure. At this point, another antiarrhythmic agent, particularly a class IB agent, could be added to attempt termination of the tachycardia.

RECURRENT SUSTAINED VENTRICULAR TACHYCARDIA: ROLE OF PROCAINAMIDE THERAPY

Recurrent sustained ventricular tachycardia is often a life-threatening arrhythmia commonly seen in the setting of structural heart disease, usually coronary artery disease with associated left ventricular wall motion abnormality. Since the possibility of a proarrhythmic response or unsuccessful suppression exists when empirical antiarrhythmic therapy is used, programmed electrical stimulation should be performed to assess the efficacy of drug therapy (see the chapter *Electrophysiologic Techniques*).

PROCAINAMIDE IN COMBINATION WITH OTHER ANTIARRHYTHMICS IN THE TREATMENT OF RECURRENT SUSTAINED VENTRICULAR TACHYCARDIA

When procainamide alone is unsuccessful in preventing the induction of sustained ventricular tachycardia, it can sometimes prove an effective agent when used in combination with a class IB or III antiarrhythmic drug. Theoretically, the combination of two agents from different classes with different toxicities may yield a better efficacy rate than each agent alone, and with a lower incidence of toxic side effects.

For inducible sustained ventricular tachycardia, unsustained ventricular tachycardia, and ventricular fibrillation, a combination of a class IA and IB agent has shown the highest efficacy when compared with other combinations. The efficacy rate for a class IA-IB combination ranges from 35 to 50 percent as evaluated by electrophysiologic testing, and 94 percent as evaluated by ambulatory monitoring. The combination of a class IA and IB agent may limit the amount of Q-T interval prolongation encountered with a class IA agent alone, and this may decrease the frequency of drug-induced torsades de pointes. In the event that suppression of the ventricular tachycardia is not accomplished, a class IA-IB combination significantly prolongs the cycle length, more than either agent alone, thus rendering the arrhythmia better tolerated hemodynamically. Typically, we use a combination of slow-release procainamide hydrochloride 1,000 to 1,500 mg every 6 to 8 hours, plus mexiletine, 150 to 300 mg every 8 hours in combination for suppression of ventricular tachycardia.

LONG-TERM FOLLOW-UP OF RECURRENT SUSTAINED VENTRICULAR TACHYCARDIA WHILE ON PROCAINAMIDE THERAPY

In most cases, long-term oral procainamide therapy is well tolerated in patients with recurrent ventricular tachycardia. There appears to be little justification for performing routine Holter monitoring unless the dosage is changed or the patient is complaining of palpitations, dizziness, or syncope. Plasma levels of both procainamide and N-acetyl procainamide can be checked periodically to ensure that no change has taken place in absorption or metabolism of the drug.

Plasma levels of procainamide and N-acetyl procainamide should be assayed when a drug with a known interaction with procainamide is initiated or when renal or hepatic function declines. In the event that there is recurrence of the ventricular tachycardia, plasma levels should be checked immediately to document that subtherapeutic levels of the drug were not the cause. If recurrence of the arrhythmia takes place when there are acceptable therapeutic drug levels, procainamide should be stopped and other antiarrhythmic drugs tested.

Patients should have periodic electrocardiograms to measure P-R, QRS, and Q-T intervals. Procainamide should be discontinued if significant prolongation occurs, i.e., a greater than 25 to 30 percent increase over baseline or for Q-Tc interval more than 0.56 second. Any change in renal or hepatic function should be carefully monitored and both procainamide and *N*-acetyl procainamide levels followed. Generally the dose of procainamide need only be altered for significant renal insufficiency, i.e., when creatinine clearance is less than 50 ml per minute, in which case it should be decreased by about one-third. Also, slow-release procainamide hydrochloride generally should not be used in patients with renal insufficiency because marked and potentially life-threatening accumulation of *N*-acetyl procainamide can occur.

With long-term procainamide therapy, approximately 50 to 80 percent of patients develop positive ANA titers. When using the drug for successful management of recurrent sustained ventricular tachycardia, procainamide should not be terminated solely because of the development of a positive ANA titer without clinical evidence of a lupus-like syndrome. Only 15 to 25 percent of patients with sustained ventricular tachycardia on long-term procainamide therapy develop a clinical lupus syndrome, and in these patients procainamide use should be stopped.

SUGGESTED READING

Chung KC. Manual of cardiac arrhythmias. New York: Butterworth Publishers, 1986.

DiPalma JR. Basic pharmacology in medicine. New York: McGraw Hill, 1982.

Duff HJ, Roden D, Primm RK. Mexiletine in the treatment of resistant ventricular arrhythmias: Enhancement of efficacy and reduction of dose related side effects by combination with quinidine. Circulation 1983; 67:1124.

Greenspan AM, Horowitz LN, Spielman SR. Large dose procainamide therapy for ventricular tachycardia. Am J Cardiol 1980; 46:453.

Greenspan AM, Spielman SR, Horowitz LN. Combination antiarrhythmic drug therapy for ventricular tachyarrhythmias. PACE 1986; 9:569.

Josephson ME, Seides FS. Clinical cardiac electrophysiology—techniques and interpretations. Philadelphia: Lea & Febiger, 1979.

Knoben JE, Anderson PO. Handbook of clinical drug data. Bethesda, MD: Drug Intelligence Publications, 1983.

Marchlinski FE, Buxton AE, Vassallo JA, et al. Comparative electrophysiologic effect of intravenous and oral procainamide in patients with sustained ventricular arrhythmias. J Am Coll Cardiol 1984; 4:1247.

Physicians' Desk Reference. 44th edition. Oradell, NJ: Medical Economics Company, 1990: 1651–1653, 1695–1701.

PROPAFENONE

PHILIP J. PODRID, M.D.
JOHN S. WILSON, M.D.

Propafenone, developed in the late 1960s, is an interesting and promising antiarrhythmic agent reported to be useful for the treatment of a wide variety of both supraventricular and ventricular arrhythmias. Propafenone is a local anesthetic or membrane-stabilizing drug classified as a class IC agent, along with encainide and flecainide. Although structurally unique, it does have a similarity to propranolol (Fig. 1). Indeed, the drug exerts mild beta-blocking activity that may be clinically important and also has been shown to possess weak calcium-channel blocking effects. However, the clinical significance of this property is uncertain. The drug can be administered both orally and intravenously but is available only for oral use. This chapter discusses the drug's mechanism of action, pharmacology, clinical use, and toxicity.

ELECTROPHYSIOLOGIC EFFECTS

Similar to the other class I antiarrhythmic agents, propafenone is a potent blocker of the fast sodium channel (Table 1). As a result of the inhibition of the fast inward sodium ion currents, there is a reduction in the upstroke velocity of the fast action potential (Vmax) or phase 0. This effect can be observed in all cardiac tissue in which a fast action potential, resulting from sodium ion influxes, is generated, including the atrial and ventricular myocardium, His-Purkinje fibers, and the accessory pathway. As a result of the depressant effect on Vmax of phase 0, there is a slowing in the impulse conduction velocity within these tissues. These electrophysiologic changes caused by propafenone are more apparent in ischemic tissue as compared with normal myocardium. As expected, there is no change in the resting membrane potential.

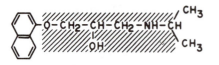

PROPRANOLOL

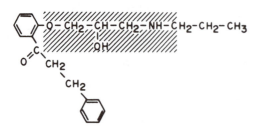

PROPAFENONE

Figure 1 Structure of propafenone compared with that of propranolol. Similarity in side chains is indicated by shaded area.

In different animal models, the effect of propafenone on the action potential duration, which represents the time for myocardial repolarization, is variable. However, in the human heart the drug produces a shortening of action potential duration in the Purkinje fibers but a slight lengthening in the

Table 1 Pharmacology of Propafenone

Electrophysiologic Actions (class IC drug)
  Local anesthetic (sodium channel blockade)
    Reduces impulse conduction velocity
    Prolongs refractory period
    Decrease automaticity
  Beta blockade (1/40 of propafenone)
  Calcium-channel blockade (1/100 of verapamil)
Electrocardiogram
  Prolongs P-R interval and QRS complex
  No change in J-Tc interval
Hemodynamics
  Negative inotrope (dose-related)
    Decreases stroke volume and cardiac output
    Increases peripheral vascular resistance
Dose
  Oral: 150–300 mg t.i.d.
Absorption
  Rapid and complete levels peak at 2–3 hours
Bioavailability
  Approximately 50%
Protein Binding
  90%
Metabolism
  Hepatic/nonlinear
Half-Life
  7 hours
Metabolites
  5-Hydroxy and *N*-depropyl propafenone
Therapeutic Level
  600–900 ng/ml

ventricular myocardium. Unlike other class IC drugs, propafenone causes a slight lengthening of the refractory period of all cardiac tissue. The antegrade and retrograde refractory periods of accessory pathway tissue are significantly increased.

In addition to its effects on sodium conductance, propafenone is a weak calcium channel blocker, estimated to be 1/100th as potent as verapamil. In vitro, propafenone eliminates delayed afterpotentials or triggered automaticity, which are generated by calcium ion fluxes into the cell. Clinically, the drug has effects on the electrophysiologic properties of those tissues that generate a slow action potential, specifically the sinus and atrioventricular (AV) node. The result is a decrease in sinus and AV nodal automaticity, a reduction in the impulse conduction velocity through the AV node, and prolongation of its refractory period. The automaticity of the sinus node and the conduction properties of the AV node are also depressed as a result of the mild beta-blocking activity exerted by propafenone. As indicated, there is a structural similarity to propranolol (see Fig. 1). The beta-blocking effect is estimated to be 1/40th of that due to propranolol. However, since the blood levels of propafenone achieved during clinical use are up to 50 times greater than those resulting from standard doses of propranolol, the beta-blocking effect of the drug may be clinically important.

On the basis of its electrophysiologic properties, it is predicted that propafenone will cause changes on the surface electrocardiogram that are typical of the class IC class of drugs. There is a dose-related increase in the P-R interval and QRS complex duration, reflecting the prolongation of depolarization time and the slowing of impulse conduction. It had been reported that changes in the P-R interval were useful for dose titration; however, prolongation reflects drug activity and not the blood level achieved. Although the sinus rate at rest is unaltered, the drug does blunt the heart rate increase attributable to exercise as a result of its beta-blocking effect. Like other class IC drugs, propafenone does not affect repolarization time or the Q-T interval. As a result of the lengthening of the QRS complex duration, the Q-Tc may be prolonged. However, the J-Tc, a more accurate measure of repolarization, is not affected, suggesting that there are no clinically important effects of the drug on the refractory periods of the Purkinje fiber or ventricular myocardium.

PHARMACOKINETICS

Although propafenone has been investigated when administered by both the intravenous and oral routes, the oral form has been more extensively studied, and most of the available data are based on this preparation (see Table 1). The intravenous dose of drug reported to be effective is a loading dose of 1 to 2.5 mg per kilogram administered over 10 minutes, followed by a constant infusion of 1 to 2 mg per minute. The usual oral dose is 150 to 300 mg three times a day, although doses of up to 1,200 mg per day have been used. When propafenone is administered by the intravenous route, the plasma drug level falls very quickly during the first 1 to 2 hours because of an initial rapid distribution to adipose tissue. When it is given by the oral route, the drug is completely absorbed from the gastrointestinal tract, and levels peak 2 to 3 hours after drug administration. However, bioavailability (which varies from 13 to 55 percent) and blood level achieved are not directly related to the dose given (150 to 450 mg). This is because propafenone has extensive presystemic hepatic clearance or a first-pass effect in the liver. The relationship between the dose administered and the blood level achieved is nonlinear because of saturable hepatic metabolism. As the dose of propafenone is increased, hepatic metabolic sites become saturated, the proportion of propafenone metabolized decreases, and there is a significant increase in blood level. It has been reported that a threefold increase in daily dose from 300 mg to 900 mg results in a ten-fold increase in the steady-state blood level of the drug. It is perhaps preferable to administer a higher dose less frequently than the same total daily dose divided into smaller amounts given more often. Approximately 90 percent of the drug in the blood is protein-bound, and because it is highly lipophilic, the steady-state volume of distribution is large, approximately 3 L per kilogram.

Propafenone is rapidly and almost completely metabolized by a saturable hepatic oxidative pathway, and less than 1 percent is excreted unchanged by the liver. The mean half-life after a single dose is 4 to 5 hours and averages 6 to 7 hours (range 2 to 17 hours) when a steady-state blood level has been achieved after multiple doses. The two major metabolites are 5-hydroxy and N-depropyl propafenone. Although the 5-hydroxy metabolite does possess minor antiarrhythmic activity, it is unclear if this is clinically important because blood levels of this metabolite are low. It has been reported that the rate of propafenone metabolism is genetically determined, similar to that of debrisoquin and other antiarrhythmic agents such as encainide. Approximately 90 percent of Caucasians exhibit rapid oxidative metabolism, and they extensively metabolize propafenone. In these patients, plasma levels of the parent compound are low and the half-life is short. In approximately 10 percent, drug metabolism is slow, and hence the blood level of propafenone is higher and the half-life of the drug is longer. In general, steady-state blood levels are achieved after 3 days of therapy regardless of the rate of metabolism.

Therapeutic blood levels of propafenone, correlated with suppression of ventricular premature complexes, vary widely from 40 to 1,800 ng per milliliter (average 830 ng per milliliter). Suppression of complex forms, however, is achieved at slightly lower blood levels, averaging from 590 to 795 ng per milliliter in different studies. Although most of the side effects are dose-related and occur more commonly at higher blood levels (average 900 to 1,460 ng per milliliter), there is marked overlap between therapeutic and toxic levels. Measurement of propafenone blood levels is generally of no clinical value.

Since propafenone is completely metabolized by the liver, hepatic dysfunction significantly reduces the rate of drug clearance and prolongs its half-life, resulting in an increase in blood levels. The dose of drug must therefore be reduced. It is possible that a reduction in hepatic blood flow, such as occurs with congestive heart failure, also affects drug metabolism. Although well-controlled studies are lacking, it does not appear that renal dysfunction affects propafenone pharmacokinetics, although the levels of the metabolites increase. One of the metabolites does have mild antiarrhythmic activity, and it may be necessary to reduce the dose. Since propafenone is highly protein-bound, it is not removed by dialysis.

DRUG INTERACTIONS

As with other antiarrhythmic agents, important drug interactions with propafenone have been reported (Table 2). Since the drug has mild beta-blocking activity, its combined use with a beta blocker may produce an excess effect on sinus and AV nodal activity. Additionally, the combined use of propafenone and a beta blocker may reduce myocardial contractility, especially in patients with left ventricular dysfunction who are at increased risk for congestive heart failure. As with several other antiarrhythmic agents, propafenone does interact with digoxin, resulting in an increase of approximately 40 percent in the steady-state plasma concentration of digoxin. Unlike the etiology for the increase in di-

Table 2 Drug Interactions with Propafenone

Warfarin	Increased warfarin levels
	Potentiation of anticoagulant effect
Digoxin	Increased digoxin levels
Beta blockers and calcium channel blockers	Potentiation of beta-blocker effect on heart rate, AV nodal conduction, left ventricular function
	Potentiation of antiarrhythmic effect
Antiarrhythmics	Additive antiarrhythmic effects
Cimetidine	Increased cimetidine and propafenone blood levels

goxin levels when combined with quinidine therapy, the elevation in digoxin level does not appear to be a result of a reduction in the renal excretion of digoxin.

Coadministration of propafenone with sodium warfarin causes an increase in propafenone levels by 24 percent, but the clinical significance is unclear. Additionally, propafenone increases warfarin blood levels, potentiating its anticoagulant effect. Therefore, the prothrombin time should be measured frequently when therapy with propafenone is begun. Food ingestion may interact with propafenone in two ways. First, the administration of the drug with a meal reduces gastric absorption and delays the time for peak blood levels, although the peak level achieved is not affected. Second, the peak levels achieved may be increased as a result of a decrease in metabolism caused by an inhibitory effect of food on first pass hepatic metabolism.

A number of interactions between propafenone and other antiarrhythmic agents have been reported. It is well established that the combined use of two antiarrhythmic agents result in additive or even synergistic antiarrhythmic effects. Increased efficacy has been reported when propafenone is used in combination with quinidine, procainamide, lidocaine, sotalol, and amiodarone. In each case, blood levels of propafenone or the other antiarrhythmic agents were not altered by their combined use, further supporting the concept of an additive effect on electrophysiologic properties.

HEMODYNAMIC EFFECTS

Propafenone is a local anesthetic agent and like other similar agents, it possesses direct negative inotropic effects. The drug has weak but clinically important beta-blocking activity, and this may contribute to its depressant effect on left ventricular contractility. In animal models, propafenone adversely affects all invasive hemodynamic measurements of left ventricular function, and as a result of the reduction in cardiac output, there is a slight increase in peripheral vascular resistance. The reduction in stroke volume and cardiac output is dose-related. In clinical studies, propafenone does not significantly depress left ventricular ejection fraction in patients without left ventricular dysfunction, although some patients with impaired left ventricular function may have a further decrease in ejection fraction. The precipitation of clinically important congestive heart failure has been reported and occurs principally in patients with a previous history of left ventricular dysfunction and congestive heart failure. The incidence ranges from 5 to 9 percent, depending on the patient population.

CLINICAL ANTIARRHYTHMIC EFFECTS
Ventricular Arrhythmia

A number of studies have been conducted in which propafenone was administered to patients with frequent ventricular premature complexes. Although doses used in these trials vary and the definition of efficacy differs, a greater than 80 percent reduction in ventricular premature complex frequency is observed in 52 to 87 percent of patients (average 70 percent), as evaluated with ambulatory monitoring. The drug is highly effective for suppressing complex or repetitive forms, and in a number of studies, runs of ventricular tachycardia are reduced overall by 95 percent, and approximately 80 percent of patients have more than 90 percent elimination of these forms. In patients with frequent ventricular arrhythmia, propafenone has been compared with quinidine and disopyramide and has been reported to be more effective than these agents for suppression of ventricular premature complexes and runs of ventricular tachycardia.

Propafenone has also been evaluated in patients with a history of a sustained ventricular tachyarrhythmia refractory to other antiarrhythmic drugs. When ambulatory monitoring is used, 55 percent of patients achieve efficacy, defined as total elimination of runs of ventricular tachycardia, a greater than 90 percent decrease in couplets, and a greater than 50 percent reduction in ventricular premature complexes. With exercise testing, these criteria are achieved in 65 percent of patients, and when both these noninvasive techniques are considered, approximately 50 percent of patients respond to propafenone (Fig. 2).

As with other antiarrhythmic drugs, propafenone is less effective when evaluated by electrophysiologic techniques, and the arrhythmias of approximately 10 to 20 percent of patients are rendered noninducible. However, in the majority of patients whose arrhythmias remain inducible, the drug significantly reduces the rate of ventricular tachycardia, usually resulting in better hemodynamic tolerance of the arrhythmia (Fig. 3). Although patients who respond to the drug remain free of recurrent arrhythmias, continued inducibility does not always predict recurrence. It has been reported that the recurrence rate is low if the arrhythmia is more difficult to induce. Additionally, significant slowing of the rate of the ventricular tachycardia by 100 msec or more may predict freedom from recurrence.

The long-term results of propafenone therapy are uncertain, as such follow-up data have been reported only infrequently. However, a few studies using invasive or noninvasive methods have reported a low arrhythmia recurrence rate and improved survival among patients with a history of a

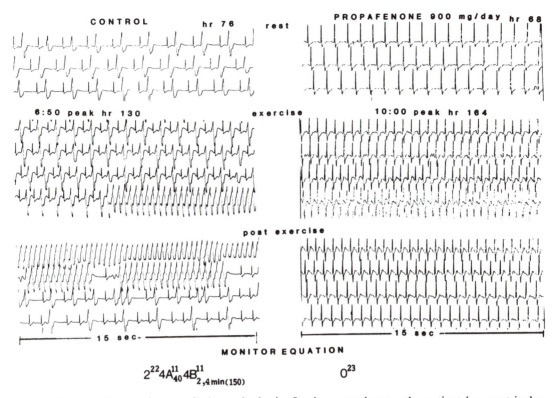

MONITOR EQUATION

$$2^{22}4A_{40}^{11}4B_{2,4min(150)}^{11} \qquad \qquad 0^{23}$$

Figure 2 Propafenone for ventricular arrhythmia. In the control state, the patient has ventricular bigeminy at rest, whereas during exercise, a brief run of ventricular tachycardia is induced. Ambulatory monitoring demonstrates frequent ventricular premature complexes for 22 hours (2^{22}), couplets during 11 hours with up to 40 episodes per hour ($4A^{11}$), and 11 hours during which ventricular tachycardia ($4B$) occurred. There were two episodes per hour lasting up to 4 minutes at rates of 150. During therapy with propafenone, arrhythmia is completely suppressed during exercise as well as during ambulatory monitoring.

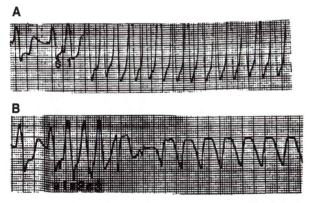

Figure 3 Effect of propafenone during electrophysiologic testing. During the control study (A), one extra stimulus (S_1) induces sustained monomorphic ventricular tachycardia with a cycle length of 220 msec (rate 270), with propafenone therapy (B), sustained monomorphic ventricular tachycardia is still induced with three extra stimuli (S_1, S_2, S_3), but the cycle length is now 375 msec (160 beats/min). The change in configuration of the ventricular tachycardia is due to the monitoring of a different lead.

serious ventricular tachyarrhythmia who respond to the drug.

Supraventricular Arrhythmia

Although this area has been less well studied, propafenone has been reported to be effective for a wide range of supraventricular arrhythmias. Intravenous propafenone reverts paroxysmal atrial fibrillation to sinus rhythm in approximately 38 percent of patients, whereas long-term orally administered therapy prevents recurrent episodes of atrial fibrillation or atrial flutter in approximately 50 percent of patients with a history of paroxysmal arrhythmias. The drug may be particularly effective for patients with atrial fibrillation provoked by catecholamines and the sympathetic nervous system. Its role in patients with chronic atrial fibrillation is unclear, although it has been reported to prevent recurrent arrhythmias once atrial fibrillation is electively reverted. As a result of its depressant effects on AV nodal conduction, propafenone does produce slowing of the ventricular response rate in patients with persistent atrial fibrillation.

Several studies have reported that intravenous propafenone terminates AV nodal reentrant tachycardia and prevents its reinduction during electrophysiologic testing in 50 to 80 percent of patients. When the oral drug is administered chronically, approximately 70 percent of responders remain free of recurrent arrhythmia or have less frequent episodes.

Propafenone is particularly effective in patients with the Wolff-Parkinson-White syndrome who have atrial fibrillation or supraventricular tachycardia. As expected from its depressive electrophysiologic effects on the accessory pathway tissue, the drug decreases the ability of the accessory pathway to conduct 1:1 as a result of prolongation of the antegrade and retrograde refractory periods, and therefore there is a reduction in the ventricular response rate during atrial fibrillation. Since propafenone affects the refractory periods of both the accessory pathway and the AV node, it is very effective for terminating and preventing recurrent AV reentrant tachycardia associated with the Wolff-Parkinson-White syndrome.

SIDE EFFECTS

Side effects from propafenone are frequent, reported in up to 50 percent of patients (Table 3). However, most are mild, well tolerated, and often dose-related, being especially frequent when a daily

Table 3 Side Effects of Propafenone

Cardiovascular
  Arrhythmia aggravation
  Congestive heart failure
  Conduction abnormalities
  Sinus node dysfunction
Neurologic
  Dizziness and lightheadedness
  Lethargy
  Paresthesias
  Headache
  Tremor
  Ataxia
  Slurred speech
Gastrointestinal
  Nausea and vomiting
  Altered taste
  Constipation
  Dyspepsia
  Abdominal pain
  Flatulence
  Anorexia
Other
  Exacerbation of chronic obstructive pulmonary disease
  Urinary frequency
  Arthralgias
  Arthritis
  Skin rash
  Blurred vision

dose of more than 900 mg is administered. Toxic side effects often respond to dose reduction, which is necessary in 12 percent of patients. Although side effects tend to be more frequent at higher doses and blood levels, there is much overlap, and therefore for the individual patient blood levels do not correlate well with toxicity.

In the majority of patients, side effects develop during the first month of propafenone therapy. Despite the frequent occurrence of nuisance side effects, drug discontinuation as a result of toxicity is necessary in only 4 to 7 percent of patients. The most common side effects resulting in drug discontinuation are related to the cardiovascular, gastrointestinal, or central nervous systems.

The most frequent side effects are those related to the cardiovascular system, reported in up to 27 percent of patients. Such toxicity is especially frequent in those patients with underlying heart disease and congestive heart failure. In patients with frequent arrhythmia but no history of a sustained tachyarrhythmia, arrhythmia aggravation, defined as the occurrence of new arrhythmia, is observed in 5 percent of patients. A statistical increase in asymptomatic ventricular premature complexes is reported in an additional 13 percent of patients. Serious arrhythmia aggravation is more frequent among patients with congestive heart failure and a history of a sustained ventricular tachyarrhythmia, and in such patients the incidence is approximately 10 percent (Fig. 4).

Congestive heart failure occurs in 4 to 7 percent of patients, but the incidence is almost 10 percent among patients with a history of congestive heart failure. Conduction abnormalities are uncommon, being observed in 8 percent of patients. Most often there is a new firstdegree AV block (prolonged P-R interval), bundle branch block, or intraventricular conduction delay. Although it is not usually serious or symptomatic, the occurrence of a new bundle branch block may be confused with recurrent ventricular tachycardia, especially if it is rate-related, occurring with exercise (Fig. 5). Serious conduction abnormalities, including complete heart block, occur in approximately 1 percent of patients. Sinus node depression and sinus bradycardia occurred in 0.9 percent.

The next most common side effects are neurologic, reported in 21 percent of patients. The majority of neurologic complaints are dose-related, being more frequent at doses higher than 900 mg per day. The incidence is substantially greater when blood drug levels are higher than 1,000 ng per milliliter. The most common complaints are dizziness and lightheadedness, ataxia, paresthesias, tremor, and slurred speech.

Gastrointestinal side effects are reported by 20 percent of patients. Most are dose-related and are especially common when blood levels of propafen-

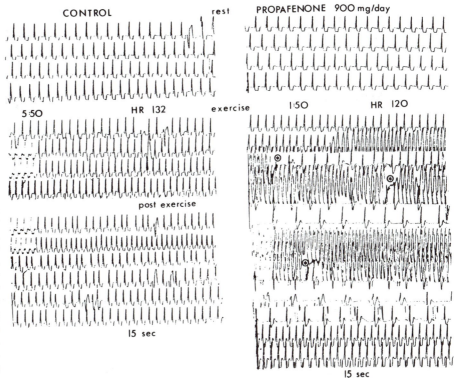

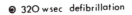

Figure 4 Aggravation of arrhythmia by propafenone. The patient had an ischemic cardiomyopathy, and ambulatory monitoring demonstrated runs of unsustained ventricular tachycardia associated with dizziness. There was no prior history of a sustained tachyarrhythmia. During therapy with propafenone, ventricular arrhythmia in the ambulatory monitor was suppressed, but during exercise testing the patient developed sustained ventricular tachycardia with syncope, requiring multiple defibrillation attempts before sinus rhythm was restored.

one are 2,000 ng per milliliter or higher. The most common complaints are nausea and vomiting, abdominal discomfort, constipation, and dyspepsia. An altered taste, usually a metallic one, is reported by many patients and is the result of secretion of the drug by the salivary glands.

Other less common side effects include skin rash (2.3 percent); visual disturbances (3.5 percent); urinary symptoms (1.4 percent); exacerbation of asthma or chronic obstructive pulmonary disease (1.7 percent); arthralgias and arthritis (1.6 percent); muscular pain (2.5 percent); chemical abnormali-

Figure 5 Development of a conduction abnormality during propafenone therapy. Prior to therapy the patient had a normal QRS complex at rest and with exercise. During therapy with propafenone, there was slight QRS complex widening, but with exercise, a complete left bundle branch block developed. This was initially thought to be ventricular tachycardia.

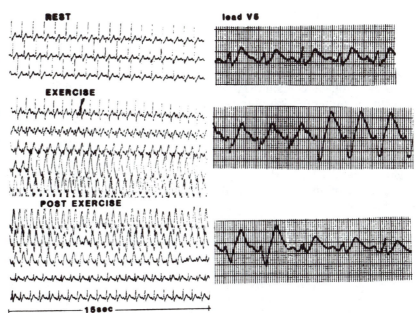

ties, including the development of a positive antinuclear antibody; an abnormal liver function test; and hematologic abnormalities. These side effects are generally not dose-related.

SUGGESTED READING

Connolly SJ, Kates RE, Lebsack CS, et al. Clinical efficacy and electrophysiology of oral propafenone for ventricular tachycardia. Am J Cardiol 1983; 52:1208.

Ludmer PL, McGowan NE, Antman EM, Friedman PL. Efficacy of propafenone in Wolff-Parkinson-White syndrome: Electrophysiologic findings and long term follow-up. J Am Coll Cardiol 1987; 9:1357–1363.

Podrid PJ, Lown B. Propafenone—a new drug for ventricular arrhythmia. J Am Coll Cardiol 1984; 4:117–125.

Podrid PJ. Special symposium on propafenone. J Electrophysiol 1987; 1:501–590.

Salerno DM, Dranrud G, Sharkey P, et al. A controlled trial of propafenone for treatment of frequent and repetitive ventricular premature complexes. Am J Cardiol 1984; 53:77–83.

Siddoway LA, Thompson EA, McAllister CB, et al. Polymorphism propafenone metabolism and disposition in man: Clinical and pharmacokinetic consequences. Circulation 1987; 75:785–791.

Zipes DP, ed. Recent advances in antiarrhythmic therapy: Symposium on propafenone. Am J Cardiol 1984; 54:1D–73D.

QUINIDINE

JOHN P. DiMARCO, M.D., Ph.D.

The use of derivatives of cinchona bark for the treatment of malaria was described in the 17th century. In 1749, Senac described the use of quinine for treating "long and rebellious palpitations." Quinidine, the dextroisomer of quinine, was isolated by Pasteur in the 19th century, and in 1918, Frey reported its effects on several different cardiac arrhythmias. By 1931, White described quinidine treatment as a "noted accomplishment in the practice of medicine." Despite the development of many other antiarrhythmic drugs, quinidine continues to hold a prominent place in modern antiarrhythmic therapy.

PREPARATIONS

Three salts of quinidine are used therapeutically (Table 1). Quinidine sulfate contains 82.8 percent quinidine base. Quinidine gluconate and quinidine polygalacturonate contain 62.3 percent and 62.0 percent of quinidine base, respectively. All three quinidine preparations have a bitter taste, but they have different solubilities in water and ethanol. Antiarrhythmic effects are dependent upon the plasma quinidine levels achieved, but some patients may tolerate one salt better than another, and the rate and percent of absorption may also differ between preparations.

ELECTROCARDIOGRAPHIC AND ELECTROPHYSIOLOGIC EFFECTS

Quinidine has numerous electrophysiologic effects. It blocks the fast inward sodium channel and decreases sodium conductance and thereby decreases the rate of rise of the action potential during phase 0. The modulated receptor model proposed by Hondeghem and Katzung has been used to explain the mechanisms by which quinidine produces these effects. In this model, membrane sodium channels may exist in resting, activated, and inactivated states with characteristic drug association and dissociation constants for each state. Resting and inactivated channels have a low affinity for quinidine, whereas the activated channel has a high affinity. With each action potential, quinidine can bind to open sodium channels, and since dissociation is delayed, progressively more Na^+ channels become blocked over time of exposure. Because dissociation occurs only during diastole, the effects of quinidine increase as cycle length shortens and firing rate increases (use dependency). Quinidine also has effects on other transmembrane ionic currents. The drug decreases delayed outward potassium currents (I_{K1}) and slowly inactivates steady-state plateau inward sodium and calcium currents.

As a result of these effects on transmembrane ionic currents, quinidine decreases action potential upstroke velocity, depresses conduction velocity, decreases excitability and automaticity slightly, and lengthens the effective refractory periods of atrial and ventricular muscles. These effects are more pronounced at faster rates and during conditions that partially depolarize tissue, such as hypoxia or ischemia.

Quinidine also has vagolytic properties that may be attributable to reflex compensation for its alpha-

Table 1 Quinidine Preparations

Compound	Dosage Sizes
Quinidine sulfate	200 mg, 300 mg extended release
Quinidine gluconate	324 mg
Quinidine polygalacturonate	275 mg

adrenergic blocking activity. In humans, electrophysiologic effects after quinidine are usually produced by a combination of both direct and indirect actions. The surface electrocardiogram usually shows little or no change in sinus rate or P-R interval, since direct depressive effects are negated by quinidine's vagolytic actions. At electrophysiologic study, there is usually no change in the A-H interval, but the H-V interval is slightly prolonged. The QRS complex may widen but usually only at higher drug concentrations or in patients with severe disease within the His-Purkinje system. The Q-T interval is usually prolonged, with increases of 25 percent common in patients with therapeutic plasma concentrations. Some patients, however, manifest idiosyncratic responses to even low concentrations and may have dramatic Q-T interval prolongation.

HEMODYNAMIC EFFECTS

Quinidine usually produces little change in cardiac contractility. Although direct negative inotropic effects can be demonstrated in isolated preparations, in clinical use aggravation of myocardial ventricular function is rare. This may be because of the offsetting of any negative inotropic effects by afterload reduction that is produced by partial alpha-adrenergic receptor blockade. Intravenous administration of quinidine is used only rarely because of the severe hypotension caused by the latter property. If intravenous quinidine is used, plasma expansion is often required to maintain adequate systemic blood pressure.

CLINICAL PHARMACOLOGY

Quinidine is usually administered orally. Intramuscular quinidine produces local necrosis, is painful, and should rarely be used. Intravenous quinidine can be used in selected circumstances, but the accompanying hypotension commonly seen is a major limitation.

The preparation of quinidine used affects absorption. Quinidine sulfate has an absorption half-time of approximately 30 minutes, and 80 to 90 percent of the administered dose enters the circulation. Peak plasma concentrations are reached within 1 to 2 hours. Both quinidine gluconate and quinidine polygalacturonate are more slowly and less completely absorbed. Peak plasma concentrations with these drugs may not be achieved for 3 to 4 hours after an oral dose. Extended-release quinidine sulfate preparations are available. These use a tablet constructed to release about one-third of the dose rapidly, with the remainder of the drug being released over 6 to 10 hours from a slowly dissolving matrix. Antacids and food may delay absorption of quinidine.

In the circulation, quinidine is 80 to 90 percent protein-bound. A high affinity binding site is present on alpha-1-acid glycoprotein, and a lower affinity site is present on albumin. The drug is widely distributed in the body, with a volume of distribution of 2 to 3 L per kilogram in adults. Concentrations of four to ten times plasma levels are seen in the heart, liver, kidneys, and skeletal muscle. The volume of distribution is decreased in the elderly and in patients with congestive heart failure. Quinidine crosses the placenta into the fetus and is also excreted in breast milk.

Quinidine is eliminated principally by means of hepatic metabolism via the mixed function oxidase system. The principal metabolites are 3-hydroxyquinidine, 2'-oxoquinidine, O-desmethylquinidine, and quinidine N-oxide. The metabolites then undergo conjugation and renal excretion. Several of the metabolites, 3-hydroxyquinidine and 2'-oxoquinidine, are known to have antiarrhythmic activity and may contribute to the actions of quinidine in selected patients.

Renal excretion of unchanged quinidine is a minor factor in the drug's elimination. Since quinidine is a weak base, excretion via an active distal tubular process shows pH-dependent properties, with patients with alkaline urine excreting little of the drug via this route.

The reported elimination half-life of quinidine in relatively healthy patients is 5 to 8 hours. This value is prolonged to some degree in cardiac patients, especially those with congestive heart failure, and in the elderly. A number of different assays for quinidine are in use. Early assays measured quinidine, contaminants, active and inactivate metabolites, and conjugates. More specific assays are now available, but they may differ in what precisely is measured, and a "therapeutic range" should be determined for each assay. Specific assays that measure quinidine only usually will yield plasma concentrations between 1 and 4 μg per milliliter (3.1 to 12.4 μmol per liter) in patients being effectively treated.

THERAPEUTIC USES

Atrial Fibrillation and Flutter

Quinidine remains a standard drug both for conversion of atrial fibrillation and atrial flutter and for maintenance of sinus rhythm after cardioversion or in patients with intermittent episodes. The arrhythmias of relatively high percentages (50 to 70 percent) of patients with recent onset of atrial fibrillation are converted after initiation of quinidine, but spontaneous conversion in such patients is also frequent. Once atrial fibrillation has become established and has persisted for more than about 10 days, lower conversion rates of 15 to 25 percent are to be expected. In patients with atrial flutter, caution must be used when quinidine therapy is begun. Since the drug slows conduction in the atrial circuit responsible for the arrhythmia and produces vagolytic effects on the atrioventricular node, 1:1 atrioventricular conduction at rates of over 200 beats per minute may be observed. It is usually wise to coadminister a second agent such as digoxin, which depresses atrioventricular nodal conduction, in order to guard against this possibility.

Paroxysmal Supraventricular Tachycardia

Quinidine has been reported to be effective in the prophylaxis of recurrent attacks of supraventricular tachycardia due to either atrioventricular nodal reentry or to atrioventricular reentry. In atrioventricular nodal reentry, it works by depressing retrograde conduction over the fast atrioventricular nodal pathway. In atrioventricular reentry, quinidine may produce or facilitate block in the accessory connection. Like procainamide, quinidine produces greater effects on accessory connection conduction and refractoriness when the pathway's effective refractory period is moderately long. This latter observation has relevance in patients with Wolff-Parkinson-White syndrome in whom quinidine may not be effective in those at highest risk for life-threatening heart rates during atrial arrhythmias. As is common to virtually all antiarrhythmic drugs, the electrophysiologic changes produced by quinidine are largely reversible by catecholamines, and a combination of a beta-adrenergic blocker with quinidine is often the best approach to therapy of patients with paroxysmal supraventricular tachycardia.

Ventricular Arrhythmias

Although quinidine has been used for years in the treatment of ventricular arrhythmias, only recently have systematically obtained data regarding its efficacy been available. In patients with chronic, stable ventricular premature beats, quinidine produces a greater than 80 percent suppression of arrhythmia in 50 to 60 percent of patients treated. This is similar to the effects reported for other class IA antiarrhythmic agents but considerably less than that observed with class IC agents or with amiodarone. Few data are available concerning long-term protection from recurrent arrhythmia in patients with sustained arrhythmias who had quinidine prescribed after serial ambulatory monitoring.

Serial electrophysiologic studies have been used to guide antiarrhythmic therapy in patients with prior sustained arrhythmias. DiMarco and colleagues reported oral quinidine to be effective in 30 of 89 (34 percent) patients tested. Rae and coworkers reported quinidine to be effective in 21 percent and partially effective in 14 percent of their patients. Duff and associates found intravenous quinidine to

be effective in 9 of 21 (42 percent) of their patients, but only 3 of 17 (17 percent) patients responded during oral quinidine treatment.

Quinidine may also be used in combination with other antiarrhythmic agents. Combined therapy with a beta-adrenergic blocker is frequently used, since quinidine's antiarrhythmic effects are largely reversible by catecholamines. Mexiletine is also commonly used in combination with quinidine. In one study in which programmed stimulation was used to assess drug efficacy, only 10 percent and 5 percent of patients responded to monotherapy with quinidine and mexiletine, respectively, but the arrhythmias of 35 percent of patients were controlled during combined therapy. Synergistic electrophysiologic interactions between these two drugs have been reported in animal studies. The advantage of combination therapy appears to be that lower doses of each agent may be used, thus avoiding the side effects commonly encountered with both agents.

When therapy has been selected based on suppression of inducible arrhythmia during serial drug studies, long-term survival has been excellent.

PROARRHYTHMIC EFFECTS

All antiarrhythmic agents possess the potential for proarrhythmia. Quinidine produces three distinct patterns of proarrhythmia. Rarely, initial doses of quinidine may produce dramatic prolongation of the Q-T interval and polymorphic ventricular tachycardia despite low plasma quinidine levels. A similar arrhythmia pattern is also seen in another subset of patients with normal or high plasma drug concentrations. These responses are more common in patients with one or more of the following: hypokalemia, atrial fibrillation with slow and irregular ventricular rates, atrioventricular block, left ventricular dysfunction, or long baseline Q-T intervals. A third pattern of proarrhythmic response is an increase in frequency of arrhythmia or conversion of unsustained arrhythmia to sustained arrhythmia even without marked Q-T interval prolongation or a polymorphic arrhythmia pattern. Most but not all proarrhythmic responses to quinidine occur during the first week of therapy. The incidence of proarrhythmic response has been estimated to be as low as 2 percent in patients with minimal structural heart disease and stable ventricular ectopy and as high as 16 percent in patients with more significant arrhythmias.

Quinidine may also produce heart block, may organize atrial fibrillation to atrial flutter, may allow 1:1 conduction as atrial cycle length slows in atrial flutter, and may unmask sinus node dysfunction after conversion of atrial flutter or fibrillation.

These observations suggest that in-hospital monitoring is required during the initial phases of quinidine therapy in patients in whom cardioversion from atrial arrhythmias is attempted or in any patient with one or more of the risk factors cited above. All patients with prior sustained arrhythmias should also, of course, be monitored during initiation of quinidine therapy. Even when these conditions are not present, it would seem prudent to administer at least the first dose of quinidine in a supervised setting so that the rare patient with the idiosyncratic pattern of dramatic Q-T interval prolongation after the initial dose of quinidine may be detected.

DRUG INTERACTIONS

Quinidine produces a large number of potentially important drug interactions (Table 2). It may potentiate the actions of anticholinergic drugs, anticoagulants, and neuromuscular blocking agents. Metabolism of quinidine is accelerated by drugs such as phenobarbital, rifampin, and phenytoin, which increase the activity of the hepatic mixed function oxidative pathways. Quinidine metabolism is decreased by cimetidine, verapamil, and amiodarone, with resulting increases in plasma concentrations if a constant dosage is continued. Additive effects on conduction and repolarization may be seen when quinidine and phenothiazines are used concomitantly.

An important set of interactions between quinidine and digoxin has been described. Quinidine reduces digoxin's volume of distribution by displacing it from binding sites in tissues. It also decreases renal clearance of digoxin by approximately 40 to 50 percent. A smaller decrease in nonrenal clearance may also be observed. These actions result in an approximate doubling of serum digoxin concentrations after quinidine has been added. It has been recommended that in previously digitalized patients, the digoxin dose be held for 24 hours after the initiation of quinidine and then continued at one-half the previous dosage. Since there is significant interpatient variability in the magnitude of the digoxin-quinidine interaction, careful plasma level monitoring of both drugs is indicated during the first weeks of therapy.

ADVERSE REACTIONS

Quinidine frequently produces one or more adverse reactions, and many patients cannot tolerate any effective dose of the drug. In one study, 13 of 54 patients receiving quinidine for sustained ventricular arrhythmias developed an adverse reaction that forced therapy to be discontinued. Seven additional patients in this series had less serious reactions that could be managed by dosage adjustment.

The most common side effects reported with quinidine are diarrhea, nausea, headache, and dizziness, but a large number of other adverse reactions may occur (Table 3). Quinidine may cause cinchonism, a syndrome characterized by tinnitus, hearing disturbance, visual blurring, and gastrointestinal upset. In more severe cases, confusion, delirium, and psychosis may be seen. Hypersensitivity reactions are also common. When it occurs, fever is usually seen in the first days to weeks of therapy. Thrombocytopenia, which may be profound, is seen within the first several weeks or months of treatment and is caused by the formation of drug-platelet complexes that stimulate antibody formation. Several types of hemolytic anemia may be seen. Hepatic toxicity, arthritic syndromes, dermatologic reactions, and acute hypersensitivity may also occur.

Table 2 Drug Interactions with Quinidine

Agents	Interaction	Frequency
Anticholinergics	Potentiation of effect	Common
Neuromuscular blockers	Potentiation of effect	Rare
Coumarin anticoagulants	Potentiation of effect	Rare
Phenothiazines	Additive effect	Common
Phenobarbital, rifampin, phenytoin	Decreased quinidine levels	Common
Digoxin	Increased digoxin levels	Common
Amiodarone, cimetidine, verapamil	Increased quinidine levels	Common
Carbonic anhydrase inhibitors	Decreased quinidine renal excretion	Rare

Table 3 Major Adverse Reactions to Quinidine

System	Reaction
Cardiac	Atrioventricular block
	Polymorphic ventricular tachycardia
	Hypotension
Gastrointestinal	Nausea, vomiting, diarrhea
	Hepatitis
Neurologic	Headache
	Visual disturbance
	Tinnitus
	Delirium, confusion
Hematologic	Hemolytic anemia
	Thrombocytopenia
Allergic	Skin rash
	Fever
	Anaphylaxis
	Arthritis

DOSAGE

There are marked interpatient differences in response to quinidine, and plasma concentration monitoring is essential for guiding therapy. For chronic treatment, long-acting preparations should be used. The usual doses employed are quinidine sulfate, 300 to 600 mg three times a day, quinidine gluconate, 324 to 648 mg three times a day, and quinidine polygalacturonate, 275 to 550 mg three or four times a day. Loading doses of quinidine have been used but should only be given when there is continuous electrocardiographic monitoring. Intravenous quinidine gluconate (7 to 10 mg per kilogram) may be administered in conjunction with careful blood pressure and electrocardiographic monitoring, but the hypotension this frequently causes makes intravenous use valuable only in selected situations.

SUGGESTED READING

Bauman JL, Bauernfeind RA, Hoff JV, et al. Torsades de pointes due to quinidine: Observations in 31 patients. Am Heart J 1984; 107:425–430.

Bigger JT Jr. The Arrhythmia Control Unit. The quinidine-digoxin interaction. Modern Concepts of Cardiovascular Disease 1982; 51:73–78.

DiMarco JP, Garan H, Ruskin JN. Quinidine for ventricular arrhythmias: Value of electrophysiologic testing. Am J Cardiol 1983; 51:90–95.

Duff HJ, Mitchell LB, Manyari D, Wyse DG. Mexiletine-quinidine combination: Electrophysiologic correlates of a favorable antiarrhythmic interaction in humans. J Am Coll Cardiol 1987; 10:1149–1156.

Duff HJ, Wyse DG, Manyari D, Mitchell LB. Intravenous quinidine: Relations among concentration, tachyarrhythmia suppression and electrophysiologic actions with inducible sustained ventricular tachycardia. Am J Cardiol 1985; 55:92–97.

Greenblatt DJ, Pfeifer HJ, Ochs HR, et al. Pharmacokinetics of quinidine in humans after intravenous, intramuscular and oral administration. J Pharmacol Exp Ther 1977; 202:365–378.

Guentert TW, Upton RA, Holford NHG, Riegelman S. Divergence in pharmacokinetic parameters of quinidine obtained by specific and nonspecific assay methods. J Pharmacokinet Biopharm 1979; 7:303–311.

Hondeghem L, Katzung BG. Test of a model of antiarrhythmic drug action. Effect of quinidine and lidocaine on myocardial conduction. Circulation 1980; 61:1217–1224.

Nygaard TW, Sellers TD, Cook TS, DiMarco JP. Adverse reactions to antiarrhythmic drugs during therapy for ventricular arrhythmias. JAMA 1986; 256:55–57.

Rae AP, Greenspan AM, Spielman SR, et al. Antiarrhythmic drug efficacy for ventricular tachyarrhythmias associated with coronary artery disease as assessed by electrophysiologic studies. Am J Cardiol 1985; 55:1494–1499.

Roden DM, Woosley RL, Primm RK. Incidence and clinical features of the quinidine-associated long QT syndrome: Implications for patient care. Am Heart J 1986; 111:1088–1093.

Salata JJ, Wasserstrom JA. Effects of quinidine on action potentials and ionic currents in isolated canine ventricular myocytes. Circ Res 1988; 62:324–337.

Velebit V, Podrid P, Lown B, et al. Aggravation and provocation of ventricular arrhythmias by antiarrhythmic drugs. Circulation 1982; 65:886–894.

SOTALOL

BRIAN A. McGOVERN, M.D.
JEREMY N. RUSKIN, M.D.
HASAN GARAN, M.D.

Sotalol is a noncardioselective, beta-adrenergic receptor blocking agent with additional class III antiarrhythmic properties. Sotalol has about one-third the beta-blocking potency of propranolol. It is devoid of intrinsic sympathomimetic activity and is relatively lipid-insoluble. Originally studied as an anti-ischemic and antihypertensive agent, its antiarrhythmic effects have been recognized and are being intensively investigated at present.

ELECTROPHYSIOLOGIC EFFECTS

In 1970, sotalol was shown to prolong the action potential duration significantly without affecting the upstroke velocity in isolated cardiac tissue preparations. This effect, also shown by amiodarone, distinguishes these agents from other antiarrhythmic drugs and has been termed a class III antiarrhythmic action. It has been demonstrated that the dextrorotatory isomer, d-sotalol, possesses the class III effects, whereas the levorotatory isomer, l-sotalol, is a potent beta-adrenergic blocking agent. The commercially available preparation, sotalol, is a racemic mixture of these isomers.

Sotalol prolongs the effective refractory period of isolated cardiac tissues. Repolarization is concomitantly prolonged in a dose-dependent manner. At very high concentrations, however, a significant reduction in action potential upstroke velocity and a shortening of the action potential duration have been reported. The ionic mechanisms underlying these dose-dependent effects of sotalol have not been elucidated.

In whole animal studies, sotalol has been shown to be more effective than metoprolol in preventing ventricular arrhythmias following experimental myocardial infarction in dogs. Both atrial and ventricular fibrillation thresholds are increased by sotalol in a variety of animal models.

The electrophysiologic effects of sotalol in

humans have been studied in detail. Sotalol prolongs the P-R, Q-T, and Q-Tc intervals as well as the Q-T interval at a fixed atrial pacing cycle length. The R-R interval lengthens, whereas the QRS complex does not change. During intracardiac electrophysiologic studies, it has been shown that the A-H interval is lengthened by sotalol, whereas the H-V interval does not change significantly in patients with normal pretreatment values. Sotalol increases the effective refractory period of the atrium, atrioventricular node, ventricle, and accessory atrioventricular connections. The functional refractory period of the His-Purkinje system is prolonged. Prolongation of the atrial and ventricular monophasic action potential durations has been demonstrated in humans using suction electrode catheters.

HEMODYNAMIC EFFECTS

Intravenous sotalol reduces heart rate and cardiac output and modestly increases systemic vascular resistance but has little effect on stroke volume. No changes in right-sided heart pressures or left ventricular end-diastolic pressure have been reported when 0.2 to 0.6 mg per kilogram of sotalol has been given intravenously, even in patients with a history of congestive heart failure. These latter findings are surprising, given the beta-adrenergic blocking effects of sotalol, and should be interpreted with caution. Experimentally, prolongation of the action potential duration (class III antiarrhythmic effect) may increase contractility, thus providing a possible explanation for sotalol's apparent weak negative inotropic properties. Clinically however, sotalol may worsen congestive heart failure, although it can be given safely to many patients with mild or moderate left ventricular impairment.

PHARMACOKINETICS

Sotalol has very high bioavailability, with more than 90 percent of an oral dose reaching the systemic circulation. Certain foods, particularly dairy products, have been reported to decrease its absorption. Peak plasma concentrations are found 2 to 3 hours after oral intake. Sotalol's apparent volume of distribution is 1.5 times body weight. It enters the cerebrospinal fluid slowly, with a cerebrospinal fluid:plasma ratio of about 1:10, similar to that of atenolol and nadolol. Sotalol crosses the placenta freely. Sotalol is not protein-bound and is largely excreted unchanged in the urine. Renal sotalol clearance varies linearly with creatinine clearance; therefore excretion of the drug is delayed in renal failure. The elimination half-life is 7 to 8 hours in patients with normal renal function. There are no known active metabolites of sotalol; thus dosing does not

have to be altered in hepatic dysfunction. Serum levels of sotalol that correlate with suppression of ventricular arrhythmias are in the range of 1 to 2 μg per milliliter. The beta-blocking effects of sotalol are typically seen at lower doses than those producing Q-Tc interval prolongation and maximal antiarrhythmic efficacy. Electrophysiologic effects vary linearly with serum sotalol levels.

CLINICAL ANTIARRHYTHMIC EFFECTS

Both intravenous and oral sotalol have been reported to be effective in suppressing or modifying a variety of cardiac arrhythmias, both supraventricular and ventricular. Detailed, controlled studies are limited however; therefore, firm conclusions regarding the role of sotalol as an antiarrhythmic agent must await further data.

Supraventricular Arrhythmias

Sotalol has been shown to slow sinus tachycardia and to slow the ventricular response during atrial fibrillation. Using doses of 0.5 to 1.5 mg per kilogram, intravenous infusion of sotalol has been reported to revert the arrhythmias of 20 to 30 percent of patients with atrial fibrillation and up to 60 percent of patients with atrial flutter to sinus rhythm. Sotalol is more effective than metoprolol in preventing supraventricular arrhythmias following cardiopulmonary bypass. However, our experience and that of others suggest that sotalol is only modestly effective in maintaining sinus rhythm long term in patients with paroxysmal atrial fibrillation.

Sotalol has been evaluated by several investigators in patients with the Wolff-Parkinson-White syndrome. The dual actions of sotalol—beta blockade and class III effects—are theoretically advantageous in this syndrome, with both atrioventricular nodal slowing and prolonged antegrade and retrograde refractoriness of accessory pathways. Indeed, sotalol is useful in many such patients. Electrophysiologic studies have shown that sotalol, at doses of 160 to 1,280 mg daily, prolongs the antegrade and retrograde refractory periods of accessory pathways, lengthens the mean and shortest R-R intervals during preexcited atrial fibrillation, and frequently prevents the induction of orthodromic, atrioventricular reciprocating tachycardias. Short-term follow-up evaluation suggests that sotalol will be an effective antiarrhythmic agent in many patients with the Wolff-Parkinson-White syndrome.

There is little published information concerning the clinical effectiveness of sotalol for other supraventricular arrhythmias, including sinoatrial reentrant tachycardias, automatic and reentrant atrial tachycardia, and accelerated junctional tachycardia. Sotalol appears to be effective for atrioventricular nodal reentrant tachycardia in many patients, but comparative data with standard therapies are lacking.

Ventricular Arrhythmias

Sotalol is more effective than placebo in suppressing ventricular premature complexes, including repetitive forms and runs of ventricular tachycardia, as shown in several blinded, placebo-controlled trials in patients with and without structural heart disease. The efficacy of sotalol appears comparable to that of other class IA drugs, but it is more effective than equivalent doses of other beta blockers. Effective doses have ranged from 160 mg to 480 mg per day. Exercise-induced complex ventricular arrhythmias were suppressed by sotalol (320 mg per day) in one study.

The effects of sotalol in patients with ventricular tachycardia or fibrillation are currently being evaluated in several centers. Acute efficacy has been assessed both invasively and noninvasively. Most published data describe the results of programmed ventricular stimulation before starting and after loading with sotalol. Clinical studies addressing the predictive accuracy of electrophysiologic testing thus far have involved relatively small numbers of patients and have short follow-up surveillance (Table 1). Earlier studies suggested that in a high percentage of patients, ventricular tachycardia is suppressed during sotalol therapy. More recent reports, however, have shown a suppression rate of 20 to 25 percent. These later studies have used three extrastimuli in the ventricular stimulation protocol, which may explain the lower suppression rates reported. The results of serial electrophysiologic studies appear to be predictive of outcome over 1 to 2 years, although further studies in large groups of patients, with longer follow-up observation, are necessary for confirmation.

A multicenter, randomized comparison of intravenous and oral sotalol and procainamide for ventricular tachycardia or fibrillation has been reported. Sotalol and procainamide appeared similar in efficacy, although the number of patients effectively treated without adverse effects was low on both drugs. Comparative trials with other antiarrhythmic agents are lacking. In addition, studies to date, in the United States particularly, have generally addressed populations of patients with drug-refractory arrhythmias, in whom the efficacy of any antiarrhythmic agent is likely to be low.

ADVERSE REACTIONS

Adverse reactions to sotalol can be considered to fall into two groups: beta-adrenergic blocking effects and new or worsened ventricular arrhythmias.

The adverse effects of beta blockade are shared with other noncardioselective beta-blocking agents and include fatigue, depression, cold extremities, bronchospasm, impotence, and lipid abnormalities. Central nervous system reactions are infrequent because of the hydrophilic properties of sotalol. Adverse cardiovascular effects include sinus node dysfunction, atrioventricular nodal and infranodal heart block, hypotension, and worsening of congestive heart failure. Sinus bradycardia and hypotension are common dose-limiting factors in treating patients with serious ventricular arrhythmias and may necessitate permanent pacemaker implantation in order to allow continued sotalol therapy.

As discussed previously, congestive heart failure may be precipitated or aggravated by sotalol, although the frequency of this in reported series and in our experience is low. Many studies have excluded patients with low left ventricular ejection fractions (less than 20 percent), New York Heart Association Class IV symptoms, or a history of severe congestive heart failure. Because of this, the reported safety and efficacy of sotalol in patients with ventricular dysfunction may be overestimated.

The most serious adverse effect of sotalol is the

Table 1 Predictive Accuracy of Electrophysiologic Testing for Ventricular Tachycardia/Ventricular Fibrillation in Patients on Sotalol

Author	Year	No. of Patients	Coronary Artery Disease (%)	Suppressed Arrhythmias (%)	Recurrence of Suppressed Arrhythmias (%)	Recurrence If Arrhythmias Not Suppressed (%)	Mean Follow-up (Months)
Senges et al	1984	18	89	67	11	NA	16
Nademanee et al	1985	33	98	45	27	50	9
Steinbeck et al	1986	34	44	35	6	100	NA
Kopelman et al	1988	11	100	18	NA	NA	NA
Kienzle et al	1988	9	89	89	38	NA	23
Gonzales et al	1988	45	72	22	0	37	20
Ruder et al	1989	39	80	20	17	44	11
Kuchar et al	1989	42	100	24	22	0	8

NA = not available.

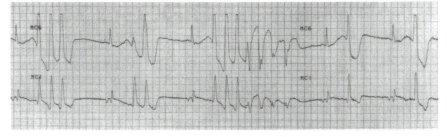

Figure 1 Sinus bradycardia, Q-T interval prolongation, and polymorphic ventricular tachycardia precipitated by sotalol in a patient with recurrent supraventricular tachycardia.

occurrence of polymorphic ventricular tachycardia in the setting of a prolonged Q-Tc interval (torsades de pointes). This has been reported most frequently in patients with a history of congestive heart failure, ventricular arrhythmias, hypokalemia, digitalis therapy, and renal failure. High serum concentrations, overdose, and concomitant therapy with other drugs that prolong the Q-T interval are contributing factors in some but not all affected patients. Torsades de pointes may rarely occur in patients without known structural heart disease who are treated for supraventricular tachycardia (Fig. 1). Torsades de pointes may result in cardiac arrest, syncope, or sudden death. New, polymorphic ventricular tachycardia may rarely occur without associated Q-Tc interval prolongation. The usual therapies are applied when torsades de pointes is seen in patients taking sotalol: withdrawal of sotalol, infusion of isoproterenol, overdrive pacing, and/or magnesium infusion (see the chapter *Proarrhythmia*).

When serial electrophysiologic studies are performed to assess the effects of sotalol on inducible ventricular tachycardia, sotalol, like other antiarrhythmic drugs, may increase the rate of the tachycardia, make the tachycardia easier to induce, or worsen the hemodynamic consequences of the tachycardia. The clinical significance of such findings is unknown, and their frequency is low.

Other rare reactions that have been attributed to sotalol include retroperitoneal fibrosis, hair loss, dry mouth, and nausea.

PRACTICAL CONSIDERATIONS IN THE USE OF SOTALOL

In practice, sotalol is used for patients in whom arrhythmias are refractory to treatment with conventional antiarrhythmic agents such as digoxin, beta-adrenergic blocking agents, or class IA or IB drugs. For patients with atrioventricular reciprocating tachycardia or ventricular tachycardia without severe ventricular dysfunction, sotalol should be used before amiodarone therapy is initiated. Our

practice is to initiate sotalol therapy in the hospital with continuous electrocardiographic monitoring in place. The initial dose of sotalol in patients with ventricular dysfunction is 80 mg twice a day, with dosage increases every 72 hours until efficacy is demonstrated, intolerable adverse reactions occur, or the Q-Tc interval reaches 550 msec. Most adverse effects of sotalol are dose-dependent and reverse promptly if the drug is stopped or the dose is reduced. Higher starting doses, e.g., 160 mg twice a day, may be used safely in many patients with good ventricular function and in whom the resting heart rate and blood pressure are normal. Adverse effects from excessive beta-receptor blockade are common at doses of 480 mg daily or higher.

SUGGESTED READING

Edvardsson N, Hirsch I, Emanuelsson H, et al. Sotalol-induced delayed repolarization in man. Eur Heart J 1980; 1:335–343.

Gonzalez R, Scheinman MM, Herre JM, et al. Usefulness of sotalol for drug-refractory malignant ventricular arrhythmias. J Am Coll Cardiol 1988; 12:1568–1572.

Kuchar DL, Garan H, Venditti F, et al. Usefulness of sotalol in suppressing ventricular tachycardia or ventricular fibrillation in patients with healed myocardial infarcts. Am J Cardiol 1989; 64:33–36.

Kunze K, Schluter M, Kuck K. Sotalol in patients with Wolff-Parkinson-White syndrome. Circulation 1987; 75:1050–1057.

McComb JM, McGovern B, McGowan JB, et al. Electrophysiologic effects of d-sotalol in humans. J Am Coll Cardiol 1987; 10:211–217.

Nademanee K, Feld G, Hendrickson J, et al. Electrophysiologic and antiarrhythmic effects of sotalol in patients with life-threatening ventricular tachyarrhythmias. Circulation 1985; 72:555–564.

Ruder MA, Ellis T, Lebsack C, et al. Clinical experience with sotalol in patients with drug-refractory ventricular arrhythmias. J Am Coll Cardiol 1989; 13:145–152.

Singh BN, Deedwania P, Nademanec K, et al. Sotalol: A review of its pharmacodynamic and pharmacokinetic properties, and therapeutic use. Drugs 1987; 34:311–349.

Singh BN, Vaughan William EM. A third class of antiarrhythmic action. Effects on atrial and ventricular intracellular potentials, and other pharmacological actions on cardiac muscle, of MJ1999 and AH3474. Br J Pharmacol 1970; 39:675–687.

Strauss HC, Bigger JT, Hoffman BF. Electrophysiologic and beta receptor blocking effects of MJ1999 on dog and rabbit cardiac tissue. Circ Res 1970; 26:661–678.

TOCAINIDE

DAN M. RODEN, M.D.

Tocainide is a primary amine analogue of lidocaine that can suppress ventricular arrhythmias. Unlike lidocaine, tocainide's pharmacokinetics make it suitable for use in chronic oral therapy. Dose-related lidocaine-like side effects, such as tremor or nausea, are common during tocainide therapy. In many patients, these side effects prevent administration of sufficiently high doses to suppress arrhythmias. More important, tocainide has also been associated with agranulocytosis; this is reversible if detected early, but it can be fatal.

A usual starting dose of tocainide is 200 to 400 mg every 8 hours. Because of the drug's elimination half-life of 13 to 19 hours in patients with arrhythmias, steady-state plasma concentrations are approached in 2 to 4 days (four to five elimination half-lives). Once steady state conditions are approached, tocainide effects can be reevaluated using Holter monitoring, exercise testing, and/or programmed electrical stimulation, depending on which modality was used at baseline. If an acceptable clinical response is not achieved and side effects are absent, the dosage may be increased and drug effects reevaluated at the new steady state. The usual dosages are 200 to 600 mg every 8 hours. Neither the time needed to achieve steady state nor the ultimate steady-state plasma concentration is altered by the use of a loading dose; moreover, loading doses can result in transient adverse effects and therefore should be avoided. Arrhythmia suppression generally requires plasma concentrations greater than 3 to 5 μg per milliliter.

Side effects are common during tocainide therapy and include nausea, tremor, dizziness, and paresthesias. In many patients, these side effects occur especially frequently if the drug is given when the patient has not eaten; tocainide should be given with food, which decreases peak plasma concentrations but does not alter the extent of its absorption. Changes in mental status, including frank psychosis, can also occur. Side effects develop more frequently in patients receiving doses higher than 1,800 mg per day or in whom plasma concentrations higher than 10 μg per milliliter are achieved.

Cardiac side effects, such as exacerbation of heart failure, exacerbation of arrhythmias, or provocation of advanced conduction system abnormalities, are uncommon during tocainide therapy. Agranulocytosis has been estimated to occur in 0.2 percent of patients receiving the drug. It is recommended that weekly white blood cell counts be performed during the first several weeks of treatment.

Tocainide has no active metabolites and no known major drug interactions. Tocainide clearance is reduced and its elimination half-life is prolonged (to 22 ± 5 hours) in patients with renal disease. In this setting, lower dosages should be used.

Tocainide is a sodium channel blocking drug with lidocaine-like (class IB) electrophysiologic properties. Like lidocaine and mexiletine, tocainide does not cause major changes in electrophysiologic indices. Similarly, aggravation of congestive heart failure is not a major problem during tocainide therapy. Those with chronic ventricular arrhythmias constitute the target population for whom tocainide therapy is a consideration. At the usual dosages, tocainide can decrease the frequency of chronic unsustained ventricular arrhythmias by 50 to 75 percent. However, at this time, no evidence supports the use of any antiarrhythmic drug in patients with this arrhythmia. Hence, given the side-effect and efficacy profile of tocainide, its use in this population is inappropriate. In patients with sustained ventricular tachycardia whose management is being guided by programmed electrical stimulation, clinically tolerated doses of tocainide are rarely (about 10 percent) effective when used alone. In occasional patients, combining an agent with quinidine-like electrophysiologic properties with a lidocaine analogue such as tocainide or mexiletine can result in enhanced efficacy with reduced side effects. When such a strategy is contemplated, mexiletine may be preferable to tocainide because of its lack of reported potential for causing serious organ toxicity. Tocainide has also been reported to be effective in atrioventricular nodal and/or bypass tract-mediated tachycardias, presumably by blocking fast ventriculoatrial conduction. Again, the risk:benefit ratio for the use of tocainide in this setting is not usually as favorable as that for other available therapeutic strategies.

SUGGESTED READING

Barbey JT, Thompson KA, Echt DS, et al. Tocainide plus quinidine for treatment of ventricular arrhythmias. Am J Cardiol 1988; 61:570–573.

Roden DM, Reele SB, Higgins SB, et al. Tocainide therapy for refractory ventricular arrhythmias. Am Heart J 1980; 100:15–22.

Roden DM, Woosley RL. Tocainide. N Engl J Med 1986; 315:41–45.

Thompson KA, Barbey JT, Kopelman HA, et al. Mexiletine and tocainide: A comparison of antiarrhythmic efficacy, adverse effects, and predictive value of lidocaine testing. Clin Pharmacol Ther 1989; 45:553–561.

IX NONPHARMACOLOGIC MANAGEMENT

CATHETER ABLATION

GERHARD HINDRICKS, M.D.
MARTIN BORGGREFE, M.D.
WILHELM HAVERKAMP, M.D.
GÜNTER BREITHARDT, M.D.

Antiarrhythmic drugs, antitachycardia pacemaker devices, and the automatic implantable cardioverter defibrillator provide useful "palliative" therapy for many patients with cardiac arrhythmias. However, selected patients with symptomatic and/or life-threatening cardiac tachyarrhythmias cannot be adequately treated by these therapeutic modalities. In these cases, a more aggressive therapy has to be applied. Definitive treatment of these patients has previously required surgery ranging from cervical sympathectomy for the treatment of long Q-T syndrome to surgical interruption of accessory pathways and open-heart, electrophysiologically guided antitachycardia surgery. The observation that in some cases limited surgical procedures directed precisely to the target tissue provided effective treatment has stimulated interest in the possibility of the use of intracardiac electrode catheters for the delivery of electrical energy for destruction of potentially arrhythmogenic structures of the heart.

In 1982, the first clinical application of catheter ablation was to create complete heart block in patients with drug-refractory supraventricular tachycardia. More recently, this was followed by attempts of catheter ablation of foci of ventricular tachycardia and ablation of accessory pathways. This chapter provides a brief review of the current role of catheter ablation techniques in the management of patients with drug-refractory tachyarrhythmias.

METHODOLOGY OF CATHETER ABLATION

The goal of catheter ablation is to interrupt or modify permanently conduction in a limited area of the heart from which the arrhythmia originates or which is an essential part of the reentrant circuit. The target tissue for catheter ablation depends on the type of underlying arrhythmia. In the setting of ectopic atrial tachycardia, atrial flutter/fibrillation, or atrioventricular (AV) nodal reentrant tachycardia, the AV conduction system may be target tissue. However, a direct approach to the ectopic focus in atrial tachycardia or the reentrant circuit in atrial flutter is also conceivable. In AV tachyarrhythmias, ablation of the accessory pathway is the appropriate approach, although occasionally indirect approaches with interruption of AV nodal conduction have been used. In the case of ventricular tachycardia, a direct approach with the aim of interrupting the reentrant circuit or destroying an ectopic focus has been used.

Different techniques of catheter ablation have been introduced and are still under intense experimental and clinical investigation. The technique first introduced and most widely used is the high voltage–direct current (DC) ablation technique (fulguration). More recently, radiofrequency alternating energy has been used. Independent of the energy source applied, a prerequisite for catheter ablation is the precise localization of the target tissue by means of electrode catheters. In the setting of AV tachycardia or ventricular tachycardia, this requires that the tachycardia be inducible in the electrophysiology laboratory by programmed stimulation or pharmacologic interventions. In addition, the induced arrhythmia has to be hemodynamically tolerable in the catheter laboratory so as to allow exact localization of the structures involved. If the tachycardia is too fast or not well tolerated, it should at least be easy to induce and terminate by pacing.

Transcatheter ablation of cardiac arrhythmias, no matter which technique is applied, is a very complex procedure that requires close collaboration of physicians, nurses, and physicists to understand and successfully apply these techniques. Therefore knowledge of the physical aspects and mechanisms of ablative techniques is a prerequisite for the effective and safe application of the technique.

HIGH VOLTAGE–DIRECT CURRENT ABLATION

A standard defibrillator cardioverter is usually used as the energy source for the DC ablation technique. In the unipolar mode, the distal electrode of an electrode catheter is connected to the anode or cathode of the defibrillator (active electrode). The electrical shock is delivered between the intracardiac lead and an external pad electrode. In the bipolar mode, shocks are delivered between the electrodes of catheters, with different poles serving as anode and cathode.

During a DC discharge via electrode catheters, the stored energy of the defibrillator is delivered within only a few milliseconds, causing a flash-like appearance. Because of this biophysical phenomenon, the technique has also been called the fulguration procedure (from Latin fulgus or fulgar — flash). Depending on the DC generator used and the selected energy, current and voltage can exceed 50 A and 3,000 V, respectively. It is important to note that only few catheters can withstand this high energy shock. Complex physical and physicochemical phenomena related to the amount of energy, the size of electrodes, and the waveform of the electrical impulse during and immediately after the electrical shock determine the tissue effects. Probably the most important mechanisms for the induction of tissue injury are the flow of current through tissue and the voltage applied. A rise in temperature at the catheter tip and mechanical barotraumatic effects caused by the development of shock waves resulting from gas bubble formation at the catheter tip might be less important. The relative contributions of electrical and thermal effects and of barotrauma for the induction of tissue injury are not fully understood at present.

Compared with radiofrequency ablation techniques, DC electrical ablation is considered the more effective technique, especially for ablation of ventricular tachycardia foci. However, the incidence of side effects of DC electrical ablation seems to be higher when compared with that of radiofrequency ablation. In addition, because the delivery of intracardiac fulguration shocks is painful, general anesthesia is required.

RADIOFREQUENCY CURRENT ABLATION

High frequency or radiofrequency alternating currents are defined as electrical currents of changing polarities in frequencies ranging between 30 kHz and 300 MHz. As with DC fulguration, the energy is delivered in either uni- or bipolar configuration via catheter electrodes. In general, the mechanism of action of radiofrequency currents can be attributed to electrolytic effects, faradic components, and most important, conversion of electrical energy into heat, which cause either coagulation or cutting of tissue. When radiofrequency alternating current flows through tissue, ions in solution are accelerated and resistive heating occurs. Heating occurs when cur-

rent density is high and electrical conductivity is relatively low. Both factors are achieved at the contact point of the "active" electrode(s) and the tissue surface. Maximal heat develops at the tissue electrode interface and decreases at increasing distances as a function of current density. The extent of tissue injury depends on multiple variables (e.g., delivered power, current density, duration of the coagulation, contact of the electrode to the tissue, and heat transfer properties of the tissue) that govern the effects of radiofrequency energy at the point of transition between active electrode(s) and tissue surface.

When compared with DC electrical ablation, major advances of radiofrequency alternating current application are (1) no general anesthesia is required during the procedure; (2) the incidence of proarrhythmic effects and hemodynamic complications seems to be lower; (3) no barotrauma occurs during radiofrequency pulse delivery, thereby decreasing the risk of perforation; and (4) energy is delivered over a longer period of time, thus being more maneuverable to achieve modification rather than complete destruction of the target tissue. This may be of particular importance for ablation of the AV conduction system. However, at present the clinical efficacy of the procedure for ablation of the AV conduction system and accessory pathways seems to be lower than that of DC electrical ablation. In addition, because experience with radiofrequency ablation for ventricular tachycardia foci is limited and published data reveal only moderate success, this procedure is far from being established.

CLINICAL EFFICACY, RISKS, AND INDICATIONS
General Considerations

Although the knowledge of the mechanisms, efficacy, and complications of catheter ablation techniques has substantially improved since the first clinical application of catheter ablation in 1982, the technique must still be considered experimental. In the light of continuously increasing experience with ablation techniques, any given indication for their application may change fast. Further studies and experience may extend or even restrict the range of indications for catheter ablation procedures. In addition, at present there is no general agreement among the different centers as to the indications for using catheter ablation techniques as a therapeutic tool. In an attempt to standardize ablation techniques and to provide a creditable scientific forum on which to judge the experience with this experimental procedure as to its efficacy and complications when tested in a large number of patients, the PCMAR (Percutaneous Catheter Mapping and Ablation Registry), a large international database, has been introduced as a pilot project to allow physicians to assess the risks and benefits of ablation procedures. This project was followed by the ongoing CAR (Catheter Ablation Registry), which prospectively analyzes the risk-benefit ratio of various ablation procedures.

Ablation of the AV Conduction System

Clinical Efficacy and Risks

The clinical efficacy of catheter ablation of the AV conduction system is high. The success rate reported from different centers ranges from 60 to 90 percent. Good results have been reported for both DC and radiofrequency catheter ablation techniques. At present, the DC technique seems to be more effective.

Data collected in the PCMAR, including more than 550 patients, revealed a mean success rate of induction of complete and persistent AV block of 65 percent. In another 8 percent of patients, an improvement of tachycardia-related symptoms caused by modification of AV conduction was observed. In 12 percent of patients, AV conduction resumed; however, these patients could be effectively treated with antiarrhythmic drugs. Thus, the cumulative success rate was 84 percent. The procedure was considered unsuccessful in only 16 percent of cases.

The incidence of severe complications associated with the ablation procedure is relatively low, ranging from between 2 and 5 percent. For DC electrical ablation, major hazards during and soon after the procedure are perforation and subsequent cardiac tamponade, hypotension, embolization, and thrombus formation. Perforation can also occur at the site of temporary electrode catheters that have been positioned in the apex of the right ventricle for pacing. One of the conditions favoring penetration of the wall by an electrode catheter is the relative fixed course, with fixation of the catheter by cardiac structures. A rare but worrisome observation has been the occurrence of sudden death after AV junction ablation. It is not clear whether this occurred because of bradycardias (despite implanted pacemakers) or because of ventricular tachycardia related or unrelated to the procedure. So far, no significant complications related to radiofrequency ablation have been reported.

Indications

Catheter ablation of the AV conduction system should be considered only in patients with severe and symptomatic supraventricular tachyarrhythmias that are refractory to antiarrhythmic drugs, which do not sufficiently slow the rate of tachycardias or prevent them (Table 1). In addition, drug-related side effects are an important consideration, although bradycardias may be counteracted by pacemakers. Catheter ablation should also be considered

Table 1 Possible Indications for Catheter Ablation of the AV Conduction System

Recurrent symptomatic and/or life-threatening supraventricular tachycardia and
1. Ineffective antiarrhythmic drug therapy,
2. Severe side effects of antiarrhythmic drug therapy,
3. Antitachycardia pacemaker not adequate,
4. Cardiac surgery not adequate.

if antitachycardia pacing is ineffective or not appropriate or if surgical procedures are not appropriate.

The symptoms of supraventricular tachyarrhythmias usually do not result from fast atrial rates but are mainly attributable to fast ventricular excitation via the AV node. Thus, possible indications for catheter ablation of the AV conduction system include a variety of supraventricular tachyarrhythmias originating from or being conducted through the AV system. However, before catheter ablation is considered in patients with supraventricular tachycardia, it has to be verified that the symptoms of the patient are in fact related to rapid ventricular rate rather than to loss of AV synchrony.

In the case of atrial fibrillation with rapid ventricular rate despite administration of antiarrhythmic drugs, today catheter ablation is preferable to surgical interruption of AV conduction. In patients with AV nodal reentrant tachycardia, the implantation of antitachycardia pacemaker devices or in some selected patients cardiac surgery represents an alternative that should also be considered. AV reciprocating tachycardia due to concealed or overt accessory pathways, ablation of the AV conduction system is usually not an adequate therapy. Instead, ablation of the accessory pathway should be considered if possible because this would not require pacemaker implantation and would eliminate the still possible risk of rapid antegrade conduction during atrial fibrillation over the accessory pathway. Ablation of the normal AV conduction system may be considered only in patients with concealed accessory pathways who are not appropriate candidates for surgery and ablation of the accessory pathway or for antitachycardia pacemakers, although in some patients a concealed pathway may become conductive in an antegrade direction after successful AV node ablation. Patients with drug-refractory ectopic atrial tachycardia may be considered for catheter ablation of the AV conduction system if they have multiple tachycardia foci, because experience with direct ablation of atrial focus is limited. In many cases, surgery may be preferable.

However, because most patients are permanently dependent on pacemakers after successful ablation, the indications for AV ablation should be made carefully and on an individual basis. Factors such as patient age, physical fitness, occupation, concomitant diseases, or preexisting pacemaker implantation should be considered in each patient. Thus, ablation of the AV conduction system cannot replace antiarrhythmic therapy but should be reserved for drug-refractory selected patients.

Ablation of Accessory Pathways

Clinical Efficacy and Risks

Catheter ablation of accessory pathways has been attempted in only a limited number of patients. In experienced centers, approximately 50 to 70 percent of patients with right-sided free wall or posteroseptal accessory pathways can be successfully treated. Because experience is still very limited, at present the risk of the procedure cannot be estimated reliably and needs further investigation.

Ablation of left-sided accessory pathways via the coronary sinus has been shown to be only moderately effective and to be associated with a high incidence of severe side effects. The most frequent complication is perforation of the coronary sinus and cardiac tamponade. New catheter ablation approaches such as energy application to the ventricular insertion of accessory pathways or bipolar radiofrequency energy application between the coronary sinus and the mitral valve annulus (so-called "epiendocardial ablation") seem to be more efficacious and less dangerous. However, because the experience with these new approaches is very limited, further exposure is necessary to delineate their efficacy and side effects.

Indications

In patients with atrioventricular tachyarrhythmias involving an accessory pathway, catheter ablation should be considered only if (1) the arrhythmia has been shown to induce severe symptoms, and/or (2) an invasive electrophysiologic study has demonstrated fast ventricular rates owing to short refractoriness of the accessory pathway, (3) antiarrhythmic therapy is not tolerated or has been insufficiently effective, as indicated by electrophysiologic evaluation and/or spontaneous recurrences, and (4) the arrhythmia can be controlled by antiarrhythmic therapy but the patient prefers catheter ablation (Table 2).

If the patient meets the above-mentioned criteria, catheter mapping to assess the location of the bypass tract precisely must be performed. Catheter ablation can be expected to be effective if a short local ventriculoatrial conduction time of less than 80 msec is found during orthodromic reciprocating tachycardia, because this represents a location of the electrode catheter close to the site of atrial insertion of the bypass tract. In addition, recordings of accessory pathway potentials, mostly with closely spaced electrodes, hint at a position close to the bypass tract.

Table 2 Possible Indications for Catheter Ablation of Accessory Pathways

Recurrent symptomatic tachycardia and/or rapid ventricular response during atrial fibrillation:
1. Ineffective antiarrhythmic drug therapy,
2. Intolerable side effects of antiarrhythmic drug therapy,
3. Effective antiarrhythmic therapy but patient prefers catheter ablation,
4. Antitachycardia surgery not adequate.

At present catheter ablation can be recommended only in patients with AV accessory pathways of the Kent type; there is a lack of experience with ablation of Mahaim's fibers, for example.

In selected patients, catheter ablation is an attractive therapeutic alternative to other treatment modalities if the bypass tract is located at the right free wall or posteroseptally. In contrast, catheter ablation of left-sided accessory pathways via the coronary sinus has only a moderate success rate and a significant incidence of severe complications, because coronary sinus rupture and pericardial tamponade have been reported in approximately 10 to 15 percent of patients. However, in one electrophysiologic center, successful catheter ablation of left-sided accessory pathways at the ventricular site of insertion was performed in a large number of patients without severe side effects. Greater improvements in the technology can be expected within the next few years, which might make catheter ablation a reasonable alternative to surgical interruption of accessory pathways. Patients with nodoventricular, atriofascicular, or para- or intranodal accessory pathways are not adequate candidates for catheter ablation because of a high risk of permanent destruction of the regular AV conduction accompanying ablation of the accessory pathways.

It should be stressed that surgical treatment of accessory pathways can be performed with a higher success rate and a low incidence of complications, thus representing the gold standard by comparison with catheter ablation. The major advantages of catheter ablation are that it obviates the need for thoracotomy and has a much shorter convalescence time. At present patient selection for catheter ablation of accessory pathways depends, in large part, on the anatomic location of the pathway and on the experience of a specific electrophysiologic center.

Ablation of Ventricular Tachycardia

Clinical Efficacy and Risks

The indications for catheter ablation of ventricular tachycardia are listed in Table 3. The clinical success rate of ablation of ventricular tachycardia reported from different centers ranges from approximately 30 to 90 percent. The reasons for these dif-

Table 3 Possible Indications for Catheter Ablation of Ventricular Tachycardia

---

Recurrent symptomatic and/or life threatening ventricular tachycardia and
1. Ineffective antiarrhythmic drug therapy,
2. Intolerable side effects of antiarrhythmic therapy,
3. Antitachycardia surgery not adequate or failed,
4. Previous cardiac surgery (= increased risk of complications),
5. Antitachycardia pacemakers and/or automatic implantable cardioverter defibrillator not adequate,
6. Ventricular tachycardia in right ventricular disease,
7. Incessant ventricular tachycardia.

---

ferences are multiple and seem to depend on varying criteria of patient selection, different definitions of study end points, and different electrophysiologic approaches used to localize the target tissue using activation mapping, pace mapping during sinus rhythm, and pacing during ventricular tachycardia to identify either the site of origin of ventricular tachycardia or the area of slow conduction. Furthermore, interpretation of the results of those mapping studies may be different and thus may influence the decision as to where to ablate. Recent evidence suggests that the success rate depends on delivering energy to areas that represent zones of slow conduction that are critical for the maintenance of the reentrant circuit. These areas are characterized by early, often middiastolic potentials during ventricular tachycardia. Pacing of these areas during ventricular tachycardia may result in an identical QRS complex with a long stimulus to QRS complex latency.

The PCMAR has collected retrospective data of more than 160 patients in whom catheter ablation of ventricular tachycardia foci has been attempted. The overall success rate was 59 percent; 18 percent of patients were successfully treated without additional antiarrhythmic therapy, whereas 41 percent of patients required antiarrhythmic drugs after the ablation procedure that had been ineffective before catheter ablation. In 41 percent of patients, the procedure was considered unsuccessful. Our own experience is based on a total of 80 patients with drug-refractory ventricular tachycardia. In 65 patients DC ablation and in the remaining 15 patients radiofrequency ablation were performed. The procedure-related in-hospital mortality rate was 3.8 percent (3 of 80 patients). Following DC ablation ($N = 65$) the arrhythmias of 70 percent of patients were successfully controlled. In the remaining patients, nonpharmacologic interventions often were performed additionally, such as antitachycardia surgery or implantation of an automatic cardioverter defibrillator. After radiofrequency ablation ($N = 15$), the success rate was 47 percent if it was performed alone, but it increased to 73 percent if an additional DC ablation was used. The additional ablation was considered necessary in 6 of 14 patients, whereas in

the remaining patients, radiofrequency ablation was followed by map-guided surgery.

As evident from several published reports, DC ablation of ventricular tachycardia foci has significant potential for severe side effects that occur in approximately 10 to 15 percent of patients. Lethal complications have been reported in up to 7 percent of patients. In our experience perioperative mortality is 3.8 percent (3 of 80 patients).

Major hazards are procedure-related pump failure and hypotension, pericardial tamponade, cerebral embolism, and ventricular tachycardia or ventricular fibrillation induced by the ablation shock (either immediately following energy application or induction of new ventricular tachycardia foci during follow-up).

Indications

Patients with symptomatic sustained ventricular tachycardia should be considered for catheter ablation only in cases of failure of antiarrhythmic drug therapy (spontaneous recurrence of tachycardia on antiarrhythmic drugs and/or failure to respond to antiarrhythmic drugs during serial electrophysiologic testing or if untolerable side effects occur during otherwise effective antiarrhythmic therapy) (see Table 1). Because of the experimental character of the technique, catheter ablation should be considered only if neither antitachycardic surgery nor implantable cardioverter defibrillators are appropriate for a specific patient.

The appropriate candidate for catheter ablation should have only one type of monomorphic, hemodynamically tolerable ventricular tachycardia that is inducible in the electrophysiology laboratory. Electrophysiologic localization procedures should include activation mapping, pace mapping, and stimulation during tachycardia from various sites (e.g., entrainment mapping) to identify the structures involved in the genesis and maintenance of ventricular tachycardia. Most important findings include (1) presystolic endocardial activity or mid-diastolic fractionated potentials during ventricular tachycardia and (2) correspondence between morphology of spontaneous and paced QRS complexes (during ventricular tachycardia) and (3) long stimulus-to-QRS complex delay when pacing during ventricular tachycardia from the site of origin is performed. These criteria may help to identify the area of slow conduction that probably represents the appropriate target for catheter ablation.

A patient with sustained ventricular tachycardia after myocardial infarction with left ventricular aneurysm and heart failure (with or without an additional indication for coronary artery bypass graft) is not a candidate for catheter ablation but would profit more from cardiac surgery. On the other hand, monomorphic sustained ventricular tachycardia in a patient with severely depressed left ventricular function or with concomitant severe noncardiac disease such as renal or pulmonary disease that may increase the risk of surgery is an appropriate indication for catheter ablation.

Catheter ablation should also be considered in patients with incessant ventricular tachycardia that is refractory to antiarrhythmic drugs and electrical therapy. Patients with right ventricular dysplasia represent another group in whom catheter ablation might be preferable to surgery because of late recurrences resulting from progression of the underlying disease. Surgical results have been shown to be poor in such patients. Whether catheter ablation should be performed in patients displaying different morphologies of ventricular tachycardia with multiple sites of origin is uncertain.

By taking the risk-benefit ratio of antitachycardia surgery and catheter ablation into consideration, it must be stressed that catheter ablation of ventricular tachycardia foci should be reserved for a highly selected subgroup of patients. The overall 5-year experience from the PCMAR gives evidence that the range of indications for catheter ablation of ventricular tachycardia foci should not be extended.

CURRENT STATUS AND FUTURE PERSPECTIVES OF CATHETER ABLATION

Ablation of the AV conduction system can be performed with a high success rate and an acceptable incidence of procedure-related side effects. However, pacemaker dependency after successful ablation limits the extension of indications. Major challenges for the future are the development of ablation techniques that allow predictable "modification" of the AV conduction system, e.g., induction of first-degree AV block rather than complete AV block. A prerequisite for predictable modification of the AV conduction system is the ability to guide energy delivery in order to be able to induce controlled tissue effects. Based on current knowledge, it is unlikely that DC electrical ablation is feasible for modification of con-

duction, but it seems possible that ablation by radiofrequency alternating current can be improved to achieve controlled modification.

Catheter ablation of right free wall and posteroseptal accessory pathways has been successfully performed in a limited number of patients. These initial results are encouraging. DC electrical ablation within the coronary sinus for the treatment of left-sided accessory pathways is not an alternative to surgery because of an unacceptable benefit-risk ratio. The development of new catheter ablation techniques such as DC electrical ablation at the ventricular insertion of the accessory pathway or the recently introduced epiendocardial ablation technique might be more feasible. However, further studies are needed to ascertain the efficacy and safety of these new techniques.

The role of catheter ablation as a nonpharmacologic therapeutic tool for the treatment of ventricular tachycardia is far from established. Despite a growing number of patients in whom the benefit of catheter ablation has been clearly demonstrated, many problems remain. Prerequisites for an increase in efficacy and a decrease in patient risk are the improvement of energy delivery systems and of the electrophysiologic methods for tachycardia localization. Transcatheter ablation of ventricular tachycardia should be reserved for a highly selected subset of patients in whom it has been clearly demonstrated that their disease is not responsive to all other palliative therapeutic tools and who are not candidates for antitachycardia surgery.

SUGGESTED READING

Breithardt G, Borggrefe M, Zipes DP, eds, Nonpharmacological therapy of tachyarrhythmias. Mount Kisco, NY: Futura Publishing Co, 1987.

Fontaine G, Scheinmann MM, eds. Ablation in cardiac arrhythmias. Mount Kisco, NY: Futura Publishing Co, 1987.

Proceedings of the IVth World Congress on Cardiac Ablation. PACE 1989; 12:131–267.

Saksena S, Goldschlager N, eds. The electrical therapy of cardiac arrhythmias. Philadelphia: WB Saunders Co, 1989.

ANTIARRHYTHMIC SURGERY: SUPRAVENTRICULAR ARRHYTHMIA IN PATIENTS WITH PREEXCITATION

GERARD M. GUIRAUDON, M.D.
GEORGE J. KLEIN, M.D.
RAYMOND YEE, M.D.
ARJUN D. SHARMA, M.D.
RAJ R. KAUSHIK, M.D.

Wolff, Parkinson, and White originally described paroxysmal tachycardia in patients with a characteristic electrocardiographic pattern of a short P-R interval and a wide QRS complex with a slurred initial deflection labeled as the delta wave. The syndrome is associated with an accessory atrioventricular (AV) connection that preexcites the ventricle by bypassing the normal AV nodal His bundle conduction system. Currently, preexcitation syndrome encompasses all electrophysiologic entities associated with accessory AV conduction, whatever the associated electrocardiographic pattern (variant preexcitation). Paroxysmal AV reciprocating tachycardia utilizing the accessory pathway as an obligatory segment of the circuit is the most common associated arrhythmia. Atrial fibrillation with fast ventricular responses via the accessory pathway is a less prevalent but more severe arrhythmia. Ventricular fibrillation and sudden cardiac death may be associated with the latter arrhythmia. Electrophysiologic studies using programmed electrical stimulation and intracardiac multicatheter recording identify the mechanism of arrhythmia and the role and location of the accessory pathway. The current surgical correction is aimed at ablating the problematic accessory pathway.

INDICATION FOR SURGERY

Antiarrhythmic drug therapy is generally the initial option in low-risk patients when a selected drug is efficacious, free of significant side effect, and inexpensive, and when good patient compliance is anticipated (see the chapters *Paroxysmal Atrioventricular Reentrant Tachycardia: Pharmacologic Therapy* and *Atrial Fibrillation in The Wolff-Parkinson-White Syndrome*).

Implanted antitachycardia devices detect the occurrence of the arrhythmia and deliver a pacing treatment. This is an acceptable option in selected patients with accessory pathways capable of only retrograde AV conduction, although curative intervention is generally preferable (see the chapter *Paroxysmal Atrioventricular Reentrant Supraventricular Tachycardia: Nonpharmacologic Therapy*).

His bundle ablation is currently rarely indicated when surgical cure is not feasible.

Catheter ablation of accessory pathways using a broad variety of energy delivery is used with increasing success, although it is still investigational. This technique may become the primary option with surgical coverage for treatment of potential complications and/or secondary ablation (see the chapter entitled *Catheter Ablation*).

Surgical ablation of the accessory pathway generally is the recommended nonpharmologic curative therapy because of its high efficacy and low morbidity.

Patient selection for surgery is based on the clinical presentation and results of electrophysiologic studies. Surgical ablation for accessory AV pathways is recommended for the following groups of patients: (1) patients with out-of-hospital cardiac arrest, (2) patients with pathways capable of fast antegrade conduction during atrial fibrillation, (3) patients with recurrent, disabling arrhythmia, (4) patients with problematic pathways who undergo cardiac surgery for other cardiac abnormalities, (5) women who desire to become pregnant, (6) patients with tachycardia-induced cardiomyopathy and/or incessant tachycardia, (7) patients who cannot accept lifelong antiarrhythmic therapy, and (8) patients whose lifestyles or occupations are jeopardized or limited by the arrhythmia. There are no specific guidelines for the timing of surgery, although there is no reason to delay a curative intervention when indicated.

PREOPERATIVE ASSESSMENT

An in-depth patient history documents the consequences of the arrhythmia on the patient's lifestyle. All patients have preoperative electrophysiologic studies to document the anatomy and electrophysiologic properties of the pathway and to identify associated arrhythmias. Associated structural heart disease is identified using routine echo-Doppler studies. Left-sided heart catheterization and cineangiography are requested in men over 40 years of age and women over 45.

CHOICE OF PROCEDURE

Surgical technique is selected on standard criteria of high efficacy and low morbidity. A surgical intervention comprises several steps, each with inherent mortality and morbidity. Five steps can be identified as follows: (1) exposure, generally via a median sternotomy incision, (2) cardiopulmonary bypass, (3) cold cardioplegic cardiac arrest or other myocardial preservation techniques, (4) cardiotomy, and (5) operative therapy. Only two steps are unavoidable: surgical exposure and operative therapy. These considerations led us to develop an "epicardial approach" aimed at avoiding "unnecessary" steps if possible, i.e., cardiotomy, cardiac arrest, and cardiopulmonary bypass. The endocardial approach, pioneered by Sealy and perfected by Gallagher and Cox, routinely requires opening of the heart, cardiac arrest, and cardiopulmonary bypass, although it is associated with a high rate of efficacy.

THE EPICARDIAL APPROACH

The epicardial approach combines epicardial exposure and cryoablation of the AV junction on the beating heart. The heart is exposed via a median sternotomy incision. Intraoperative electrophysiologic testing is performed before dissection, after dissection, and after cryoablation. Accessory pathway location is determined using epicardial activation mapping at 17 predetermined sites along the AV sulcus. Ventricular mapping is obtained during atrial pacing. Atrial mapping is performed during reciprocating tachycardia and/or ventricular pacing. The coronary sulcus is divided into four regions: left ventricular free wall, posterior septal region (posterior superior process of the left ventricle), right ventricu-lar free wall, and anterior septal region (right coronary fossa) (Fig. 1). There is no anatomic partition between adjacent regions, and transitional pathways can be difficult to classify. This classification into four regions of the coronary sulcus is of great practical value and is well correlated with delta-wave morphology on the surface electrogram, catheter mapping during electrophysiologic studies, and specific surgical approaches for each region.

Epicardial dissection of the coronary sulcus combined with continuous electrophysiologic testing has allowed identification of three possible pathway locations within a region. Most pathways are epicardial and course within the AV sulcus; subendocardial pathways course endocardially across the AV annulus; "atypical" pathways are located in the septum and are distinct to the AV sulcus. *Epicardial pathway* conduction is not present after dissection of the AV sulcus. *Subendocardial pathway* conduction is still present after dissection and is temporarily interrupted by ice mapping over the AV junction. *Atypical* intraseptal septal pathway conduction is still present after dissection but is not interrupted by ice mapping or is simultaneously interrupted by AV nodal conduction, suggesting a close proximity of the accessory pathway to the AV node. Either "anterior septal" or "posterior septal" pathways can be in an intraseptal atypical location.

Surgical strategy requires deep and wide dissection in the region of interest. Cardiopulmonary by-

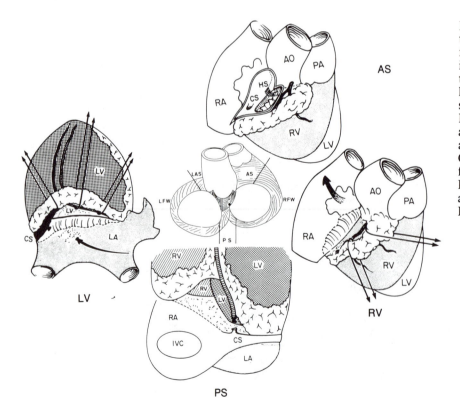

Figure 1 Schematic depiction of the epicardial approach in the four regions. The central drawing is a posterior view of the base of the ventricles with the tentative limits of each region of the AV sulcus. RV = right ventricle, LV = left ventricle, RA = right atrium, LA = left atrium, AO = aorta, PA = pulmonary artery, CS = coronary sinus, LFW = left free wall, RFW = right free wall, PS = posterior septal, LAS = left anteroseptal, AS = anteroseptal, HS = bundle of His.

pass is currently essential for anterior septal pathways that are intraseptal in the paraHissian region. Cardiopulmonary bypass is also used in patients with atypical posterior septal pathways, coronary sinus diverticula, and rare subendocardial left free wall pathways. In all, cardiopulmonary bypass is required in about 20 percent of patients.

Epicardial dissection of the AV fat pad is carried out using either the "en bloc" approach or the "direct" approach. The en bloc approach constitutes the dissection and mobilization of the entire AV fat pad and its vascular contents. The epicardium is incised along the atrial limit of the fat pad. A plane of dissection between the atrial wall and the fat pad is identified. The dissection is extended to the AV annulus and encompasses the adjacent ventricular wall. Identification and division of venous or arterial branches facilitate the mobilization of the fat pad. Large stay sutures are passed around the entire fat pad as soon as possible to facilitate dissection and exposure of the sulcus. Intramural coronary arteries should be identified and carefully mobilized.

The direct approach exposes the AV annulus via an incision of the epicardium along the ventricular wall. The fat pad is entered using blunt dissection. A plane of cleavage is found over the ventricular wall, and the AV annulus is identified. Cardiac veins may be divided. Coronary arteries and their ventricular branches are isolated and mobilized only to obtain adequate exposure of the AV annulus. Electrophysiologic testing is carried out after completion of the epicardial dissection. The accessory pathway ablation is completed accordingly using epicardial cryoablation of the AV junction for epicardial pathways, endocardial cryoablation of the AV junction for subendocardial pathways, and atriotomy combined with right or left septal atrial dissection for atypical septal pathways.

Surgical technique is adapted to each region. Ablation of the left free wall pathways can be carried out without using cardiopulmonary bypass when the region is exposed by dislocating the heart in a sling passed via the transverse sinus (sling exposure). Adequate exposure is obtained without hemodynamic impairment. The left AV junction is dissected using the direct epicardial approach and cryoablated accordingly. The posterior septal pathway region is easily exposed, and pathways are ablated using an en bloc epicardial approach. The division of the mid-cardiac vein is the key step to attaining adequate dissection. Rare atypical intraseptal posterior septal pathways require an endocardial approach to the septum. Right free wall pathways are easily approached and ablated using closed heart endocardial cryoablation when necessary. Most anterior septal pathways in the parahissian region are atypical and require endocardial dissection of the membranous septum to achieve uniform ablation.

Multiple accessory pathways are defined as widely separated into two distinct regions (7 percent of patients). Preoperative electrophysiologic study identifies the presence of multiple pathways in about 75 percent of the patients. A second pathway may become apparent only after the ablation of the dominant accessory pathway. Multiple accessory pathways are ablated in sequence.

Variant Accessory Pathways

The permanent form of junctional reciprocating tachycardia (Coumel's tachycardia) is associated with a posterior septal accessory AV pathway with decremental retrograde conduction. There is evidence that the accessory pathway characteristics with the Mahaim fiber electrophysiologic entity are right ventricular pathways with antegrade decremental conduction.

Two congenital cardiac abnormalities are related to the preexcitation syndrome: Ebstein's anomaly and the recently described coronary sinus diverticulum. Symptomatic Wolff-Parkinson-White syndrome associated with Ebstein's anomaly does not necessarily require anatomic correction, but all surgical correction for Ebstein's anomaly should be combined with ablation of the frequently associated accessory AV pathways. The coronary sinus diverticulum is a congenital abnormality of the intracardiac veins associated with posterior septal pathways.

Concomitant cardiac procedures are carried out after ablation of the accessory pathways. Before the chest is closed, four pairs of temporary pacing wires are attached onto each cardiac chamber for postoperative electrophysiologic testing. This is performed a few hours after surgery, the following day, and 5 to 7 days postoperatively. A 12-lead surface electrocardiogram is obtained daily until the last electrophysiologic study is completed.

POSTOPERATIVE COURSE

The vast majority of patients have an uneventful recovery and are discharged after 5 to 7 days. Surgical risk is minimal. We have had no deaths. Complications have been rare, essentially being confined to re-sternotomy for bleeding, and only in patients in whom cardiopulmonary bypass has been used. Other rare complications can be observed related to median sternotomy (chylopericardium), cardiopulmonary bypass (noncardiogenic pulmonary edema), or associated structural heart lesions. Efficacy of the surgical approach is high. In rare cases (1 percent) re-sternotomy is required for recurrence of accessory pathway conduction. A second undetected problematic pathway can become manifest in rare instances (less than 1 percent). The risk of permanent heart block is minimal.

Based on our experience with more than 450 patients, the success rate is higher than 99 percent, with no mortality and no long-term complications.

Surgery for preexcitation syndrome is currently an accepted curative intervention for patients with problematic accessory pathways. Although the endocardial approach is associated with high efficacy, we prefer the epicardial approach for the following advantages: surgery on the beating heart allows continuous monitoring of the accessory pathway conduction during dissection, facilitates identification of multiple pathways, and decreases the risk of inadvertent heart block in most patients. Epicardial dissection does not require the use of cardiopulmonary bypass, cardioplegic arrest, or cardiotomy with their inherent associated morbidity in about 80 percent of patients. Only a surgical technique with high efficacy and minimal morbidity can endure as a preferred alternative to other nonpharmacologic interventions.

SUGGESTED READING

Gallagher JJ, Sealy WC, Cox JL, et al. Results of surgery for preexcitation caused by accessory atrioventricular pathways in 267 consecutive cases. In: Josephenson ME, Wellens HJJ, eds. Tachycardias—mechanisms, diagnosis, treatment. Philadelphia: Lea & Febiger, 1984:259.

Guiraudon GM, Guiraudon CM, Klein GJ, et al. The Coronary sinus diverticulum—a pathological entity associated with the Wolff-Parkinson-White syndrome. Am J Cardiol 1988; 62:733–735.

Guiraudon GM, Klein GJ, Sharma AD, et al. Closed-heart technique for Wolff-Parkinson-White syndrome: Further experience and potential limitations. Ann Thorac Surg 1986; 42:651–657.

Guiraudon GM, Klein GJ, Sharma AD, et al. Surgery for the Wolff-Parkinson-White syndrome—the epicardial approach. Semin Thorac Cardiovasc Surg 1989; 1:21–33.

Guiraudon GM, Klein GJ, Sharma AD, et al. "Atypical" posterior septal accessory pathway in the Wolff-Parkinson-White syndrome. J Am Coll Cardiol 1988; 12:1605–1608.

Sealy WC, Hattler BG Jr, Blumenschein SD, Cobb FR. Surgical treatment of Wolff-Parkinson-White syndrome. Ann Thorac Surg 1969; 8:1–11.

ANTIARRHYTHMIC SURGERY: VENTRICULAR ARRHYTHMIAS

T. BRUCE FERGUSON, JR., M.D.
JAMES L. COX, M.D.

Both the nonsurgical and surgical management of life-threatening ventricular tachyarrhythmias has progressed considerably in recent years. Advances in pharmacologic, pacemaker, and defibrillator therapies have affected the patient population ultimately presenting for surgical treatment of these arrhythmias. Concomitantly, advances in surgical technique, in intraoperative mapping, and in understanding the fundamental electrophysiologic nature of these arrhythmias have likewise had an impact on the patient population presenting for surgical treatment. This chapter briefly outlines the current approach at Barnes Hospital, Washington University in St. Louis, to the preoperative evaluation, selection, and operative intervention in this particular patient. The encouraging results with surgical intervention suggest that surgery should play an increasing role in the management of these most common and lethal of arrhythmias.

PREOPERATIVE ELECTROPHYSIOLOGIC AND HEMODYNAMIC EVALUATION

Patients with both ischemic and nonischemic ventricular tachycardias who are surgical candidates undergo complete electrophysiologic, angiographic, and ventriculographic evaluation. The catheter electrophysiologic study is performed (1) to confirm that the arrhythmia is ventricular and not supraventricular in origin, (2) to demonstrate that the arrhythmia is reentrant by induction and termination with programmed electrical stimulation techniques, and (3) to identify the earliest site of origin of all morphologically distinct tachycardias using catheter mapping techniques. From a surgical point of view, it is convenient to distinguish between simple monomorphic ventricular tachycardia and other more complex types, including the multiple monomorphic and polymorphic forms. Polymorphic unsustained ventricular tachycardia that quickly deteriorates into ventricular fibrillation must be distinguished from primary ventricular fibrillation. This latter arrhythmia is characterized by the absence of any type of induced ventricular tachycardia prior to the onset of ventricular fibrillation following programmed electrical stimulation and is not yet amenable to direct surgical therapy.

Angiographic and ventriculographic evaluation is particularly helpful in the evaluation of three of the nonischemic forms of ventricular tachycardia. In patients with *diffuse cardiomyopathy* attributable to patchy myocardial fibrosis, angiographic and hemodynamic data usually indicate some type of abnormal myocardial contractility associated with recurrent tachycardia. Ventriculography demonstrates diffuse dilatation of both ventricles. This same finding on ventriculography can also be present in cases of *idiopathic ventricular tachycardia* owing to repeated bouts of tachycardia; however, in this latter entity, pathologic evidence of primary cardiac disease is absent. In *arrhythmogenic right ventricular dysplasia* caused by transmural infiltration of adipose tissue resulting in weakness and aneurysmal bulging of three areas of the right ventricle, ventriculography demonstrates diffuse dilatation, depressed contractility, and delayed emptying of the right ventricle. Frank aneurysms of the infundibulum, apex, and/or posterior basilar region are seen, and hypertrophic muscular bands in the infundibulum and anterior right ventricular wall result in a feathering appearance of the outflow tract. Because the origin of the tachycardia is the right ventricle, the 12-lead electrocardiogram shows a pattern consistent with left bundle branch block during the tachycardia, and right-sided ventriculography should be performed in any patient with ventricular tachycardia and this QRS complex configuration.

SURGICAL INDICATIONS AND CONTRAINDICATIONS

The final decision regarding surgical therapy for ventricular tachycardias of both ischemic and nonischemic origin is based on a variety of preoperative and clinical factors. The primary indication for surgery is refractoriness to medical therapy. Our current algorithm for the optimal surgical treatment of refractory *ischemic* ventricular tachycardia is shown in Figure 1. With this algorithm as a guide, the following points can be emphasized:

1. The evaluation regarding surgical intervention for medically refractory ischemic ventricular tachycardia should be made prior to the institution of amiodarone therapy. The depressant effect of amiodarone on left ventricular function is aggravated by ischemic cardioplegic arrest in the majority of patients, and thus therapy with the drug prior to surgical intervention can significantly complicate the operative procedure.

2. The evaluation for surgical intervention should be based primarily on the determination that the patient has a sufficient degree of normal left ventricular function to survive operative intervention. In a review of the available literature, the only preoperative variables shown to increase operative mortality are (1) in a patient with a left ventricular aneurysm, a nonaneurysmal portion of the left ventricle so dysfunctional that class III or IV heart failure exists prior to surgery; (2) in a patient without a ventricular aneurysm, global dysfunction so severe that class III or IV heart failure exists prior to surgery; and (3) if emergency surgical intervention is required. Because most patients with ischemic ventricular tachycardia have a left ventricular aneurysm, accurate determination of the ejection fraction is difficult, and the absolute number is not an accurate predictor of operative mortality. Patients with discrete apical or posterior aneurysms and myocardium that contracts in a normal or near-normal fashion in the remainder of the heart are the best candidates for surgery from a functional point of view.

3. If the patient has a prohibitive degree of left ventricular dysfunction, amiodarone therapy should be initiated. If this therapy is unsuccessful, an automatic implantable cardioverter defibrillator (AICD) should be implanted, provided that the episodic rate of the patient's tachycardia is low enough so as not to exhaust the battery supply of the device or to make the patient's life prohibitively uncomfortable because of an excessive number of device discharges.

4. If the patient's tachycardia is uncontrolled on amiodarone with an AICD, cardiac transplantation should be considered. If the patient is not a transplant candidate, surgery for ventricular tachycardia is the only therapeutic option available.

5. If the patient's left ventricular function is sufficient for surgery, the surgical approach outlined below is performed.

INTRAOPERATIVE MAPPING: ROLE IN VENTRICULAR TACHYCARDIA SURGERY

The role of intraoperative mapping is closely related to the type of procedure that can be performed. With the advent of intraoperative mapping systems, the concept existed that localization of the region of origin of the tachycardia would enable a relatively limited resection procedure to be performed. The *localized* procedures that were developed on this concept include the subendocardial resection procedure, endocardial cryoablation, laser photoablation, and the partial encircling endocardial ventriculotomy. To reduce the dependence of the operative procedure on intraoperative mapping results, *generalized* procedures have also been developed, including the original encircling endocardial ventriculotomy, the extended endocardial resection procedure, and procedures that completely encircle the visible scar with contiguous cryolesions or laser photoablations. A number of authors have argued that performance of a procedure that resects more potentially arrhythmogenic tissue (i.e., a generalized procedure) would minimize the assumed benefit associated with intraoperative mapping. No difference

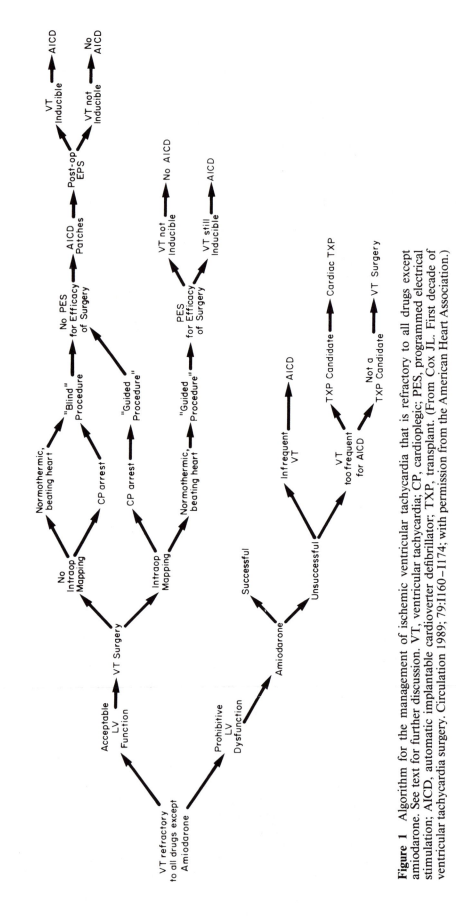

Figure 1 Algorithm for the management of ischemic ventricular tachycardia that is refractory to all drugs except amiodarone. See text for further discussion. VT, ventricular tachycardia; CP, cardioplegic; PES, programmed electrical stimulation; AICD, automatic implantable cardioverter defibrillator; TXP, transplant. (From Cox JL. First decade of ventricular tachycardia surgery. Circulation 1989; 79:I160–I174; with permission from the American Heart Association.)

in operative mortality between "map-guided" or "visually guided" procedures exists when the available literature is reviewed, indicating that the performance of intraoperative mapping does not adversely affect the outcome of the operative procedure.

The data regarding the reinducibility rate of tachycardia and intraoperative mapping are inconclusive, but the following generalizations can be made. Preoperatively, surgical failure is associated with the presence of complex (polymorphic or multiple monomorphic) ventricular tachycardia and with the anatomic-electrophysiologic characteristics of the tachycardia. Computerized, multichannel intraoperative mapping systems have made the intraoperative localization and treatment of complex tachycardias possible, as outlined below. Ventricular tachycardias associated with a posteroinferior infarct or aneurysm have in the past been more difficult to eradicate than those arising in the anterior portion of the left ventricle, but this has been due in part to difficulties associated with intraoperative mapping using single-point systems. Again, multichannel computerized systems appear to be making the surgical treatment of these infarcts/aneurysms somewhat less difficult.

Analysis of the intraoperative factors that affect the reinducibility rate of ventricular tachycardia suggests that the use of intraoperative mapping to guide surgical procedures for ventricular tachycardia results in a higher cure rate than can be attained with visually guided procedures alone, particularly when mapping is used to direct a generalized type of procedure. Certainly, the development of more sophisticated computerized mapping systems, including a potential distribution mapping system developed in our laboratory, will undoubtedly produce an overall beneficial effect on the results of ventricular tachycardia surgery. The potential distribution system appears to be as precise in localizing the earliest site of activation as conventional isochronous systems but does not require editing of the individual electrograms. Thus a complete activation map for the 256-channel system can be recorded and generated in under 5 minutes.

The computerized mapping system currently used in the operating room at Barnes Hospital was developed by Witkowski and Corr in 1984. The system can record 160 unipolar or bipolar signals simultaneously, analyze the data, and display it in various forms within 2 minutes after data acquisition for editing (Fig. 2). Analog data recorded from

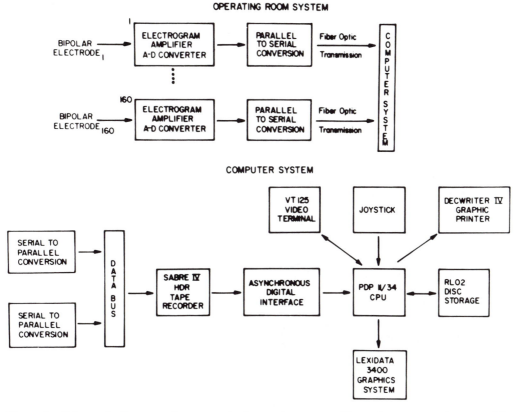

Figure 2 Schematic diagram of computerized mapping system illustrating separate data acquisition and analysis components. See text. (From Cain ME, Cox JL. Surgical treatment of supraventricular arrhythmias. In: Platia EV, ed. Management of cardiac arrhythmias—the nonpharmacologic approach. Philadelphia: JB Lippincott, 1987; with permission.)

the heart enter the front-end system located in the operating theater, where each electrogram is individually filtered and digitized. The digitized data are transferred across a fiberoptic cable to a remote computer facility located approximately 1,500 meters away. The personnel in the operating room and computer facility are connected by both audio and video display systems, allowing constant communication during the mapping procedure.

The detailed intraoperative mapping procedure is performed as follows in our institution. All 160 channels of the computerized system are used to map the heart in patients with ventricular tachycardia. An epicardial map employing a 96-electrode sock array (Fig. 3) is recorded, and this information is used to guide the subsequent placement of plunge needle electrodes in order to delineate further the specific site of arrhythmogenesis (Fig. 4). The epicardial map is also most useful in characterizing nonclinical arrhythmias that may be induced during programmed electrical stimulation. As mentioned, the availability of a computerized mapping system that permits the accurate localization of arrhythmogenic myocardium has resulted in the amenability of unsustained polymorphic ventricular tachycardia to surgical therapy with predictably excellent results.

Subsequently, multiple plunge needle electrodes containing four bipolar pairs of electrodes are inserted into the ventricle in the region of earliest epicardial activation (Fig. 5). If the tachycardia appears to arise from the intraventricular septum, a right atriotomy is performed, and up to 15 plunge needle electrodes are inserted into the septum from the right side. A total of up to 160 endocardial, intramural, and epicardial data points can be recorded simultaneously from the septum and free wall. A ventriculotomy, which can prevent further inducibility

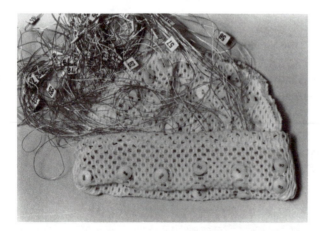

Figure 3 The "sock electrode." The material used is flexible nylon mesh that is contoured to fit the heart and can be slipped over the ventricles and positioned in a matter of seconds. The sock records 96 unipolar and bipolar electrograms simultaneously such that a global epicardial activation sequence can be obtained from a single beat.

of the ventricular tachycardia and necessitate performance of a procedure that is not map-guided, does not have to be performed in order to obtain an endocardial map.

OPERATIVE APPROACH FOR ISCHEMIC VENTRICULAR TACHYCARDIA

The operative procedure that we employ is based on the following analysis. The preoperative variables of amiodarone therapy, evidence of severe left ventricular dysfunction, and the requirement for emergency surgical intervention are associated with an increased operative risk. The intraoperative variables known to represent an incremental risk factor for operative death are the use of the standard encircling endocardial ventriculotomy and the inability to perform an aneurysmectomy. Significantly, aortic cross-clamping time, cardiopulmonary bypass time, intraoperative mapping, and the avoidance of cardioplegic arrest do not correlate with the operative mortality for ventricular tachycardia surgery. With regard to reinducibility rate, the data suggest that intraoperative mapping in combination with a wide excision or exclusion of the arrhythmogenic tissue yields the best results. In addition, we feel that ventricular tachycardia surgery performed in the normothermic, beating heart probably results in a higher cure rate than surgery performed under cardioplegic arrest. The ability to induce ventricular tachycardias during the postoperative electrophysiologic study has a profound effect on subsequent prognosis, thus emphasizing the importance of effecting a surgical cure at the time of operation if at all possible. In the postoperative population with inducible tachycardia on reexamination, the incidence of spontaneous ventricular tachycardia/sudden death is sixfold higher than in those patients in whom cure is obtained.

Our current technique, then, involves the initial intraoperative mapping sequence described above, usually with the patient on cardiopulmonary bypass. With the heart in the normothermic beating state, and preferably during ventricular tachycardia, the ventricle is opened through the infarct or aneurysm and all of the associated endocardial fibrosis is resected except that which extends onto the base of the papillary muscles (Fig. 6). Approximately 10 percent of patients still have inducible tachycardia following resection of the endocardial fibrosis, indicating that the actual site of origin of the tachycardia in these patients is deeper in the myocardium than the visible gross border of the fibrosis. Endocardial cryolesions are applied with a 2.5-cm nitrous oxide cryoprobe to the site(s) of origin of the tachycardia(s) as determined by the intraoperative mapping, thus ablating the myocardium beneath the visible fibrosis that is responsible for the tachycardia (Fig. 7). Resection of

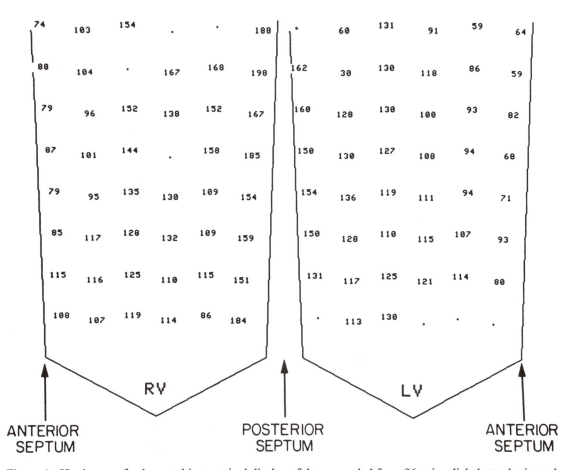

Figure 4 Hard copy of color graphics terminal display of data recorded from 96 epicardial electrodes in sock electrode array during induced ventricular tachycardia. Epicardial data show that the earliest area of epicardial breakthrough is over the upper anterior ventricular septum. These data were used to guide subsequent placement of multiple plunge needle electrodes in the ventricular septum and the anterior right and left ventricular free walls to obtain data from 160 endocardial, intramural, and epicardial sites in and around this region of early epicardial breakthrough. RV = right ventricle, LV = left ventricle. (From Cox JL. Intraoperative computerized mapping techniques. In: Brugada P, Wellens HJJ, eds. Cardiac arrhythmias: Where to go from here? Mount Kisco, NY: Futura, 1987; with permission.)

Figure 5 One bay of four needle electrodes. Each needle shaft contains four bipolar electrodes to record data from four different layers of ventricular free wall or septum, or both; thus, this one bay carries signals recorded from 16 individual sites in the heart. By inserting multiple needle electrodes, endocardial maps of the left or right ventricle or of both (in addition to intramural and epicardial maps) can be constructed without ventriculotomy. (From Cox JL. Intraoperative computerized mapping techniques. In: Brugada P, Wellens HJJ, eds. Cardiac arrhythmias: Where to go from here? Mount Kisco, NY: Futura, 1987; with permission.)

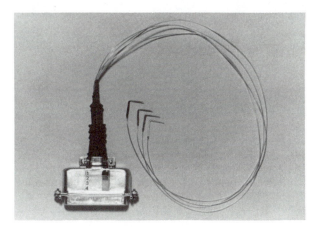

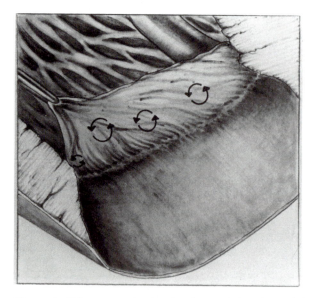

Figure 6 Diagrammatic sketch of extended endocardial resection procedure in an anterior left ventricular aneurysm. The principle involved in this procedure is the same as that for the localized endocardial resection procedure, but in this procedure all of the endocardial fibrosis associated with the aneurysm is resected except that involving papillary muscle. Circles = arrhythmogenic subendocardial tissue. (From Cox JL. Surgical treatment of ischemic and non-ischemic ventricular tachyarrhythmias. In Cohn LH, ed. Modern technics of surgery. Mount Kisco, NY: Futura, 1985; with permission.)

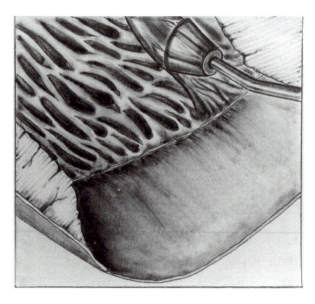

Figure 7 After resecting all endocardial scar as a preliminary measure, endocardial cryolesions are placed at the site or sites of ventricular tachycardia as determined by intraoperative mapping. In addition, any remaining scar on papillary muscle is cryoablated as shown. (From Cox JL. Surgical treatment of ischemic and non-ischemic ventricular tachyarrhythmias. In: Cohn LH, ed. Modern technics of surgery. Mount Kisco, NY: Futura, 1985; with permission.)

endocardial fibrosis extending onto the base of the papillary muscles is not performed; instead, one or more cryolesions are placed directly on the base of the involved papillary muscle. The clinical and laboratory experience with this method of dealing with fibrosis extending onto the base of the papillary muscle argues strongly against the practice of resecting papillary muscles for ventricular tachycardia, as has been recommended by some authors in the past. These techniques are applicable to both anterior and posteroinferior infarcts and aneurysms (Fig. 8).

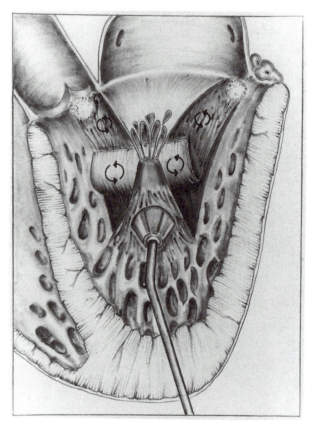

Figure 8 Extended endocardial resection of fibrosis associated with posterior myocardial infarction or aneurysm and cryoablation of the lower two-thirds of the posterior papillary muscle. Endocardial fibrosis is resected to within 5 mm of aortic and mitral value anuli. Because the site of origin of ventricular tachycardia is frequently adjacent to the junction of the aortic and mitral valve anuli, endocardial cryolesions (white circles) are applied at the base of the aortic and mitral valve anuli to ablate any reentrant circuits that might reside in remaining endocardial fibrosis immediately beneath valve anuli. In addition, endocardial cryolesions are applied to the site or sites of origin of ventricular tachycardia, as determined by intraoperative mapping, but only after removal of all endocardial scar. Circles = arrhythmogenic subendocardial tissue. (From Cox JL. Surgical treatment of ischemic and non-ischemic ventricular tachyarrhythmias. In: Cohn LH, ed: Modern technics of surgery. Mount Kisco, NY: Futura, 1985; with permission.)

Following completion of the extended endocardial resection and cryoablation of the endocardium, septum, and occasionally epicardium as required, programmed electrical stimulation is applied in an attempt to reinduce the arrhythmia. If ventricular tachycardia is still inducible, mapping is again performed and the remaining arrhythmogenic myocardium is again cryoablated. If the arrhythmia is no longer inducible at this time in the procedure, there is a 98 percent chance that it has been permanently ablated. If coronary artery bypass grafting or other procedures are required, they are performed after completion of the antiarrhythmic portion of the operation. The reason for the strict insistence that cardioplegic solution not be administered until the

antiarrhythmic portion of the operative procedure has been successfully completed is that the cardioplegia itself may temporarily alter the delicate reentry circuits causing the tachycardia. If the antitachycardia procedure is performed under cardioplegic arrest, it is impossible to determine intraoperatively whether or not the surgical procedure has ablated the arrhythmias.

The following recommendations can be made as additions to the treatment algorithm outlined in Figure 1:

1. If an institution does not have the capability of performing computerized intraoperative mapping or cryosurgery and a procedure that is not dependent upon intraoperative mapping is performed or the

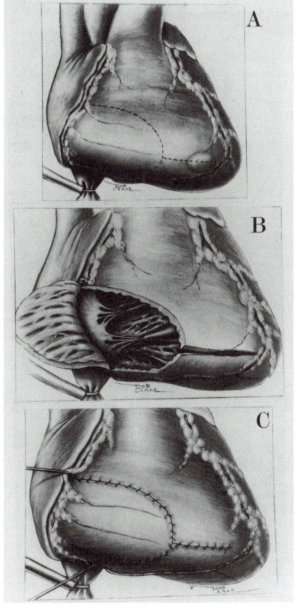

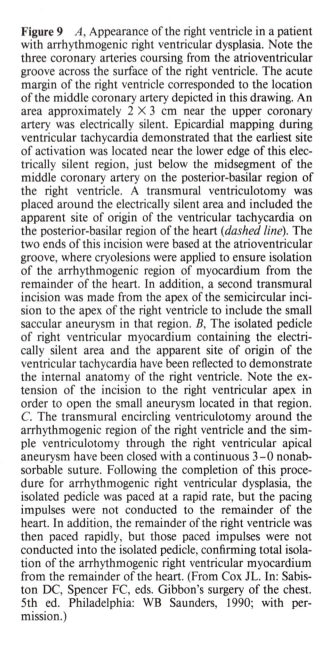

Figure 9 *A*, Appearance of the right ventricle in a patient with arrhythmogenic right ventricular dysplasia. Note the three coronary arteries coursing from the atrioventricular groove across the surface of the right ventricle. The acute margin of the right ventricle corresponded to the location of the middle coronary artery depicted in this drawing. An area approximately 2×3 cm near the upper coronary artery was electrically silent. Epicardial mapping during ventricular tachycardia demonstrated that the earliest site of activation was located near the lower edge of this electrically silent region, just below the midsegment of the middle coronary artery on the posterior-basilar region of the right ventricle. A transmural ventriculotomy was placed around the electrically silent area and included the apparent site of origin of the ventricular tachycardia on the posterior-basilar region of the heart (*dashed line*). The two ends of this incision were based at the atrioventricular groove, where cryolesions were applied to ensure isolation of the arrhythmogenic region of myocardium from the remainder of the heart. In addition, a second transmural incision was made from the apex of the semicircular incision to the apex of the right ventricle to include the small saccular aneurysm in that region. *B*, The isolated pedicle of right ventricular myocardium containing the electrically silent area and the apparent site of origin of the ventricular tachycardia have been reflected to demonstrate the internal anatomy of the right ventricle. Note the extension of the incision to the right ventricular apex in order to open the small aneurysm located in that region. *C*. The transmural encircling ventriculotomy around the arrhythmogenic region of the right ventricle and the simple ventriculotomy through the right ventricular apical aneurysm have been closed with a continuous 3–0 nonabsorbable suture. Following the completion of this procedure for arrhythmogenic right ventricular dysplasia, the isolated pedicle was paced at a rapid rate, but the pacing impulses were not conducted to the remainder of the heart. In addition, the remainder of the right ventricle was then paced rapidly, but those paced impulses were not conducted into the isolated pedicle, confirming total isolation of the arrhythmogenic right ventricular myocardium from the remainder of the heart. (From Cox JL. In: Sabiston DC, Spencer FC, eds. Gibbon's surgery of the chest. 5th ed. Philadelphia: WB Saunders, 1990; with permission.)

surgical procedure is performed under cardioplegic arrest, it is appropriate to implant AICD patches in these patients at the time of the ventricular tachycardia surgery. The rationale for this recommendation is that under these circumstances, approximately 25 percent of patients will have inducible tachycardia following the surgical procedure.

2. If the tachycardia is inducible at the time of the postoperative electrophysiologic study, implantation of the AICD device should be performed. However, if the rationale recommended here for surgical intervention is employed, this would then be necessary only in the small number of patients with an unsuccessful operative procedure and inducible tachycardia postoperatively.

3. The operative and long-term follow-up results for ventricular tachycardia surgery argue strongly against routine implantation of the AICD device and performance of coronary bypass surgery as the primary therapeutic modalities for ventricular tachycardia in patients who are otherwise candidates for a map-directed, wide-resection/cryoablative procedure as described above.

4. It should be recognized that the AICD device provides a viable therapeutic option for those patients in whom performance of ventricular tachycardia surgery has been fraught with an excessive mortality, namely, patients with extreme degrees of ventricular dysfunction. Judicious selection of these patients for the AICD should reduce the operative mortality rate in this subset of ventricular tachycardia patients, thereby reducing the overall operative mortality rate for ventricular tachycardia procedures as well.

SURGICAL TECHNIQUES FOR NONISCHEMIC VENTRICULAR TACHYCARDIAS

These tachycardias usually arise in the right ventricular free wall or septum and in general are extremely resistant to medical therapy. Localized surgical isolation techniques are usually employed for tachycardias arising in the right ventricular free wall, whereas multipoint map-guided cryoablative techniques are used for arrhythmias localized to the septum.

The surgical procedure developed for arrhythmogenic right ventricular dysplasia is designed to isolate the arrhythmogenic myocardium from the remainder of the heart. For well-localized ventricular tachycardias, focal isolation or ablation procedures are recommended. When the area of arrhythmogenic myocardium is larger, a transmural encircling ventriculotomy is created with the surgi-

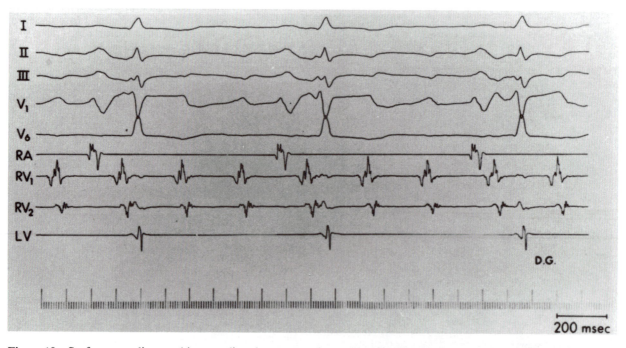

Figure 10 Surface recordings and intracardiac electrograms in a 16-year-old boy during an episode of right ventricular (RV) tachycardia following right ventricular isolation procedure. Limb lead (I through III) and precordial lead (V₁ and V₆) electrograms demonstrated normal sinus rhythm in the remainder of heart, documented by right atrial (RA) activity preceding each left ventricular (LV) complex. RV₁ = high right atrial electrogram; RV₂ = low right atrial electrogram. (From Cox JL. The surgical management of cardiac arrhythmias. In: Sabiston DC, Spencer FC, eds. Gibbons surgery of the chest. 5th ed. Philadelphia: WB Saunders, 1989; with permission.)

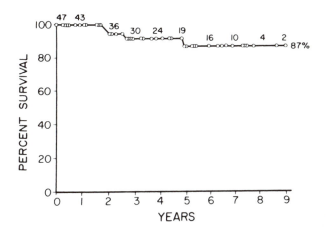

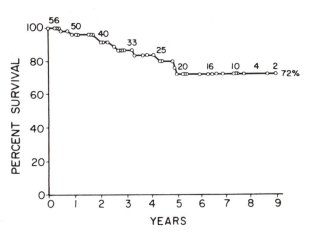

Figure 11 Freedom from recurrent ventricular tachycardia and/or sudden death curve (%) during a 9-year follow-up period in the author's series of patients undergoing an extended endocardial resection followed by cryoablation at the site(s) of origin of the ventricular tachycardia(s). (From Cox JL. First decade of ventricular tachycardia surgery. Circulation 1989; 79:I160–I174; with permission from the American Heart Association.)

Figure 12 Actuarial survival curve (%) minus operative mortality during a 9-year follow-up period in the author's series of patients undergoing an extended endocardial resection followed by cryoablation at the site(s) of origin of the ventricular tachycardia(s). (From Cox JL. First decade of ventricular tachycardia surgery. Circulation 1989; 79:I160–I174; with permission from the American Heart Association.)

cally isolated pedicle based on a vascular supply originating from the right coronary artery (Fig. 9). Two cryolesions are placed at the proximal and distal aspects of the incision at the level of the tricuspid annulus to ensure complete separation of all ventricular muscle fibers on either side of the incision. Successful isolation has been demonstrated in a small number of patients (Fig. 10). In certain instances, intraoperative mapping has suggested that the entire right ventricular free wall may be arrhythmogenic, giving rise to multiple morphologic types of tachycardia. In such cases, surgical isolation of the entire right ventricular free wall has been performed in the past. Postoperatively, however, the right ventricle has on occasion undergone a progressive dilatation, and today cardiac transplantation in a suitable patient with this arrhythmia is the most feasible surgical approach.

Patients with ventricular tachycardia occurring in association with the long Q-T interval syndrome frequently have torsades de pointes as the manifestation of their tachycardia. Medical therapy consists of beta-adrenergic blockade, and this recently has been coupled with permanent atrial or ventricular pacing. Surgical therapy has consisted of left cervicothoracic sympathectomy with removal of the left stellate ganglion and the first three to four left thoracic sympathetic ganglia. Our experience has found this procedure to be associated with early success but late failure, and as a result implantation of an AICD is now recommended at the time of sympathectomy to serve as back-up therapy in those patients with a history of life-threatening arrhythmias.

The long-term success rate for patients who survive ventricular tachycardia surgery is 87 percent at 9 years in our series of patients operated on for ischemic ventricular tachycardia (Fig. 11). Long-term survival in this series is 72 percent at 9 years following successful operative intervention (Fig. 12). These promising results have provided an extremely strong impetus to optimize the preoperative evaluation, operative selection, and intraoperative management of this critically ill but potentially curable group of patients.

SUGGESTED READING

Cox JL. Surgery for cardiac arrhythmias. Curr Probl Cardiol 1983; 8:46.

Cox JL. Intraoperative computerized mapping techniques. In: Brugada P, Wellens HJJ, eds. Cardiac arrhythmias: Where to go from here? Mount Kisco, NY: Futura, 1987.

Cox JL. A decade of ventricular tachycardia surgery. Circulation 1989; 79 (Suppl I):I160–I177.

Cox JL, Ferguson TB Jr. Cardiac arrhythmia surgery. Curr Probl Surg 1989; 26:199.

X MANAGEMENT WITH ELECTRONIC DEVICES

TEMPORARY PACEMAKERS

CHARLES NYDEGGER, M.D.
STEVEN P. KUTALEK, M.D.

Temporary pacemakers can be used for control of bradyarrhythmias of acute onset, prophylactically in patients at high risk for bradyarrhythmias, and for the treatment of supraventricular or ventricular tachyarrhythmias. A variety of pulse generators provide single-chamber pacing (atrial or ventricular), dual-chamber pacing (atrioventricular [AV] sequential), or rapid overdrive pacing. Corresponding pacing electrodes are available for percutaneous insertion with or without fluoroscopy as well as for invasive or noninvasive transthoracic pacing.

Selection of the appropriate temporary pacing system takes into account the type of arrhythmia, the effect of pacing on hemodynamics, ease of placement of the pacing catheter, safety, comfort, reliability of the catheter and pulse generator, therapeutic objectives, and long-term goals. Temporary pacemakers can provide definitive therapy for arrhythmias of a transient nature or act as a bridge to implantation of a permanent device. When properly used, temporary pacemakers represent a safe and effective form of therapy.

PATIENT SELECTION AND INDICATIONS

Temporary pacemakers may be categorized into those intended for treatment of bradyarrhythmias and those intended for treatment of tachyarrhythmias. The clinical situation dictates selection of the type of pacemaker.

Bradycardia temporary pacing is often required on an emergency basis. Acute indications include those in which hemodynamic compromise has developed or is likely to occur, such as complete heart block with a slow ventricular escape mechanism; prolonged sinus pauses with associated hypotension; or any degree of persistent bradyarrhythmia or heart block that results in symptoms of lightheadedness, syncope, acute exacerbation of heart failure, or progressive angina. Temporary pacemakers are especially beneficial in patients with bradyarrhythmias caused by drugs that affect the sinus or AV nodes, such as digitalis or beta-adrenergic blockers, since resultant slow ventricular rates may resolve as drug levels decrease.

More frequently, however, prophylactic temporary pacing is used to control intermittent or anticipated bradyarrhythmias. Pacing may be applied to patients with frequently occurring Mobitz II AV block, new bifascicular block following acute anterior wall myocardial infarction, or intermittent symptomatic sinus pauses. In cases in which prophylactic pacing is being considered, one must carefully weigh the risks versus the benefits of temporary pacemaker placement. It is in these patients that noninvasive prophylactic transthoracic pacing may be most useful. Indications for temporary bradycardia pacing are listed in Table 1.

Table 1 Indications for Bradycardia Pacing

Indicated
Acquired complete heart block with bradycardia
Heart rate less than 30 beats per minute
Symptomatic bradycardia of any cause
New bifascicular block after anterior myocardial infarction.
Immediately after cardiac surgery (wires implanted in operating room)

Indicated Depending on Clinical Situation
Acquired complete heart block without bradycardia
Intermittent Mobitz I or Mobitz II heart block
Medication overdose with intermittent bradycardia

Not Indicated
Congenital complete heart block without symptoms
Intermittent atrioventricular dissociation without bradycardia or heart block

Temporary antitachycardia pacing can be used to terminate supraventricular or ventricular arrhythmias. Overdrive pacing is an effective mode for termination of atrial flutter and can be accomplished by pacing through temporary transthoracic atrial wires left in place at the time of surgery. Rhythm conversion may be more easily performed and sinus rhythm better maintained by overdrive pacing after the patient has been given a class IA antiarrhythmic medication, such as procainamide or quinidine. Overdrive pacing may also be useful for termination of intraatrial or AV nodal reentry as well as for management of AV reciprocating bypass tract tachycardias.

Insertion of a temporary electrode catheter for overdrive pacing is indicated if supraventricular tachyarrhythmias cannot be terminated with drugs or occur very frequently in an acute setting, especially if they are associated with hemodynamic compromise. Temporary pacing electrodes can provide a means to evaluate extensively the efficacy of various antitachycardia modes if a permanent antitachycardia device is being considered.

Temporary pacing can also be used for termination of recurrent ventricular tachycardia, especially tachycardia that is incompletely responsive to antiarrhythmic drugs. Attempts at overdrive pacing for ventricular tachycardia are feasible only if the arrhythmia is monomorphic and slow enough to be tolerated hemodynamically while the pacing impulses are delivered. Since there is a risk of acceleration of ventricular fibrillation, resuscitative equipment must be available when ventricular tachycardia overdrive pacing is attempted.

Torsades de pointes may be suppressed by temporary pacing; however, since this arrhythmia is paroxysmal, polymorphic, and short-lived, overdrive pacing for termination is not useful. Patients with torsades de pointes and a prolonged Q-T interval, especially if the result of a transient cause such as therapy with a class IA antiarrhythmic drug, may benefit from continuous atrial or ventricular pacing at a rate above the sinus rate (usually 100 to 120 beats per minute) to shorten the ventricular refractory period and suppress the intermittent ventricular arrhythmia. Although ventricular pacing widens the QRS complex, a ventricular catheter has better long-term stability than an atrial catheter for this rhythm disorder. Antitachycardia temporary pacing indications are summarized in Table 2.

HARDWARE SELECTION

The choice of the pulse generator and pacing catheter is dictated by the clinical situation. For bradycardia pacing, two decisions must be made: (1) single- versus dual-chamber pacing and (2) catheter type and insertion site.

Table 2 Indications for Temporary Antitachycardia Pacing*

Atrial overdrive to terminate supraventricular tachycardia
  Atrial flutter
  Intraatrial reentry
  AV nodal reentry
  AV reciprocating bypass tract tachycardia

Ventricular overdrive pacing to terminate ventricular tachycardia

Atrial or ventricular pacing at a rate faster than sinus to suppress torsades de pointes

*Antiarrhythmic medications and cardioversion may also be effective for treatment of these rhythm disorders.

Most temporary pacing systems are single-chamber devices and involve placement of one electrode catheter, usually for ventricular pacing. This combines the advantages of stability, reliability, and maintenance of ventricular depolarization. Dual chamber AV sequential pacing can, however, improve hemodynamics in patients with decreased left ventricular compliance or critically low cardiac output.

Despite the availability of AV sequential pacing catheters, most temporary external dual-chamber pacing generators do not track atrial activity. This requires AV pacing at rates above the intrinsic sinus rate to maintain AV synchrony. Dual-chamber units may require placement of two catheters if a jugular or subclavian approach is unavailable for a combined AV system. Temporary dual-chamber pulse generators can also be attached to pacing wires implanted at cardiac surgery.

The Noninvasive Transthoracic Pacemaker

Noninvasive transthoracic pacing can be accomplished with an external pacemaker connected to the patient by two large cutaneous patch electrodes placed on the anterior and posterior chest walls. Pacing pulses pass between the patches, depolarizing the heart, resulting in ventricular contraction. This unit is generally effective, noninvasive, and can be applied rapidly in emergency situations; however, it may be difficult to maintain adequate pacing because of high thresholds. Further, the high energy of the delivered pulse causes chest wall muscle stimulation and can be quite uncomfortable. This device is best suited for patients who require immediate institution of temporary ventricular pacing as well as for those who refuse placement of a transvenous catheter or are at high risk for the procedure. Transthoracic pacing should *not* be considered a long-term substitute for a stable transvenous electrode in patients who require temporary bradycardia pacing, especially if the patient is dependent on the pacemaker to maintain ventricular activity.

The Single-Chamber Pacemaker

Single-chamber pacemakers are generally used in the ventricle for bradycardia pacing but also can be used in either the atrium or ventricle for temporary antitachycardia pacing. A single-chamber atrial electrode can provide AV synchrony in patients with sinus nodal dysfunction and intact AV conduction; however, temporary atrial wires tend to be less stable than ventricular electrodes. Generally, if AV synchrony is required, it is preferable to place a dual-chamber system to ensure ventricular depolarization, especially if any question arises regarding the adequacy of the AV conduction system.

Single-chamber bradycardia pulse generators allow asynchronus (AOO or VOO) or demand (AAI or VVI) operation, with fixed pulse width but adjustable pulse amplitude, sensitivity, and pacing rate. Pacing rates range from 30 to 180 beats per minute, and the devices connect directly to the standard 1-mm pin connectors found on temporary pacing catheters. Manual antitachycardia overdrive pacemaker generators can deliver higher pacing rates (to 800 beats per minute) with adjustable pulse amplitude, but these often do not have a demand mode.

A variety of catheters may be used in conjunction with single-chamber pacemaker generators (Table 3), and nearly all catheters can be adapted for use with any external pulse generator. The clinical situation (e.g., emergency insertion, bedside insertion) often determines the most appropriate catheter, although the physician doing the procedure must also consider venous access and the availability of fluoroscopy. In elective situations, a transvenous bipolar No. 5 or 6 French electrode catheter positioned in the right ventricular apex provides the greatest stability.

Table 3 Temporary Pacing Catheters

Catheter Type	Uses
Balloon-tipped bipolar	Acute initiation of ventricular pacing when fluoroscopy is unavailable
"Hard-wire" bipolar	Atrial or ventricular pacing with fluoroscopic guidance
Pace-Port Swan-Ganz	Prophylactic ventricular pacing in low-risk patients who need pulmonary artery pressure monitoring
Preformed atrial J wire	Atrial pacing via subclavian or jugular approach
AV sequential	Atrial and ventricular pacing via subclavian or jugular approach
Transthoracic (external)	Prophylactic ventricular pacing
Transthoracic (internal)	
Postoperative indwelling wires	Atrial or ventricular postoperative pacing
Acutely placed by right ventricular puncture	Acute ventricular pacing in emergency situations

In the first few days following cardiac surgery, temporary transthoracic right atrial and ventricular wires provide a reliable pacing system. These electrodes can also assist in the diagnosis and treatment of postoperative arrhythmias. Their sensing and pacing thresholds gradually deteriorate over a period of days to weeks, requiring daily evaluation to ensure consistent capture. This system may need to be replaced with transvenous electrodes for continued pacing.

In emergency situations, any unipolar ventricular lead can be grounded to the skin (with a surface electrode) or subcutaneous tissue (with a needle) for acute pacing. If a skin electrode is used, dermal abrasion is required to reduce the electrode to skin resistance. The cardiac pole may be a surgical wire or transvenous catheter. Additionally, invasive transthoracic pacemakers may be placed by the subcostal or left anterior thoracic approach directly into the right ventricle as a lifesaving procedure; however, because of the risk of cardiac tamponade, this should be considered only as a last resort when other transvenous or noninvasive pacemakers fail to capture.

The Dual-Chamber Pacemaker

Dual-chamber, AV sequential temporary pacemakers are useful for patients with hemodynamic compromise in conjunction with AV conduction disorders or sinus nodal disease as well as for patients with reduced left ventricular compliance who require temporary pacing. The most common application for temporary dual-chamber pacing occurs following cardiac surgery. AV synchrony may significantly improve hemodynamics in postoperative patients, decreasing their reliance on catecholamine infusions or on intraaortic balloon counterpulsation.

The temporary dual-chamber pulse generator is similar to the single-chamber device with the addition of controls for AV delay, separately adjustable atrial and ventricular output amplitudes, and attachments for two pairs of pacing leads. Most units do not allow full DDD operation, since atrial sensing is not generally available; these units function in the DVI mode.

The dual-chamber pulse generator can be connected to a variety of lead systems, including pairs of transthoracic postoperative wires; individual atrial and ventricular bipolar electrode catheters inserted through separate transvenous sites; combined AV sequential pacing systems that allow individual positioning of an atrial J electrode and a ventricular electrode via a single sheath; and Berkovits-Castellano hexapolar electrode catheters advanced via subclavian or jugular access to be positioned proximally against the lateral right atrial wall and distally in the right ventricular apex.

TEMPORARY PACEMAKER INSERTION

The physician implanting the pacemaker should ensure that the nursing staff and other physicians understand the nature and use of the pacemaker system. Although the risks involved with temporary pacemaker insertion and the subsequent use of an indwelling catheter are relatively small, they must be explained to the patient and family, as should the limitations of the device and what can be expected from its use. This is especially important for patients who receive antitachycardia and noninvasive transthoracic pacemakers.

Prior to placement of a temporary electrode catheter, the coagulation status and activity level of the patient must be evaluated. If the patient is thrombocytopenic or on anticoagulants or thrombolytic agents, peripheral venipuncture (e.g., antecubital) or noninvasive transthoracic pacing is preferable to central venous access to reduce the risk of bleeding; however, central venipuncture sites (femoral, subclavian, internal jugular) provide more stability than do peripheral sites. Combined AV sequential systems, atrial J wires, and Berkovits-Castellano catheters must be placed from superior sites (e.g., jugular or subclavian) to function properly. Swan-Ganz pacing wires can also be positioned most easily from above. Subclavian, jugular, and antecubital locations maximize patient mobility, whereas femoral locations require bed rest. Subclavian sites should be avoided if possible in patients in whom a permanent device is anticipated in order to prevent hematoma or infection at the permanent implant site.

A well-equipped procedure room should be used for temporary pacemaker insertion, providing a sterile environment and adequate lighting and emergency equipment, including oxygen, a cardiac monitor, a defibrillator, and cardiac medications for acute conditions. A selection of electrode catheters provides flexibility in the event that there is difficulty in catheter manipulation or in obtaining venous access. The availability of fluoroscopy is desirable, and it is required to position some pacing catheters.

Electrode Catheter Placement

The procedure is conducted in a sterile manner, with the operator and assistant gowned and gloved. The venipuncture site is prepared with an iodine solution or equivalent, and the area is draped. It is important that a large sterile work area be available to ensure that the pacing catheter remains sterile. The skin is anesthetized locally, and venipuncture is performed with either a Cournand or Cook needle. A flexible guidewire is advanced into the vein, and its position is verified fluoroscopically. The needle is removed, and a tiny skin incision is made so that an introducer can be passed over the wire into the vein. We prefer an introducer with an internal diameter of

the same French size as the catheter. After the catheter is positioned, the sheath can be withdrawn out of the skin over the electrode catheter.

Unless it is balloon-tipped, a standard bipolar electrode catheter used for atrial or ventricular pacing requires fluoroscopy for proper placement. The electrode catheter should be positioned in a stable location. Atrial leads can be placed in the right atrial appendage or along the right lateral atrial wall, and ventricular leads should be placed in the distal right ventricular apex. Recording a rhythm strip during cough and deep breathing while pacing ensures that the catheter position will not change with these maneuvers. Figure 1 shows the proper position of atrial and ventricular leads in a temporary AV sequential pacing system.

If fluoroscopy is not available, a balloon-tipped pulmonary artery catheter with provision for a pacing catheter (such as a Swan-Ganz Pace-Port) can be used. The pacing wire can be directed by proper positioning of the catheter. The pacemaker port of the catheter is connected to a pressure transducer, and the catheter is advanced 1 cm beyond the point at which the pressure waveform shows that the pacing port has entered the right ventricle. This positions the exit site of the pacing port below the tricuspid valve. The pacing catheter, connected to an electrocardiographic monitor, is then advanced until it contacts the right ventricular wall, producing an

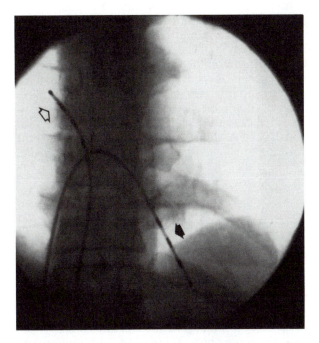

Figure 1 Fluoroscopic view of two temporary quadripolar electrode catheters positioned in the high lateral right atrium (*open arrow*) for atrial pacing and in the right ventricular apex (*closed arrow*) for ventricular pacing. Catheters were inserted via a femoral venous approach.

injury current on the electrogram. Although it is not required, fluoroscopy is useful for this procedure.

Electrode position can always be verified noninvasively by recording a unipolar electrogram from the electrode (using lead V_1 of a standard electrocardiographic recorder connected to the electrode). Acutely, the electrogram recorded from the tip of the catheter should show an injury potential, and the electrogram recorded from the proximal electrode of a bipolar catheter should show a Q-S pattern without an R wave or injury potential. The lack of an injury potential at the tip or the presence of an R wave at the proximal or distal electrode suggests perforation and an epicardial position. A 12-lead electrocardiogram recording during ventricular pacing shows a left bundle branch block morphology for catheters in the right ventricular apex. A right bundle branch pattern also suggests perforation.

After lead position has been verified and tested for stability, threshold and sensing functions are evaluated using the pacemaker generator. The capture threshold is determined by increasing pacing output and rate to a level at which continuous pacing occurs, then slowly decreasing output amplitude until capture is lost. The pacing threshold in the ventricle at the wide pulse width delivered by temporary external generators should be less than 1.0 mA. Atrial thresholds tend to be slightly higher but usually less than 2.0 mA. Capture threshold should be recorded at implant to allow comparisons on subsequent days and should be checked at least daily. Sensing function can be evaluated by reducing the pacing rate below the patient's intrinsic heart rate and placing the unit at maximal sensitivity (lowest millivolt setting). The sensitivity is gradually decreased (higher millivolt setting) until inappropriate pacing occurs. R wave amplitudes of greater than 5.0 mV are optimal for temporary ventricular pacemakers. After adequate capture and sensing are confirmed, the electrode catheter is secured in place with nonabsorbable suture and dressed with a transparent covering to allow visualization of the insertion site.

COMPLICATIONS

Complication rates of temporary electrode catheter placement are low. Most problems arise during insertion; these include bleeding, infection, pneumothorax, cardiac perforation, pericardial tamponade, air embolism, complete heart block, and development of tachyarrhythmias. Caution is also required to avoid complications of chronic pacing catheters, particularly thrombophlebitis and infection. Meticulous technique during insertion and appropriate choice of catheter and insertion site minimize complications. Monitoring vital signs during and after

Table 4 Temporary Pacemaker Complications

Acute (Implant) Complications
  Pneumothorax
  Bleeding
  Arterial injury
  Cardiac perforation
  Pericardial tamponade
  Air embolism
  Ventricular or atrial tachyarrhythmia
  Heart block
  Dislodgement of intracardiac thrombus

Chronic (Postimplant) Complications
  Infection
  Venous thrombosis
  Cardiac perforation
  Pulmonary embolism
  Loss of capture

the procedure is essential, and a postinsertion chest x-ray film should be obtained. Antibiotics are not routinely required.

Full dose intravenous anticoagulation may decrease the incidence of venous thrombosis, especially with femoral access. The risk of bleeding is slight after insertion; however, bleeding into central sites is often not visible until late into the episode. Late bleeding is uncommon but can be unrecognized if it is intrapleural or retroperitoneal. The more common complications of temporary pacemaker placement are listed in Table 4.

ALTERNATIVES

Very few alternatives to the use of a temporary pacemaker exist. Atropine and isoproterenol can be used in emergency situations for bradyarrhythmias and heart block; however, unless an easily correctable metabolic derangement is present, medications generally provide only transient relief until the temporary electrode catheter can be placed. Very transient or sporadic bradyarrhythmias may best be monitored and controlled with an external noninvasive pacing system.

SUGGESTED READING

Haffajee CI. Temporary cardiac pacing: Modes, evaluation of function, equipment, and troubleshooting. Cardiol Clin 1985; 3:515–526.

Hynes JK, Holmes DR Jr, Harrison CE. Five-year experience with temporary pacemaker therapy in the coronary care unit. Mayo Clin Proc 1983; 58:122–126.

Madsen JK, Meibom J, Videbak R, et al. Transcutaneous pacing: Experience with the Zoll temporary pacemaker. Am Heart J 1988; 116:7–10.

PERMANENT PACEMAKERS: INDICATIONS FOR PLACEMENT AND DEVICE SELECTION

CLIFFORD S. STRAUSS, D.O.
SCOTT R. SPIELMAN, M.D.

Since implantation of the first asynchronous pacemaker in 1958, a technologic explosion has occurred in device complexity and capacity. Pacemakers have progressed from asynchronous systems to multilead, multiprogrammable devices capable of maintaining atrioventricular synchrony over a wide range of cardiac rates as well as responding to physiologic parameters such as motion and temperature. With these advances, the indications for permanent pacing have broadened from simple heart block to sinus node dysfunction, certain types of bi- and trifascicular block, and even many supraventricular and ventricular tachyarrhythmias.

New pacemaker implants may now exceed 120,000 a year, resulting in an annual expenditure approaching $2 billion. Figures of this magnitude ultimately attract the attention of the federal government and indeed were the subject of a congressional inquiry in 1982. The United States Senate Special Subcommittee on Aging concluded that up to one-half of the Medicare outlay in 1982 for pacemakers may not have been justified. This led to the development of implant guidelines by a joint commission of the American Heart Association (AHA) and American College of Cardiology (ACC) in 1984, which now constitute the basis for Medicare reimbursement for pacemakers (Table 1).

All physicians must be familiar with the true indications for pacemaker implantation and be able to choose wisely among the various devices available. The purpose of this chapter is to review the indications for permanent pacemaker implantation for various bradycardia diagnoses, using both electrocardiographic and electrophysiologic parameters, and to examine specific device selection criteria.

Table 1 Implant Guidelines—AHA/ACC

Class I	Conditions in which there is general agreement that permanent pacemakers should be implanted
Class II	Conditions in which permanent pacemakers are frequently used but there is divergence of opinion as to their necessity
Class III	Conditions in which there is general agreement that pacemakers are not necessary

SINUS NODE DYSFUNCTION

Because the diagnosis of sick sinus syndrome now accounts for as many as one-half of all pacemaker implants, one must distinguish between true manifestations of sinus node dysfunction and normal physiologic responses. For instance, sinus bradycardia with a heart rate of 30 beats per minute may be of no consequence to a 20-year-old long-distance runner but may be associated with severe neurologic symptoms in a 75-year-old patient with poor ventricular function.

Electrocardiographically, sinus node dysfunction is a clinical syndrome that includes (1) severe sinus bradycardia, (2) sinus exit block, (3) sinus arrest, (4) brady-tachy syndrome, and (5) carotid sinus hypersensitivity. Cerebral symptoms usually accompany any or all of these abnormalities when asystolic periods exceed 3 seconds. Frequently pauses of this magnitude occur while patients are taking medications (e.g., calcium antagonists, beta blockers, amiodarone) for other cardiac conditions, and it is obviously important to determine whether or not these medications can be eliminated or their dosages decreased before a pacing device is implanted.

In most patients, sinus node dysfunction can be diagnosed and a symptom correlation made using noninvasive methods, including a 12-lead electrocardiogram, a 24-hour Holter monitor, and/or in-hospital telemetric monitoring. In 30 to 40 percent of patients in whom sick sinus syndrome is suspected, however, symptoms are paroxysmal, leaving the physician uncertain that there is a correlation with the observed sinus abnormality rather than some other arrhythmic etiology or sinus node dysfunction is truly latent. In such individuals, electrophysiologic testing is warranted and should include measurements of the sinus node recovery time and the sinoatrial conduction time, the effects of pharmacologic intervention, and a search for other electrophysiologic causes of syncope or presyncope such as intra- or infra-His disease or supraventricular and/or ventricular tachyarrhythmias (see the chapter *Electrophysiologic Studies*).

The sinus node recovery time is a measure of the automatic firing capability of the sinus node. It is determined by pacing the atrium at incremental rates above the basic cycle length for 30 seconds to 1 minute, a period usually sufficient to depress phase 4 automaticity in the sinus node, and then measuring the time to the first sinus return beat. A normal sinus node recovery time is less than 2 seconds, with a normal corrected recovery time (sinus node recovery time − basic cycle length) of greater than 550 msec. One can also calculate the total recovery time, which is measured from the last paced beat to the return of a stable basic cycle length (normal more than 5 seconds).

Conduction properties out of the sinus node are more difficult to assess, especially as sinus node function worsens. Our only method currently is the sinoatrial conduction time, which can be measured in two ways. The first is the Strauss method, which uses single atrial extrastimuli during normal sinus rhythm, and the second is the Narula method, which uses atrial pacing of short duration just above the sinus cycle length. In either case, the pause from the last paced beat to the first return sinus beat is measured, and this interval is subtracted from the basic cycle length. This is thought to represent the time it takes to get into and out of the sinus node and back to the recording site. Dividing this number in half gives the sinoatrial conduction time, which should be less than 125 msec. The limitations of this technique are obvious when one realizes that there is no a priori reason why conduction times should be equal entering and exiting the perinodal tissue.

Because the sinus node is under heavy autonomic influence, one can try to distinguish patients with intrinsic sinus node disease from those in whom abnormalities result from marked vagal tone by administering intravenous atropine during electrophysiologic testing. A normal response to 0.04 mg per kilogram of drug is an increase in basal heart rate to 90 beats per minute or more or a 50 percent increase over baseline. Patients with intrinsic sinus node disease manifest a blunted rate response and occasionally a paradoxically prolonged sinus node recovery time. Complete autonomic blockade can be achieved with the addition to intravenous atropine of intravenous propranolol, at 0.2 mg per kilogram. The resultant rate is termed the intrinsic heart rate; normal responses fall above a nomogram calculated by subtracting 0.53 times the heart rate, after administration of atropine and propranolol, from 117.

Table 2 lists the ACC/AHA guidelines for pacemaker implantation in sick sinus syndrome. Devices are allowed if the patient's abnormality occurs on an essential medication and are best implanted when a strong symptom correlation can be made.

CAROTID SINUS HYPERSENSITIVITY

Carotid sinus hypersensitivity is defined as dizziness, presyncope, or syncope resulting from an extreme reflex response to carotid sinus stimulation. Its incidence in the adult population is approximately 10 percent. We normally include carotid sinus hypersensitivity within the spectrum of sinus node dysfunction, although it has been considered separately in the ACC/AHA guidelines (Table 3).

Carotid sinus hypersensitivity is composed of two physiologic processes that may occur together or separately: (1) a cardioinhibitory response characterized by extreme bradycardia caused by sinus arrest, marked sinus bradycardia, sinus exit block, and/or atrioventricular nodal block, and (2) a vasodepressor response resulting from a reduction in sympathetic activity followed by marked peripheral vasodilation and hypotension. Permanent pacing obviously does not affect the vasodepressor component, which may actually be worsened by VVI pacing.

Clinically, patients with carotid sinus hypersensitivity present with sudden syncope frequently precipitated by a tight collar, shaving, or sudden head turning. If the cardioinhibitory response is present, it can be documented by brief (i.e., less than 3 seconds) carotid sinus massage during electrocardiographic monitoring. Pauses longer than 3 seconds are usually sufficient to cause cerebral symptoms. However, it is extremely important to correlate the findings with the patient's clinical milieu, as many more patients have positive responses to carotid sinus pressure than have syncope secondary to carotid sinus hypersensitivity. In fact, we believe, especially in patients with bundle branch block and/or ventricular dysfunction, that electrophysiologic testing is essential to rule out other potential arrhythmic causes of syncope before ascribing the patient's symptoms to carotid sinus hypersensitivity based solely on a positive response to carotid sinus massage. This approach

Table 2 Pacing in Sinus Node Dysfunction

Class IA	Sinus node dysfunction with documented symptomatic bradycardia with or without essential drug therapy
Class IIA	Sinus node dysfunction with symptoms and with heart rates <40 beats per minute, either spontaneous or with essential drug therapy, but without documented symptom correlation
Class IIIA	Sinus node dysfunction in asymptomatic patients, including those with drug induced rates <40 beats per minute
IIIB	Sinus node dysfunction in patients with symptoms of another etiology

Table 3 Pacing in Hypersensitive Carotid Sinus Syndrome

Class IA	Recurrent syncope associated with events typically producing carotid sinus stimulation and with >3-sec pauses with carotid sinus pressure in the absence of medications that depress sinus node or atrioventricular conduction.
Class IIA	Recurrent syncope without typical provocative clinical events but with a positive response to carotid sinus pressure
Class IIIA	Positive response to carotid sinus pressure without symptoms
IIIB	Positive response to carotid sinus pressure with vague symptoms (dizziness or lightheadedness)
IIIC	Cerebral symptoms with predominant vasodepressor response

would only be obviated by the direct observation of a bradycardic event during a clinical episode. In addition, one must be extremely cautious about interpreting positive responses to carotid sinus massage in the presence of drugs such as beta blockers and/or calcium blockers. If possible, such agents should be discontinued and carotid sinus massage repeated before a pacemaker is placed.

CHRONIC BI- AND TRIFASCICULAR BLOCK

Electrocardiographically, the spectrum of bi- and trifascicular block includes right bundle branch block–left anterior hemiblock, right bundle branch block–left posterior hemiblock, left bundle branch block, and alternating bundle block either with or without first degree atrioventricular block. In 1972, Narula evaluated a series of patients with chronic bifascicular block and found that progression to second- or third-degree block occurred in 42 percent of patients with prolonged H-V intervals (defined as greater than 55 msec) over a mean follow-up period of 3 years. In addition there was a significantly higher mortality in patients with prolonged H-V intervals, and it was suggested that this excess mortality could be markedly reduced by permanent pacemaker implantation. Narula's data led to the placement of many temporary and permanent pacemakers in asymptomatic patients with bifascicular block and mildly prolonged H-V intervals.

Subsequent studies in large patient populations followed in "heart block clinics" refuted Narula's data, documenting that the annual progression of patients with bi- and trifascicular block to complete heart block was in fact low. Although patients with H-V intervals of 70 msec or longer were shown to have a four-time increase in the incidence of progression to complete heart block over patients with H-V intervals of less than 70 msec, this incidence was still less than 15 percent overall and far too low to warrant routine pacemaker implantation, particularly in asymptomatic patients. Each of these later studies did confirm the presence of a high sudden-death mortality rate in patients with long H-V intervals that could not be reduced by permanent pacing, strongly implicating ventricular tachyarrhythmias as the true cause of death.

Currently, therefore, we approach clinical bi- and trifascicular block quite differently from the way we did in the early 1970s. Because of the low incidence of progression to complete heart block in such patients, we neither perform electrophysiologic testing nor implant pacing systems in asymptomatic individuals. In patients *with* symptoms, including dizziness and syncope, we recommend electrophysiologic testing to examine sinus node function and the propensity to sustained tachyarrhythmias as well as to measure the H-V interval. In patients with H-V

intervals of 70 msec or longer in whom all other cardiac and noncardiac causes of syncope have been ruled out, placement of a permanent pacing device is warranted. We find it particularly helpful in these patients to stress the infra-His system pharmacologically and/or with atrial pacing. If intra- or infra-His block develops with intravenous procainamide infusion or with atrial pacing, this provides further evidence to support placement of a permanent pacemaker. In the small subset of patients with intra-His block and split-His potentials or with H-V intervals of 100 msec or longer, several studies have shown a very high rate of progression to complete heart block. Placement of a permanent pacemaker in these individuals is therefore allowable even when symptoms are absent.

ACC/AHA guidelines (Table 4) to some extent reflect these considerations, but we feel strongly that the addition of electrophysiologic testing helps to clarify pacing indications labeled as class II.

ACUTE MYOCARDIAL INFARCTION

Following an acute myocardial infarction, changes in the electrophysiologic milieu may occur for several days after initial presentation. One must therefore differentiate between clinical situations that require only observation or a temporary pacemaker as opposed to those that necessitate placement of a permanent device (Table 5). In inferior infarction, for example, patients may even develop complete heart block and remain hemodynamically stable. In most of these instances, block is at the atrioventricular nodal level and resolves spontaneously. Temporary pacing is therefore only indicated for persistent hypotension or heart failure and permanent pacing only for heart block that persists for more than 7 days.

In anterior infarction, on the other hand, temporary pacing is clearly indicated in patients who present with or develop second- or third-degree block, as the site of block is invariably infra-His. The

Table 4 Pacing in Bifascicular and Trifascicular Block

Class IA	Bifascicular block with intermittent complete heart block and symptomatic bradycardia
IB	Bifascicular block with intermittent type II second-degree block and associated symptoms
Class IIA	Bi- or trifascicular block with intermittent type II second-degree block without symptoms
IIB	Bi- or trifascicular block with syncope of unproven cause in which other etiologies have been excluded
IIC	Pacing-induced infra-His block
Class IIIA	Fascicular block without atrioventricular block or symptoms

Table 5 Pacing After Myocardial Infarction

Class IA	Persistent advanced second-degree atrioventricular block or complete heart block
Class IIA	Persistent first-degree atrioventricular block in the presence of bundle branch block not previously documented
IIB	Transient advanced atrioventricular block and associated bundle branch block
Class IIIA	Transient atrioventricular conduction disturbances without persistent intraventricular conduction defects
IIIB	Transient atrioventricular block with persistent isolated left anterior hemiblock
IIIC	Acquired left anterior hemiblock in the absence of atrioventricular block

more subtle clinical decision-making issue arises in patients with new-onset bi- or trifascicular block. Unlike chronic bi- or trifascicular block, several studies have shown that patients with new-onset bi- or trifascicular block in anterior myocardial infarction have a greater than 20 percent rate of progression to at least transient complete heart block and therefore warrant placement of a temporary pacemaker. If no progression to complete heart block occurs over several days, the temporary wire can be removed, since the late incidence of development of complete heart block is extremely low. However, if the patient does develop even transient complete heart block and then reverts to bi- or trifascicular block, a permanent pacemaker should be placed because the late, posthospitalization rate of development of recurrent complete heart block is almost 30 percent.

ACQUIRED ATRIOVENTRICULAR BLOCK

Electrocardiographically, acquired atrioventricular block is characterized as first, second, or third degree. Second-degree atrioventricular block is further subclassified as type I with progressive P-R prolongation before a blocked QRS complex, i.e., Wenckebach block, or type II with no prolongation before a nonconducted P wave. Electrophysiologic testing is primarily of historical interest in these patients, as it is well established that first-degree and type I second-degree blocks are almost always attributable to block at the supra-His or atrioventricular nodal level and that type II second-degree and third-degree blocks usually are caused by intra- or infra-His disease. H-V interval measurements are occasionally useful in clinical situations where the site of block is uncertain and could be the determining factor in recommending a permanent device.

Permanent pacing is certainly warranted in patients with advanced forms of intra- or infra-His block given the inherent instability of such states, provided of course that the block is not related to a nonessential medication, e.g., tricyclic antidepressants or class IA antiarrhythmic drugs. Pacing is also warranted in patients with block at any level who become symptomatic or hemodynamically compromised, as indicated in Table 6. Permanent devices are acceptable as well in patients with chronic atrial fibrillation or flutter and slow ventricular rates, a phenomenon usually due to atrioventricular nodal delay, provided again that the slow rate is not produced by nonessential drugs, e.g., digitalis, calcium blockers, and/or beta blockers.

DEVICE SELECTION

Given the development of dual-chamber pacemakers and now of rate-responsive single- and dual-chamber pacemakers, choosing the type of device best suited for any individual patient has become a much more complex issue than in prior years. In fact, devices to be released within the next 6 months will alter selection criteria dramatically as we enter the 1990s. Although today the vast majority of implanted units are still simple VVI pacemakers, dual-chamber and rate-responsive device implants will probably garner more than 50 percent of the marketplace within 5 to 10 years.

We currently recommend standard VVI pacemakers only in patients in whom pacing simplicity is

Table 6 Pacing in Acquired Atrioventricular Block

Class IA	Permanent or intermittent complete heart block at any anatomic level associated with (1) symptomatic bradycardia, (2) congestive heart failure, (3) ventricular ectopy and other conditions requiring drug therapy that might suppress escape foci, (4) asystole of ≥3 sec, (5) escape rates below 40 beats per minute, and/or (6) confusional states that clear with temporary pacing
IB	Second-degree atrioventricular block, permanent or intermittent, regardless of the site of the block, with symptomatic bradycardia
IC	Atrial fibrillation/flutter or rare cases of supraventricular tachycardia with complete or advanced atrioventricular block and bradycardia plus any of the conditions listed under class IA
Class IIA	Permanent or intermittent asymptomatic complete heart block at any anatomic site with rates >40 beats per minute
IIB	Permanent or intermittent asymptomatic type II second-degree atrioventricular block
IIC	Asymptomatic type I second-degree atrioventricular block at intra- or infra-His levels
Class IIIA	First-degree atrioventricular block
IIIB	Asymptomatic type I second-degree atrioventricular block at the atrioventricular nodal level

of overall importance regardless of the indication for implant. This group includes patients who are older than 75 years of age, lead particularly sedentary lives, have a known limited life expectancy, live far from a follow-up center, or suffer from limited mental capacity (e.g., those with senile dementia). We particularly avoid VVI pacers in patients who have intermittent bradycardic states, known hypotension with temporary ventricular pacing, and/or left ventricular hypertrophy such as idiopathic hypertrophic subaortic stenosis or severe hypertension, in whom atrial contribution to cardiac output is likely to be critical. These individuals are particularly prone to the development of "pacemaker syndrome" and frequently end up requiring conversion to a dual-chamber device later on. Moreover, in patients about to undergo pacer replacement for battery depletion of an existing VVI system, symptoms of pacemaker syndrome should obviously be looked for before another fixed-rate device is implanted. Nonetheless, VVI pacing remains adequate for many patients, and it is not warranted to change over to a dual-chamber or rate-responsive device before pacemaker "end of life," unless the patient is clearly symptomatic from an adverse hemodynamic state created by a single-chamber and/or fixed rate system.

Single-chamber rate-responsive systems seem most appropriate in patients with chronic atrial fibrillation/flutter or atrial quiescence and a slow ventricular response in whom a dual-chamber system is not feasible. Certainly at this point there is reasonable evidence that such devices improve exercise capacity and decrease symptoms associated with single-chamber fixed-rate systems. These devices are also an acceptable alternative in patients who are in sinus rhythm with sinus node dysfunction and/or atrioventricular block in whom technical considerations simply prevent proper placement of an atrial lead. Patients whose atrial appendages have been amputated in open heart surgery may be in this category. It is probably also acceptable to implant a single-chamber rate-responsive system in the atrium of patients with sinus node dysfunction and intact atrioventricular conduction proved by electrophysiologic testing, although one must be extremely cautious in this regard because patients with sinus node disease usually have atrioventricular nodal disease as well.

Standard dual-chamber pacing systems seem particularly suited to patients with atrioventricular block and intact atrial chronotropic responsiveness. Such individuals may be returned to a near-normal physiologic state and, having never suffered through the adverse hemodynamics of VVI pacing, they fortunately may never fully appreciate the substantial disadvantages of a single-chamber system. Dual-chamber pacing is also of major importance in patients with left ventricular hypertrophic states in which the loss of atrial kick can be devastating, as noted previously, and in carotid sinus hypersensitivity, in which multiple authors have shown that patients have fewer recurrent cerebral symptoms with dual-chamber as opposed to single-chamber pacing systems. Although many clinicians performing implants and referring physicians are still dissuaded from recommending dual-chamber devices because of technical considerations, the ease of use of atrial leads and programmers for follow-up have reduced these concerns substantially.

We are currently entering a new era of rate-responsive pacing that will allow application of this technology to dual-chamber devices. In our view these pacemakers are particularly suited to patients with sinus node dysfunction and abnormalities of atrioventricular conduction who can then be provided with atrioventricular synchrony as well as chronotropic competence. This advance conquers the last major problem in pacing for bradycardic states, leaving only arguments as to the optimal type of sensor for rate adaptivity.

SUGGESTED READING

Dhingra RC, Palileo E, Strasberg B, et al. Significance of the HV interval in 517 patients with chronic bifascicular block. Circulation 1981; 64:1265–1271.

Frye RL, Collins JJ, DeSanctis RW, et al. Guidelines for permanent cardiac pacemaker implantation. Circulation 1984; 70:331A–339A.

Greenspan AM, Kay HR, Berger BC, et al. Incidence of unwarranted implantation of permanent cardiac pacemakers in a large medical population. N Engl J Med 1988; 318:158–163.

Hindman MC, Wagner GS, JoRo M, et al. The clinical significance of bundle branch block complicating acute myocardial infarction. 2. Indications for temporary and permanent pacemakers. Circulation 1978; 58:689–699.

Ludmer PL, Goldschleger N. Cardiac pacing in the 1980's. N Engl J Med 1984; 311:1671–1680.

Peters RW, Scheinmann MM, Modin G, et al. Prophylactic permanent pacemakers for patients with chronic bundle branch block. Am J Med 1979; 66:678–1985.

PERMANENT PACEMAKERS: TECHNIQUES OF IMPLANTATION

HAROLD R. KAY, M.D.

Techniques of permanent pacemaker implantation have evolved considerably since the days when all pacemakers were implanted using a transthoracic approach and epicardial electrodes. The latest changes in techniques of implantation reflect improved lead technology and other nonpacemaker considerations (e.g., concurrent need for an automatic implantable cardioverter defibrillator).

We favor a transvenous technique using an active fixation, unipolar lead in the vast majority of patients. Procedures are performed in a designated electrophysiology/pacemaker laboratory using local anesthesia with or without intravenous sedation. All procedures are performed with the same team of physicians, technicians, and nurses.

Pacemaker leads can be placed using one of four surgical techniques: (1) transvenous (endocardial), (2) subxiphoid (epicardial), (3) transthoracic (epicardial), or (4) sternotomy (epicardial).

TRANSVENOUS APPROACH

The advantages of a transvenous approach include lower pacemaker thresholds, improved lead longevity, a less invasive procedure (local anesthesia, small incision), more convenient generator location (prepectoral region versus abdominal wall), more options for optimal intracardiac electrode position, and fewer postoperative complications.

Implants are performed in a designated laboratory for two reasons: (1) availability of good, reliable overhead fluoroscopy, and (2) centralization and maintenance of pacemaker-related instruments, supplies, and accessories. A dedicated team of nurses, technicians, and physicians promotes familiarity with equipment and consistency of approach. Prior to and during pacemaker procedures, the laboratory is treated like an operating room, with complete preprocedure room cleaning and intraoperative sterile precautions. The incidence of pacemaker-related infections is less than 1 percent.

On the day prior to operation, patients are prepared and shaved using an antiseptic solution, kept on nothing by mouth after midnight except for essential medications, and intravenous antibiotics (a cephalosporin or vancomycin) are started before the procedure.

On arrival at the laboratory, patients are positioned on the fluoroscopy table; limb lead electrocardiographic electrodes are connected for six-channel monitoring, a pulse oximeter is attached to a fingertip to monitor oxygen saturation and peripheral pulse, an automatic blood pressure cuff is placed around the patient's upper arm, oxygen is given via a nasal cannula, and the patient's arms are secured at his or her sides. Patients receive a 3-minute povidone preparation, including the bilateral upper chest wall and neck (both sides).

Local anesthesia (a combination of 1 percent lidocaine mixed with 0.25 percent bupivacaine) is administered in the incision site, and a field block is created to anesthetize an area for the generator box. Many patients also require additional intravenous sedation (fentanyl or Midazolam).

The preferred incision is curvilinear, starting parallel and 2 to 3 cm inferior to the clavicle and curving laterally to a point just inferior and lateral to the deltopectoral groove. This incision allows access to both the cephalic and subclavian veins.

The generator pocket is created superficial to the pectoralis muscle and located such that the lateral aspect of the generator is at least 2 to 3 cm medial to the axilla and the superior aspect of the generator lies 2 cm below the inferior border of the clavicle.

The cephalic vein is identified in the adipose tissue of the deltopectoral groove. The vein is gently dissected, a venotomy is made, and electrode(s) are introduced into the central venous circulation. The anatomy of the venous system as well as the optimal position of the pacemaker pocket are illustrated in Figure 1.

The cephalic vein approach is associated with fewer complications (e.g., hemorrhage, pneumothorax), less friction between leads, and easier lead fixation. However, in patients with inadequate cephalic veins (small, not easily accessible, or occluded), electrodes are introduced through the subclavian vein.

When the subclavian vein is used, central venous pooling is improved by elevating the legs. A floppy J wire is introduced through the needle in the subclavian vein, and a No. 10.5 French sheath and dilator are passed over the J wire. The dilator and J wire are removed, and the lead is introduced through the sheath. If two leads are used, the J wire is again passed through the sheath, the first sheath is removed (keeping one lead and one J wire in the vein), and a second sheath is introduced over the J wire. The second lead is then introduced through the second sheath.

Rarely, venous access is obtained via the external or internal jugular vein. If the jugular vein is used, the lead is passed superficial to the clavicle (deep to the clavicle only if there is excellent operative exposure) into the pacemaker pocket. Rather

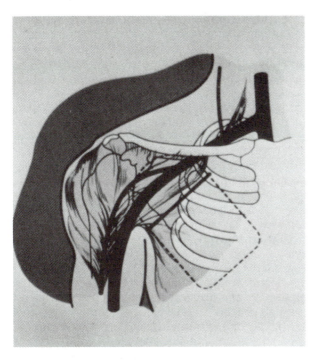

Figure 1 Venous anatomy of the shoulder with overlay of appropriate position for permanent pacemaker.

than use a jugular vein (incidence less than 0.2 percent in our institution), we close the incision and use the contralateral cephalic or subclavian vein.

The choice of implant side (left versus right) is based on the patient's handedness (i.e., the left side is used for right-handed patients). However, the high incidence of venous distortion and left innominate vein position anomalies after open heart operations has led us to use the right side in patients who have had previous sternotomies.

POSITIONING OF LEADS

Ventricular Lead

Once the lead is within the venous system, the straight stylet is partially withdrawn and the lead is allowed to "flop" across the tricuspid valve into the pulmonary artery. Having the patient take a deep breath facilitates passing the lead through the tricuspid valve. If the lead does not advance into the pulmonary artery easily, inserting a curved stylet usually allows the lead to be positioned. Confirmation of position in the pulmonary artery guarantees that the wire is not in the coronary sinus. Once the wire is stabilized in the pulmonary artery, 2 to 3 inches of the tip of the lead are made "floppy." Then, gentle withdrawal of the lead allows the tip to stay along the intraventricular septum to its inferior aspect, after which the tip points downward toward

the right ventricular apex. When the tip "falls off" the septum and points downward, the stylet is advanced and the lead is advanced into the inferior wall or apex of the right ventricle. An appropriate position of the ventricular wire is one in which it is on the left side of the spine, below the diaphragm, and with its tip pointing downward and anteriorly (Figs. 2 and 3).

Once the lead is in place, preliminary thresholds are measured. With a screw-in lead, the electrode surface area is initially low (just the tip of the corkscrew) and therefore resistance is high (usually over 1,200 ohm).

The corkscrew is then extruded, and thresholds are again measured. An active fixation device frequently produces a current of injury in the electrogram recorded from the electrograde. This causes a temporary decrease in the R wave and an increase in the voltage threshold, which almost invariably resolves over 3 to 4 minutes. Once the current of injury has resolved, acceptable parameters are an R-wave amplitude greater than 5 mV, pacing thresholds of 0.7 V (pulse duration 0.5 msec), a resistance of approximately 700 ohm, and a current of approximately 1 mA.

If an atrial lead is to be positioned, it is done at this point. Otherwise, the stylet is removed, and final

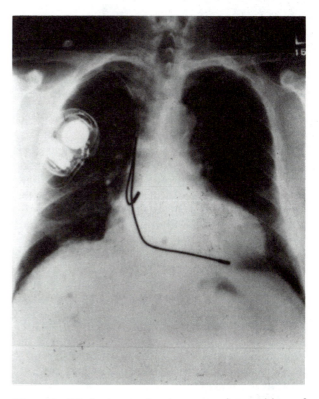

Figure 2 PA chest x-ray showing appropriate positions of atrial and transvenous permanent pacing wires.

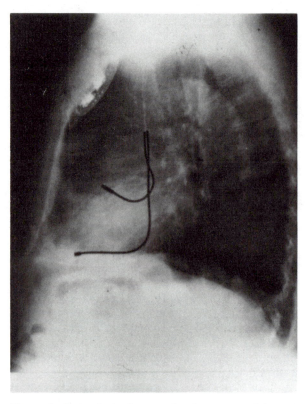

Figure 3 Lateral chest x-ray showing appropriate positions of atrial and transvenous permanent pacing wires.

extruded, and thresholds are measured. Final atrial thresholds should indicate P-wave sensing in excess of 2.2 mV and atrial capture of 1 V or less at a pulse duration of 0.5 msec with a resistance of approximately 700 ohm and, therefore, a current of 1.3 mA.

Once the leads are positioned within the heart (see Figs. 2 and 3), they are secured to the prepectoral fascia with permanent (silk) sutures. It is important to secure these leads over the tying sleeve in order to prevent injury to the lead. The pocket is irrigated with antibiotic solution, the leads are connected to the pacemaker generator, and the generator is placed in the pocket. If necessary, pacemaker function is tested with a sterile magnet. The wound is closed in layers of absorbable suture.

Postoperatively, patients receive antibiotics every 6 hours for four doses. They are restricted to bed rest for 24 hours, a portable chest x-ray film and an electrocardiogram are obtained soon after the procedure, and a repeat posteroanterior and lateral chest x-ray study is taken in 24 hours. All patients are placed on continuous telemetric monitoring.

Patients are discharged between 24 and 36 hours after the procedure. Unless there is a specific contraindication, the generator is left in its nominal settings. Patients are seen in 6 weeks, at which time their pacemaker parameters are adjusted to capture at three times chronic thresholds.

CHOICE OF LEADS

The choice of a transvenous lead is highly individual. We have been using one specific unipolar screw-in lead in both the atrium and the ventricle for the past 8 years. This lead seems to have the best "feel," is easy to position precisely, and has a dislodgement rate of less than 0.4 percent. It is also one of the easiest to remove because it has no tines, and it can be positioned at almost any part of the atrium, even in an atrium in which numerous previous operations have been performed.

The lead has several theoretical disadvantages: (1) it is stiffer than some of the newer, more flexible leads; (2) any unipolar lead system has an increased incidence of myoinhibition (sensing skeletal muscle motion as cardiac depolarizations); and (3) some of the target tip or steroid-eluding leads have low implant thresholds and therefore allow generator output to be lowered, with a resultant increase in generator life.

We have found that myoinhibition that cannot be controlled by decreasing the sensitivity (assuming good lead placement) is a problem that occurs in less than 1 percent of our implants. Second, although the lower thresholds are theoretically advantageous, the average implant threshold of the screw-in lead is 0.7 V. Our experience over 8 years has shown that thresholds in these leads do not increase dramati-

thresholds are measured. In its final position, the ventricular lead should take a gentle curve, lie along the inferior wall of the right ventricle, have a small impression in its course made by the tricuspid valve, and not straighten during deep inspiration.

Atrial Lead

The atrial lead is introduced with a straight stylet to allow it to advance through the central venous circulation. Once the tip of the lead is in the right atrium, a J stylet is substituted for the straight stylet. The short limb of the J wire is positioned anteriorly, and the lead is gently withdrawn until the tip of the J wire catches the right atrial appendage. Good position in the appendage is usually associated with a lateral motion of the tip during atrial systole. If an anteroposterior orientation is not effective, a more lateral orientation is tried. If the atrial appendage cannot be located easily (for example, after open heart surgery), alternative positions for the atrial lead include the lateral wall of the right atrium and the intraatrial septum. The positive fixation lead is particularly valuable in patients who have had previous open heart surgery.

Acceptable atrial lead parameters include a P-wave amplitude greater than 2 mV and voltage thresholds of 1 to 1.3 V. The corkscrew is again

cally after 4 or 5 years, as had originally been thought. Therefore, when all factors are considered, the advantages of the unipolar, screw-in, positive fixation lead exceed its disadvantages.

There are certain situations in which we routinely use bipolar, positive fixation leads. These include patients in whom a bipolar device is required (than with a history of myoinhibition, those for whom there are current or future plans for an automatic implantable cardioverter defibrillator, or those in whom a bipolar antitachycardia pacemaker is required). Our experience with these bipolar screw-in leads is that they are more difficult to position but still have advantages over passive fixation (tined) bipolar leads.

ALTERNATIVES TO THE TRANSVENOUS APPROACH

There are few instances in which a transthoracic approach is preferred for placement of pacemaker leads: inability to secure adequate lead position using the transvenous approach (because of anomalous course or stenotic central veins, "slippery" endocardium, or other technical reasons) or in a patient who is undergoing sternotomy for other reasons. In patients undergoing open heart surgery, the indication for a permanent pacemaker must be obvious prior to the sternotomy; that is, patients who come off cardiopulmonary bypass in complete heart block are not candidates for immediate permanent pacemaker implantation.

Other than sternotomy, the most commonly employed epicardial approach is a subxiphoid incision. The xiphoid process is removed, and the sternum is retracted. A small incision is made in the pericardium, and two screw-in epicardial electrodes are placed. Pacing thresholds are usually found to be higher than those obtained during transvenous electrode placement. Two screw-in electrodes are implanted even though a unipolar generator is used, so that easy options are available for subsequent generator replacement. A pocket is made superficial to the rectus sheath. One lead (the one with the higher thresholds) is capped and placed in the pocket and the lead with the better threshold is connected to the pulse generator.

An alternative approach to a subxiphoid incision (for example, in patients who have previously had upper abdominal surgery) is a left anterior thoracotomy incision. This incision is made in the sixth or seventh intercostal space on the left side. The pericardium is opened, and the screw-in leads are placed directly on the left ventricle. The leads are then tunneled to the upper abdomen where a second incision is made, and the generator is placed in a position superficial to the rectus sheath. In this procedure, a chest tube is frequently necessary, and the patient has the additional morbidity associated with recovering from a thoracotomy incision.

In patients undergoing pacemaker implantation through a sternotomy incision, two screw-in electrodes are placed in the wall of the left ventricle and two atrial "hook" electrodes are used in the right atrium. We have not been happy with any of the permanent atrial epicardial electrodes, but the hook electrodes seem to provide the best long-term thresholds. Two electrodes are used because of the high early failure rate (2 to 3 years) of epicardial atrial leads.

A major disadvantage in the transthoracic approach (other than the sternotomy approach) is that although either atrial or ventricular leads can be placed, both leads cannot be placed using either a subxiphoid or a single thoracic incision.

In patients in whom epicardial electrodes are placed after cardiopulmonary bypass, thresholds during the first 2 to 3 days frequently are very variable, probably as a function of myocardial edema. Therefore, the generators are programmed to maximal sensitivity and output. The patient is seen in 6 weeks, at which time the pulse generator parameters are adjusted appropriately.

SUGGESTED READING

Chung EK. Artificial cardiac pacing: Practical approach. 2nd ed. Baltimore: Williams & Wilkins, 1984.

Furman S, Hayes DL, Holmes DR Jr. A practice of cardiac pacing. 2nd ed. Mount Kisco, NY: Futura Publishing, 1989

Gillette PC, Griffin JC eds. Practical cardiac pacing. Baltimore: Williams & Wilkins, 1986.

Riegel B, Purcell JA, Brest AN, Driefus LS. Driefus' pacemaker therapy: An interprofessional approach. Philadelphia: F.A. Davis, 1986.

CARDIAC PACING IN CHILDREN AND YOUNG ADULTS

PAUL C. GILLETTE, M.D.
VICKI ZEIGLER, B.S.N.
JOHN KRATZ, M.D.
PAUL OSLIZLOK, M.D.

Cardiac pacing is being used with increasing frequency in children and young adults with both bradycardias and tachycardias. This is not only because of a better understanding of the mechanisms and prognosis of arrhythmias but also because of major improvements in the size, technology, and reliability of cardiac pacemakers and leads. The use of the transvenous subpectoral implantation technique and the ability of pacemakers to sense the atrial rate to provide both atrioventricular (AV) synchrony and rate increase during exercise have improved the usefulness of pacemakers in children. Pacemakers that sense either activity or a physiologic variable and pace the atrium, the ventricle, or both are also useful in selected patients.

INDICATIONS

The indications for cardiac pacing in children are varied. They are put forward in the joint American College of Cardiology/American Heart Association Task Force report. Most children who need pacemakers are symptomatic. The symptoms range from syncope to excessive fatigue and inability to keep up with their peers. One syncopal episode in a child with significant bradycardia is an indication for pacing.

Congenital complete AV block is one of the most common conduction disturbances requiring a pacemaker. If the ventricular rate is less than 55 beats per minute in a neonate, a pacemaker is indicated. A ventricular rate of 65 beats per minute in a neonate with significant congenital heart disease is considered an indication for a pacemaker. Most deaths in patients with congenital complete AV block occur in infants with significant heart defects in the first year of life. The fetus with complete AV block and congenital heart disease—particularly AV valve regurgitation—is also at risk for death and should be considered a candidate for pacing.

In older children with congenital complete AV block, one syncopal spell or near-syncopal spell should indicate a permanent pacemaker. It is not necessary to correlate an excessively slow rate with the symptoms. A ventricular rate of less than 45 beats per minute has been strongly correlated with early syncope in older children with congenital complete AV block and thus is considered a pacemaker indication. Frequent or complex ventricular premature complexes at rest or with exercise in a patient with complete AV block are also indications for a permanent pacemaker.

Excessive fatigue, recent onset of poor school performance, or inability to keep up with peers may be indications for pacemaker insertion. Periods of 2:1, 3:1, or greater block out of the focus controlling the ventricular rate or lack of rate variability have been said to predict symptoms. We are often told by patients and parents about great improvements in lifestyle after DDD pacemaker implantation in patients with congenital complete AV block. We are probably waiting too long to perform implantation in many patients.

Surgical complete AV block that persists for longer than 10 to 14 days is an indication for permanent pacing in children. The ventricular rate is often surprisingly fast early in this period because of high adrenergic and low vagal tone, but it usually decreases later after surgery. The repaired heart does better with a faster rate, AV synchrony, and rate variability. Complete AV block associated with myocarditis should probably be managed as surgical block.

Surgical sinus bradycardia associated with tachycardias often requires pacing. In the brady-tachy syndrome, the use of an antiarrhythmic drug other than digoxin or phenytoin requires the implantation of a pacemaker. Often an atrial antitachycardia pacemaker is useful in this situation. Any syncope, near-syncope, or excessive fatigue in a postoperative patient with sinus bradycardia or junctional rhythm may be effectively treated by pacing. Clinical congestive heart failure or increasing cardiac size according to chest x-ray study or echocardiogram will respond to cardiac pacing.

Sinus node dysfunction rarely causes symptoms in patients with normal hearts, but when it does, pacing results in symptomatic improvement. Other situations occur rarely and are covered in the American College of Cardiology/American Heart Association report.

PACING MODE

The decision of pacing mode is as important as the decision to implant a pacemaker (Table 1). The restoration of normal physiology should always be our goal, although it is not yet possible in every case. In the patient with AV block, the use of an atrial synchronous pacemaker will nearly restore normalcy in most patients. Some patients with either congenital or surgical AV block develop later chronotropic incompetence and are not able to increase

Table 1 Indications for Pacing Mode

Clinical Situation	Pacing Mode
CCAVB	DDDCO
CCAVB with SSS	DDDRO
SCAVB	DDDCO
SCAVB with SSS	DDDRO
SSSS with tachycardia	AAICP
SSSS without tachycardia	AAICP
SSS without adequate rate with exercise	AAIRO
Transient infrequent AVB	VVICO
Premature infant	VVICO
Atrial fribrillation with bradycardia	VVIRO

CCAVB = congenital complete AV block; SSS = block sinus syndrome; SCAVB = surgical complete AV block; AVB = atrioventricular block.

Pacing modes are in the NASPE, British pacing group code.

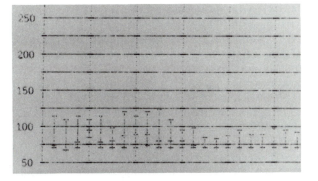

Figure 2 Demonstration of maximal, median, and low heart rates from a patient with a rate-responsive pacemaker using a piezoelectric crystal. The lower rate limit is set at 70 beats per minute. Each vertical bar represents 1 hour. The top crossbar is the maximal rate, the middle crossbar is the median rate, and the lower crossbar is the lower rate. It can be seen that both the maximal and the mean heart rate vary considerably from hour to hour, being higher when the patient is awake (to the left of the graph) and less when the patient is asleep (to the right of the graph).

their sinus rate to normal during exercise. In these patients, rate response may be restored by adding a sensor (Figs. 1 and 2).

In patients with sinus bradycardia and intact AV conduction, an atrial pacemaker is significantly more physiologic than ventricular pacing. If AV conduction is maintained 1:1 at rates of 100 beats per minute or higher during atrial pacing, we have found there is no incidence of progression to AV block. If AV conduction is inappropriate or if the patient has had repair of a ventricular septal defect, a dual-chamber pacemaker is used. Following atrial surgery (for atrial septal defect, atrial repair of transposition of the great arteries, or Fontan operation), an atrial automatic antitachycardia pacemaker

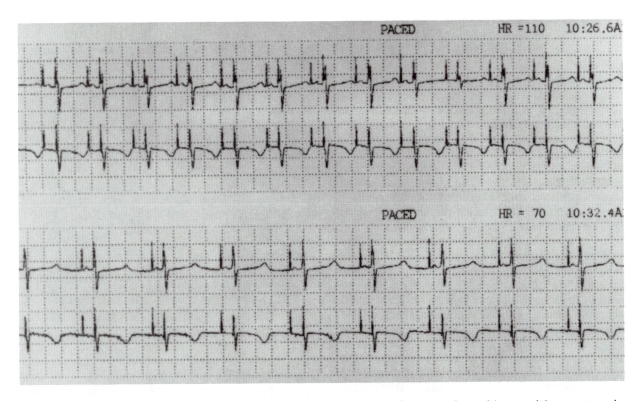

Figure 1 Simultaneous lead II and chest lead electrocardiogram taken from a patient with an atrial rate-responsive pacemaker using a piezoelectric crystal as a sensor. At 10:26 the atrial paced rate is 110 beats per minute, whereas at 10:32 the atrial paced rate is 70 beats per minute, the lower rate limit.

should be used because of the high frequency of atrial arrhythmias in this group. As sensors become more available and have more appropriate parameters for atrial pacing, they will be used more frequently for both atrial and dual-chamber applications.

Ventricular pacemakers are reserved for very small premature infants and patients with very infrequent bradycardia. It is not yet clear whether sensor-driven pacemakers will work in infants. Sensor-driven pacemakers should only be used when necessary because they use energy to run the sensor.

IMPLANTATION TECHNIQUE

Most pacemakers in children are implanted by the transvenous technique, and are now routinely implanted transvenously in infants as small as 8 kg. Indications for epicardial pacing are right-to-left shunt, lack of access from the superior vena cava to the chamber to be paced, inexcitable right atrium, and newborn or premature infants.

The technique of implantation of a pacemaker in a child is not dissimilar from the technique for adults (see the chapter *Permanent Pacemakers: Techniques of Implantation*). It should be performed by an operator familiar with pediatric catheterization techniques who does a sufficient number of implants to keep his or her technical skills honed. The left infraclavicular area is the preferred site for venous access. Lead manipulations seem to be easier from this site. An exception may be in patients with dextroverted ventricles. The subclavian puncture technique is used with a retained guidewire to avoid a second puncture. In most patients, a catheter is placed from the groin into the axillary vein, and the subclavian puncture is made fluoroscopically at the edge of the rib cage.

Screw-in leads are used in an increasing percentage of pediatric patients because of their security and theoretically improved likelihood of removability. Leads with porous surfaces are preferred.

The ventricular lead is placed not in the apex of the right ventricle (Fig. 3) but one-quarter to one-third of the way up the septum (Fig. 4) to avoid diaphragmatic pacing. The atrial lead is placed anywhere in the right atrium. Following repair of transposition of the great arteries (Senning or Mustard procedure), the atrial lead should be positioned in the roof of the anatomic left atrium, away from the radiographic border of the left side of the heart to avoid the left phrenic nerve (Fig. 5). High-output (10 V, 2 msec) pacing should be performed on both leads during implant in order to predict stimulation of noncardiac structures.

The pulse generator is positioned under the pectoralis major muscle. The muscle is spread by blunt

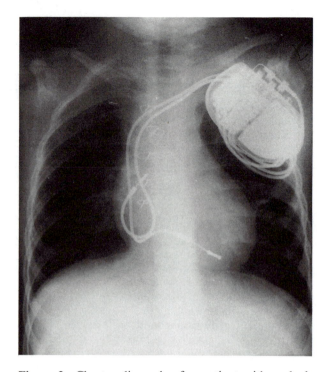

Figure 3 Chest radiograph of a patient with a dual-chamber pacemaker implanted from the left subclavian approach. The atrial lead is coiled in the right atrium, with a screw-in electrode attached to the base of the right atrial appendage. The ventricular lead is placed too low in the right ventricular apex, and if the output has to be turned up, diaphragmatic pacing may result.

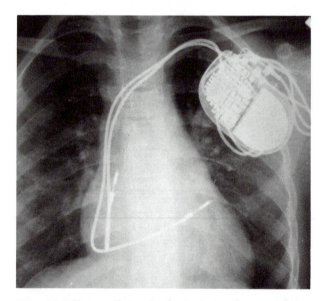

Figure 4 Chest radiograph of a dual-chamber pacemaker implanted in a pediatric patient. The pacemaker is placed by the subclavian technique from the left shoulder. The atrial lead is coiled in the right atrium, and the screw-in lead is attached to the base of the right atrial appendage. The ventricular bipolar screw-in lead is appropriately placed about halfway up the ventricular septum to avoid diaphragmatic pacing.

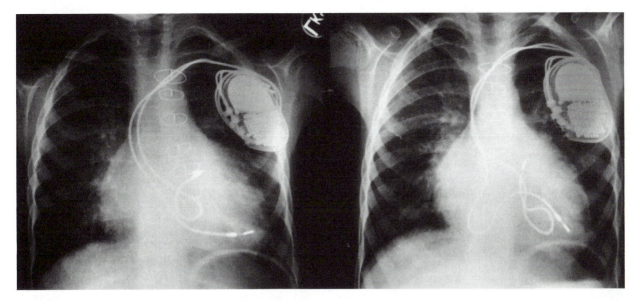

Figure 5 Early and late chest radiographs of a patient following Senning repair of transportation of the great arteries and tricuspid valve replacement, with resultant sick sinus syndrome and AV block. *A*, A 3-day postoperative chest x-ray film after implantation of the dual-chamber pacemaker by the left subclavian technique. The ventricular lead is placed on the free wall of the left ventricle using a bipolar screw-in lead, whereas the atrial lead is implanted in the roof of the anatomic left atrium, with a loop left for potential growth. The leads were sutured with an absorbable suture. *B*, The 6-month postoperative chest radiograph shows that both leads have advanced from the pocket into the heart, giving more room for growth. Although the loop of the atrial lead has advanced into the left ventricle, it has not caused any ventricular ectopy. The belly of the ventricular lead outlines the Senning repair of the transposition. The use of an absorbable suture as a tie-down may allow a lead to be taken into the heart in pediatric patients to avoid a need for repositioning leads with growth. The atrial lead should always be kept away from the radiographic border of the left side of the heart in patients with D-transposition of the great arteries to avoid pacing the phrenic nerve.

dissection and sutured with 2–0 absorbable suture. The lead is tied down with a 2–0 absorbable suture to allow some amount of lead to advance with growth.

PHYSIOLOGY

We now have a variety of ways to attempt to maintain a physiologic response that is as normal as possible with a pacemaker. Pacemakers that sense the atrium and pace the ventricle after a programmable AV delay have been available for several years (Fig. 5). These pacemakers require that the patient's sinus node have a normal or acceptable response to exercise and other stresses that require a response in heart rate. Alternatively, we now have single-chamber devices that sense bodily functions such as activity, temperature, or minute ventilation, and increase their pacing rate in response. Atrial synchronous pacemakers improve cardiac performance and the sense of well-being in adults and probably in children. It is not certain yet how closely ventricular pacemakers that increase their rate will come to achieving this response. Clearly, they allow a greater exercise performance for adults than does a single-rate ventricular pacemaker.

Because our experience with dual-chamber atrial synchronous pacemakers has been excellent, and because we have not seen a significant number of problems in children caused by a two-lead system, we continue to use DDD pacemakers in most children. The advent of dual-chamber modulated rate pacemakers will allow us to test exercise responses in the same patient in two modes.

Atrial pacing is a viable option in children with sinus node dysfunction and intact AV conduction, as occurs frequently after the Senning, Mustard, and Fontan operations. In this setting there are often isolated sinus node abnormalities, although the AV node is spared. There does not seem to be a significant amount of progression to AV block in these patients. Thus, a simpler, smaller, less expensive pacing system can be used. In Fontan procedure patients this allows a transvenous approach, whereas ventricular or dual-chamber pacing would require an epicardial approach. The early postoperative Fontan procedure patient presents a special challenge because thresholds are often higher than in other clinical settings.

LEADS

The pacing lead has evolved tremendously in the last decade. From the pediatric perspective, a major advance is in size. The size of either bipolar or unipolar leads is now acceptable for children of all sizes. Polyurethane insulation may help prevent thrombosis, although this has not been a problem in pediatric transvenous pacing. Noninvasive screening for subclavian thrombosis has failed to reveal any abnormalities.

Although tined leads have prevented almost all lead dislodgements for ventricular leads, screw-in leads are attractive in children who have had previous heart surgery. They may also be easier to remove after many years, which is an important consideration in children. The advantage is partially lost if the entire lead is not isodiametric, since sheaths that develop where the lead touches the vascular wall may impede removal. The shape of commercially available tined J leads is not appropriate for children.

The in-line bipolar connector has been a major advance as well, since it saves bulk not only on the lead but also on the pulse generator header. Some of this advantage is currently lost because as yet there is no standardization of the in-line connectors, which require bulky adapters in some situations (Fig. 6).

The use of a small quantity of steroid released from the lead tip has been useful in patients with repeated high stimulation thresholds. It also improves stimulation thresholds and flattens the acute peak in thresholds. Other innovations such as porous tips and grooved platinized tips have also resulted in improved stimulation and sensing thresholds.

We currently use bipolar porous-tipped screw-in or grooved, platinized electrodes with in-line bipolar connectors. Our average stimulation threshold at 6 months after implantation is 0.07 msec at 5 V. We then usually set the pulse generators at 2.7 V at 0.3 or 0.4 msec, resulting in a large saving in energy when compared with nominal settings.

Bipolar leads offer many advantages over unipolar ones, more than outweighing their size disadvantage. Atrial bipolar leads have a smaller far field R wave than do unipolar leads (Fig. 7). They are less sensitive to pectoral muscle sensing and other unwanted sensing. They allow a subpectoral pocket that improves the cosmetic result and may minimize erosion and trauma. The use of two bipolar leads has never led to a clinical problem with venous thrombosis or embolus in children as small as 12 kg. No damage to the tricuspid valve has been noted.

It is now clearly proved that epicardial leads are less desirable than endocardial ones. This is especially true in atrial applications, but it is also true for ventricular ones. The incidence of fracture is clearly higher, chronic stimulation thresholds are higher, and the incidence of excessively high thresholds is greater. In addition, postpericardiotomy syndrome with a need for pericardiocentesis is not an uncommon problem with epicardial leads. We reserve epicardial leads for patients without venous access, for tiny newborn babies, and for those with right-to-left shunts.

PULSE GENERATORS

We currently use bipolar, multiprogrammable telemetric DDD (atrial synchronous) pulse generators (Fig. 8). For children, we believe each pulse

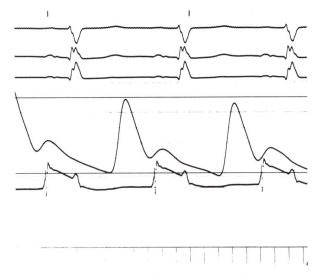

Figure 7 Demonstration of three surface electrocardiographic leads together with femoral artery blood pressure and an atrial electrogram taken from an acutely implanted bipolar screw-in lead. Each division represents 2 mV. The atrial electrogram has a rapid upstroke and an approximate 3 mV voltage, whereas the far field R wave from this bipolar lead is approximately 1.5 mV with a very slow upstroke.

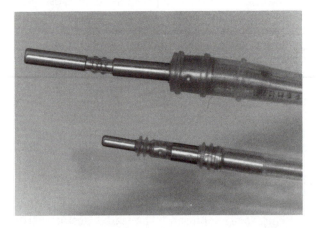

Figure 6 Example of two manufacturers' in-line bipolar leads showing the gross incompatibility of these two bipolar leads and the pacemakers intended to be used with them.

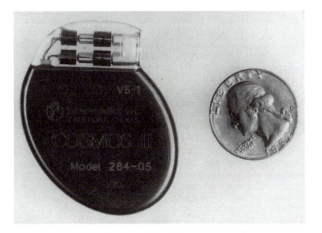

Figure 8 Demonstration of the size of a currently available DDD bipolar pulse generator alongside an American quarter. This very small pulse generator allows implantation even in the smallest infants. A second version is available for use with epicardial unipolar leads.

generator should have an upper rate limit of 175 beats per minute. The upper rate response should probably be gradual second-degree AV block, not 2:1 AV block. The atrial refractory period must be programmable in order to prevent pacemaker mediated tachycardia. The maximal atrial sensitivity should be at least 0.6 mV. With bipolar units, these high sensitivities are usable. Telemetry is essential. It allows confirmation and documentation of programmed settings at the beginning and end of non-invasive pacemaker evaluations. In many units, measurement of lead and battery parameters is possible. Telemetry can also be used to confirm programming changes. Event counters have also proved useful but are not essential.

Single-chamber pulse generators should be capable of all the same appropriate programming as dual-chamber devices. When used in an atrial application, as we usually do, high sensitivity and programmable refractory periods are very useful.

The degree of programmability available in current pulse generators has obviated the need for "special order" pediatric pulse generators, because any pulse generator can be programmed to pediatric specifications.

ANTITACHYCARDIA PACING

Atrial antitachycardia pacing is a useful modality in children. The two most frequent clinical situations in which it is used are the postoperative brady-tachy syndrome and atrioventricular nodal reentry. The fact that antiarrhythmic drugs often worsen sinus bradycardia is particularly important in postoperative patients. The additive negative effect of an AV dissociation on cardiac output caused by junctional escape rhythm is also important. Each of these

problems is addressed by atrial antitachycardia pacing. Marked improvement in symptoms and in objective indices of cardiac performance is the rule after implantation of these pacemakers. The transvenous bipolar route of implantation is particularly important in these patients because of the marginal size of atrial electrograms both in sinus rhythm and during tachycardia.

The most common tachycardia we have treated is atrial flutter. Aggressive tachycardia reduction algorithms are sometimes necessary. For example, one patient required 100 beats per minute beginning at 85 percent of the tachycardia cycle length and decreasing by 2 msec each beat. Another patient has repeatedly had successful tachycardia termination with two beats at 70 percent of the tachycardia cycle length. It is now becoming clear that repeated successful rapid termination of atrial flutter in a patient with a good hemodynamic result from reparative surgery results in fewer and fewer episodes of atrial flutter. In our first patient, there were more than 255 tachycardia overdrives recorded by the pacemaker counter during the first 3 months after implant, but no episodes recorded from $2\frac{1}{2}$ to $4\frac{1}{2}$ years after implant. This type of pacing has resulted in some of the greatest symptomatic improvement noted in any of our patients.

In patients after atrial septal defect or transposition repair, digoxin is usually the only drug necessary after antitachycardia pacing. In patients following the Fontan procedure, other powerful antiarrhythmic drugs must often be used.

Tachycardia recognition is accomplished by setting a recognition rate and a change of rate. Using these two criteria, we have not been able to fool the second-generation antitachycardia pacemaker with sinus tachycardia.

FOLLOW-UP

The aim of follow-up is to detect pacing system malfunction or normal battery depletion while the patient is in the asymptomatic stage without giving the patient or family pacemaker psychosis or neurosis. The techniques are essentially the same as in adults. To this end, we use transtelephonic and hands-on follow-up techniques. We see patients at 6 weeks, 6 months, and then yearly. Transtelephonic follow-up is performed monthly for the first year and then every 3 months. The threshold is tested within 25 percent of output energy automatically at each telephone check by decreasing the output energy on the fourth magnet beat. Atrial sensing can usually be seen in DDD and atrial antitachycardia units, but atrial capture is hard to detect for DDD units transtelephonically (see Fig. 7).

At the first (6 weeks) hands-on visit, we test capture thresholds and adjust pulse generator output to two times threshold for the atrial channel and three times threshold for the ventricle. The absence of pacemaker dependency if present is demonstrated to the patient at each visit by completely inhibiting the pulse generator for 2 to 3 minutes. This results in a significant improvement in the patients' and families' feelings of well-being. The use of the subpectoral pocket, with its resultant improvement in cosmetic results, may also make the patient feel better about the pacemaker (see Fig. 8). In the last 4 years, we have not detected a pulse generator malfunction. Lead problems are still encountered.

The effect of growth on lead position is of great importance in pediatric pacing. As much extra lead as possible is left in the right atrium at implant. The lead is sutured at the subclavian vein entrance with an absorbable suture in the hope that lead may be "played out" of the pocket. Periodic advancements of the lead may be necessary, but this has rarely been the case.

Patients are encouraged to lead a normal life. Only tackle football and hockey are proscribed. Very little psychopathology is noted in patients treated in this manner.

SUGGESTED READING

Dewey RC, Capeless MA, Levy AM. Use of ambulatory electrocardiographic monitoring to identify high-risk patients with congenital complete heart block. N Engl J Med 1987; 316:835–839.

Fry R, Collins JJ, DeSanctis RW, et al. Guidelines for permanent cardiac pacemaker implantation. A report of the Joint American College of Cardiology/American Heart Association Task Force on Assessment of Cardiovascular Procedures (Subcommittee on Pacemaker Implantation). Circulation 1984; 70:331A–339A.

Gillette PC. Atrial sensing pacemakers. In: Gillette PC, Griffin JC eds. Practical cardiac pacing. Baltimore: Williams & Wilkins, 1986:87–103.

Gillette PC. Transvenous implantation technique. In: Gillette PC, Griffin JC eds. Practical cardiac pacing. Baltimore: Williams & Wilkins, 1986:45–62.

Gillette PC, Wampler DG, Shannon C, Ott D. Use of atrial pacing in a young population. PACE 1985; 8:94–100.

Gillette PC, Zeigler V, Bradham GB, Kinsella P. Pediatric transvenous pacing: A concern for venous thrombosis? PACE 1988; 11:1935–1939.

Hayes DL, Holmes DR Jr, Maloney JD, et al. Permanent endocardial pacing in pediatric patients. J Thorac Cardiovasc Surg 1983; 85:618–624.

Karpawich PP, Garson A, Gillette PC, et al. Congenital complete atrioventricular block: Clinical and electrophysiologic prediction of need for pacemaker insertion. Am J Cardiol 1981; 48:1098–1102.

King DH, Gillette PC, Shannon C, Cuddy T. A steroid eluting endocardial pacing lead for treatment of exit block. Am Heart J 1983; 106:1438–1440.

Michaelsson M, Engle MA. Congenital complete heart block: An international study of the natural history. Cardiovasc Clin 1972; 4:86–101.

Ott DA. The epicardial approach to cardiac pacing. In: Gillette PC, Griffin JC eds. Practical cardiac pacing. Baltimore: Williams & Wilkins, 1986:63.

Shannon CE. Pacing system follow-up. In: Gillette PC, Griffin JC eds. Practical cardiac pacing. Baltimore: Williams & Wilkins, 1986:137–160.

ANTITACHYCARDIA PACING

JOHN D. FISHER, M.D.

Antitachycardia pacing is grossly underutilized in the acute or temporary setting, may be approaching its peak for use in termination of supraventricular tachycardias using implanted devices, and is approaching a period of profusion for long-term treatment of ventricular tachycardias (VTs).

PREVENTION OF TACHYCARDIAS

More than two decades ago, it was recognized that some sustained arrhythmias could be prevented by "overdrive suppression" of frequent premature complexes. In this technique, the pacemaker is set at the minimum rate required to suppress premature complexes, typically under 100 beats per minute.

Modern automated versions of this technique continually adjust the pacing rate up and down to ensure that the minimal overdrive rate is being used. The technique has been useful in coronary care units and in postoperative situations in patients who have had frequently recurring tachycardias. The effectiveness of the technique has been confirmed in recent studies in which levels of ectopy were compared in the same patient and on the same medications in two successive 24-hour periods, one without pacing and the other during overdrive suppression pacing. Not all patients respond to the technique, and not all those who respond initially show a long-term response; implanted pacemakers for overdrive suppression should therefore be used only if efficacy can be proved during multiple Holter monitoring periods, both paced and unpaced, in a manner analogous to testing of antiarrhythmic drug efficacy.

For patients with torsades de pointes, overdrive suppression is one of the mainstays of therapy. Torsades de pointes is a polymorphic VT whose axis appears to spiral around a central point; many episodes terminate spontaneously, but death may occur if the rhythm degenerates to ventricular fibrillation. The rhythm occurs in patients with hereditary syndromes but more frequently as an idiosyncratic proarrhythmic drug effect, particularly in the presence of hypokalemia.

More complex forms of preventive antitachycardia pacing have been described but are less generally applicable. In some patients with atrioventricular nodal reentrant tachycardia or the Wolff-Parkinson-White syndrome, sustained tachycardia can be prevented if an atrial or ventricular premature complex is immediately answered by stimulation in the opposite chamber (DDT pacing). Stimulation at a "choke point" in a tachycardia circuit, such as an accessory pathway or the atrioventricular conduction system, can prolong local refractoriness and prevent initiation or perpetuation of a tachycardia. A pacemaker programmed to recognize the pattern of abnormal complexes that typically results in a sustained tachycardia can also be programmed to respond with preventive pacing. The techniques described in this paragraph are not yet applicable to the everyday setting.

HEMODYNAMIC IMPROVEMENT DURING INTERMINABLE TACHYCARDIAS

As discussed in a subsequent section, most organized tachycardias can be terminated by pacing techniques, but others cannot be terminated or recur incessantly after termination. In some instances, pacing can be used to ameliorate the effects of persistent tachycardias.

Pacing-Enhanced Atrioventricular Block

Although pacing is most often thought of as a treatment for atrioventricular block, it can also be used to create or worsen block for therapeutic purposes. The most common settings for such scenarios are in the postoperative patient or in a patient with a proarrhythmic drug effect. When such a patient begins to show hemodynamic compromise from a persistent supraventricular tachycardia at, for example, 150 beats per minute, then pacing at 180 to 200 beats per minute may create 2:1 atrioventricular block with a resulting ventricular response under 100 beats per minute and consequent hemodynamic improvement. Bursts of rapid atrial pacing can also be used to precipitate atrial fibrillation, a rhythm in which the ventricular response is often easier to control pharmacologically. Although this approach is most commonly used in the acute setting, implanted pacers designed to precipitate or perpetuate atrial fibrillation have also been used. Pacing to slow the ventricular response in various supraventricular arrhythmias is one of the underutilized techniques that should be employed much more frequently.

Improved Hemodynamics During Incessant VT

In slower VTs, a properly timed atrial stimulus can result in provision of an "atrial kick" that can improve blood pressure by 15 to 25 mm Hg. Although this AVT pacing mode requires sophisticated equipment, it should be considered in patients with incessant VT, particularly that related to proarrhythmic drug effects that may gradually abate. The occasional patient will benefit from pacing at multiple ventricular sites, possibly through improvement of the sequence of ventricular contraction; some patients who show such improvement have a narrower QRS complex during effective pacing.

The effective ventricular rate can also be slowed during sustained VT by inserting a premature stimulus at a point where insufficient filling has occurred, so that the aortic valve does not open during electrical systole. This allows additional time to complete ventricular filling during an additional cycle, and the effective ventricular rate may be halved with consequent hemodynamic benefit. These benefits occur, however, at a metabolic price that may be difficult to pay in a patient with coronary artery disease or cardiomyopathy. Additionally, the concept of placing an extra stimulus on the T wave of a VT complex carries a substantial risk of precipitation of ventricular fibrillation. Indeed, the experience at our institution is that coupled pacing of this type is more likely to fail than succeed and should be kept in reserve for special cases. This, together with special equipment needed, make coupled pacing a relatively small contributor to antitachycardia pacing.

The technique of paired pacing is similar to that of coupled pacing outlined above but can be performed with only slightly special equipment. In paired pacing, both the first complex and the extra complex are stimulated by the pacemaker. For use during a persisting tachycardia, the basic pacing rate must be faster than the tachycardia in order to achieve capture, and the premature complex is introduced at a coupling interval approximating 250 msec. This can be accomplished using a standard and widely available temporary atrioventricular sequential (DVI) pacemaker, set to the asynchronous mode (DOO) and with both outputs connected to the ventricular pacing wire. These units generally have an upper rate setting of approximately 180 beats per minute and are therefore limited to somewhat slower tachycardias (and at faster rates would be likely to wreak havoc anyway).

PACING FOR TERMINATION OF TACHYCARDIA

General Concepts

Most tachycardias susceptible to pacing termination are caused by reentry. Automatic mechanisms may be less susceptible to pacer termination, and any apparent termination of fibrillation is in fact coincidental. Interruption of a tachycardia circuit may be accomplished with one or more stimuli, depending on the duration of the excitable gap, the tachycardia rate, the physical or physiologic distance between the site of stimulation and the tachycardia circuit, and other factors.

The general concepts are similar for atrial and ventricular tachycardias. Acceleration of VT or precipitation of atrial fibrillation in some patients with the Wolff-Parkinson-White syndrome can be disastrous. It is therefore mandatory that temporary pacing be performed with adequate back-up and that extreme care be taken in selection of patients for implantable antitachycardia pacemakers.

Site of Stimulation

In general, VT responds to ventricular pacing far more often than to atrial pacing. The right ventricular apex is more stable than other pacing sites and is equal in efficacy to the right ventricular outflow or left ventricle in most cases. It is occasionally possible to achieve ventricular stimulation using esophageal pacing, but this should not be relied upon in emergency situations. Transthoracic pacing using large patch electrodes may be suitable for use in the emergency room, critical care unit, and similar settings and can be accomplished promptly without the need for an invasive procedure. Many of the high amplitude–long pulse duration units designed for transthoracic pacing provide the capability of rapid stimulation in excess of 200 beats per minute. Units without this capability are probably no longer suitable for purchase unless they have special features of particular interest to individual physicians. The epicardial wires commonly left in place after open heart procedures can also be used for both diagnosis and antitachycardia pacing, a frequently overlooked option.

Supraventricular tachycardias generally respond best to atrial stimulation. Some patients with atrioventricular node reentry tachycardia respond equally well to ventricular stimulation, but the risks may not outweigh the benefits. The atrioventricular reentrant tachycardias associated with the Wolff-Parkinson-White syndrome typically respond well to atrial pacing, but there are many individuals in whom ventricular pacing is more effective.

For atrial stimulation using temporary pacemakers, we have found that the coronary sinus offers the most stable position in the event that the wire is to be retained for use during repetitive episodes. Temporary atrial J electrodes and catheters with special fronds are also available, but others have apparently enjoyed greater success with these wires, particularly in terms of long-term stability, than we have. Atrial tachycardias are common in postoperative patients, and pacer termination is ideal for these.

Esophageal pacing and transthoracic pacing are also effective in terminating atrial tachycardias. The esophageal technique has the advantage of being able to record atrial and ventricular depolarizations clearly and may therefore be helpful in diagnosis of some tachycardias. Esophageal pacing can be accomplished using specially designed electrode catheters that can be inserted like a nasogastric tube. A gelatin encapsulated "pill electrode" with a very tiny wire attached is designed to be swallowed with a gulp of water and may be a preferable approach for some patients, although others are unable to swallow them.

From the patient's standpoint, many find transthoracic pacing or the insertion of an esophageal catheter unpleasant and experience discomfort with the high-amplitude pacing required. However, the procedures are noninvasive and can be performed at the bedside or in the emergency room.

If fluoroscopy is available (primarily to negotiate the shoulder area), insertion of a small No. 4 French wire via an antecubital vein is very benign, relatively comfortable for the patient, and painless during stimulation; it also offers the flexibility of atrial or ventricular stimulation.

Antitachycardia Pacing Patterns

Great effort has been expended by many investigators to develop the perfect tachycardia-terminating stimulation pattern. Both the patterns and the equipment needed to carry them out range from simple to highly complex. Burst pacing remains the gold standard because of its combination of simplicity and efficacy.

Toxic:Therapeutic Ratios

Faster and longer pacing is more likely to achieve both termination and acceleration of tachycardias. A single stimulus or slow pacing for brief periods is less likely to result in either termination or acceleration. If a tachycardia is well tolerated, pacing efforts should begin with those least likely to cause acceleration, working gradually toward more aggressive stimulation patterns. For patients in whom a previously placed pacer wire is being used in a last desperate attempt to avoid countershock, more aggressive techniques should be employed without delay. In these latter patients, a slow stepwise progression is likely to result in hemodynamic deterioration followed by countershock, even if the tachycardia is not accelerated.

Underdrive Pacing

Asynchronous pacing is initiated at a rate below that of the tachycardia. If the tachycardia rate is not a multiple of the pacing rate, the pacemaker stimuli will gradually "scan" the tachycardia cycle, resulting in termination of susceptible arrhythmias. Single programmed extrastimuli delivered in the electrophysiology laboratory or with certain sophisticated implantable pacemakers also use this scanning technique.

Multiple Programmed Extrastimuli

This technique is not readily available without special equipment and offers little, if any, advantage over rapid pacing techniques described below.

Burst Pacing

This is the gold standard technique for termination of tachycardia. In stable patients, the objective is to achieve termination without acceleration, keeping the rate and duration of the burst to the lowest possible levels. One approach is to begin pacing 10 to 20 beats per minute faster than the tachycardia until five successive captures are achieved. If the arrhythmia is not terminated, pacing is reinitiated at the same rate, but the duration is increased to 10 and then if necessary to 15 captures. If the tachycardia (and hence the initial burst rate) is not too high, substantially longer bursts may prove effective. Otherwise, the rate can be increased in steps of 10 to 20 beats per minute, and the previous sequence of changes in duration can be repeated until termination or acceleration occurs.

"Tune Down" Rate Decremental Pacing

This is a variation of the long–slow burst technique, in which pacing is begun at a rate sufficient to achieve consistent capture of the myocardium, and then after a few seconds, the rate is gradually decreased for a period of many seconds until the pacer rate is lower than that of the tachycardia. Failure is usually heralded by the appearance of fusion beats as the rate is decreased, but this may occur at rates well below those of the original tachycardia. In some cases the technique may therefore be used to decrease the ventricular rate when the tachycardia cannot be terminated.

Incremental Ramp (Cycle Length Decremental) Pacing

Pacing is initiated at a rate slightly above the tachycardia and quickly increased over a total of five to six captures. If this is ineffective, the procedure is repeated with additional stimuli and gradually increasing rates. Implantable pacemakers capable of such "autodecremental pacing" have been developed, as has a related technique in which the cycle

length decreases initially and levels off, although additional stimuli continue to be delivered with each successive attempt.

Entrainment

In patients whose tachycardia circuits have a wide excitable gap, rapid pacing can invade the circuit. At increasingly rapid rates, a larger portion of the circuit is invaded by the stimulated wavefront, so that the fusion between the paced and tachycardia morphologies (constant at any given rate) becomes more pacer-like as the rate is increased. Cessation of pacing during this period of transient entrainment results in prompt resumption of the original tachycardia rate. At a critical pacing rate, the circuit becomes refractory, with a consequent and often sudden change in the paced morphology. Cessation of pacing at this point often reveals that the tachycardia has been terminated. The technique of entrainment is particularly useful in postoperative patients with atrial flutter, in whom a high success rate can be anticipated with the relatively low incidence of precipitation of atrial fibrillation. The phenomenon of transient entrainment has also been observed with many other arrhythmias but is frequently difficult to demonstrate. From a practical viewpoint, the technique remains most useful in postoperative patients with atrial flutter.

IMPLANTED PACEMAKERS FOR TERMINATION OF TACHYCARDIA

Our group has been interested in antitachycardia pacing since the early 1970s. Nevertheless, only 7 percent of patients with supraventricular tachycardia and 3 percent of patients with VT have met the rigorous criteria that we have established for implantation of such devices. When a decision is made to consider an antitachycardia pacemaker, the patient is placed on the antiarrhythmic drug regimen (if any) expected to be used chronically, and 100 episodes of tachycardia are induced over a period of 2 to 3 days, with the patient in different body positions and with the drug at peak and trough serum blood levels. A passing score during such testing varies with the patient and the arrhythmia being treated. Occasional failure to terminate or precipitation of atrial fibrillation with a slow ventricular response may be acceptable in some patients with supraventricular tachycardia. Acceleration of VT even once during the trial series is unacceptable, unless the patient is also provided with a back-up implantable defibrillator or (rarely) a manually activated unit is implanted, for use only in an emergency room setting. Implantation of the device is followed by a series of 100 trials prior to discharge.

Long-Term Results With Implanted Antitachycardia Pacemakers

For the first 2 years following implantation, results are generally fair to good, with continued efficacy of 86 percent for supraventricular tachycardia and 72 percent for VT. In following years, there is a decrease in efficacy, reaching 68 percent for supraventricular tachycardia and 55 percent for VT at 5 years. For patients with supraventricular tachycardia, most of the late failures are caused by precipitation of atrial fibrillation or other atrial arrhythmias combined with an increasing frequency of arrhythmia. Few of these patients die, but many go on to other therapy, such as catheter ablation. For VT patients, long-term follow-up is marred by sudden death; this occurs even in patients who have never previously suffered cardiac arrest and in whom the pacemaker was not activated at the time of sudden death, and it emphasizes the need for a back-up implanted defibrillator. Progressive deterioration of the myocardium also contributes to the late mortality in these patients.

IMPLANTED PACEMAKERS FOR LONG-TERM ELECTROPHYSIOLOGIC STUDIES AND INCIDENTAL ANTITACHYCARDIA PACING

In some patients Holter monitoring does not provide satisfactory guidance regarding the continuing efficacy of an antiarrhythmic regimen. These are patients whose treatment has been devised using serial electrophysiologic studies. Since many have potentially progressive myocardial disease, there is well-justified concern over gradual loss of efficacy of the chosen therapy. The conventional way to test this is to admit the patient for periodic invasive electrophysiologic studies. Because this is impractical, only selected patients actually undergo such testing. The value of an implanted pacemaker capable of performing noninvasive electrophysiologic studies is immediately apparent.

At present, there are several implantable pacemakers capable of performing noninvasive electro-physiologic studies. We feel that it is important that such a pacemaker be chosen for arrhythmia patients who also require antibradycardia pacing. We have had several patients in whom a worsening of spontaneous ventricular arrhythmias was "predicted" more than a year in advance through the use of an implanted pacemaker.

Many of the pacemakers capable of performing noninvasive electrophysiologic studies can also be used as manually activated antitachycardia pacemakers, and patients receiving such units should be tested for the potential efficacy of this approach.

The author acknowledges the assistance of Ms. Stephanie Olsen and of other members of the Arrhythmia Group.

SUGGESTED READING

Charos GS, Haffajee CI, Gold RL, et al. A theoretically and practically more effective method for interruption of ventricular tachycardia: Self-adapting autodecremental overdrive pacing. Circulation 1986; 73:309–315.

den Dulk K, Bertholet M, Brugada P, et al. A versatile pacemaker system for termination of tachycardias. Am J Cardiol 1983; 52:731–738.

Fisher JD. Electrical devices for the treatment of tachyarrhythmias. Cardiol Clin 1986; 4:527–542.

Fisher JD, Furman S, Kim SG, et al. DDD/DDT Pacemakers in the treatment of ventricular tachycardia. PACE 1984; 7:173–178.

Fisher JD, Johnston DR, Furman S, Mercando AD. Long-term efficacy of antitachycardia pacing for supraventricular and ventricular tachycardias. Am J Cardiol 1987; 60:1311–1316.

Fisher JD, Johnston DR, Kim SG, et al. Implantable pacers for tachycardia termination: Stimulation techniques and long-term efficacy. PACE 1986; 9:1325–1333.

Fisher JD, Kim SG, Matos JA, et al. Comparative effectiveness of pacing techniques for termination of well-tolerated sustained ventricular tachycardia. PACE 1983; 6:915–922.

Fisher JD, Kim SG, Waspe LE, et al. Mechanisms for the success and failure of pacing for termination of ventricular tachycardia: Clinical and hypothetical considerations. PACE 1983; 6:1094–1105.

Fisher JD, Teichman SL, Ferrick A, et al. Antiarrhythmic effects of VVI pacing at physiologic rates: A crossover controlled evaluation. PACE 1987; 10:822–830.

Waldo AL, MacLean WA, Karp RB, et al. Entrainment and interruption of atrial flutter with atrial pacing: Studies in man following open heart surgery. Circulation 1977; 56:737–745.

AUTOMATIC IMPLANTABLE CARDIOVERTER DEFIBRILLATOR

DAVID S. CANNOM, M.D.

During the past decade, the most striking development in the field of clinical electrophysiology has been new, highly effective devices for the treatment of life-threatening ventricular arrhythmias. The safety and efficacy of the automatic implantable cardioverter defibrillator (AICD)* are now beyond doubt. In the past 4 years there has been a striking increase in the number of devices implanted (Fig. 1). The clinical success of the device is redefining our approach to high-risk patients.

PATIENT SELECTION

Many factors affect the selection of proper therapy for patients with life-threatening arrhythmias. These factors include clinical history, electrophysiologic data, and arteriographic and hemodynamic studies. Also important are the skills and interests of the attending electrophysiologists and surgeons and the availability of both standard and experimental devices.

Between 1980 and 1982, during the initial clinical trial of the automatic implantable defibrillator (AID) device, the eligibility criteria were stringent; the patient had to have survived at least two episodes of cardiac arrest not associated with infarction. Clinical criteria for implantation have broadened in the past few years. Newly published data have established improved survival of AICD patients compared with patients treated with other therapies.

Clinical and electrophysiologic criteria that warrant AICD implantation (Table 1) are

1. A clinical episode of cardiac arrest caused by a ventricular arrhythmia (not clinically due to an acute infarction).
2. Recurrent ventricular tachycardia (VT) with inducible VT or ventricular fibrillation (VF) at electrophysiologic study despite conventional antiarrhythmic therapy. These first two indications are the current Food and Drug Administration approved criteria.
3. Recurrent arrest or clinical VT in a patient

*The AICD is currently the only device available for implantation; it is manufactured by Cardiac Pacemakers Inc., St. Paul, Minnesota.

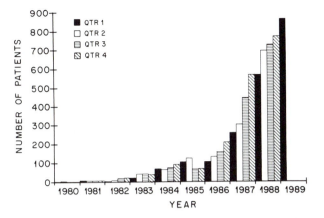

Figure 1 The bar graph shows the number of new implants of the AICD by quarter. The first automatic implantable defibrillator (AID) in humans was implanted in 1980. In 1982, cardioverting capability was added (AICD). In 1985, the first fully integrated circuit was built (Ventak). In October 1985, the Food and Drug Administration approved the device for clinical use. Despite this growth in implantation numbers, only a small percentage of survivors of sudden death each year receive an AICD. (Data provided by Cardiac Pacemakers, Inc., St. Paul, Minnesota.)

without inducible arrhythmia. This may be single arrest due to long Q-T syndrome, primary electrical disease, associated with poor left ventricular function. There is a 13 percent 1-year incidence of recurrent cardiac arrest in the patient in whom no arrhythmia is inducible in the electrophysiology laboratory after a cardiac arrest.

4. Surgical ablation of VT. AICD leads are implanted at the time of surgery, and an AICD is used for those patients whose arrhythmia remains inducible postoperatively.
5. Syncope in a patient who has inducible VT. Approximately 20 percent of cardiac arrest survivors have had a prior episode of syncope.

The criteria for AICD selection have become independent of the results of electrophysiologic test-

Table 1 Indications for the AICD

Cardiac arrest caused by ventricular arrhythmia (not during an acute infarction)
Recurrent VT with inducible VT or VF at electrophysiologic study despite conventional antiarrhythmic drugs
Recurrent arrest or VT owing to long Q-T syndrome or primary electrical disease or associated with poor left ventricular function in a patient without inducible VT/VF
In a patient undergoing surgical ablation of VT whose arrhythmia remains inducible postoperatively
In a patient with syncope and inducible VT

417

ing. Only patients with good left ventricular function (ejection fraction greater than 40 percent), in whom VT/VF is suppressed or noninducible at electrophysiologic study do as well over the long term as do AICD patients (Fig. 2). All other groups of patients undergoing electrophysiologic study have shorter survival than groups treated with AICD. Groups with shorter survival using routine therapy include (1) patients whose VT/VF is inducible at baseline study but suppressed by drug therapy, (2) patients whose arrhythmias are inducible but not suppressed, and (3) patients whose VT/VF is noninducible. Empirical amiodarone therapy is the best single drug for sudden death survivors, but the population treated with amiodarone alone has a 1-year mortality rate five times that of the AICD population.

Map-directed surgical resection is an alternative to AICD implantation. We recommend surgical ablative therapy only in the ideal candidate. The best patients for surgical resection are young people who have anteroapical aneurysms and ejection fractions greater than 30 percent and who require coronary artery bypass surgery. Such patients constitute only 10 percent of the population who have survived sudden cardiac death. The operative mortality of this surgery is approximately 10 percent even in the "ideal" case, providing a serious deterrent to surgical intervention. If successful, however, the operation is curative in 80 percent of patients, and recurrent cardiac arrest rates are as low as 5 to 10 percent during 2 to 3 years of follow-up.

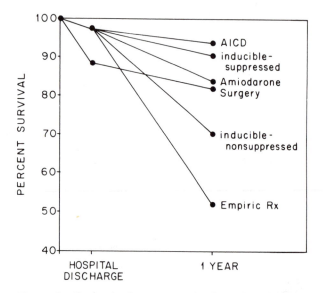

Figure 2 Shown is the percentage of survival obtained using a particular therapy on the y axis plotted against time on the x axis in patients with ventricular fibrillation or hemodynamically significant ventricular tachycardia. Survival estimates for each therapy are taken from representative literature citations. Survival of the AICD-treated patients is superior to that of any other therapy.

Because of the high risk of arrhythmic death in end-stage cardiomyopathy, many centers use the AICD as a "bridge to transplantation" in patients who have serious ventricular arrhythmias and are awaiting heart transplantation. We have used this approach and do not view a low ejection fraction as a contraindication to AICD implantation in this population.

PREOPERATIVE EVALUATION

Preoperatively, all AICD candidates undergo a similar evaluation. The preoperative evaluation of a candidate for AICD implantation is less complicated than it was 2 to 3 years ago. Each step is important in determining the type of operation done and the pulse generator parameters chosen.

The patient must be stabilized before the diagnostic phase of the work-up is begun. Arrhythmias, congestive heart failure, and ischemia are treated as thoroughly as possible. Any spontaneously occurring, unsustained ventricular tachycardia or paroxysmal atrial fibrillation must be suppressed by empirical drug therapy.

A treadmill exercise test is done to determine the peak sinus rate with exercise and the presence of ischemia. Sinus tachycardia greater than 140 beats per minute usually must be treated with beta blockade or a higher device rate cutoff must be chosen. Holter monitoring is done with the patient on antiarrhythmic drugs to ensure that the maximum number of device-activating supraventricular and ventricular tachycardias is suppressed.

All patients undergo a complete diagnostic left-sided heart catheterization to identify the need for concomitant coronary artery bypass grafting. Ventriculograms are done in two projections to find patients who will benefit from incidental aneurysmectomy (for hemodynamic reasons) or mitral valve replacement during coronary artery bypass grafting.

In the electrophysiology laboratory, we assess the inducibility of the patient's arrhythmia, document the rate and morphology of the provoked rhythms, and test the response to stimulation after administration of intravenous procainamide. The device cutoff rate is selected for the clinical rhythm that caused the arrest. AICD implantation is now generally recommended after a single electrophysiologic test demonstrating the failure of procainamide. Only in the patient with an ejection fraction over 40 percent do we recommend serial electrophysiologically guided drug testing to find drugs to suppress inducibility.

We favor concomitant coronary artery bypass surgery with AICD patch implantation if there is a reasonable possibility that a cardiac arrest (especially a VF arrest) was caused by an episode of acute ischemia. The data from the Coronary Artery Surgery

Table 2 Preoperative Evaluation

Initial stabilization and treatment of ischemia and congestive heart failure
Treadmill stress test
Holter monitor, signal-averaged electrocardiogram, and 12-lead electrocardiogram
Cardiac catheterization with ventriculography
Electrophysiologic study
Empirical treatment of significant supraventricular and ventricular arrhythmias
Education of patient and family

Study show that coronary revascularization reduces the risk of recurrent arrest even if the patient has poor left ventricular function. Many of our patients have had previous coronary artery bypass grafting surgery, and we determine the need to redo one or more grafts at the time of AICD implantation.

Usually a full day is necessary for the nurses, cardiologists, and surgeons to teach the patient and family fully about the AICD and the associated procedures. Surgery is often delayed further to optimize arrhythmia control and to deal with other medical issues such as pulmonary function. As more programmable options for the AICD become available, it is important to determine which equipment is required in the operating room (pulse generators of varying rates, energies and programmability, compatible pacemakers). Most important is having the entire implant team scheduled early in the day to work in an operating room routinely designated for AICD implantation.

In some parts of the country, reimbursement issues currently impede more widespread use of the AICD. This therapy is expensive: Hospital inpatient charges for new implants average approximately $50,000.

CHOICE OF PROCEDURE

The choice of the appropriate lead system and pulse generator and its proper implantation are crucial in assuring the long-term survival of the high-risk patient.

Two lead configurations are available. One system employs a superior vena caval helical electrode as the anode and a titanium mesh patch as the cathode; patch leads are either "small" (13.9 cm^2) or "large" (27.9 cm^2). This system was historically the most popular and was called the spring-patch configuration. Subsequent experience has shown that a two-patch system reduces the necessary defibrillation energy by 10 J on the average. We use two large patches placed epicardially, with the anterior patch overlying the septum and anterior left ventricle and the posterior patch over the posterior lateral left ventricle. Myocardial screw-in leads are closely placed

in healthy-appearing muscle for R-wave (rate) sensing. An endocardial lead system for rate sensing is also available.

Two models of the AICD are available that detect arrhythmias differently. A very early model of the device and the current Ventak series are shown in Figure 3. The size of the device has been reduced, but it remains bulky. One nonprogrammable model (Ventak 1520) uses rate alone to sense and initiate a shock and will give a shock for any rhythm above the preprogrammed rate cutoff (typically 155 beats per minute, although units with rate cutoffs of up to 200 beats per minute can be ordered). Inappropriate shocks for rapid supraventricular tachycardia are inevitable with this unit. The other generator (Ventak 1510) uses a separate morphology analysis in addition to rate criteria before calling a rhythm VT. This unit is less likely to shock a narrow QRS supraventricular tachycardia mistakenly but will call supraventricular tachycardia with aberration VT. We favor this unit, but either is satisfactory if its limitations are known. Shocking energies of the device are preprogrammed at manufacture and vary between 28 and 31 J. The device will deliver up to four shocks during each sensed tachyarrhythmia or 100 total shocks before battery depletion occurs. A newer model of the device, the Ventak AICD 1550, is programmable for rate and detection criteria (rate only or rate and morphology). It is quickly gaining wide acceptance. The investigational Ventak P also has programmable first shock energy.

We favor a midline sternotomy for AICD lead system implantation even in the young patient who may later need a second open chest operation. Exposure is excellent, which is an advantage if multiple patch configurations are to be tested. We also find postoperative healing faster and less painful than with a left thoracotomy. We feel that the subxiphoid approach gives inadequate exposure for patch lead placement. The patches are placed epicardially unless concomitant bypass surgery is done. We tunnel the leads through the diaphragm and make a horizontal abdominal pocket at the level of the umbilicus. If an associated coronary artery bypass grafting procedure, aneurysmectomy, or valve replacement is done, the AICD system is placed while the patient is coming off cardiopulmonary bypass.

Careful testing of the defibrillating lead system must be done at surgery to assure that adequate energy will be available via the implanted pulse generator to convert the arrhythmia. Alternating current delivered to the heart is used to induce VF, approximately 10 seconds is allowed to elapse, and the energy required to defibrillate the heart via an external cardioverter is measured (Fig. 4). We require at least a 10 J safety margin between the defibrillation threshold and the first high-energy shock of the device. This usually means that a defibrillation threshold value of 20 J or less must be obtained

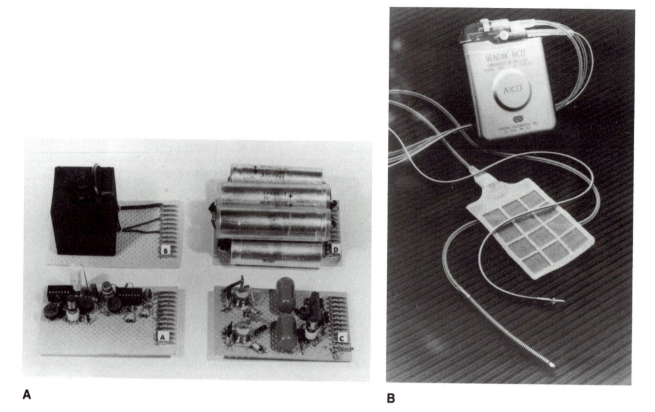

A

B

Figure 3 Panel *A* shows the component boards of the initial breadboard device tested on dogs at the Sinai Hospital of Baltimore in 1969. *A* = sensing circuit. *B* = direct current converter, *C* = high-voltage switching circuit, *D* = capacitor bank. The components of the modern AICD are basically the same as those in this very early model. (Photo courtesy of Dr. Morton W. Mower.) Panel *B* shows the pulse generator and lead system of the currently used device. A right atrial spring lead, right ventricular sensing lead, and large apical patch are shown. Two large patches have emerged as the preferred sensing and shocking system in most centers.

at testing, or the patch configuration is changed. We begin testing defibrillation thresholds at 15 J, measure three successful conversions at each value, and work down to the lowest defibrillation threshold obtainable. We also attempt to induce the patient's clinical VT but find that cardioverting energies for VT are lower than for VF. The previously selected AICD generator is then attached to the lead system, turned on, and also tested. Most experienced centers note a learning curve for patch placement and with experience can find a patch position giving satisfactory defibrillation thresholds in nearly all patients.

If a permanent pacemaker is implanted during or after an AICD system, the unit must be bipolar (see the chapter *Permanent Pacemakers: Techniques of Implantation*) and placed far from the AICD rate-counting electrodes. Pacemakers can cause both over- and undercounting of the true ventricular rate by the AICD and must be carefully tested at surgery to ensure that they do not affect AICD function. Unipolar pacemakers are contraindicated with the AICD. A large unipolar pacing spike may inhibit the proper sensing of VT and VF by the AICD. This is also possible but less so with bipolar pacemakers, and careful intraoperative testing is mandatory to recognize this potential interaction.

POSTOPERATIVE COURSE

The operative mortality rate is ~1.0 percent for AICD implantation alone in our hands. Patients recover in the coronary care unit, allowing easier management of the complicated postoperative arrhythmias. The AICD generator is not turned on until the patient is moved to the telemetry ward (approximately 2 days after implant). After implantation, fully two-thirds of patients require antiarrhythmic agents to control VT, and a similar number require AV nodal blocking drugs.

We perform postoperative electrophysiologic studies in the following circumstances: (1) if the defibrillation thresholds at operation were borderline (15 to 20 J), (2) if the patient has a permanent pacemaker, or (3) if a new antiarrhythmic drug (especially amiodarone) is added. Posthospital care of

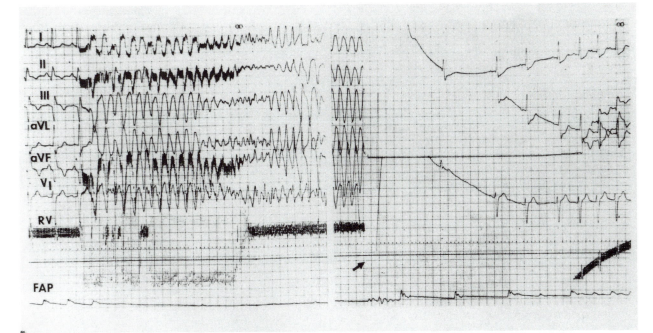

Figure 4 Shown is the first conversion of VT by an implanted device (AID) in a patient. The procedure was performed in 1980 at Johns Hopkins Hospital by Mirowski and colleagues. Shown are surface electrocardiograms (leads I to V_1), a right ventricular endocardial lead (RV), and a femoral arterial pressure line (FAP). Coarse VT is induced by alternating current on the lefthand side of the figure, and a defibrillating pulse is delivered at the *arrow* (noted above the FAP line), with prompt resumption of sinus rhythm. The basic method of arrhythmia detection and conversion has changed little in the ensuing 10,000 patients. (Courtesy of Dr. Morton W. Mower.)

the patient is usually simplified if the patient experiences an AICD shock in the electrophysiology laboratory while moderately sedated before going home.

Each patient has a treadmill stress test and Holter monitoring before discharge from the hospital. We enroll all patients in an arrhythmia surveillance system based in the coronary care unit. With this system, patients can transmit their rhythm via the telephone after a discharge of the AICD.

The AICD patient must be followed carefully every 2 months by a physician experienced in follow-up testing. Noninvasive magnet testing is performed to assure that the device is turned on and to determine battery life (charge time) and the number of shocks delivered since the last visit of the patient. Generator replacement indices are exceeded at approximately 19 ± 4 months, although these indices appear overly conservative for both the AID-B and Ventak series. Generator replacement is done under general anesthesia, as defibrillation thresholds must be rechecked.

COMPLICATIONS

The most serious long-term complication of device implantation has been infection. The incidence is 2 to 3 percent and appears to be caused by initial surgical contamination, although the infection may not be manifest for months postoperatively. Gallium and computed tomographic scanning of the patches help in the diagnosis; the organism is usually *Staphylococcus aureus* and occurs more commonly in diabetics. If device infection is diagnosed, the entire device, including the patches, must be explanted. Lead fractures and insulation breaks are rare. Other surgical complications are the same as for any other patient undergoing median sternotomy.

FOLLOW-UP

Approximately 60 percent of the patients we follow have received shocks from their devices. The existing device has no stored telemetry, so judgment is necessary to decide whether the shock was "appropriate" and delivered for VT/VF or merely "problematic" and delivered for supraventricular tachycardia or sinus tachycardia. One-half of our patients have received "appropriate" shocks; this is also the experience in the literature. Determining whether a shock is true or false will continue to involve guesswork until there are devices with stored telemetry. Twenty percent of patients with VT proved by Holter monitoring who receive true shocks are asymptomatic just before the device fires. Patients with a low ejection fraction and easily induced VT are most apt to receive a shock. Most patients receive their first shock within 6 months of implant, but 20 percent do not receive a shock until after 1 year of implant. We instruct patients to transmit their electrocardiogram after a shock, but we do not see the patient or consider hospitalization unless there are multiple shocks and a change in antiarrhythmic drugs is needed. Some antiarrhythmics, e.g., amiodarone, raise defibrillation thresholds, and their use often necessitates a rechecking of the defibrillation threshold at surgery. We do this if the initial defibrillation threshold was over 15 to 20 J.

Patients with an AICD rarely suffer fatal cardiac arrest. The 1-year sudden death incidence is approximately 1.0 percent, and the 5-year cumulative incidence is approximately 4.0 percent. A recent study showed that most of the sudden deaths were caused by unsuccessful termination of arrhythmias by the AICD device. However, many of these deaths (up to 45 percent) were the result of preventable technical errors, including device deactivation or battery depletion, borderline defibrillation thresholds at surgery or the recent addition of antiarrhythmic drugs without rechecking defibrillation thresholds.

AICD patients need careful postoperative psychological support. Our patients meet every 2 to 3 months with the implanting team, which includes active involvement of a psychiatrist and psychologist. We do not allow our patients to drive for 6 months unless they have a nonsyncopal AICD discharge before that time. Patients who lose consciousness during shocks should never drive.

FUTURE DEVELOPMENTS

The next generations of the device will have many desirable features that will substantially improve this mode of therapy. Most important is the capability of doing antitachycardia pacing. Other desirable features include programmable shocking energies and sensing times, back-up ventricular pacing, telemetered electrograms of each clinical shock, and noninvasive methods of performing electrophysiologic tests. These devices are compared in Table 3. In theory, these units are similar. Their relative effectiveness and popularity with physicians and patients depends on reliable function and ease of use. A new nonthoracotomy lead system employing a single transvenous sensing and shocking system is currently in clinical trials and shows great promise. It will not be a suitable choice for all patients because of unacceptably high defibrillation thresholds in some patients. (Fig. 5).

Table 3 Automatic Defibrillator Models for the 1990s

	Ventak PRX	Ventritex Cadence	Guardian ATP	Medtronic 7216
Size (g)	220	240	270	280
Output (pulse)	Biphasic	Monophasic Biphasic	Monophasic	Monophasic Sequential
(energy)	0.1–30 J	0.1–38 J	0.5–35 J	0.2–34 J
Programmable rate cutoff (for VT sensing)	Yes	Yes	Yes	Yes
Automatic gain control	Yes	Yes	Yes	Yes
Backup bradycardia pacing	Yes	Yes	Yes	Yes
Antitachycardia pacing (for VT conversion)	Yes	Yes	Yes	Yes
Telemetry (real time)	Yes	Yes	Yes	Yes
(stored)	Yes	Yes	Yes	Yes
Patient electrogram (stored)	No	Yes	No	No
Noninvasive electrophysiologic testing	Yes	Yes	Yes	Yes
Longevity (nonshocking)	5 Years	5 Years	5 Years	5 Years

The characteristics of the devices were supplied by the manufacturers. The intent is to compare devices available to patients in late 1989 or early 1990. Ventak PRX is manufactured by Cardiac Pacemakers Inc., Cadence by Ventritex Inc., Guardian ATP by Teletronics, and Medtronic 7216 by Medtronic, Inc.

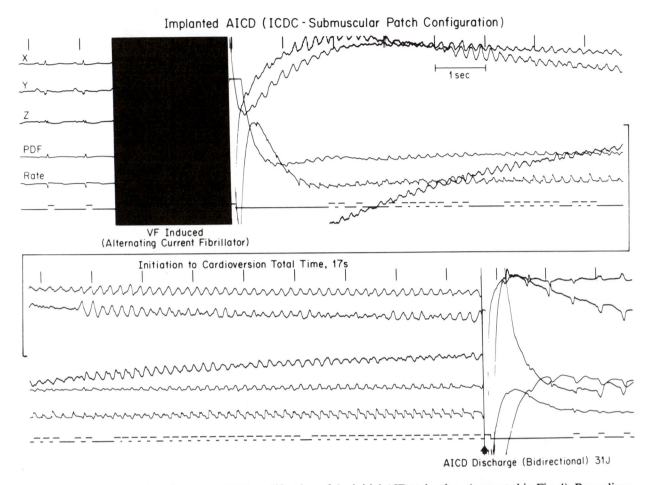

Figure 5 A VT conversion that uses a 1988 modification of the initial AID technology (presented in Fig. 4). Recordings are from the final testing of an Endotak transvenous nonthoracotomy lead system (manufactured by Cardiac Pacemaker Inc., St. Paul, Minnesota) in a patient. The sensing function is contained in a single lead, and the shock is delivered between the right ventricle and a subcutaneous patch on the left side of the chest. Alternating current induced VF which is appropriately sensed with defibrillation occurring within 17 seconds. This system is the only nonthoracotomy device in clinical trials. Labeled are three surface ECGs (*X, Y, Z*), the device morphology sensing lead (*PDF*), and the device rate sensing lead (*Rate*). ICDC stands for Intec Cardioverter Defibrillator Catheter.

SUGGESTED READING

Cannom DS, Winkle RA. Implantation of the automatic implantable cardioverter defibrillator (AICD): Practical aspects. PACE 1986; 9:793–809.

Mirowski M. The automatic implantable cardioverter defibrillator: An overview. J Am Coll Cardiol 1985; 6:461–466.

Mower MM, Nisam S. AICD indications (patient selection): Past, present and future. PACE 1988; 11:2064–2070.

Wilber DJ, Garan H, Finkelstein D, et al. Out-of-hospital cardiac arrest. Use of electrophysiologic testing in the prediction of long-term outcome. N Engl J Med 1988; 318:19–24.

Winkle RA, Mean HR, Ruder MA, et al. Long-term outcome with the automatic implantable cardioverter-defibrillator. J Am Coll Cardiol 1989; 13:1353–1361.

A page number in bold indicates an illustration
A "t" following a page number indicates a table